Second Edition

HEALTH
PROMOTION
IN
MULTICULTURAL
POPULATIONS

This book is lovingly dedicated to Anita

—M. V. K.

To Kathryn, Eric, and Erin

—R. M. H.

Second Edition

HEALTH
PROMOTION
IN
MULTICULTURAL
POPULATIONS

A Handbook for Practitioners and Students

Michael V. Kline • Robert M. Huff
California State University, Northridge

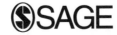

Los Angeles • London • New Delhi • Singapore

For information:

SAGE Publications, Inc.
2455 Teller Road
Thousand Oaks, California 91320
E-mail: order@sagepub.com

SAGE Publications Ltd.
1 Oliver's Yard
55 City Road
London EC1Y 1SP
United Kingdom

SAGE Publications India Pvt. Ltd.
B 1/I 1 Mohan Cooperative Industrial Area
Mathura Road, New Delhi 110 044
India

SAGE Publications Asia-Pacific Pte. Ltd.
33 Pekin Street #02–01
Far East Square
Singapore 048763

Printed in the United States of America

Library of Congress Cataloging-in-Publication Data

Health promotion in multicultural populations: A handbook for practitioners and students/[edited by] Michael V. Kline, Robert M. Huff. —2nd ed.
        p. cm.
Rev. ed. of: Promoting health in multicultural populations. c1999.
Includes bibliographical references and indexes.
ISBN 978-1-4129-3911-9 (cloth : alk. paper)
ISBN 978-1-4129-3912-6 (pbk. : alk. paper)
    1. Health promotion—United States. 2. Minorities—Medical care—United States. 3. Transcultural medical care—United States. I. Kline, Michael V. II. Huff, Robert M. III. Promoting health in multicultural populations.
    [DNLM: 1. Ethnic Groups—United States. 2. Health Promotion—United States. 3. Cultural Diversity—United States. 4. Minority Groups—United States. WA 300 H43396 2008]

RA427.8.H497515 2008
s362.108900973—dc22   2007052933

Printed on acid-free paper

08   09   10   11   12   10   9   8   7   6   5   4   3   2   1

Acquiring Editors:	Erik Evans and Cheri Dellelo
Editorial Assistant:	Lara Grambling
Production Editor:	Sarah K. Quesenberry
Copy Editor:	QuADS Prepress (P) Ltd
Typesetter:	C&M Digitals (P) Ltd.
Proofreader:	Wendy Jo Dymond
Indexer:	Michael Ferreira
Cover Designer:	Candice Harman
Marketing Manager:	Stephanie Adams

ntents

Foreword

Some paradoxes face those seeking to promote health in multicultural institutions, communities, and societies in which equity stands as a central value. Some of these paradoxes arise from the inherently competitive, if not sometimes contradictory, goals that multiculturalism and equity seem to pursue. We prize diversity, but we loathe disparities, at least in matters of health. Can we protect and even promote diversity in ethnicity or culture while seeking to eliminate disparities in health? Is the culture of a practitioner bound to limit his or her ability to understand and promote a vision of health and to find a way of achieving health within another culture? This handbook for practitioners should help the practitioner bridge this cross-cultural divide.

A second paradox arises from the global, to national, to regional and local, to family and individual lenses through which multiculturalism and equity are variously viewed and the sometimes contradictory actions taken at these various ecological levels to achieve equity. At the global, national, and state levels, we seek uniform policies that are legislated at these centralized levels to ensure equity across regions, while recognizing that the essence of diversity and multicultural sensitivity depends on local, family, and even individual autonomy. Can practitioners reconcile the policies they are required to implement with the social realities, histories, and cultural variations that they find locally? This handbook for practitioners should help them do so.

A third paradox is that the only way to achieve equity in the face of inherited social, economic, and political inequalities and inequitable societal forces is to treat people or populations differently. The provinces of Alberta, British Columbia, and Ontario, for example, pay higher taxes than some other provinces to subsidize the Canadian commitment to health equity and universal health care through revenue sharing and income transfers to the poorer provinces. More affluent people must pay higher taxes to subsidize essential social and health services to the less affluent. Whole classes and regions, then, must be treated unequally in the name of equity. The only alternative to this strategy is to limit the concept of equity more severely to include only equality of economic opportunity and to ignore history, political traditions, prejudice, catastrophic illness, and conditions of birth and inheritance that give people unequal circumstances and starting points in availing themselves of their otherwise equal economic opportunities. This handbook will help make practitioners more sensitive to the histories, traditions, and sociocultural circumstances that matter.

A fourth paradox arises for individuals in a multicultural society. Each of us must act toward other people of different ethnic origins with recognition and respect for their differences while treating them equally in every other way. But where do we draw the line in our behavior between differences and equality to achieve equity? In what ways should we be equal, and what are the "every other" ways? We face this daily in our relations between genders. Affirmative action in hiring or building ramps for disabled people to have equal access; avoiding sexual harassment in gender relations between teachers and students or between colleagues; and recognizing the disadvantages an employee, client, or student had at the beginning of a professional encounter, all reflect our efforts to reconcile these paradoxes.

These instances of societal adjustments to inherent or inherited differences while seeking to achieve equity hold lessons for the health professions and other sectors seeking to promote health in multicultural populations. Cultural differences related to health can be obvious or subtle; malleable or rigid; prescribed or proscribed; and dictated by religious or secular traditions, edicts, norms, customs, or ideologies. The variable forms and sources of the differences can be a partial guide to how they should be treated in planning, implementing, and evaluating health promotion programs. But beyond these partial guides, the humanity of multiculturalism cannot and should not claim a science as its only compass. Some combination of philosophical commitment, cultural knowledge, human sensitivity, and open communication must be brought to bear in achieving the balance and proper trade-offs between distinctiveness and equality that multiculturalism and equity demand.

Besides the paradoxes, the diversity issue presents another challenge for the practitioner. The tendency of those who produce "best-practice" guidelines too often generalize too glibly from the theories and evidence generated in mainstream populations or from the experiences of successful health promotion programs in one population. As guidance for practice in another population, especially another culture, this has led many programs

down a primrose path of misplaced precision and misguided certainty about practices. The editors of this book, in the previous edition and in this new edition, have wisely avoided the overgeneralization or external-validity trap by addressing the question of promoting health for each of the major ethnic populations separately.

With the addition of a chapter on the ethics of multicultural health promotion and one on the nature of the disparities in this second edition of their book, Professors Kline and Huff expand the perspectives on multicultural issues. As in the previous edition, the book presents the experience of health promotion professionals in their work with specific racially, ethnically, and culturally identified populations. Each chapter can be read for the lessons it may hold for other professionals working with the same populations. Each can be read, with some greater caution, for the lessons it may hold for working with other populations. Generalizability may be the least appropriate scientific construct to be brought to bear in multicultural health promotion.

Even within the culturally identified categories used in the chapter titles, such as Latino, African American, American Indian, Alaska Native, Asian American, and Pacific Islander, one finds vastly varied populations. One must exercise similar caution in generalizing from these categories to their counterparts living under national conditions other than the United States. The American Indian and Alaska Native counterpart "First Nations" populations of Canada and Aboriginal populations of Australia, for example, have some common historical colonization, economic disadvantage, and cultural characteristics vis à vis their respective majority neighbors. But each has distinct features and circumstances that would make some generalization from the American experiences in this book misguided if not hazardous for health promotion professionals working cross-culturally in other countries.

These cautions notwithstanding, the authors of the chapters in this anthology of multicultural experience offer a wealth of insight and a treasure of stories and case studies that can enlighten the cultural knowledge and awaken the cultural sensitivity of practitioners everywhere. As a handbook for practitioners, this volume promises to serve health promotion well.

One overriding lesson, principle, or prediction to be drawn from the multicultural experiences reflected in this handbook would be that promoting health in multicultural populations must ultimately be from within the cultures intended to benefit from the health promotion. Yes, collaboration between an ethnic minority population and professional practitioners from the majority culture can be helpful and productive, but such collaboration must be in the spirit of participatory research. Why participatory research? Because the health promotion task in every community is first to understand itself, second to communicate that understanding with consistency and credibility, and third to produce action from the understanding and commitment mobilized by its communication. These are the three elements of participatory research: systematic investigation or self-study, colearning, and action. Practitioners working cross-culturally can only participate in the self-study, learning, and action process effectively if the population affected by the issues is actively engaged in all three.

Each of the chapters in this book brings a unique set of perspectives from the multicultural encounters represented by it. Each represents such encounters within the American context of multiculturalism, except one. The chapter by Frankish, Lovato, and Poureslami

from Canada reminds us that we risk falling into another level of ethnocentrism if we view the issues of multiculturalism strictly through the American lens of health promotion or of interethnic encounters in the United States. The very naming of the ethnic groups as African American, Asian American, and Native American, for example, might lull us into parochialism about these ethnic populations. Thus, we would miss the opportunity to study and understand their counterparts in Canada, Australia, and other countries absorbing immigrant and indigenous populations and seeking to nurture the maintenance of their cultural heritages together with the inevitable experience of acculturation and assimilation into their mainstreams. The Canadian First Nations and the Australian Aboriginal populations, for example, have much to teach us about the multicultural experiences in health promotion, and the comparative study of these experiences can enlighten the efforts in all countries that must grapple with them. The contemporary European experience of immigration from Muslim countries and the massive refugee movement across the borders of war-torn countries in Africa and the Middle East make the subject addressed by this book all the more urgent in the broader global perspective.

—*Lawrence W. Green, DrPH*
Adjunct Professor, Department of
Epidemiology and Biostatistics
School of Medicine
Co-Leader, Society, Diversity
and Disparities Program
Comprehensive Cancer Center
University of California at San Francisco

Preface

It has been over seven years since the release of the first edition of *Promoting Health in Multicultural Populations*. In that period, the United States has become more ethnically diverse than ever before. The editors recognize that ethnicity is a rather broad way in which to examine special populations. However, categorization by ethnicity does make it possible to focus on the unique characteristics of ethnic groups and their subgroups with respect to their cultural values, beliefs, customs, and mores and how these may affect programs addressed to improving their health and well-being. Regardless of the special populations being treated, we recognize that with the passage of time, many of these special populations have produced second generations of native-born children of native-born parents. In most instances, with or without mixed marriages, they straddle two or more cultures and face the challenges of living in both while seeking their own identities and lifestyle patterns. In addition, the number of recent and new immigrants coming from a myriad of countries has brought forth a variety of old and new health problems that now must be addressed. These problems and needs will require health practitioners to think and act in new ways to effectively address the health care needs of these special population groups. There are, obviously, a number of difficulties associated with defining special population groups that present some challenges to a book such as ours. These include issues such as gender and age differences as well as generational differences in which adoption of Western health practices might be in conflict with more traditional practices. The editors also recognize that special populations can be defined on the basis of shared similarities, including chronic or acute health problems, disabilities, sexual orientation, and almost anything else one might consider when trying to categorize people. It is not the aim of this book to try to address all these issues. Rather, we seek to combine theory, practice, and ethnic considerations that address the broad range of special population characteristics in the belief that, through this approach, practitioners can adapt these to their particular needs and issues.

The editors recognize that the book is heavily "swayed" to U.S. practitioners and practice settings and that making generalizations from the American experiences and practices covered in the text to other multicultural populations outside the United States should be done with caution. Even so, we certainly want to encourage health promotion students and professionals working in other countries (outside the United States) to use the book because it does contain many methods, approaches, and take-off points that can be of value regardless of national differences. But, again, there must be an awareness of the differences and limitations as they attempt to transfer the information and experiences into their multicultural settings particularly in light of major system differences–that is, in political, economic, ecological, health care, and social/cultural climates and in the confusing use of different labels and categories by which target populations are described.

Lawrence Green, in the Foreword to this second edition wrote, "promoting health in multicultural populations must ultimately be from within the cultures intended to benefit from the health promotion. Yes, collaboration between an ethnic minority population and professional practitioners from the majority culture can be helpful and productive, but such collaboration must be in the spirit of participatory research." Participatory research should occur in all multicultural settings regardless of geographical locale. The need for intensive collaboration between the target group, community members, and practitioners should be emphasized from the outset of a program or intervention. This book, throughout, strongly encourages collaborative processes that can better ensure that any programs or interventions ultimately developed must be tailored to the needs of each specific target group.

In the time period that has elapsed since our first edition, there have been many advances and improvements in theory and practice in health promotion and disease prevention (HPDP). There has been, with this phenomenon, increased awareness by practitioners, instructors, and students of the impact of culture, cultural diversity, cultural competency, national differences, and health disparities. They continually voice their need for greater access to improved theories of health behavior change and models for guiding the development of more culturally sensitive and responsive assessment activities for achieving more effective program-planning processes. This increased awareness by practitioner, instructor, and student constituencies concerning the importance of these areas has increased their need to learn more about current best practices and processes used in the field when working across multicultural population groups.

This book has been written for a variety of health practitioners representing the many disciplines involved in the fields of health promotion and education, public health, nursing, medicine, psychology, sociology, social work, dentistry, physical therapy, radiologic technology, and all other helping professions that are in daily contact with culturally diverse population groups. It also has been written for students training in these professions to help them develop perspectives and foundations on cultural differences and on how these affect HPDP programs and services.

Health practitioners in the field are consistently reporting that it is becoming more demanding in all communities to effectively initiate and facilitate systematically designed and culturally specific activities for promoting health in special populations where issues of ethnicity, nontraditional health beliefs and practices, and other factors are encountered with increasing frequency.

OVERVIEW OF THE BOOK

This book is grounded in the premise that working within multicultural settings to promote health and prevent disease requires an understanding of the basics of program planning and an in-depth understanding of the cultural group and locale being targeted. The awareness of who these people are requires knowledge of their history and immigration patterns, cultural values and norms, cosmology and religious practices, social and political systems, health disparity status, health beliefs and practices, and other culture-specific demographic variables that characterize the population and/or subpopulations of interest.

The structure and format of the second edition has been improved and expanded, with increased attention directed to students and instructors as to how the text can best be used by them. This includes chapter objectives at the beginning of each chapter and suggested discussion topics and/or exercises following each chapter to guide the reader and instructor in the classroom use of the book. Also, the second edition is arranged to achieve a clearer and more consistent transition between its chapters. Such transitions better enable the reader to cross-reference material and apply later specific chapter information by building on the knowledge of the earlier foundation chapters.

As a classroom text, the authors offer the following suggestions for how this book can be used. Some of these guidelines come from their personal experiences with using the book in their own public health education classes. Because the text is a handbook and includes a number of sections that highlight diverse cultural and ethnic groups, having students read the entire text may not be the best way to use this book. Rather, the book should be used as a sampler where students seek out information and skills about different cultural groups that can be used as a basis for classroom discussion and related activities. That is, depending on the focus of the course the book is to be used in, the instructor may have the class concentrate on the opening section of the book that lays the foundation for everything else that follows and then break the class into small groups to explore other sections as a group work assignment. Then, groups can come together to share their readings, compare and contrast similarities and differences between the multicultural groups that were assigned, and then look at how they might design health education and promotion interventions for specific problems the instructor might identify. This provides students with an opportunity to delve more deeply into their assigned multicultural group by studying the pertinent literature in depth on that group and the HPDP interventions that have been employed and reported on in the literature. This could lead to classroom presentations and or papers that explore their assigned multicultural group in

much greater depth than the book is able to do.

In the course we teach, students are required to read Part 1 of the book over several weeks. Issues are then discussed in class using exercises that deal with subjects such as stereotyping, personal cultural competence assessments, and related issues. Then, all members of the class are given an opportunity to select a multicultural group they are interested in for their individual research projects. We then focus on health disparities, cultural assessment and program planning, implementation, and evaluation using the chapters in the book as the basis for these discussions. As the semester progresses, students are required to prepare short presentations about their target group, including a historical overview of the target group, its migration and immigration to the United States, and its acculturation and assimilation practices; the health beliefs and practices relevant to that target group; suggestions for how to intervene with that group; and tips that others in the class could use if they found themselves working with that population group. Clearly then, there are many ways a text such as this one can be used in the classroom to help students develop a sense of cultural competence and the steps they will need to take once they are in the field. We have also included discussion questions and suggested exercises at the end of each chapter so that the instructor can move beyond what was presented to further explore issues and concerns presented in each chapter. As in the first edition, there are substantial "tips" chapters following each major part of the book. Each of these six chapters provides many take-off points for questions, exploration, and discussion. We did not include any student objectives or discussion questions/exercises in these chapters. Instructors are encouraged to make their own decisions as to ways of using the "tips" subject matter to enhance their students' learning.

Detailed references that have been deemed valuable in the first edition have been expanded in the process of chapter updating. Some selected Web sites for increasing the student and the practitioner's knowledge of valuable resources and supplementary materials are also included. We believe these changes would also appeal to health professionals using the book as a handbook or reference guide and make it easier for them to access important information they may need in their practice settings.

The book is divided into seven major parts. Several new chapters have been added to help lay a stronger foundation for the other six parts that follow. These new chapters include one that is focused on health disparities among multicultural groups across the United States and one that looks at ethical concerns and considerations when working cross-culturally. The book is intended to serve as a handbook of concepts, methods, tips, and suggestions for working with multicultural peoples. The editors recognize that no single book can possibly present all of the issues related to multicultural HPDP. But we do hope that readers will find this book useful in helping them organize their thinking about working with culturally diverse populations and more appropriately plan health promotion and education programs within a variety of special population groups.

The first part of the book seeks to establish a foundation for the parts that follow and includes eight chapters that define and consider (1) health disparities among different population groups in the United States; (2) concepts of culture and cultural competence; (3) ethical issues when working with multicultural population groups; (4) traditional concepts of health and disease; (5) an overview of current theories and models of behavior change as they relate to health promotion with multicultural populations and groups; (6) an overview of health promotion and education planning models, theories, and practice issues; (7) a presentation and discussion of the cultural assessment framework; and (8) "tips" for the practitioner who is engaged in designing and implementing HPDP programs for multicultural populations.

The next five parts consider five specific multicultural groups: the Hispanic/Latino, African American, American Indian and Alaska Native, Asian American, and Pacific Islander population groups. Each of these parts includes three chapters followed by a customized "tips" chapter. The first chapter in each part presents an overview devoted to understanding this special population from a variety of perspectives and includes terms used to define the subgroups within the broader population, historical and demographic characteristics, immigration patterns, health and disease issues and concerns, and health beliefs and practices. The second chapter is concerned with how to assess, plan, implement, and evaluate programs for each of the specific groups, including tips, models, and suggestions for more effective program design. The third chapter presents a case study to emphasize the points made in the overview and planning chapters.

The final part of the book considers several issues and needs raised in earlier chapters of the text that are of special concern to the editors. Discussion centers on future dilemmas and concerns that will be faced by practitioners working with multicultural populations in a variety of community health care settings.

Acknowledgments

The editors deeply thank all those who helped in the preparation of this book. We especially thank our Sage team of editors, Cheri Dellelo, Erik Evans, and Lara Grambling; our production editor, Sarah Quesenberry; our current marketing manager, Stephanie Adams; and Helen Salmon, Marketing Director, Books Division. We also want to thank Shamila Swamy and her team from QuADS Prepress (P) Ltd. for their diligent copyediting of the entire draft. Finally, we thank our families for their support, encouragement, and patience during the preparation of this second edition.

PUBLISHER'S ACKNOWLEDGMENTS

Sage Publications gratefully acknowledges the contributions of the following reviewers:

Dawn Doutrich, *Washington State University*

Lucille Eller, *Rutgers University*

Julie Gast, *Utah State University*

Kristie E. Holt, *California State University–Long Beach*

Beth Lanning, *Baylor University*

Tonya Manselle, *University of Illinois*

Ester Shapiro, *University of Massachusetts at Boston*

Susan Wilkinson, *Angelo State University*

PART I

Foundations

1

Health Promotion in the Context of Culture

ROBERT M. HUFF

MICHAEL V. KLINE

Chapter Objectives

On completion of this chapter, the health promotion student and practitioner will be able to

- Define and discuss the concepts of health education, health promotion, and disease prevention as these relate to working with multicultural population groups

- Define and discuss at least five common terms associated with working with diverse population groups, including the terms *culture*, *ethnicity*, *acculturation and assimilation*, *ethnocentrism*, and *cultural competence*

- Identify and discuss at least five potential barriers to multicultural health promotion and disease-prevention activities designed for diverse cultural groups

Activities for promoting health and preventing disease in any population, whether directed at individuals, groups, or communities, are a formidable task! Such endeavors require an organized effort characterized by an understanding that *culture* and *cultural forces*, among other social forces, are powerful determinants of health-related behaviors. Culture, in any group or subpopulation, can exist as a total or partial system of interrelationships of human behavior guided and influenced by the organization and the products of that behavior. Indeed, the beliefs, ideologies, knowledge, institutions, religion, and governance, as well as nearly all activities (including efforts to achieve health-related behavior change), are

3

affected by the forces of culture that guides one's group or subgroup.

Culture is a complex force in the lives of individuals, groups, and communities. And it is this complexity that has made it difficult to formulate a universally accepted definition of "culture." Kreuter, Lukwago, Bucholtz, Clark, and Sanders-Thompson (2003) note that no single definition of culture is universally accepted. But there is "general agreement that culture is learned, shared, and transmitted from one generation to the next, and it can be seen in a group's values, norms, practices, systems of meaning, ways of life, and other social regularities" (p. 133). The definition of "culture" will be dealt with in greater depth later in the chapter. It is also important, where possible, to be aware that ethnic and cultural factors may be connected with a target group's vulnerability to certain communicable and chronic diseases and other health-related problems. Such knowledge can provide the planner with many clues during the assessment process. Students and practitioners should be aware that many of a target group's health risk factors are amenable to behavior change, thus reducing risk. Efforts to promote health and prevent disease within culturally different ethnic subgroups, as in any target group, will entail influencing the health behavior of individuals, families, groups, or communities. This will require identifying and changing those factors that are associated with accomplishing the desired health-related behavior. Also, these efforts probably will require some type of sustained collaboration between the public, private, and voluntary sectors and the people most directly affected by a defined health concern or problem. Cultural considerations ultimately may determine whether a particular population or target group will choose to participate in health promotion and disease prevention (HPDP) programs. There will need to be a continuing communication between these stakeholders that establishes and maintains working relationships characterized by mutual understanding, trust, and respect.

There are many settings in the community where activities are conducted for promoting health for preventing disease in a population. These include myriad work sites, schools, health care program sites, and the community itself. Comprehensive health promotion activities at a work site consisting of a large, culturally diverse employee population may, for example, carry out employee-risk assessments (including screenings and appraisals) as well as establish and maintain an appropriate variety of educational programs, services, and activities to reduce or eliminate identified areas of health risk. In this setting, a work site must carry out culturally sensitive and effective interventions that meet the needs of the employees. This sensitivity must be carried over in the group as well as in one-to-one counseling or educational encounters. Awareness and sensitivity to cultural diversity, then, must be reflected in the planning, design, and implementation phases of such a complex undertaking.

HPDP efforts in multicultural populations are very demanding undertakings involving a combination of activities associated with achieving desired outcomes. There is, then, a need at the outset of this chapter to distinguish between the concepts of health promotion and health education and to briefly examine the implications and impact of culture at these two overlapping levels. This chapter also provides an overview of culture, particularly as cultural differences affect HPDP efforts, and discusses current paradigms that have been proposed to improve practitioner skills in working in multicultural health care settings (including the barriers to effective multicultural HPDP efforts).

HEALTH PROMOTION AND DISEASE PREVENTION

The terms *health promotion* and *disease prevention,* when used in this text, encompass a similar range of interests and concerns as expressed long ago in the Joint Committee on Health Education Terminology (1991) report. The committee defined HPDP as "the aggregate of all purposeful activities designed to improve personal and public health through a combination of strategies, including the competent implementation of behavior change strategies, health education, health protection measures, risk factor detection, health enhancement, and health maintenance" (p. 102). Central to this conceptualization, it should be noted, is the need to achieve different levels of outcomes (e.g., individual, family, group, organization, community) through a combination of health promotion and health education strategies and intervention activities.

Another ageless definition of health promotion is "any planned combination of educational, political, regulatory, and organizational supports for actions and conditions of living conducive to the health of individuals, groups, or communities" (Green & Kreuter, 1991, p. 432). Explicit in this definition is the need for interventions that respond to a broad level of community concern relating to stimulating, establishing, and sustaining an appropriate combination of educational, organizational, and political support needed to facilitate actions aimed at achieving desired community health outcomes. These definitions of health promotion provided above serve the purpose of this text well because they are valid in today's context; they are succinct, readily understandable, multidimensional; and they focus on the reality and need for several different levels of specific and needed program activities and outcomes (e.g., individual, family, group, organization, community) in HPDP program planning.

Health education has been defined as "any planned combination of learning experiences designed to predispose, enable, and reinforce voluntary behavior conductive to heath in individuals, groups, or communities" (Green & Kreuter, 1991, p. 432). Intervention efforts

from this particular vantage point concentrate on facilitating the voluntary acquisition of specific health-related knowledge, attitudes, and practices associated with achieving specific health-related behavior changes. Health education is mentioned here because health promotion emerged out of health education and designates a broader level of outcome than does health education. However, health education is considered a primary instrumentality for achieving health promotion outcomes. For example, the focus of health education interventions in a cervical cancer education and screening program targeting African American women living in a certain geographical area may be concerned with making educational programs more available and accessible to this group. Such programs can enable the target group to develop skills for carrying out defined voluntary screening behaviors related to reducing the risk of this life-threatening disease. However, the planning of interventions and related activities at this level, then, usually focuses on reaching only one target group among the many possible groups of women at risk in need of specified educational programs. On the other hand, the planning of strategies and interventions at the health promotion level goes beyond single cervical cancer education program focus. For example, interventions may focus on the need to establish and sustain a more accessible and equitably distributed system of women's health screening and education programs for enhancing the overall health of all poor and underserved women in that particular community. The complexity of health promotion program efforts requires a greater scope of coordination, participation, commitment, and expense than does the cervical cancer education and screening aimed at a single target group. Indeed, many community participants representing a plethora of public, private, and voluntary agencies, organizations, and institutions will need to be involved in this endeavor.

Health promotion efforts also may be conducted at a broader community level and may seek health and health-related behavior changes or social outcomes through ecological or environmental approaches intended to result in permanent structural changes or supports in the form of policies, regulations, and expanded access to resources affecting people where they work and live (Green & Kreuter, 1991, 2005; Green, Richard, & Potvin, 1996; McLeroy, Bibeau, Steckler, & Glanz, 1988; Richard, Potvin, Kischuk, Prlic, & Green, 1996).

It is seen, then, at one level, health education programs, for example, might concentrate on facilitating the voluntary acquisition of specific health-related knowledge, attitudes, and practices for reducing the specific target group's health risk for certain chronic or communicable diseases. It is important to recognize that interventions designed to achieve change on only the individual level will not be as effective as those that can achieve broader change on the community level. Thus, program efforts at other levels (i.e., the health promotion level) may seek social or environmental changes (supportive structures) for reducing population health risk. These changes are in the form of new risk-reducing policies, laws, and regulations and new or increased organizational or structural arrangements that encourage, enable, and reinforce the acquisition and practice of certain health-related behaviors (Green & Kreuter, 1991, 2005).

HPDP programs, through their assessment and diagnosis processes of community needs (discussed in Chapters 6 and 7 of this volume), must be able to identify at-risk target groups in the community and specifically the kinds of *disease prevention* efforts (by particular target group) that need to be included in their health promotion activities. The following identifies the specific focus and types of activities generally conducted under the different levels of *disease prevention*: (1) the *primary prevention level* (providing specific protection that prevents the onset of the disease itself or reduces exposure or risk levels to the disease processes, e.g., immunizations against a variety of childhood diseases, disease screening, smoking prevention and cessation programs, HIV/AIDS education and screening programs); (2) *the secondary prevention level* (providing activities related to early diagnosis and prompt treatment of a disease that is already present, e.g., syphilis, HIV/AIDS, gonorrhea, diabetes, cervical cancer); and (3) *the tertiary level of prevention* (activities through treatment and rehabilitation efforts to minimize disability after the damage has been done from existing illness, e.g., alcoholism, diabetes, cirrhosis of the liver, chronic obstructive pulmonary disorder, emphysema, high blood pressure) (Turnock, 2001).

Finally, the focus of all HPDP efforts must of necessity include an awareness and sensitivity to culture and the many cultural differences reflected in the population to be targeted. And within their own cultural milieu all planning participants (e.g., planners and community participants) need to recognize that any HPDP interventions contemplated must consider the personal experiences, knowledge, health practices, and problem-solving methodologies that are acceptable within the framework of the individual, group, or community.

HEALTH PROMOTION AND CULTURE

What we see as science, the Indians see as magic. What we see as magic, they see as science. I don't find this a hopeless contradiction. If we can appreciate each other's views, we can see the whole picture more clearly. To heal ourselves or to help heal others, we need to reconnect magic and science, our right and left brains. (Hammerschlag, 1988, p. 14)

Promoting health and preventing disease is a noble goal that, to many, might seem straightforward, logical, and highly scientific. After all, we know about germ theory, diseases of lifestyle, medications, radiation, surgery, and other Western approaches to preventing and/or diagnosing and treating health problems in the general population. What Hammerschlag (1988) is pointing out, however, is that this process is not always what it seems. Indeed, there are many different ways of perceiving, understanding, and approaching health and disease processes across cultural and ethnic groups with which health practitioners need to become better acquainted.

Cultural differences can and do present major barriers to effective health care intervention. This is especially true when health practitioners overlook, misinterpret, stereotype, or otherwise mishandle their encounters with those who might be viewed as different from them in their assessment, intervention, and evaluation-planning processes.

There is not a day that goes by that we are not exposed to a variety of sights, sounds, and tastes reflecting influences coming at us from a multitude of sources including the news media, our work settings and contacts in the community, and the foods we choose to eat. From these, we form opinions, make judgments, and take actions perceived to be appropriate to the situation and setting in which we find ourselves. When these choices involve our efforts to improve the health of the many "publics" we encounter in our health care roles, our perceptions of how these publics relate to and respond to our efforts may be colored by our own ethnocentric views of the world. In turn, we may be viewed by our "publics" in a similar manner. That is, whereas we might view a client as delusional if the individual comes to us for help and tells us he or she has been seeing a traditional folk healer because they believe someone has put a "hex" on him or her, that client might view us as ignorant and inexperienced when we offer him or her counseling and medication as the treatment for the problem. In both cases, cultural beliefs and practices born out of years of

enculturation and socialization in divergent world views have gotten in the way of the communication and treatment possibilities.

Brislin and Yoshida (1994) note that health care professionals' lack of knowledge about health beliefs and practices of culturally diverse groups and problems in intercultural communication has lead to significant challenges in the provision of health care services to multicultural population groups. They also observed that the cultural diversity of the health care workforce itself can present problems that can disrupt the provision of services because of competing cultural values, beliefs, norms, and health practices in conflict with the traditional Western medical model. For example, Putsch (1985) describes a situation in which an elderly Navaho patient with a mild senile dementia has returned for an outpatient visit after several long hospitalizations. He greets his physician in Navaho, shakes hands, and embraces him. He then turns to greet the nurse's aide, who will act as an interpreter, and extends his hand to her. She flees from the room visibly frightened. When later questioned about her behavior, she relates that she had been warned by her mother never to shake hands with gray-haired people because they might "witch you." She also noted that she knew about this man through her husband's family and that he was "no good" (p. 3346). In exploring cultural differences in more detail, a discussion of what we mean by *culture, ethnicity, acculturation,* and other related terms will help set the scene for how these may affect our ability to assess, plan, implement, and evaluate HPDP programs for a variety of multicultural population groups.

CULTURE

The term *culture* has been defined in many ways over the years and continues to be a concept that is hotly debated among anthropologists even today. In 1871, E. B. Tylor defined culture as "that complex whole which includes knowledge, belief, art, morals, law, custom and any other capabilities and habits acquired by man as a member of society" (quoted in Bock, 1969, p. 17). Stein and Rowe (1989) define culture as "learned, nonrandom, systematic behavior that is transmitted from person to person and from generation to generation" (p. 4). Kagawa-Singer and Chung (1994) describe culture as "a tool which defines reality for its members" (p. 198) and note that within this perception of reality, the individual's purpose in life emerges through a process of socialization in which he or she learns the appropriate beliefs, values, and behaviors shared by society. Thus, culture is seen as both integrative and functional in that the beliefs and values transmitted to the individual provide a sense of identity as well as the rules the individual must follow to enable his or her culture to survive over time.

Slonim (1991) identifies five basic criteria for defining a culture: having a common pattern of communication, sound system, or language unique to the group; similarities in dietary preferences and preparation methods; common patterns of dress; predictable relationship and socialization patterns between members of the culture; and a common set of shared values and beliefs. No matter how it may be defined, culture can be seen as a dynamic template or framework a society uses to view, understand, behave, and pass on its culture to each succeeding generation. Culture helps specify what behaviors are acceptable in any given society, when they are acceptable, and what is not acceptable. It also provides some guidance for dealing with the basic problems of life. Anderson and Fenichel (1989) caution, however, that this cultural framework is only a set of tendencies or possibilities for behavior and individuals within any given society are essentially free to choose from all the available possibilities within this frame.

What do the above issues have to do with HPDP? Consider, if you will, what possible barriers one might encounter if they were designing a health program for a community primarily composed of first-generation Hmong who were recent immigrants to the United States. Certainly, language could be a problem, but so too could the many cultural differences at nearly every level, from the basic nuances of communication to the significant differences in their worldview of what constitutes health and disease, from cause and prevention to treatment and cure. In fact, the Hmong health belief system is primarily based on the supernatural, and much of their traditional treatment is based on spiritual appeasement (Brainard & Zaharlick, 1989). A failure to understand and appreciate these "differences" would have serious implications for the success of any HPDP effort.

ETHNICITY

Ethnicity relates to the sense of identity an individual has based on common ancestry, national, religious, tribal, linguistic, or cultural origins. It generally implies that there are shared values, lifestyles, beliefs, and norms among those claiming affiliation to a specific ethnic group (Nunnally & Moy, 1989; Office of Minority Health, 2001; Paniagua, 1994; Spector, 2004). Ethnic identity provides a sense of social belonging and loyalty for the individual and often is used by others outside the ethnic group to identify or label "difference" (Kagawa-Singer & Chung, 1994). Unfortunately, ethnicity also is used to stereotype diversity in human populations and frequently leads to misunderstanding and/or distrust in all sorts of human interactions. In fact, the use of an ethnic label by someone outside the ethnic group may lead to a partial or complete shutdown of the learning curve for both parties to this process. For example, it can be seen that once the stereotype has been identified, one or both parties often cease to look beyond the stereotype to find out who each really is.

Slonim (1991) distinguishes between culture and ethnicity but notes that they tend to overlap with respect to how they are defined and used. She notes that culture is concerned with symbolic generalities and universals about social and family groups, whereas ethnicity is concerned with one's sense of identification and belonging to a specific reference group within any given society. Ethnicity, then, helps shape the way we think, relate, feel, and behave within and outside our reference group and defines the patterns of behavior that provide an individual with a sense of belonging and continuity with his or her ethnic group over time.

Ethnicity is a word that often is used in the same breath as the term *race*. It is important, however, not to confuse ethnicity with race, the latter of which is a biological term used to describe ethnic groups on the basis of physical characteristics such as skin color or shape of the eyes, nose, and mouth (Montague, 1964). Nelson and Jurmain (1988) note that *race* is an ancient concept that in more recent times has been used by scientists to place human populations into "racial" categories for purposes of classification. This form of classification, although convenient, ignores the issue of genetics, which is concerned with heredity and biological variation in all living things. Nelson and Jurmain regard the term *race* as a socio-cultural concept rather than a biological one. Thus, people often are classified along racial lines regardless of their genetic traits, and these racial categories have long been used as a basis for promoting discrimination, hatred, and divisiveness among human groups all around the world. In this book, the term *race* is not used to describe the various multicultural groups discussed. The exceptions are where contributors are reporting epidemiological data presented by federal, state, or local health agencies that gather and report health statistics using race as a variable. The terms *ethnic, multicultural,* and *culturally diverse* are preferred

by the editors, who believe that these terms reflect a more accurate description of human populations. For the health practitioner, reframing the term *race* to *multicultural, ethnic,* or *culturally diverse* may serve to promote a greater sensitivity to the challenges, potentialities, and rewards of working with diverse cultural groups in HPDP activities.

ACCULTURATION AND ASSIMILATION

Acculturation is a term used to describe the degree to which an individual from one culture has given up the traits of that culture and adopted the traits of the dominant culture in which he or she now resides. Locke (1992) identifies four levels of acculturation: the "bicultural" individual, who can function equally well in his or her own culture and the dominant culture; the "traditional" individual, who holds on to most, if not all, of his or her traits from his culture of origin; the "marginal" individual, who seems not to have any real contact with traits from either culture; and the "acculturated" individual, who has given up most of his or her traits of origin for those of the dominant culture. Locke notes the importance of assessing the degree of acculturation when working in a multicultural setting as there is a natural tendency on the part of many culturally diverse individuals to resist acculturation. This resistance can lead to significant misunderstandings and the inability to establish meaningful and mutually beneficial working relationships between the health care practitioner and those he or she may be seeking to help or influence. An example might be the practitioner who encounters a Latina mother with a newborn who feels that the child is ill because of the *mal de ojo* (evil eye)—that is, the belief that a sudden change in the emotional or physical health of an infant or young child is caused by the jealousy (or admiration) of a person with powerful eyes (de Paula,

Lagana, & Gonzales-Ramirez, 1996). A failure to recognize the significance of this problem for the patient, and the prescribing of a treatment that seems out of order in the mind of the mother, might result in her not following through or even engaging in an active way in the clinical encounter.

Assimilation is a closely related process to acculturation and is viewed as the social, economic, and political integration of a cultural group into a mainstream society to which it may have emigrated or otherwise been drawn (Casas & Casas, 1994). Generally, for assimilation to occur, there must be at least some minimal acculturation with respect to the language, values, laws, customs, and other major features of the dominant society. As Locke (1992) notes, however, there may be a genuine resistance and rejection of many of the values of the dominant culture with only a minimal level of cultural assimilation into mainstream society. Like acculturation, then, the level of an ethnically diverse client's assimilation into mainstream society might need to be assessed by the health practitioner to better understand and perhaps predict how well that person will accept and/or participate in HPDP recommendations and behaviors. One has only to pay a visit to areas of his or her city where recent immigrants have settled or where there is a long established but insular population characterized by the maintenance of the culture-of-origin behaviors, language, customs, food practices, and other social conventions that keeps its members isolated from mainstream society.

ASSESSMENT OF ACCULTURATION

The measurement of acculturation levels in the clinical setting has been the focus of a number of investigators studying a diversity of multicultural groups (Cuellar, Harris, & Jasso, 1980; Hoffman, Dana, & Bolton, 1985; Mendoza, 1989; Milliones, 1980; M. Ramirez,

1984; Smither & Rodriguez-Giegling, 1982; Suinn, Rickard-Figueroa, Lew, & Vigil, 1987). Paniagua (1994) comments on the variety of acculturation scales that can be used, depending on the ethnic group in which one is interested, and describes the Brief Acculturation Scale suggested by Burnam, Hough, Karno, Escobar, and Telles (1987). This Scale uses three variables: generation in the United States, preferred language, and preferences for who the individual most often socializes with. The assumptions underlying these variables hold that (a) the longer the individual is exposed to the dominant culture or the younger the individual is at the time he or she enters this culture, the more the individual communicates in the language of the dominant culture and (b) the more the individual socializes outside his or her primary cultural group, the more acculturated the individual is likely to become within the dominant society.

In general, assessment of acculturation has been used in clinical research settings rather than in HPDP programs but this has been changing in recent years as researchers and interventionists look more closely at the effects of acculturation on other variables influencing HPDP activities (Abraido-Lanza, Armbrister, Florez, & Aguirre, 2006; Clark & Hofsess, 1998; Dolhun, Munoz, & Grumbach, 2003; Rojas-Guyler, Ellis, & Sanders, 2005). Incorporating assessment of acculturation in the formative stages of HPDP program planning could prove quite valuable to the practitioner. For example, A. G. Ramirez, Cousins, Santos, and Supic (1986) devised and tested a four-item Media Acculturation Scale (MAS) for use with Mexican Americans that focused on media and language preferences and were able to demonstrate that the instrument could identify subsets of their study group by their distinct media usage patterns and demographic characteristics. The ability to identify specific target group media preferences and sources is a much more efficacious way to reach one's audience than guessing at them and expending resources that might have little payoff. Marin and Gamba (1996) developed and validated a Bidimensional Acculturation Scale (BAS) for use with Hispanics that they note works very well with Mexican Americans and Central Americans. They argue that acculturation is bidirectional in that as the individual is learning and taking on characteristics of the new culture, the individual is simultaneously doing the same within his or her culture of origin. Marin and Gamba note that understanding this process can help the practitioner be more aware of what Hispanics go through as they acculturate. It also would seem that the practitioner who is aware of where his or her target group is with respect to acculturation might be better able to tailor interventions that integrate health-promoting strategies into the learning that is occurring in both the culture of origin and the new culture as that acculturation process proceeds.

Although acculturation scales have been primarily used in research and clinical settings, what seems clear is that these scales have the potential to be included within needs assessment instruments used in the early stages of program plan development. For example, Castro, Cota, and Vega (1999) present a scale that they have found quite useful in a variety of settings working with Hispanics in health-promoting efforts. Thus, the use of acculturation scales for HPDP activities represents a relatively new and innovative tool the practitioner can employ to better understand the culturally diverse population groups with which he or she may be working.

ETHNOCENTRISM

Ethnocentrism is a concept that often plays a part in confusing an already difficult situation when working with ethnically diverse individuals or cultural groups. Ferguson and Brown (1991) describe ethnocentrism as the assumption an individual makes that his or her way of believing and behaving is the most preferable and correct one. She notes that often the health practitioner is unaware of his or her own ethnocentric behavior and that this can lead to dysfunctional treatment encounters. Leddy (2003) terms this behavior *medicocentrism*, that is, "the bias produced by viewing health through the lens of medicine as it is currently found in modern society" (p. 100). For example, the practitioner may directly or indirectly discount or ignore the client's cultural orientation and belief system, considering them unimportant, incorrect, or in conflict with their own perceptions or worldview of how best to treat the clients health problem or issue. This can leave the client feeling angry, frustrated, and uncooperative. Of equal importance is the awareness that whereas health care practitioners may be caught in their own ethnocentric dance, so too may be the culturally diverse client they are serving. That is, the culturally diverse client may view the health professional as foreign, ignorant of illness or disease causality, or uneducated to proper social customs, forms of address, and nonverbal behaviors deemed appropriate by the client for dealing directly or indirectly with his or her health problem or concern. For example, Kramer (1992) notes that Native American elders find such behaviors as getting right down to business; speaking to strangers in loud, confident tones; and frequently interrupting the speaker as intolerably rude. This, in turn, may lead to the withholding of important information the health professional needs for an accurate assessment and intervention plan.

One can argue, then, that there is a need for both the health professional and the culturally diverse client to develop a modicum of cultural sensitivity and cultural competence with respect to each other's values, beliefs, and health practices. This would be a major step forward in achieving a more balanced and respectful partnership in any health-related encounter.

CULTURAL COMPETENCE AND ETHNOSENSITIVITY

There is a large body of literature emerging from the social, behavioral, and health sciences promoting a philosophy of cross-cultural competence to which all persons working with multicultural groups should subscribe. Cross, Bazron, Dennis, and Isaacs (1989), examining how health care agencies serve culturally diverse clients, view the process of cultural competence among these agencies on a continuum ranging from "culturally destructive" to "culturally competent." On this continuum, agencies that provide health care services may be seen as moving through a number of phases as they become increasingly more aware of how it is that they serve culturally diverse groups. Agencies that do not consider that culture is an important factor when delivering services can be seen as "culture blind," whereas agencies that accept, respect, and work with cultural differences can be seen as being "culturally competent."

Campinha-Bacote (1994) defines cultural competence as "a process for effectively working within the cultural context of an individual or community from a diverse cultural or ethnic background" (pp. 1–2). She proposes a Culturally Competent Model of Health Care, which encompasses four levels: Cultural Awareness, Cultural Knowledge, Cultural Skill, and Cultural Encounter. Cultural Awareness is concerned with the process of becoming more sensitive to differences manifest in culturally diverse clients and of the health professional's own biases and prejudices toward different cultural groups. Cultural Knowledge is the process of gaining an understanding of different cultural groups, including their beliefs, values, lifestyle practices, and ways of solving problems in their world. Cultural Skill is concerned with the process of cultural assessment as the first step in designing treatment interventions for culturally diverse clients. Through this process, the practitioner seeks to identify his or her client's specific values, beliefs, and practices in an effort to include these in the planning of a mutually acceptable treatment plan. Cultural Encounter is the last stage of the model and is the process of directly relating to culturally diverse groups in an effort to refine one's knowledge and skills for working in culturally diverse settings. The model reflects a process that is ongoing in that the health professional always should be on a continuous quest to increase and improve his or her abilities to work in a variety of cross-cultural settings.

In concert with cultural competence is the concept of *ethnosensitivity*, which is concerned with the process of becoming more sensitive and respectful of cross-cultural differences. Borkan and Neher (1991) describe a Developmental Model of Ethnosensitivity, which can be used to help train physicians to improve their cross-cultural communication and practice skills. Their model proposes a seven-stage developmental continuum that can be used to assess a health care provider's ethnosensitivity. These stages range from fear or mistrust of different cultural groups, denial of cultural differences, feelings of superiority over other cultural groups, minimization of cultural differences, cultural relativism (acceptance and respect for differences), empathy, and cultural integration in which the practitioner becomes a multicultural person able to relate well to several different cultural groups. For example, once the developmental stage is identified, specific interventions can be tailored to help the physician move forward in the learning process. This is only one of a number of models being used in medical school– and hospital-based training programs that hold promise for improving the cross-cultural skills of health care providers (Dolhun et al., 2003; Purnell & Paulanka, 2003; Spector, 2004). For those interested readers, the following brief exercise is offered as a way to begin looking at one's own ethnosensitivities. Consider the last time you saw or interacted with someone you categorized as representing a particular ethnic group. How did you come to categorize that individual as representing a particular ethnic group? How have you come to your knowledge of the specific characteristics you employed to categorize that individual? How accurate do you think these characteristics are with respect to that specific individual? What do you actually know or not know about that specific individual in terms of his cultural heritage, lifestyle, and the like? What more did you seek to learn about that individual? How would you feel knowing that others may be categorizing you in similar ways? Your honest answers to these questions may provide a better understanding about how easy it is to stereotype or otherwise categorize people whom you know little. Often, these categorizations are quite inaccurate and insensitive. As noted earlier, once they are employed, they generally decrease one's interest in learning much more about a particular individual or group.

The need to develop an awareness of one's own interpersonal and communication style is of equal importance in becoming competent and sensitive to cultural differences. These areas have been identified by a number of investigators as potential barriers to working with culturally diverse population groups (Helman, 2007; Luckmann, 1999; Spector, 2004). Bell and Evans (1981) discuss the need for the practitioner to become aware of the interpersonal style he or she is operating from when dealing with persons from other cultures. They note five interpersonal styles: overt hostility, covert prejudice, cultural ignorance, color blindness, and cultural liberation. The first four of these styles fail to respect or openly consider cultural differences in the health care consultation, whereas cultural liberation reflects a lack of fear of cultural differences, awareness of one's own attitudes toward different cultural groups, acceptance of and encouragement of client expressions regarding his or her feelings about their ethnicity, and

the ability to use these feelings as shared learning experiences.

It is easy for practitioners to quote models and recommendations, and even easier to pay lip service to their value in becoming more culturally competent and sensitive. However, if practitioners are to improve their skills in these areas, then they must be willing to step their of our current frames of reference and take the risk of discovering their own biases and stereotypes and to open themselves up to new and perhaps quite divergent points of view about the world in which they live. In taking these steps, practitioners will also need to consider the challenge of learning to communicate across cultures.

CROSS-CULTURAL COMMUNICATION

Brislin and Yoshida (1994) comment that the typical Western medical model for communication in the health care encounter is the direct question-and-answer method, which seeks to quickly establish the facts of the case and often relies on the use of negative and double negative questions, for example, "You don't want to get heart disease, do you?" For the culturally diverse individual (or family), this approach to the communication process may be seen as cold and too direct or otherwise in conflict with his or her more traditional beliefs, values, and ways of seeking, communicating, and receiving health care. For example, Kramer (1992) notes that there are significant differences in how Native Americans perceive the initial visit with a health care provider. They might expect the initial visit to begin with a brief, light handshake rather than the typical firm handshake of the Westerner, which is seen as a sign of aggressiveness. Furthermore, behaviors such as staring, excessive eye contact, and direct questioning are considered rude and an invasion of privacy and dignity.

Northouse and Northouse (1992) and others (Dainton & Zelley, 2005; Rothwell, 2004) have defined communication as a process of information sharing in which those involved in the communication share a common set of rules. These rules may prescribe how the communication will take place, through what channels, when it will occur, and even how feedback may or may not be provided between the message communicator and the message receiver. For example, in a traditional Japanese family, it is often the head of the household who will be the primary individual communicating with the health care practitioner in the event a family member needs medical care. Likewise, the head of the household is the one who will make the decisions about treatment options and even what the ill family member should be told about his or her medical condition. Northouse and Northouse further divide communication into two subsets: human communication and health communication. Human communication relates to the interactions between and among people through the use of common symbols and language. Health communication is human communication primarily concerned with health-related interactions and processes. Here, the common symbols and language may be obscured by special professional jargon, including the use of medical terms to describe the condition and treatment options available to a client or patient. All these communication processes are dynamic, ongoing, and ever-changing transactions that involve human feelings, attitudes, knowledge, and behavior. Thus, in an interaction between two or more individuals representing divergent cultural orientations and where different rules may govern the communication process, the opportunity for miscommunication is significant.

A review of the many models of interpersonal communication advanced over the past 40 to 50 years suggest that there are a variety of factors affecting communication in general and in cross-cultural encounters specifically. These factors include the communication skills, attitudes, knowledge, social systems, and culture of both the sender and the receiver of communication transactions; the framing of the communication with respect to structure, content, and coding; the communication channel that will involve one or more of the five senses; "noise," which refers to auditory, perceptual, or psychological factors that can affect and influence the communication anywhere along the channel; and feedback mechanisms, which ensure that all parties to the communication transaction heard and understood the communication as it was intended. In addition, human interaction factors including dominance-submission or love-hate relationships, communication transactions, and the contexts in which they occur have all been identified as important to understanding and improving the communication process (Brislin & Yoshida, 1994; Dainton & Zelley, 2005; Kreps & Kunimoto, 1994; Northouse & Northouse, 1992; Rothwell, 2004). Given the incredible diversity of multicultural populations in the world today, the potential for miscommunication in any human encounter is staggering.

For the health professional seeking to develop an increased sense of cultural competence and sensitivity as well as improved communication skills, the task might seem daunting. However, patience and persistence are the keys to unlocking these skills, and many recommendations have been posited in the literature for improving the entire cross-cultural experience in health care. Among these are a series of recommendations made by Kreps and Kunimoto (1994). They urge health professionals to develop a genuine interest in and respect for cultural differences, including the development of communication attitudes and skills that demonstrate an appreciation for and sensitivity to cultural differences. This process can begin by reading about other cultural groups, learning a new language, attending multicultural events, or spending time in communities representative of the cultural or ethnic group of interest. Kreps and Kunimoto also recommend that health professionals become aware of the many different interpretations of reality that exist in the world, especially where health and health care issues are concerned. Here again, a patient's interpretation of what might be causing his or her problem (e.g., a witch, ghost, fate) might run totally counter to what the health care professional thinks is going on. Reading about different cultures and talking with willing members of the group of interest can provide valuable insights into these multiple realities. Finally, the practitioner should be ready and willing to endure uncertainty and discomfort when working in cross-cultural health care settings. It is, after all, those times we are most uncomfortable that we have the greatest opportunity for learning and growth. We just have to be open to that possibility.

BARRIERS TO MULTICULTURAL HPDP

As it will no doubt be evident to the reader by this time, there are a multitude of factors that can act as barriers or impediments to successful HPDP efforts. For purposes of this discussion, a *barrier* is defined as any obstacle that might interfere with the ability of the health practitioner or his or her culturally diverse client (to whom they are intending to provide interventions) to be able to fully achieve the intended assessment, intervention, and/or evaluation objectives. The range of potential barriers is extensive and not necessarily easily categorized, though some attempt will be made here to cluster some of these variables for purposes of discussion. Table 1.1 presents a partial listing of demographic, cultural, and health care systems barriers that have been identified in the literature as having the potential to impede HPDP efforts.

As can be seen in Table 1.1, there are a variety of demographic factors that can play a role in impeding multicultural health-promoting efforts, and no doubt the reader can add many more items to this list. It is important to recognize that many of the barriers identified heretofore will be mediated by the degree of acculturation and assimilation of the client being targeted for health promotion interventions, and it is incumbent on the health practitioner to assess these levels before implementing programs. Although many of these barriers are fairly self-explanatory, a quick look at several of these might help highlight the importance of demographics when working with or planning health promotion programs and services for the culturally diverse. For example, gender may become an issue when seeking to provide health promotion services such as screening mammography. Mo (1992) describes the problems that arise in providing this type of service to Chinese women and notes that cultural values associated with modesty and sexuality, coupled with institutional barriers such as the unavailability of educational materials written in Chinese, and a lack of female physicians played a significant role in the low number of women in her study who accessed breast health services. Ohmans, Garrett, and Treichel (1996) recognize that social class can be a significant barrier, particularly for new immigrants where their social status or class distinction may have been radically altered since leaving their country of origin. They caution that we should be particularly careful with health education and not assume that immigrant or refugee status equates with poverty or lack of education. Kramer (1992) comments that older Native Americans report a fear of non–Native American health professionals, expect to be treated unfairly by them, and anticipate negative contact experiences when they do encounter these health professionals. Uba (1992) reports that many Southeast Asians have difficulties in accessing health care services (even if they know about them) because of language difficulties associated with making appointments or even understanding the process. Furthermore, they often lack health insurance benefits because many of these people are poor and are working in low-paying jobs. Stevens and Cousineau (Chapter 5, this volume) present an extensive discussion of

Table 1.1   Potential Barriers to Health Promotion and Disease Prevention

Demographic Barrier	Cultural Barrier	Health Care System Barrier
Age	Age	Access to care
Gender	Gender, class, and family dynamics	Insurance or other financial resources
Ethnicity	Worldview/perceptions of life	Not always valued as useful
Primary language spoken	Time orientation	Orientation to preventive health services
Religion	Primary language spoken	Perceptions of need for health care services
Educational level and literacy level	Religious beliefs and practices	Ignorance and/or distrust of Western medical practices and procedures
Occupation, income, and health insurance	Social customs, values, and norms	Cultural insensitivity and competence
Area of residence	Traditional health beliefs and practices	Western vs. folk health beliefs and practices
Transportation	Dietary preferences and practices	Poor doctor-patient communications
Time and/or generation in the United States	Communication patterns and customs	Lack of bilingual and bicultural staff

health disparities and barriers to access that the reader might like to review. Geographic factors including a lack of hospitals or private physician offices in their communities, as well as difficulties in accessing public transportation or getting a driver's license, also complicate their access problems. By now the reader may have noticed how these demographic factors cross over into the other categories identified in Table 1.1. There are, in fact, many shades of gray to be considered when looking at barriers, and this makes the process that much more difficult to understand.

Cultural barriers include a number of factors of importance to the HPDP process. Like the demographic barriers, some of these seem readily understandable whereas others need clarification. For example, Uba (1992) notes

that many Southeast Asians are reluctant to seek health care services because of their attitudes regarding the nature of life and the inevitability of suffering. She comments that suffering and illness are seen as an unavoidable part of life, so seeking health care services early may be considered inappropriate. She cites the Hmong as an example of a cultural group who believe that life is predetermined, so lifesaving medical intervention is worthless. With respect to communication patterns and customs, Ramakrishna and Weiss (1992) describe nonverbal communication patterns among East Indian patients where the patient may not know how to respond to the American physicians' social smiles or may use lateral motions of the head to indicate a positive affirmation. In India, smiles are only exchanged between social equals, and East Indians use head shaking to denote "yes" which might confuse a Western physician.

Health beliefs and practices are the subject of Chapter 2, but a few brief comments might be of value here. Uba (1992) comments that many Southeast Asians view disease and illness etiology as arising from a variety of possible sources. These include organic problems, an imbalance between the yin and yang, an obstruction of *chi* (life energy), failure to be in harmony with nature, a curse from an offended spirit, or a punishment for immoral behavior. Riser and Mazur (1995) discuss folk illnesses among Hispanics and comment that the most common ailment in their study population was *mal ojo*. This folk illness was attributed to someone with "strong eyes" looking at a child (often unintentionally). The result of this "look" was felt to heat up the child's blood and lead to inconsolable crying, fever, diarrhea, vomiting, and gassy stomach. They also described *empacho*, a folk illness attributed to certain foods such as swallowed gum, grape skins, and poorly mixed powdered milk or formula that sticks in the intestines. Obviously, there are significant differences in perception of disease causality as well as treatment that must be understood and worked with if health-promoting efforts are to be effective. In addition, there are a variety of common yet divergent values among multicultural groups that the health promotion practitioner might find to be useful in his or her practice efforts. Schilling and Brannon (1986) developed a list of these common values that are presented in Table 1.2.

It is obvious that the practitioner engaged in health promotion efforts is likely to be confronted by any number of divergent viewpoints regarding the nature of life and social interaction. As May (1992) notes, this will require the practitioner to be flexible in their design of programs, policies, and services to meet the needs and concerns of the diverse cultural groups he or she is likely to encounter.

Health care system variables present yet another level of potential barriers that the health promotion practitioner will need to be aware of when working in multicultural contexts. As Table 1.1 demonstrates, access to health care services, insurance or financial resources, and other demographics play a role in health care systems barriers but as Mull (1993) comments, there are a number of other systems issues that need to be considered. For example, the concept of preventive health is not one that is well known or understood among peoples from developing countries. Although they may know about immunization, the rationale for Pap smears, mammography, and other screening procedures might elude them. In fact, they may not even perceive that there is a need for preventive or other health care services unless more traditional methods of care have been found to be ineffective in dealing with a health issue or problem. Fear of Western medical procedures, including common practices such as drawing blood, can also present as a barrier. Among people from Third World countries, the fear of loss of blood is quite real. They believe that this blood cannot be replaced and will result in weakening the body. Uba (1992) comments that among Southeast Asians, such as rural Cambodians, there is a strong distrust of Western medicine that is often associated with death. This attitude can be traced to accessing health care services late in the course of an illness often resulting in death at the point the patient enters the health care system for treatment. Uba also notes that services, such as dietary counseling, that discuss typical Western food choices will be considered irrelevant or inappropriate by many whose cultural or ethnic preferences conflict with the recommendations they may be given.

Given the number of potential barriers that may be encountered in HPDP efforts, what can be done to help overcome some of these impediments?

Table 1.2   Comparison of Common Values From Dominant and Nondominant Perspectives

Anglo-American	Other Ethnocultural Groups
Mastery over nature	Harmony with nature
Personal control over the environment	Fate
Doing/activity	Being
Time dominates	Personal interaction dominates
Human equality	Hierarchy/rank/status
Individualism/privacy	Group welfare
Youth	Elders
Self-help	Birthright inheritance
Competition	Cooperation
Future orientation	Past or present orientation
Informality	Formality
Directness/openness/honesty	Indirectness/ritual/"face"
Practicality/efficiency	Idealism
Materialism	Spiritualism/detachment

SOURCE: Adapted from Schilling and Brannon (1986, p. 4).

STRATEGIES TO OVERCOME BARRIERS

As noted in earlier sections of this chapter, improving one's cultural competence and sensitivity to differences can be a significant step forward in overcoming many of the problems that have been identified in this chapter. This includes learning about and practicing cross-cultural communication skills and adding questions to the usual assessment tools that seek to better understand the target group's orientation toward health, disease, and folk treatment practices; acculturation levels; and other related assessment items (see Chapter 6 for questions and strategies that can be incorporated into the assessment process). In addition, taking more time to explain Western concepts of health, disease, prevention, and treatment in terms that are culturally understandable and relevant to the target group, designing and employing educational materials that are relevant and culturally appropriate to the target group, using well-trained bilingual/bicultural staff, employing indigenous health workers when working in and with diverse multicultural communities, and seeking ways to improve access to services for multicultural populations are but a few strategies that can be used to overcome barriers to HPDP efforts. Chapter 2 will expand on some of the issues presented in this chapter as well as to lay a foundation focused on traditional concepts of health and disease among a variety of multicultural populations discussed in this text.

CHAPTER SUMMARY

The United States often has been described as a melting pot in which immigrants arrive, become acculturated, and assimilate into American society and culture. As May (1992) points out, however, this blending is a very inaccurate and potentially destructive way to view American culture and society. A more accurate metaphor would be to view America as a rich and complex tapestry of colors, backgrounds, and interests. Having an understanding of this tapestry and its implications on health and disease patterns can enable the health promotion practitioner to be much more effective in reducing morbidity and mortality among the many multicultural population groups residing in the United States and elsewhere in the world.

This chapter has not sought to provide a comprehensive overview of culture; rather, it has sought to provide insights into the complex nature of culture with respect to the potential impact of cultural diversity on HPDP efforts. Culture was defined as a template or framework that a society uses to make sense of and to organize its world. A variety of terms including *acculturation, assimilation, ethnocentrism, cultural competence, ethnosensitivity,* and *cross-cultural communications* were defined and discussed to make overt the implications of these factors on HPDP practices. Barriers to promoting health among multicultural populations were described and a number of recommendations were made for improving the efficacy of health-promoting efforts when working with multicultural population groups.

Chapter 2 that follows will expand on the concept of culture presented in this chapter and will focus on health-related cultural concepts as defined by the "explanatory models" that different multicultural groups use to describe and make sense of health, illness, and disease. It will also include a brief discussion of health beliefs associated with traditional peoples living in the United States and elsewhere. This foundational information can help in better understanding of the relationship of culture to health beliefs and practices in a variety of multicultural settings. This information has great relevance in later planning rational and sensitive HPDPs.

DISCUSSION QUESTIONS AND ACTIVITIES

1. Find a journal article that reports on a HPDP project and look for how terms related to working with diverse cultural groups are defined. What barriers to HPDP were reported, and how were these overcome? Report your findings to the class or write an abstract to be turned in to the course instructor.

2. Consider the family you were raised in. What values, traditions, languages, religious practices, and related ways of living were you enculturated to? How, if at all, did these ways of living conflict with the broader culture you were raised in? How did you compromise or otherwise adapt your family's cultural traditions to those of the broader culture?

REFERENCES

Abraido-Lanza, A. F., Armbrister, A. N., Florez, K. R., & Aguirre, A. N. (2006). Toward a theory-driven model of acculturation in public health research. *American Journal of Public Health, 96*(8), 1342–1346.

Anderson, P. P., & Fenichel, E. S. (1989). *Serving culturally diverse families of infants and toddlers with disabilities.* Washington, DC: National Center for Clinical Infant Programs.

Bell, P., & Evans, J. (1981). *Counseling the black client.* Center City, MN: Hazelden Education Materials.

Bock, P. K. (1969). *Modern cultural anthropology: An introduction.* New York: Alfred A. Knopf.

Borkan, J., & Neher, J. (1991). A developmental model of ethnosensitivity in family practice training. *Family Medicine, 23*(3), 212–217.

Brainard, J., & Zaharlick, A. (1989). Changing health beliefs and behaviors of resettled Laotian refugees: Ethnic variation in adaptation. *Social Science and Medicine, 29*(7), 845–852.

Brislin, R. W., & Yoshida, T. (Eds.). (1994). *Improving intercultural interactions: Modules for cross-cultural training programs.* Thousand Oaks, CA: Sage.

Burnam, M. A., Hough, R. L., Karno, M., Escobar, J. I., & Telles, C. A. (1987). Acculturation and lifetime prevalence of psychiatric disorders among Mexican Americans in Los Angeles. *Journal of Health and Social Behavior, 28,* 89–102.

Campinha-Bacote, J. (1994). Cultural competence in psychiatric mental health nursing: A conceptual model. *Nursing Clinics of North America, 29*(1), 1–8.

Casas, J. M., & Casas, A. (1994). The acculturation process and implications for educational services (pp. 26–27). In *The multicultural challenge in health education.* Santa Cruz, CA: ETR Associates.

Castro, F. G., Cota, M. K., & Vega, S. C. (1999). Health promotion in Latino populations: A sociocultural model for program planning, development, and evaluation. In R. M. Huff & M. V. Kline (Eds.), *Promoting health in multicultural populations: A handbook for practitioners* (pp. 137–168). Thousand Oaks, CA: Sage.

Clark, L., & Hofsess, L. (1998). Acculturation. In S. Loue (Ed.), *Handbook of immigrant health* (pp. 37–69). New York: Plenum Press.

Cross, T. L., Bazron, B., Dennis, K. W., & Isaacs, M. R. (1989). *Towards a culturally competent system of care.* Washington, DC: CASSP Technical Assistance Center at Georgetown University Child Development Center.

Cuellar, I., Harris, L. C., & Jasso, R. (1980). An acculturation scale for Mexican American

normal and clinical populations. *Hispanic Journal of Behavioral Sciences, 2,* 199–217.

Dainton, M., & Zelley, E. D. (2005). *Applying communication theory for professional life: A practical introduction.* Thousand Oaks, CA: Sage.

de Paula, D., Lagana, K., & Gonzalez-Ramirez, L. (1996). Mexican Americans. In J. G. Lipson, S. L. Dibble, & P. A. Minarik (Eds.), *Culture and nursing care: A pocket guide.* San Francisco: UCSF Nursing Press.

Dolhun, E. P., Munoz, C., & Grumbach, K. (2003). Cross-cultural education in U.S. medical schools: Development of an assessment tool. *Academic Medicine, 78*(6), 615–622.

Ferguson, B., & Browne, E. (Eds.). (1991). *Health care and immigrants: A guide for the helping professions.* Sydney, Australia: McLennan & Petty.

Green, L. W., & Kreuter, M. W. (1991). *Health promotion planning: An educational and environmental approach.* Mountain View, CA: Mayfield.

Green, L. W., & Kreuter, M. W. (2005). *Health program planning: Educational and ecological approach* (4th ed.). New York: McGraw-Hill.

Green, L. W., Richard, L., & Potvin, L. (1996). Ecological foundations of health promotion. *American Journal of Health Promotion, 10*(4), 270–281.

Hammerschlag, C. A. (1988). *The dancing healers: A doctor's journey of healing with Native Americans.* San Francisco: Harper.

Helman, C. (2007). *Culture, health and illness* (5th ed.). London: Hodder Arnold.

Hoffman, T., Dana, R., & Bolton, B. (1985). Measured acculturation and MMPI-168 performance of Native American adults. *Journal of Cross-Cultural Psychology, 16,* 243–256.

Joint Committee on Health Education Terminology. (1991). Report of the 1990 Joint Committee on Health Education Terminology. *Journal of Health Education, 22,* 97–108.

Kagawa-Singer, M., & Chung, R. (1994). A paradigm for culturally based care in ethnic minority populations. *Journal of Community Psychology, 22,* 192–208.

Kramer, B. J. (1992). Health and aging of urban American Indians. In Cross-cultural medicine:

A decade later [Special issue]. *Western Journal of Medicine, 9*(157), 281–285.

Kreps, G. L., & Kunimoto, E. N. (1994). *Effective communication in multicultural health care settings.* Thousand Oaks, CA: Sage.

Kreuter, M. W., Lukwago, S. N., Bucholtz, D. C., Clark, E. M., & Sanders-Thompson, V. (2003). Achieving cultural appropriateness in health promotion programs: Targeted and tailored approaches. *Health Education and Behavior, 30*(2), 133–146.

Leddy, S. K. (2003). *Integrative health promotion: Conceptual bases for nursing practice.* Thorofare, NJ: Slack.

Locke, D. C. (1992). *Increasing multicultural understanding: A comprehensive model.* Newbury Park, CA: Sage.

Luckmann, J. (1999). *Transcultural communication in nursing.* Albany, NY: Delmar.

Marin, G., & Gamba, R. (1996). A new measurement of acculturation for Hispanics: The Bidirectional Acculturation Scale for Hispanics (BAS). *Hispanic Journal of Behavioral Sciences, 18*(3), 297–316.

May, J. (1992). Working with diverse families: Building culturally competent systems of health care delivery. *Journal of Rheumatology, 19*(33), 46–48.

McLeroy, K. R., Bibeau, D., Steckler, A., & Glanz, K. (1988). An ecological perspective on health promotion programs. *Health Education Quarterly, 15*(4), 351–378.

Mendoza, R. H. (1989). An empirical scale to measure type and degree of acculturation in Mexican-American adolescents and adults. *Journal of Cross-Cultural Psychology, 20,* 372–385.

Milliones, J. (1980). Construction of a black consciousness measure: Psychotherapeutic implications. *Psychotherapy: Theory, Research and Practice, 17,* 175–182.

Mo, B. (1992). Modesty, sexuality, and breast health in Chinese-American women. In Cross-cultural medicine: A decade later [Special issue]. *Western Journal of Medicine, 9*(157), 260–264.

Montague, A. (Ed.). (1964). *The concept of race.* London: Collier Books.

Mull, J. (1993). Cross-cultural communication in the physician's office. *Western Journal of Medicine, 159,* 609–613.

Nelson, H., & Jurmain, R. (1988). *Introduction to physical anthropology* (4th ed.). St. Paul, MN: West Publishing.

Northouse, P. G., & Northouse, L. L. (1992). *Health communications: Strategies for health professionals* (2nd ed.). Norwalk, CT: Appleton & Lange.

Nunnally, E., & Moy, C. (1989). *Communication basics for health service professionals.* Newbury Park, CA: Sage.

Office of Minority Health. (2001). *National standards for culturally and linguistically appropriate services in health care.* Washington, DC: U.S. Department of Health and Human Services.

Ohmans, P., Garrett, C., & Treichel, C. (1996). Cultural barriers to health care for refugees and immigrants: Providers' perceptions. *Minnesota Medicine, 5*(79), 26–30.

Paniagua, F. A. (1994). *Assessing and treating culturally diverse clients: A practical guide.* Thousand Oaks, CA: Sage.

Purnell, L. D., & Paulanka, B. J. (2003). *Transcultural health care: A culturally competent approach.* Philadelphia: F. A. Davis.

Putsch, R. W., III. (1985). Cross-cultural communication: The special case of interpreters in health care. *Journal of American Medical Association, 254,* 3344–3348.

Ramakrishna, J., & Weiss, M. G. (1992). Health, illness, and immigration: East Indians in the United States. In Cross-cultural medicine: A decade later [Special issue]. *Western Journal of Medicine, 9*(157), 265–270.

Ramirez, A. G., Cousins, J. H., Santos, Y., & Supic, J. D. (1986). A media-based acculturation scale for Mexican-Americans: Application to public health programs. *Family and Community Health, 9*(3), 63–71.

Ramirez, M. (1984). Assessing and understanding biculturalism-multiculturalism in Mexican-American adults. In J. L. Martinez & R. H. Mendoza (Eds.), *Chicano psychology* (pp. 77–94). Orlando, FL: Academic Press.

Richard, L., Potvin, L., Kishchuk, N., Prlic, H., & Green, L. W. (1996). Assessment of the ecological approach in health promotion programs. *American Journal of Health Promotion, 10*(4), 318–328.

Riser, A., & Mazur, L. (1995). Use of folk remedies in a Hispanic population. *Archives of Pediatric and Adolescent Medicine, 149,* 978–981.

Rojas-Guyler, L., Ellis, N., & Sanders, S. (2005). Acculturation, health protective sexual communication, and HIV/AIDS risk among Hispanic women in a large midwestern city. *Health Education & Behavior, 32*(6), 767–779.

Rothwell, J. D. (2004). *In mixed company: Communicating in small groups and teams* (5th ed.). Victoria, Australia: Thomson-Wadsworth.

Schilling, B., & Brannon, E. (1986). *Strategies for working with culturally diverse communities and clients.* Washington, DC: Association for the Care of Children's Health, Maternal and Child Health Bureau.

Slonim, M. (1991). *Children, culture, and ethnicity: Evaluating and understanding the impact.* New York: Garland.

Smither, R., & Rodriguez-Giegling, M. (1982). Personality, demographics, and acculturation of Vietnamese and Nicaraguan refugees to the United States. *International Journal of Psychology, 17,* 19–25.

Spector, R. E. (2004). *Cultural diversity in health and illness* (6th ed.). Upper Saddle River, NJ: Pearson Prentice Hall.

Stein, P. L., & Rowe, B. M. (1989). *Physical anthropology* (4th ed.). New York: McGraw-Hill.

Suinn, R. M., Rickard-Figueroa, K., Lew, S., & Vigil, S. (1987). The Suinn-Lew Asian Self-Identity Acculturation Scale: An initial report. *Education and Psychological Measurement, 47,* 401–407.

Turnock, B. J. (2001). *Public health: What it is and how it works* (2nd ed.). Gaithersburg, MD: Aspen.

Uba, L. (1992). Cultural barriers to health care for Southeast Asian refugees. *Public Health Reports, 107,* 545–548.

2

Cross-Cultural Concepts
of Health and Disease

ROBERT M. HUFF

SOHEILA YASHARPOUR

Chapter Objectives

On completion of this chapter, the health promotion student and practitioner will
be able to

- Describe the relationship of culture to health beliefs and practices in a variety of
  multicultural settings

- Describe and provide examples of explanatory models used by different
  ethnic/cultural groups living in the United States

- Identify and discuss four lay theories of illness with at least one example for each
  theory

- Identify and discuss at least three different types of traditional healers who can
  be found practicing in the United States

Health is one consequence of the balance between yin and yang energy forces, which rule the world, and an imbalance between these two forces can result in illness (Seidel, Ball, Dains, & Benedict, 1995). So begins one explanation for health and disease that characterizes traditional Chinese beliefs about disease causation. As this explanation implies, the relationship of culture to health beliefs and practices is highly complex, dynamic, and interactive. Often these explanations involve family, community, and/or supernatural agents in cause, effect, placation, and treatment rituals to prevent, control, or cure illness across a variety of multicultural groups. In contrast, the Western biomedical model explains illness in terms of the presenting pathophysiology. Sickness is often reduced to disease, and the focus is on the body rather than on the whole person within the context of his or her culture.

This chapter seeks to expand on the concept of culture presented in the previous chapter but with a focus on health-related cultural concepts as defined by the "explanatory models" that different multicultural groups use to describe and make sense of health, illness and disease. A brief discussion of health beliefs associated with traditional peoples living in the United States and elsewhere is included. The authors recognize that trying to cover these issues in a few pages is an impossible task but hope that the brief sketches provided will present a glimpse of some of the traditional concepts of health and disease held by the peoples who are being addressed in this book.

CONCEPTS OF HEALTH AND DISEASE

Landrine and Klonoff (1992) noted that many multicultural groups in the world view health and illness as fluid and continuous manifestations of the long-term and changing relationships and dysfunctions the individual has with his or her family, community, and environment. They observe that the health concepts of many of these cultural groups involve macrolevel, interpersonal, and supernatural agents of illness and disease causality. Many of those holding these views may choose not to seek Western medical treatment procedures because they do not view the illness or disease as coming from within themselves. In fact, Dimou (1995) observes that among many Eastern cultures and other cultures in the developing world, the locus of control for disease causality often is centered outside the individual, whereas in Western cultures, the locus of control tends to be more internally oriented. That is, in Eastern cultures, the illness or disease may be perceived as retribution coming from an angry spirit for some

transgression or violation of a person's role within his or her family or social group rather than the result of the person's lifestyle choices and associated behaviors over which he or she has some control. Landrine and Klonoff (1992) note that if the more traditionally entrenched person does seek Western medical treatment, he or she might be labeled as a *poor historian*, a *difficult patient*, or a mentally ill *somaticizer* because this person cannot provide or describe his or her symptoms in precise terms so that the Western medical practitioner can readily treat them. This person also might not follow through with the treatment recommendation because he or she perceives the medical encounter as a negative, and perhaps even hostile, experience.

Kleinman (1980) describes a process for explicitly distinguishing the explanations that individual patients and health care practitioners have about health and disease causality. He calls these "explanatory models" and defines them as "the notions about an episode of sickness and its treatment that are employed by all those engaged in the clinical process" (p. 105). He comments that the explanatory models of patients and health practitioners are important in helping us understand how each player perceives, understands, and treats illness and can help illuminate the real or potential problems that might occur in a clinical or other health care communication encounter. Kleinman also distinguishes explanatory models from general beliefs about sickness and health care, noting that general health beliefs are part of the health ideology of the patient, whereas explanatory models, although they draw from the basic health ideology, are much more specific to a particular episode of an illness. He distinguishes five major concerns that explanatory models seek to answer for illness episodes. These include the etiology, the time and mode of onset of symptoms, the pathophysiology of the illness, and the course of the illness, including severity, sick role behaviors, and treatment. Kleinman comments that

Western health care practitioner models tend to answer all or most of these questions, whereas patient or family models address only the most important concerns for them. Paying attention to these patient explanations can help disclose the significance of the illness for the patient (or family), including their desired treatment goals.

Pachter (1994) notes that most clinical encounters can be viewed as an interaction between two cultures: the culture of the patient and the culture of medicine. Both are likely to have divergent perceptions, knowledge, attitudes, behaviors, and communication styles relative to the illness or health issue as a result of their explanatory models of health, disease, causality, and treatment. An individual's model is generally a conglomeration of his or her ethnocultural beliefs and values; personal beliefs, values, and behaviors; and understanding of biomedical concepts. In fact, Pachter suggests that there is a range or spectrum of illness beliefs, with one end encompassing illnesses defined within the Western biomedical model. Here also can be found lay/popular explanatory models that are more closely aligned with Western models (e.g., cancer as an abnormal growth). In this case, the sickness episode is acknowledged by both systems, and there is high potential for a good exchange of ideas between the systems with regard to mutually acceptable treatment options. In the middle of this spectrum are other illness categories where the incompatibility between lay/popular beliefs and biomedical beliefs is much wider (e.g., the belief that high blood pressure is caused by too much blood). On the far end of the spectrum can be found the illness explanations that are the most widely discrepant between the lay/popular beliefs and the biomedical model. These illnesses often are classified as folk illnesses commonly recognized or associated with specific cultural groups, such as the illness *empacho* (e.g., food sticking to the inside of the stomach or intestines) among Latino population groups. Obviously, the more widely

disparate the differences between the biomedical model and the lay/popular explanatory model, the greater is the potential for encountering resistance to Western medical assessment, treatment, and adherence to treatment recommendations. Thus, it would seem appropriate for the health promoter to take the time in his or her initial needs assessment efforts to explore the explanatory models of the cultural or ethnic group(s) with which the health promoter will be working. This can serve to uncover potential barriers to the programs and services the health promoter is planning and even to suggest intervention approaches more acceptable to his or her target audiences.

TRADITIONAL CONCEPTS OF ILLNESS CAUSALITY

Helman (2007) describes folk illnesses as syndromes that individuals from particular cultural groups claim to have and from which they define the etiology, diagnostic procedures, prevention methods, and traditional healing/curing practices. He notes that folk illnesses are more than just a cluster of signs and symptoms the patient experiences; they also have symbolic meaning to the individual and culture from which the folk illness arises. These meanings may be moral, social, or psychological and often link the illness of the patient to changes in the natural world or the workings of the supernatural realm. Helman offers a caveat to all those working with different cultural groups. He observes that folk illnesses can be, and often are, learned. For example, the child who sees and learns to respond to a range of illness symptoms (e.g., physical, social, and emotional) in culturally patterned ways will, over time, come to exhibit these in response to specific episodes of illness. Thus, the health practitioner working with diverse cultural groups must make himself or herself aware of how these groups acquire, display, and typically define and treat their traditional folk illnesses.

A number of researchers (Buchwald, Panwala, & Hooton, 1992; Helman, 1984, 2007; Jack, Harrison, & Airhihenbuwa, 1994; Landrine & Klonoff, 1992; Seidel et al., 1995; Spector, 1991, 2004; Uba, 1992) have sought to place illness causality into a series of categories as a way of helping to make sense of and classify lay theories of illness. Helman (2007) describes four categories: the individual, the natural world, the social world, and the supernatural world. He notes that lay illness explanatory models may arise from any one or a combination of these. At the individual level, illness may result from malfunctions of the body as a result of factors such as diet or behavior over which the person has some control. This is a common explanation used in Western societies, where illnesses associated with health behaviors such as smoking, drinking, or lack of exercise are commonly cited as personal choices the individual makes and for which he or she might have to pay a health-related price over time. This category also recognizes hereditary, social, economic, and other personality factors that may play a role in illness causality and response. Here, it is important to determine the individual's locus of control to determine whether the person will take responsibility for his or her own health or see it as lying outside of the person.

The natural world includes both animate and inanimate factors believed to cause illness. For example, causality might be attributed to microorganisms such as bacteria or viruses (e.g., flu or tuberculosis); parasitic infections, such as those caused by pinworms; and injuries caused by animals, birds, or fish. Other factors include environmental irritants such as smog, pollens, and poisons; natural disasters where physical injuries may occur, such as earthquakes, floods, and fires; and climatic conditions such as extremes of heat, cold, wind, rain, or snow.

The social world is concerned with interpersonal conflicts that include physical injuries inflicted by people on others (i.e., personal assaults resulting from gang violence, war, and other similar causes). Stresses resulting from conflicts with family, friends, and employment are also part of this social causality. In more traditional non-Western cultures, illness is often ascribed to sorcery or witchcraft, in which certain people have the power to cast spells, create potions, or carry out rituals that can result in illness or death for individuals against whom the sorcerer or witch has a personal vendetta.

The supernatural world includes ancestral and other spirits and gods who can directly intercede in human life and cause personal difficulties, illness, and death. Illnesses inflicted from the supernatural world include things such as spirit possessions, spirit aggression, and soul loss as retribution for behavioral lapses (e.g., not thanking a particular god for a blessing, sinful behavior such as getting drunk, offending a particular ancestor's spirit, or breaking a particular social taboo). Where supernatural causes of illness are suspected, neither traditional home remedies nor Western medical practitioners are considered useful in treating and curing the illness. Such situations call for repentance, prayer, and/or the intercession of a shaman, priest, or other spiritual advisor or healer. As Helman (2007) observes, however, most cases of lay illness have multiple causalities and may require several different approaches to diagnosis, treatment, and cure. For the health promoter, an awareness of how the cultural or ethnic group perceives and defines disease causality and the appropriate treatment interventions can help him or her tailor programs, services, and/or medical treatment recommendations that consider and incorporate these cultural differences in the health promoter's planning and intervention processes.

TRADITIONAL MODELS OF HEALTH CARE DELIVERY

Folk illnesses, which are perceived to arise from a variety of causes, often require the services of a folk healer who may be a local *curandero*, shaman, native healer, spiritualist, root doctor, or other specialized healer. These traditional healers are believed to be capable of prescribing specific teas, ointments, and compresses to cure illness. They may also be consulted to carry out spiritual rituals and ceremonies or other magical practices to promote health and prevent or cure disease. Murray and Rubel (1992) discuss practices that fall under the rubric of alternative medicine and identify five categories of practitioners who may be found practicing alternative medicine. The first category consists of "spiritual and psychological" practitioners, including religious faith healers, psychics, and mystics, who may use a variety of psychological techniques to heal or cure their patients. The second category is "nutritional" and includes those persons who use herbal remedies and special diets for healing. The third category includes "drug and biological" specialists who employ various chemicals, drugs, and vaccines to cure or prevent disease. The fourth category includes those who employ treatment with physical forces and devices (e.g., chiropractors, massage therapists). The fifth category includes those who use other techniques that do not seem to fit the other categories of healer (e.g., aroma therapists, iridologists). The use of these traditional or alternative models of health care delivery is widely varied and may come into conflict with Western models of health care practice. An understanding of these differences may help the health promoter be more sensitive to the special beliefs and practices of his or her target group when planning a program for a particular multicultural population group. It goes without saying that the health practices of any population group will be mediated by a variety of factors, including level of acculturation, socioeconomic status, education, and access to Western health care services. With these thoughts in mind, the following discussion explores some of the traditional health beliefs, practices, and folk healers used by the population groups described in this book.

Latino Americans

Within the traditional Latino American community, with its highly diverse population groups, the explanatory models for health and illness are generally associated with the social, psychological, or physical domains. For example, among Brazilians, illnesses may be attributed to divine intervention or fate. They may also result from changes in temperature, food ingestion, activity, or very strong emotions (Hilfinger Messias, 1996). Among Central Americans (e.g., Guatemalans, Salvadorans, Nicaraguans), illness may be the result of an imbalance between the individual and his or her environment (thus a concern with hot, cold, weak, and strong forces), extremes of emotion, and outside sources including evil eye, ghosts, a witch's curse, and other similar agents (Boyle, 1996; Helman, 2007; Spector, 2004). For Cubans, the concept of equilibrium and balance between the individual and his or her environment and the germ theory of disease are well accepted as explanations for illness, although other causes such as stress, extreme nervousness, evil spells, or voodoo-type magic also are included in their explanatory models (Lassiter, 1995; Varela, 1996). Mexican Americans also view ill health as an imbalance between the individual and his or her environment, with variables such as emotions and social, physical, and spiritual factors accounting for sickness (de Paula, Lagana, & Gonzales-Ramirez, 1996; Spector, 2004). For Puerto Ricans, illness may be attributed to heredity, lack of personal attention to health, punishment from God for a sin, or evil or negative environmental forces (Juarbe, 1996; Spector, 2004). In general, these belief systems constitute a folk medical system called *curanderismo*.

Curanderismo as a system has evolved from a variety of elements drawn from spiritualistic, homeopathic, Aztec, and Spanish and other Western scientific foundations (Kiev, 1968; Lassiter, 1995; Roeder, 1988; Spector, 1991, 2004). Within this system, folk healers can be either male or female and may arrive at their calling by being born into it, serving an apprenticeship, or being called to it through a vision, trance, or dream. de Paula et al. (1996) and others (Kiev, 1968; Roeder, 1988; Spector, 2004) identify a number of different types of folk healers within the curanderismo system. These include the *curandero* or *curendera*, who generally uses rituals, prayers, pledges, and herbal baths to effect healing; the *yerbalista*, who employs herbal prescriptions that are brought home by the patient (or family) and brewed into a broth or tea; the *sobador* (male) or *sobadora* (female), who uses massage and may manipulate bones and joints if no physician is available; the *partera* (midwife), who is a woman skilled in pregnancy care and delivery; the *tendor* or *tendora*, who is a birth assistant who holds or supports the woman in labor; *bruja*, *brujo*, and *hechicero* (witch, warlock, and sorcerer), who practice black magic and who may be asked to counteract it; and *espiritista* and *espiritualista* (spiritualist and spiritist medium), who go into trances and may call on the assistance of a well-known deceased healer (e.g., don Pedro Jaramillo) to effect a cure.

Although illness causality has many explanations among Latino population groups, one major concept within the system that is important to recognize is that of "hot" and "cold" illnesses and remedies. That is, it is believed that certain illnesses are hot and must be treated with a cold remedy to restore balance (e.g., tonsillitis is a hot illness, which would be treated with cold tomatoes). Cinnamon (a hot food) is used to treat respiratory infections, which are cold illnesses. Also, certain foods should not be mixed because they might bring about an imbalance in the body and cause illness, such as eating fish and drinking milk (Roeder, 1988; Spector, 2004).

As might be expected, those who use the curanderismo system might be less inclined to volunteer information about their beliefs in the Western system of care unless a high degree of trust has been established between themselves and their health care provider. The degree of acculturation also plays a role in how often or how much the system is used in the United States today, although in personal interviews with Latinos who are at least third generation, they have confided that they still remember and occasionally use folk medical treatments before seeking, or in concert with, Western medical services.

Spector (1991, 2004) notes that when compared with the Western medical approach to healing, with its more formal, expensive, and businesslike methods, the curandero or other specialized healer is generally less expensive, shares the worldview of his or her patient, maintains a more informal and friendly relationship with the family, and will come to the patient's home day or night. Velez, Chalela, and Ramirez (Chapter 9, this volume) provide a more comprehensive overview of Latino population groups, which will help readers expand their understanding of this diverse population group, including its health beliefs and practices, its access to care, and related issues.

African Americans

Among African American communities, the use of folk healers and folk remedies continues to be carried on in place of, or in a complementary manner with, Western treatment modalities. Lassiter (1995) and others (Ashley & Harris, Chapter 14, this volume; Hopp & Herring, Chapter 13, this volume; Spector, 2004) observe that beliefs about health and health practices vary widely and are highly dependent on the degree of adherence to traditional ideas, geographic locale, education, scientific orientation, and socioeconomic status. They also observe that most African Americans retain a holistic philosophy of health and perceive the mind and body as inseparable, with balance and harmony in one's life central to maintaining health. Jack et al. (1994) comment that folk-healing practices among African Americans is centuries old and that the use of folk healers in modern society might be a reflection of their greater emotional, physical, and financial accessibility. They note that traditional African American healers include spiritualists who rely on prayer, ritual, magic, or other related practices and herbalists who may prescribe teas, herbs, and warm medicated compresses to heal or cure. These practitioners may be chosen for their calling by being born with a "veil" over their faces (the amniotic sacs that surround the babies during pregnancies), or they may be apprenticed to folk healers, from whom they learn the secrets of the trade (Haskins, 1990; Hopp & Herring, Chapter 13, this volume). Those born with the veils are believed to be able to summon spirits or communicate with the dead.

Voodoo, a belief system directly traceable to West Africa and that is associated with the practice of white or black magic, still is believed to have some influence among some African Americans today (Haskins, 1990; Spector, 2004). *Hoodoo*, a term believed to be derived from the term *juju* (to conjure), refers to both complex magical practices and simple medicinal procedures and superstitions associated with African American life that have evolved since the time slavery was first introduced into North America (Haskins, 1990). Haskins (1990) provides a number of examples to demonstrate the differences between voodoo and hoodoo, although the boundary between them still seems quite gray. For instance, a hoodoo procedure might involve placing a charm or hiding an object in someone's yard to bring about or ward off evil, or it might involve reading a sign such as a bird that has gotten into the house (which can portend the death of an immediate family member, often within a week's time). A voodoo procedure might involve casting a spell or a hex on an enemy to cause trouble or even to bring death to him or her. For example, practices such as the burning of different-colored candles (black candles to cause a slow death or red to cause an accidental death) or the brewing of a special concoction to harm a

person would reflect the dark side of voodoo. Haskins observes that the distinctions between voodoo and hoodoo have become blurred and the terms are frequently used interchangeably. He comments that voodoo practitioners want to get away from the images of dolls stuck with pins and serpent rites and prefer to use the term *spiritualist* in referring to themselves. He also notes that modern practitioners of hoodoo and voodoo are not easily identified in the black community and might only be known by observing the numbers of visitors going into and out of their homes each day.

Hopp and Herring (1999; Chapter 13, this volume) provide an excellent overview of African American health beliefs and practices. They note that blacks tend to attribute illness to two major categories: natural and unnatural. Within the natural category are illnesses caused by stress; drinking or eating too much; fighting with friends or neighbors; impurities in air, food, and water; cold air and winds; and other related factors. Natural illnesses can occur at any time and are often viewed as a punishment from God visited directly on the persons or their children. Unnatural illnesses are caused by evil influences that may have been induced by witchcraft and are not amenable to self-treatment or the usual traditional or Western treatment modalities. In this situation, the use of a voodoo practitioner is required to remove the spell, curse, or hex.

In general, traditional models of health care delivery (faith and root healers) are often used in conjunction with Western approaches, although the use of folk healers might not be readily disclosed to the Western health care practitioner (Hopp & Herring, Chapter 13, this volume; Locks & Boateng, 1996). Lassiter (1995) points out that prayer often is the first treatment method employed to counter a health problem. This often is followed by a folk health treatment and then the professional health care system if necessary. As Hopp and Herring (1997; Chapter 13, this volume) also observe, it is important to understand that folk healers often are the only health care providers available to low-income blacks.

Asian Americans

Among Southeast Asians, illness may arise from physical, metaphysical, or supernatural forces and may require the services of a shaman, a spirit medium, an astrologer, a herbalist, an acupuncturist, a Buddhist monk, or other specialists to effect a cure or healing. Chan (1992) and others (Kagawa-Singer & Han, Chapter 21, this volume; Spector, 2004) discuss the evolution of ancient Chinese medicine and note that it is an extremely well-organized medical system that has had an impact on the medical concepts of a number of Asian peoples, including the Koreans, the Japanese, and other Southeast Asians. Underlying traditional Chinese medicine is the concept of *Tao* (the harmony between heaven and earth), the forces of yin and yang, and the five elements (i.e., wood, fire, earth, metal, and water). Following the Tao (the way or path) helps the individual to be in balance with the laws of nature and the universe. Yin and yang represent the dualism of the universe and can be seen as opposite ends of a mutually complementary and interacting system. Yin represents the passive or negative female force (i.e., moon, earth, water, poverty, sadness), which produces cold, darkness, and emptiness. Yang is the active, male force (i.e., sun, heaven, fire, goodness, wealth) and is reflected in warmth, light, and fullness (Chan, 1992). To be healthy, the individual must seek to adjust himself or herself completely within the environment (the five elements) and balance the forces of yin and yang. A violation of this harmony can lead to chaos, one manifestation of which is illness.

Spector (2004) elaborates on these Chinese concepts, noting that various parts of the body correspond to the principles of yin and yang. That is, the inside of the body is yin, whereas the outside is yang. The front of the body is yin, while the back of the body is yang. The five elements correspond to the liver, heart, spleen, lungs, and kidneys and are considered yin, whereas the gallbladder, stomach, large intestine, small intestine, and bladder are considered yang. The diseases of winter and spring are considered yin, whereas those of summer and fall are yang. For example, yin conditions include cancer, pregnancy, and postpartum care and are treated with yang foods (e.g., chicken, beef, eggs, and spicy foods). Yang conditions include infections, hypertension, and venereal diseases and are treated with yin foods (e.g., pork, fish, fresh fruits, and vegetables). Chan (1992) comments that for traditional Chinese, the hot/cold classification of disease is a means for diagnosing and treating illness.

In addition to the hot-cold polarity, there are several other concepts relating to health and disease that are important to understand. The first is the concept of breath (*hay*), which resides in the respiratory system and provides resistance, strength, and freedom from illness. Next is the concept of blood, which may be weak or strong and, based on how well it is circulating, can contribute to atherosclerosis and hypertension. Finally, wind (*foong*) is associated with being bloated, passing gas, and having foam in the sputum. *Foong* is used to describe illnesses that have a fast onset and questionable outcomes (Lassiter, 1995). For the Chinese, a variety of healing methods may be used, including acupuncture, acupressure, meditation, acumassage, moxibustion, cupping, coining, herbology, shamanistic rituals, and Western medicine if necessary (Chan, 1992; Lassiter, 1995; Spector, 2004).

Among traditional Southeast Asian population groups, illness may arise from a variety of causes, some of which closely parallel those of the Chinese. For the Hmong, mild illnesses are generally attributed to organic causes, whereas more serious illness is caused by supernatural forces including spirit attacks, soul loss, and other metaphysical manifestations that can only be treated by a shaman using a variety of ritualistic ceremonies and practices, such as tying strings around the wrists in a *baci* ceremony to symbolically keep protective spirits within one's body (Brainard & Zaharlick, 1989; Fadiman, 1997; Johnson, 1996; Livo & Cha, 1991; Uba, 1992).

Livo and Cha (1991) and Kagawa-Singer and Han (Chapter 21, this volume) observe that with the resettlement of many Hmong in the United States and in other areas in the world, many of their traditional habits and practices are changing. They note, however, that the more traditional Hmong people continue to hold to animistic beliefs (i.e., a belief that spirits inhabit rocks, ponds, rivers, valleys) and to use the shaman (*tu-au-neng*), who is a combination medical doctor, psychologist, holy man, spiritual healer, and advisor. Typical shamanic healing practices may involve the use of rattles, gongs, finger bells, pieces of buffalo horn, and herbs and plants to restore patients to psychic balance and health. Livo and Cha also comment that some Western medical practices such as surgery and autopsy frighten the traditional Hmong and that other practices such as "coining" (vigorously rubbing the edge of a coin against the skin, which leaves bruises) with sick children are also avoided because they might be interpreted as child abuse by Western medical practitioners and could lead to the shaman's arrest.

The Vietnamese perceive magic, ancestors or natural spirits, and natural organic causes as agents of illness. Western biomedical explanations involving "germs" may also be accepted. Treatment for illness may require offerings and prayers to the spirits, the involvement of a powerful sorcerer, the use of treatment modalities derived from the Chinese medical system, or Western biomedical interventions (Brainard & Zaharlick, 1989; Chan, 1992; Farrales, 1996; Kagawa-Singer & Han, Chapter 21, this volume; Spector, 2004). Laotians and Cambodians also attribute illness to natural organic causes and to supernatural agents. Like other Southeast Asian

population groups, the use of magic, prayer, medicinal potions, charms, and herbal remedies all have their place in Laotian and Cambodian health belief systems (Chan, 1992; Kagawa-Singer & Han, Chapter 21, this volume; Kulig, 1996). Brainard and Zaharlick (1989), in a study of Laotian, Cambodian, Vietnamese, and Hmong refugees in the United States, observed that Laotian refugees tended to move away from traditional healing practices to Western biomedicine, whereas Cambodians seemed to show no preference between traditional and Western approaches. Vietnamese refugees tended to use traditional methods first, with Western health care accessed only when these methods were unsuccessful. Hmong refugees were the least likely to use Western medical approaches and only when all other methods had failed.

As can be seen from this brief overview, illness causality and treatment methods are quite diverse, and the choice of the type of healer will often depend on the problem that has presented. Among traditional Southeast Asian groups, the perception of what constitutes a "good" health care provider or healer is often based on who intrudes on the body the least. That is, traditional healers generally employ four basic methods of diagnosis: looking, listening, inquiring, and feeling the pulse. Abdominal palpation may also be included in the diagnostic process (Chan, 1992; Spector, 2004). In contrast, Western health care diagnostic procedures often involve invasive procedures including removal of blood and other body fluids and extensive X-ray and related diagnostic procedures along with patient history taking and tracking of symptomology. Thus, the Western approach to medicine and health care may be perceived by some Southeast Asians as unnecessary, irrelevant, and rather excessive. It is important, however, to note that, as with the other population groups discussed in this section, the degree of acculturation, education, and socioeconomic status can play a significant role in how these groups perceive and access preventive and/or curative health care services. For a more thorough review of Asian American health care issues, the reader is directed to Chapters 21 to 24 of this volume.

Native Americans

Health beliefs and practices among American Indians and Alaska Natives are extremely varied, though they all seem to share a common belief that health is closely linked to spirituality. That is, the interconnectedness of all things, both living and nonliving, and humans is but one small piece of the fabric of the universe (Joe & Malach, 1992). Traditional American Indian medicine is holistic and focuses on the need to maintain a balance among the physical, mental, spiritual, and emotional (Hodge & Fredericks, 1999; Jack et al., 1994; Kramer, 1992; Spector, 2004). Within this framework, illness is viewed as an imbalance resulting from natural or supernatural forces, and healing may require rituals and traditional medical practices carried out by an accepted native healer (Jack et al., 1994; Spector, 2004). Natural causes include disturbances in the equilibrium of the individual resulting from accidents not brought on by witchcraft, lifestyle choices, the breaking of a cultural taboo, or other violations against the natural or spiritual laws. Supernatural causes of illness include witchcraft, ghosts, spirit loss, spirit intrusion, spells, and other unnatural events (Joe & Malach, 1992; Lake, 1993; Levy, Neutra, & Parker, 1995; Lyon, 1996).

Native American traditional healing practices encompass a holistic and wellness-oriented approach to treating the individual. As Kramer (1992) observes, the focus is on behavior and lifestyle and seeking to reestablish harmony in one's physical, mental, spiritual, and personal life. These approaches may involve a combination of methods including prayer and chanting, dancing rituals, purification ceremonies, prescribing botanical medicines,

diagnosing disharmony, and/or performing physical manipulations (Hultkrantz, 1992; Lyon, 1996; Sorrell & Smith, 1993). While carrying out these methods, the traditional healer (who may be a man or a woman) may play the role of psychiatrist/psychologist, doctor, arbitrator, diviner, and/or religious consultant.

A review of the traditional health beliefs and practices of Alaska Native populations revealed that these groups, like other Native American tribal groups, relate their religious beliefs and health practices to the environments in which they live—that is, a belief system that perceives the world as filled with spirits who inhabit the land, water, animals, and sky and who require respectful treatment (Jorgensen, 1990). Chance (1990) observes that despite the heavy influence of Western religious practices, some Alaska Native populations continue to hold to beliefs about spirit people who inhabit their environments, including monsters and other supernatural beings. He notes that among these peoples, the universe is seen as a place where the various supernatural forces were largely hostile toward humans. Through the use of ritual and magic, these forces can be influenced for the benefit of the people (e.g., improving the weather and food supply, seeking protection from illness, and curing illness when it strikes). Explanatory models for illness among Alaska Natives include both Western and traditional health beliefs and practices (Chance, 1990; Jorgensen, 1990; Lantis, 1947; Lyon, 1996; Minority Rights Group, 1994). Although many of the traditional beliefs and rituals have disappeared since the arrival of the first whites, there are still those who rely on native healers and shamans to cure illnesses, some of which are believed to arise from causes such as soul loss or the intrusion of foreign objects into the body. Traditional healing practices may include prayer, chants, dancing, divination, sucking of foreign objects from the body, physical manipulation (laying on hands), or plant and animal remedies (Chance, 1990;

Fienup-Riordan, 1991; Jorgensen, 1990; Lyon, 1996; Purnell & Paulanka, 2003; Spector, 2004).

A number of researchers and native healers have observed that many American Indians and Alaska Natives see no conflict in the use of both Western and traditional medical practices (Chance, 1990; Fienup-Riordan, 1991; Kramer, 1992; Lake, 1993; Sorrell & Smith, 1993). In fact, in recent years there has been a movement toward combining traditional and Western therapies within the hospital and other clinical settings. This includes involving medicine people in conducting traditional healing ceremonies within the hospital setting and even teaching traditional healers about diabetes so that they, in turn, can help teach about this disease within the context of their own traditional healing practices (Hardeen, 2002; Trujillo, 2002). For a more complete overview of American Indian and Alaska Native health promotion/disease prevention (HPDP) issues, the reader is directed to Chapters 17 to 20 of this volume.

Pacific Islanders

Pacific Islanders constitute a diverse population group representing three major geographic locales in the Pacific: Melanesia, Micronesia, and Polynesia. The two most populous of these groups residing in the United States are the Native Hawaiians and Samoans (Mokuau & Tauili'ili, 1992). For this reason, these two groups are the focus of this brief overview of health beliefs and practices among Pacific Islanders.

Casken (Chapter 25, this volume) observes that traditional health beliefs among native Hawaiians were focused on the spiritual aspect of illness and its relationship to the breaking of rules for how one was to live and relate to both the spiritual and physical worlds, including family, neighbors, and community. Sickness was believed to be a punishment imposed directly or indirectly by the gods for having broken their *kapus* (taboos, prohibitions, or rules) and to result in loss of *mana* (spiritual power) as well as physical illness (Bushnell, 1993). Thus, healing of the body could occur only after the sick spirit was restored, and then only if the gods were so inclined. These beliefs have carried down to the present and also have come to incorporate germ theory as another cause of ill health (Casken, Chapter 25, this volume; Loos, Chapter 26, this volume; Mokuau & Tauili'ili, 1992).

According to Mokuaru and Tauili'ili (1992), medical care in historical times often was left to the *Kahuna Lapa'au* (medical experts), who used prayers, physical massage, and medicinal plants and herbs. King (1987) comments that the term *kahuna* refers to someone who has mastered the secrets of some field of knowledge and that the term is used rather indiscriminately in modern Hawaii to denote someone who could be a priest, minister, sorcerer, psychic, healer, or shaman. Lyon (1996) describes seven types of kahunas, including the *Kahuna Lapa'au*, who conducted healing ceremonies with the support of his helping spirit (*Akua*), to which prayers and a sacrifice had been made. Sweat baths and herbs also could be used for treatment. Diagnosis of illness was done by a *Kahuna ha ha*, who felt the patient to determine what was wrong and made referrals based on whether the illness had a spiritual cause or another cause. The *Kahuna Lomiloni* was a master of massage who was skilled at manipulating sore and stiff muscles to bring relief. The *Kahuna Kahea* was a master of psychotherapy and used prayer and the power of suggestion to cure. In addition, there were a variety of sorcerers who might be consulted if the illness was diagnosed as having been caused by an evil spirit or sorcery and requiring their intercession to effect a cure. In precontact Hawaii, religious beliefs were centered on the natural environment and ancestor worship, and despite the heavy influence of Christianity, there still exists a tendency to invoke ancestral guardian spirits and to practice religious beliefs related to the individual's relationship to nature and the gods. In fact, Mokuau and Tauili'ili (1992) observe that there has been a revival of these traditional beliefs and practices among Native Hawaiians in recent years.

In Samoa, there are two coexisting medical systems: traditional and Western. Depending on whether the illness is considered indigenous (*ma'i samoa*) or foreign (*ma'i palagi*), either or both systems might be consulted (Casken, Chapter 25, this volume; Ishida, Toomata-Mayer, & Mayer, 1996; Mokuau & Tauili'ili, 1992). Traditional Samoan health beliefs are holistic (i.e., mind, body, and spirit are all interconnected), with illness viewed as a consequence of one's actions toward the living or dead (Ishida et al., 1996). Although Samoans have strong beliefs in the Christian God, they also believe in supernatural powers and attribute the events of life to these powers. Thus, they feel they have very little control over their own destinies (Mokuau & Tauili'ili, 1992). Ishida et al. (1996) comment that because of the holistic belief system of Samoans, healing practices are directed at restoring balance in the mind-body-spirit dimensions, which might require traditional or Western healing approaches, or a combination of both, to effect a cure. They also note that the concept of preventive health is not well established among Samoan population groups, an observation that Loos (Chapter 26, this volume) echoes when he comments that Samoans view health as something that cannot be promoted and sickness as something that cannot be prevented. Mokuau and Tauili'ili (1992) observe that the use of Western medical facilities can be linked with Samoan religious beliefs in that God is seen as working through hospital care or medications. If persons "do right" before God, then they will be cured. They do note, however, that preference for traditional care and treatments or advice from relatives or their pastor will take precedence over Western health care services.

Zane, Takeuchi, and Young (1994) and Stevens and Cousineau (Chapter 5, this volume), in discussing the health issues of Asians and Pacific Islanders, comment that both of these groups are affected by the same barriers to health care as other segments of society—that is, high costs for services, fragmentation of the health care system, and inadequate health care facilities in urban and rural areas. In addition, socioeconomic factors (e.g., poverty, unemployment, and lack of health insurance, education, and literacy) also are critical variables. They also perceive that the lack of cultural competence with respect to traditional health and healing practices has created a significant conflict between native peoples and the Western biomedical health care system. Chapters 25 to 28 of this volume will provide the reader with a more comprehensive overview of this multicultural population group.

Middle Eastern Cultures

Among Afghan, Arab, and Iranian Americans, the concept of health means "wholeness" or "completeness," with illness often described as resulting from natural causes and the supernatural. Natural illnesses are believed to be caused by things that exist in nature, such as germs, dirt, cold, and winds (Giger & Davidhizar, 2004).

Supernatural illnesses are believed to be caused by *jinns* or the *evil eye*, or they are a punishment from God. For example, epilepsy is believed to be caused by jinns. The devil is believed to be responsible for unacceptable wishes, feelings, and acts. The evil eye, or *nazar*, is the belief that someone can cause illness by looking at another person with the particularly powerful gaze that comes from impure or ill people. The sudden onset of *nazar* illness can be prevented by saying "in the name of God" or "with the power of God" when giving a compliment (Diversity Resources, 2004). People most susceptible to the evil eye are children, beautiful women, brides, and rich people. A number of protections are available against the evil eye and include wearing talismans or charms, such as blue stones and beads, or burning *espand* (wild rue) in the fireplace. It is believed that the sound of the popping seeds from the burning espand symbolizes the sounds of the evil eyes popping and forcing the foul spirits out (Giger & Davidhizar, 2004).

Among Middle Eastern groups, traditional health beliefs are strongly influenced by humeral theory or the "hot" and "cold" theory of diseases. When someone feels ill, that person might be asked whether he or she has eaten something that did not agree with his or her *mezaj* (personal humeral temperament). Hot and cold imbalances cause sickness, and medicinal herbs or foods representing the opposite of what caused the problem are prescribed for specific medical problems. For example, hot illnesses, such as fever or measles, would be treated with a diet emphasizing cold foods (cucumbers, yogurt), whereas a cold illness, such as arthritis or chicken pox, would be treated with hot foods or herbs. Honey and walnuts are examples of hot foods (Giger & Davidhizar, 2004).

Medical treatment choices will depend on the cause of the illness, and both folk-traditional and Western biomedical treatments are valued and often used at the same time. For example, Western biomedical treatments will not cure illness caused by supernatural forces. These must be treated via religious approaches and healers. Mild natural illnesses are often treated with home and herbal remedies, while more serious problems will require a Western biomedical approach and practitioner (Giger & Davidhizar, 2004).

PROMOTING HEALTH ACROSS CULTURES

In the Western biomedical model, illness is explained in terms of a patient's presenting pathophysiology. Sickness is often reduced to disease, and the focus is on the patient's body rather than the whole person, where illness can be seen as the person's experience of being sick and is reflected in his or her thoughts, feelings, and altered behaviors (Weston & Brown, 1989). Weston and Brown (1989) observe that "to understand a patient's experience of illness a physician must attempt to enter the patient's world, to understand the patient's beliefs about what is wrong, why it happened, and what should be done" (p. 80). Their point is well-taken and has application to any situation where efforts to promote health and prevent disease are undertaken.

Of equal importance when working in culturally diverse settings is the need for health promoters to suspend their personal biases and judgments about those for whom they may be planning HPDP activities. As Perrone, Stockel, and Krueger (1989) comment, if one is to understand healing traditions in other cultures, then one must be open to the possibility of encountering unfamiliar beliefs and concepts about health and disease and be willing to cast out personal bias. As has been discussed in this chapter, the range and variety of health beliefs and practices associated with humankind is staggering. Not seeking to understand, respect, and work with these differences may be the greatest error any health promoter can make. Finally, it is also important to recognize that in recent years, there has been a resurgence in the use of complementary and alternative medical treatment practices across the United States. This would include approaches such as aromatherapy, special diets, homeopathic and naturopathic medicine, traditional Chinese medicine, ayurveda, Qi gong, Reiki, therapeutic touch, light and sound therapy, energy healing, distant healing, and other modalities. This has led to the establishment of the National Center for Complementary and Alternative Medicine (NCCAM, 2007) within the National Institutes of Health to explore complementary and alternative medicine (CAM) practices, train CAM researchers, and share research findings with public and health professionals.

CHAPTER SUMMARY

This chapter has sought to provide a brief overview of the explanatory models that different cultural groups use to explain and make sense of health and disease. Explanatory models were considered by Kleinman (1980) to be the notions people have about sickness episodes and how these were to be treated by those engaged in the clinical process. It was noted that explanatory models often differ significantly between the Western health care provider and more traditional peoples and that these models must be considered and respected when planning HPDP programs and activities.

Folk illnesses, syndromes that define how a culture perceives, diagnoses, and treats illness, were reviewed broadly, and it was noted that these tend to be classified under four general headings: the individual, the natural world, the social world, and the supernatural world. Thus, illness causality could be attributed to malfunctions of the body, microorganisms, injuries, environmental factors, interpersonal conflicts, sorcery and witchcraft, ancestral and other spirits, and malevolent gods who send sickness as a retribution for violations of taboos, rules, and laws of the culture.

Finally, a discussion of traditional versus Western approaches to the diagnosis and treatment of illness was described for the major multicultural groups presented in this volume. It was noted that all these groups and the diverse subgroups within them employ traditional healers and healing methods for dealing with illness, including the use of medicinal plants and herbs, physical manipulation of the body through massage and other methods, acupuncture, acupressure, coining, cupping, moxibustion, prayer, chants, incantations, divining, sorcery, and other related practices. Traditional healers tend to be specialists in different aspects of the healing tradition and are often seen and used by traditional peoples as the first step in diagnosing and treating a

sickness episode. It also was observed that many cultural groups have adopted Western medical approaches where these seem appropriate or complementary to the treatment of illness and disease but that it is critical to be culturally competent when seeking to promote health and prevent disease among diverse cultural groups. Finally, a recommendation was made that the health promoter be willing to suspend his or her judgment with respect to perceptions of how others culturally different from the health promoter perceive and deal with health and disease. A failure to respect and work within these differing frameworks is likely to contribute to conflict, confusion, indifference, and poor health care outcomes for all those involved in the HPDP encounter. Chapter 3 of this volume explores the ethics of HPDP in multicultural population groups as well as elaborate on a new model for looking at cultural competence in professional health care training programs and other Western health care settings.

In Chapter 3, the ethical implications of working with culturally diverse populations in health care and health promotion settings will be studied. There are vast differences in the cultural beliefs, values, and traditions of the many different population groups residing in and outside the United States, and the potential for a health promoter/practitioner to encounter issues or concerns that contain an ethical domain is quite probable. The following chapter discusses the importance of ethics as a major feature of any culturally competent practice in the development of HPDPs. Health professions must include the domain of culture. By not doing so, they will ignore the importance of cultural differences and cultural responses to health interventions targeting diverse cultural groups.

DISCUSSION QUESTIONS AND ACTIVITIES

1. Think back to when you were growing up. When someone became ill in your immediate

family, what types of home or folk remedies were used to treat him or her? Did they work? When you become ill now, do you still use one or more of these remedies before seeking other Western medical approaches? Why or why not?

2. Conduct one or more interviews of family members representing at least two generations to explore their concepts of health, illness, and disease. Compare and contrast these with Western biomedical explanations.

REFERENCES

Boyle, J. S. (1996). Central Americans. In J. G. Lipson, S. L. Dibble, & P. A. Minarik (Eds.), *Culture and nursing care: A pocket guide*. San Francisco: UCSF Nursing Press.

Brainard, J., & Zaharlick, A. (1989). Changing health beliefs and behaviors of resettled Laotion refugees: Ethnic variation in adaptation. *Social Science and Medicine, 29*(7), 845–852.

Buchwald, D., Panwala, S., & Hooton, T. M. (1992). Use of traditional health practices by Southeast Asian refugees in a primary care setting. *Western Journal of Medicine, 156*(5), 507–511.

Bushnell, O. A. (1993). *The gifts of civilization: Germs and genocide in Hawaii*. Honolulu: University of Hawaii Press.

Chan, S. (1992). Families with Asian roots. In E. W. Lynch & M. J. Hanson (Eds.), *Developing cross-cultural competence: A guide for working with young children and their families*. Baltimore, MD: Paul H. Brookes.

Chance, N. A. (1990). *The Inupiat and Arctic Alaska: An ethnography of development*. Fort Worth, TX: Holt, Rinehart & Winston.

de Paula, T., Lagana, K., & Gonzales-Ramirez, L. (1996). Mexican Americans. In J. G. Lipson, S. L. Dibble, & P. A. Minarik (Eds.), *Culture and nursing care: A pocket guide*. San Francisco: UCSF Nursing Press.

Diversity Resources. (2004). Retrieved January 17, 2006, from www.diversityresources.com/rc_sample/me.html

Dimou, N. (1995). Illness and culture: Learning differences. *Patient Education and Counseling, 26*, 153–157.

Fadiman, A. (1997). *The spirit catches you and you fall down*. New York: Farrar, Straus & Giroux.

Farrales, S. (1996). Vietnamese. In J. G. Lipson, S. L. Dibble, & P. A. Minarik (Eds.), *Culture and nursing care: A pocket guide*. San Francisco: UCSF Nursing Press.

Fienup-Riordan, A. (1991). *The real people and the children of thunder*. Norman: University of Oklahoma Press.

Giger, J. N., & Davidhizar, R .E. (2004). *Transcultural nursing* (4th ed.). St. Louis, MO: Mosby.

Hardeen, G. (2002, January 10). Medicine men conduct research to educate patients about diabetes. *The Tuba City Indian Medical Center Newsletter, 2*(4), 1, 4.

Haskins, J. (1990). *Voodoo and hoodoo: The craft as revealed by traditional practitioners*. New York: Scarborough House.

Helman, C. G. (1984). *Culture, health and illness*. Bristol, UK: John Wright.

Helman, C. G. (2007). *Culture, health and illness* (5th ed.). London: Hodder Arnold.

Hilfinger Messias, D. K. (1996). Brazilians. In J. G. Lipson, S. L. Dibble, & P. A. Minarik (Eds.), *Culture and nursing care: A pocket guide*. San Francisco: UCSF Nursing Press.

Hodge, F. S., & Fredericks, L. (1999). American Indian and Alaska Native populations in the United States: An Overview. In R. M. Huff & M. V. Kline (Eds.), *Promoting health in multicultural populations: A handbook for practitioners* (pp. 269–289). Thousand Oaks, CA: Sage.

Hopp, J. W., & Herring, P. (1999). Promoting health among black Americans: An overview. In R. M. Huff & M. V. Kline (Eds.), *Promoting health in multicultural populations: A handbook for practitioners* (pp. 201–221). Thousand Oaks, CA: Sage.

Hultkrantz, A. (1992). *Shamanic healing and ritual drama: Health and medicine in Native North American religious traditions*. New York: Crossroad.

Ishida, D. N., Toomata-Mayer, T. F., & Mayer, J. F. (1996). Samoans. In J. G. Lipson, S. L. Dibble, & P. A. Minarik (Eds.), *Culture and nursing care: A pocket guide*. San Francisco: UCSF Nursing Press.

Jack, L., Jr., Harrison, I. E., & Airhihenbuwa, C. O. (1994). Ethnicity and the health belief systems. In A. C. Matiella (Ed.), *The multicultural challenge in health education*. Santa Cruz, CA: ETR Associates.

Joe, J. R., & Malach, R. S. (1992). Families with Native American roots. In E. W. Lynch & M. J. Hanson (Eds.), *Developing cross-cultural competence: A guide for working with young children and their families*. Baltimore, MD: Paul H. Brookes.

Johnson, S. (1996). Hmong. In J. G. Lipson, S. L. Dibble, & P. A. Minarik (Eds.), *Culture and nursing care: A pocket guide*. San Francisco: UCSF Nursing Press.

Jorgensen, J. G. (1990). *Oil age Eskimos*. Berkeley: University of California Press.

Juarbe, T. (1996). Puerto Ricans. In J. G. Lipson, S. L. Dibble, & P. A. Minarik (Eds.), *Culture and nursing care: A pocket guide*. San Francisco: UCSF Nursing Press.

Kiev, A. (1968). *Curanderismo: Mexican-American folk psychiatry*. New York: Free Press.

King, S. (1987). The way of the adventurer. In S. Nicholson (Ed.), *Shamanism: An expanded view of reality*. Wheaton, IL: Theosophical House.

Kleinman, A. (1980). *Patients and healers in the context of culture*. Berkeley: University of California Press.

Kramer, B. (1992). Health and aging of urban American Indians. In Cross-cultural medicine: A decade later [Special issue]. *Western Journal of Medicine, 157*, 281–285.

Kulig, J. C. (1996). Cambodians (Khmer). In J. G. Lipson, S. L. Dibble, & P. A. Minarik (Eds.), *Culture and nursing care: A pocket guide*. San Francisco: UCSF Nursing Press.

Lake, M. G. (1993). *Native healer: The path to an ancient healing art*. New York: Harper Paperbacks.

Landrine, H., & Klonoff, E. A. (1992). Culture and health-related schemas: A review and proposal for interdisciplinary integration. *Health Psychology, 11*(4), 267–276.

Lantis, M. (1947). *Alaskan Eskimo ceremonialism*. New York: J. J. Augustin.

Lassiter, S. M. (1995). *Multicultural clients: A professional handbook for health care providers and social workers*. Westport, CT: Greenwood Press.

Levy, J. E., Neutra, R., & Parker, D. (1995). *Hand trembling, frenzy witchcraft, and moth madness: A study of Navaho seizure disorders*. Tucson: University of Arizona Press.

Livo, N. J., & Cha, D. (1991). *Folk stories of the Hmong: Peoples of Laos, Thailand, and Vietnam*. Englewood, CO: Libraries Unlimited.

Locks, S., & Boateng, L. (1996). Black/African Americans. In J. G. Lipson, S. L. Dibble, & P. A. Minarik (Eds.), *Culture and nursing care: A pocket guide*. San Francisco: UCSF Nursing Press.

Lyon, W. S. (1996). *Encyclopedia of Native American healing*. Santa Barbara, CA: ABC-CLIO.

Minority Rights Group (Eds.). (1994). *Polar peoples: Self-determination and development*. London: Minority Rights.

Mokuau, N., & Tauili'ili, P. (1992). Families with Native Hawaiian and Pacific Island roots. In E. W. Lynch & M. J. Hanson (Eds.), *Developing cross-cultural competence: A guide for working with young children and their families*. Baltimore, MD: Paul H. Brookes.

Murray, R. H., & Rubel, A. J. (1992). Sounding board: Physicians and healers—unwitting partners in health care. *New England Journal of Medicine, 326*(1), 61–64.

NCCA. (2007). *NCCAM facts-at-a-glance and mission*. Retrieved February 5, 2007, from http://nccam.nih.gov/about/ataglance/

Pachter, L. M. (1994). Culture and clinical care: Folk illness beliefs and behaviors and their implications for health care delivery. *Journal of the American Medical Association, 271*(9), 690–694.

Perrone, B., Stockel, H. H., & Krueger, V. (1989). *Medicine women, curanderas, and women doctors*. Norman: University of Oklahoma Press.

Purnell, L. D., & Paulanka, B. J. (2003). *Transcultural health care: A culturally competent approach* (2nd ed.). Philadelphia: F. A. Davis.

Roeder, B. A. (1988). *Chicano folk medicine from Los Angeles, California*. Berkeley: University of California Press.

Seidel, H. M., Ball, J. W., Dains, J. E., & Benedict, G. W. (1995). *Mosby's guide to physical examination* (3rd ed.). St Louis, MO: Mosby-Year Book.

Sorrell, M. S., & Smith, B. A. (1993). Navajo beliefs: Implications for health professionals. *Journal of Health Education, 24*(6), 336–338.

Spector, R. E. (1991). *Cultural diversity in health and illness* (3rd ed.). Norwalk, CT: Appleton & Lange.

Spector, R. E. (2004). *Cultural diversity in health and illness* (6th ed.). Upper Saddle River, NJ: Pearson Prentice Hall.

Trujillo, M. H. (2002, March). Insights from Michael H. Trujillo. *Health for Native Life, 4, 5.*

Uba, L. (1992). Cultural barriers to health care for Southeast Asian refugees. *Public Health Reports, 107*(5), 545–548.

Varela, L. (1996). Cubans. In J. G. Lipson, S. L. Dibble, & P. A. Minarik (Eds.), *Culture and nursing care: A pocket guide*. San Francisco: UCSF Nursing Press.

Weston, W. W., & Brown, J. B. (1989). The importance of patients' beliefs. In M. Stewart & D. Roter (Eds.), *Communicating with medical patients*. Newbury Park, CA: Sage.

Zane, N. W. S., Takeuchi, D. T., & Young, K. N. J. (1994). *Confronting critical health issues of Asian and Pacific Islander Americans*. Thousand Oaks, CA: Sage.

3

The Ethics of Health Promotion Intervention in Culturally Diverse Populations

AIMIE F. KACHINGWE

ROBERT M. HUFF

Chapter Objectives

On completion of this chapter, the health promotion student and practitioner will be able to

- Define ethics and the constructs of morality and bioethics

- Discuss the importance of having and adhering to a professional code of ethics that incorporates the practice of cultural ethics

- Describe how cultural dichotomy in transcultural relationships can lead to ethical dilemmas and cultural imposition

- Define the terms *cultural sensitivity, cultural competence, cultural proficiency,* and *ethical competency*

- Discuss how the Kachingwe-Huff model of culturally proficient and ethical practice could be incorporated into the practice setting

- Discuss the components of culturally proficient practice and promotion

- Define conviction and discuss its pivotal position in the Kachingwe-Huff model

The purpose of this chapter is to discuss the ethical implications of working with culturally diverse populations in health care and health promotion settings. The ethnic profile of the United States has undergone significant change over the past 10 years (U.S. Census Bureau, 1990, 2000a), and it has been projected that ethnic diversity will only continue to increase (U.S. Census Bureau, 2000b). These population shifts will result in health care promoters working with more ethnically diverse clients in culturally diverse communities.

Culture is the accumulation of beliefs, values, customs, and behaviors that are shared by a group, used to provide meaning, interpret experience, and generate behavior, and that is passed on from generation to generation (Kachingwe, 2000). Understanding that there are vast differences in the cultural beliefs, values, and traditions of the many different population groups residing in the United States, the potential for a health promoter/practitioner to encounter issues or concerns that contain an ethical domain is quite probable. Given this concern, the ethical implications of working with culturally diverse individuals and communities, and providing culturally proficient health care, will be addressed in three major realms: (1) the fundamental principle of including cultural ethics and providing culturally proficient care into the health professions' code of ethics, (2) the ethical dilemmas that may occur if there is a dichotomy between the cultural beliefs and practices of the client and health promoter, and (3) the centrality of ethics and conviction in providing cultural proficient care. A model for providing culturally proficient and ethical health care and promotion with the overriding concepts of conviction and ethics will be presented.

DEFINING ETHICS

Ethics refers to how individuals conduct themselves in personal and professional interactions (Scott, 1998). The word ethics comes from the Greek words *ethikos,* meaning character and *ethos,* meaning custom (Scott, 1998). *Ethics* as a discipline employs methods and approaches to help one reflect on and examine moral situations (Purtilo, Jensen, & Royeen, 2005). *Morality,* a term often used interchangeably with ethics, refers to beliefs, principles, and values about what is right and what is wrong (Purtilo, 2005; Scott, 1998). According to Hinman (2002), morality is the first-order set of beliefs and practices about *how* to live our lives, and ethics is the second-order set of beliefs in which the conscious mind reflects on the adequacy of our moral beliefs. Thus, ethics offers a way to examine moral life and involves consciously stepping back and reflecting on our beliefs and practices based on what we perceive as right and wrong (Wells, 2005).

Bioethics is a term often used to describe the ethical decision making of medical professionals (Bailey & Schwartzberg, 1995; Donnelly, 2000). A synonymous term, *clinical ethics,* relates specifically to ethical problems, issues, and dilemmas associated with patient care activities in clinics and health care institutions (Jonsen, Seigler, & Winslade, 1992; La Puma, 1990).

Ethical traditions is a term used to describe the differences in ethical perceptions and practices employed by individuals and/or groups who may be different from the health promoter or practitioner (Shive & Marks, 2006). *Ethical competency* refers to the ability to be able to work with others whose ethical traditions may be different from our own.

PROFESSIONAL CODE OF ETHICS

Every health care discipline, through its professional association, has a code of ethics governing the official conduct of association members. There is some debate surrounding the necessity of professional codes of ethics. At one end of the spectrum are individuals who believe that professional codes are futile since professionals have no rights or duties above and beyond the ethics of ordinary human beings living within a moral society (Ladd, 1995; Luegenbiehl, 1983). Others argue that professional codes of ethics are important in that they provide a framework of professional responsibilities and behaviors (M. Davis, 1991; Harris, Pritchard, & Rabins, 1995). Professional codes of ethics have four primary purposes: (1) to provide a directive of mandatory behavior by members of a profession; (2) to protect the rights of patients and clients; (3) to address areas of ethical problems, issues, and dilemmas specific to the discipline; and (4) to provide a document for how codes are enforceable and enforced (Scott, 1998).

Professional codes of ethics contain two types of provisions: directive and nondirective (Scott, 1998). Directive provisions address required conduct and usually contain the words *shall* or *will* or the converse negatives *shall not* or *will not*. Nondirective provisions address permissive conduct and/or recommended conduct. Directives of permissive conduct use the word *may*, whereas recommended conduct uses the words *should* or *should not*(Scott, 1998).

A review of various health professions' code of ethics reveals many similar principles across disciplines. Ethical principles are statements of human obligations or duties that are generally accepted (Purtilo, 2005; Scott, 1998). The most common bioethical principles include autonomy (an individual's right to make his or her own decisions and self-determination), beneficence (duty to do good in the client's best interest), confidentiality (duty to respect privacy of information), nonmaleficence (duty to cause no harm), respect for persons (duty to honor others and their rights), and justice (duty of equity or fair treatment) (Kenyon, 1999; Purtilo, 2005; Scott, 1998; Turner, 2003). These bioethical codes are centered in the concept of *respect for the person*— focusing on the individual who is affected by the ethical choices made by another

(A. J. Davis, Aroskar, Liaschenko, & Drought, 1997; Haddad, 2005; Jensen & Richert, 2005).

Although it is inarguably important to concentrate health care ethics on respecting the individual, this focus overlooks *cultural ethics* in decision making. That is, respecting, valuing, and understanding how cultural diversity and cultural differences can affect the ethical standards employed by a practitioner or health promoter whether in a clinical, community, or other health care or health promotion setting (Donnelly, 2000; Eliason, 1993; Erlen, Lebeda, & Tamenne, 1993). Most health care providers, however, are trained in bioethical principles that largely ignore cultural differences (Iwama, 2003; Sheikh, 2001; Turner, 2003). Since decisions of morality and ethics are founded within our own cultural beliefs and practices, and the lens through which we examine, interpret, judge, and subsequently act on another's actions is grounded within our own personal cultural identity, it is vital that health promoters are attentive to the influences of a client's culture when working with diverse clients and within ethnically diverse communities (Hinman, 2002; Wells, 2005).

INCORPORATION OF CULTURE INTO HEALTH PROFESSIONS' CODE OF ETHICS

There are a small number of health professions whose code of ethics directly addresses the importance of client culture. Principle 8 of the American Public Health Association Code of Ethics states, "Public health programs and policies should incorporate a variety of approaches that anticipate and respect diverse values, beliefs, and cultures in the community" (American Public Health Association, 2002). The Society for Public Health Education Code of Ethics includes numerous references to culture and diversity. For example, in the preamble, "By acknowledging the value of diversity in society and embracing a cross-cultural approach, Health Educators support the worth, dignity, potential, and uniqueness of all peoples" (Society for Public Health Education, 2006). The code of ethics of the National Association of Social Workers (2006) has a principle stating that social workers must "respect the inherent dignity and worth of the person" and should "treat each person in a caring and respectful fashion, mindful of individual differences and cultural and ethnic diversity." The American Occupational Therapy Association (2005) Code of Ethics Principle 1A states,

> Occupational therapy personnel shall provide services in a fair and equitable manner. They shall recognize and appreciate the cultural components of economics, geography, race, ethnicity, religious and political factors, marital status, sexual orientation, gender identity, and disability of all recipients of their services.

Other health professions do not specifically refer to the ethics of culture, but may infer its inclusion through general statements of respecting individualism. Principle 1 of the American Medical Association (2006) code of ethics states, "A physician shall be dedicated to providing competent medical care, with compassion and respect for human dignity and rights." Provision 2.1 of the American Nurses Association (ANA) Code refers to a commitment to the uniqueness of the individual in the nursing plan of care. As yet another example, the Physical Therapy Code of Ethics, Principle 1 states,

> A physical therapist shall respect the rights and dignity of all individuals and shall provide compassionate care . . . and shall recognize that each individual is different from all other individuals and shall respect and be responsive to those differences. (American Physical Therapy Association, 2005)

If the health professions are to continue the advancement of providing culturally competent care with diverse individuals and communities, it is vital that professional codes of ethics reflect this commitment. Thus, the first tenet to the discussion of ethics and of providing culturally appropriate care is a mandate from each respective professional association that their codes of ethics must *directly and specifically* address the ethics of working with diverse cultural groups.

ETHICAL DILEMMAS IN THE CLIENT-PRACTITIONER RELATIONSHIP

It is important to consider that current ethical principles prevalent in health care may be in direct conflict with the cultural values and beliefs of culturally diverse clients (Elliot, 2001; Hyun, 2002; Ludwick & Silva, 2000; Turner, 2003). As an example, autonomy, which refers to an individual's right to self-determination, may be in direct conflict with cultural value systems that place the family, community, or society above that of the individual and may result in distancing clients from their families, religious practices, and/or cultural values (A. J. Davis, 1999; Kaufert & Putsch, 1997; Ludwick & Silva, 2000). Another example is the bioethical principle of informed consent that requires health care providers to disclose risks of treatment to the patient. This principle violates the Navajo ideal that one should only think and speak in a positive way as thought and language have the power to shape and control the future (Carrese & Rhodes, 1995). Thus, advanced care planning and advance directives are in violation of these traditional practices and values (Carrese & Rhodes, 1995).

Health promoters need guidelines or rules of conduct for how to ethically respond to cultural problems, issues, or dilemmas. Ethical problems involving questions of professional conduct are relatively uncomplicated and easily solved (Scott, 1998). One example of an *ethical problem* is if a client comes to his or her appointment 10 minutes late on four consecutive occasions. Perhaps the client comes from a culture with a different perception of time. Although the traditional Anglo perception is that time is measured and controlled, many cultures have a "present oriented" perception of time where time is given, not measured, and there is less emphasis on future consequences (Brown & Segal, 1996; Graham, 1981; Lynch, 1998a). This dichotomy between the practitioner's and the client's perception of time can lead to a cultural problem. Perhaps the problem can be resolved by making the appointment time more flexible. In other situations, it may be necessary for the health practitioner to sit down and explain to the client that clinic schedules depend on everyone coming on time and thus need to operate on a more rigid schedule. This discussion may facilitate the client's understanding of the significance of coming on time and subsequently the ethical problem may be resolved.

An *ethical issue,* also referred to as *ethical distress,* occurs when there is controversy with strong sentiments on opposing sides of an issue and which must be resolved through compromise (Purtilo, 2005; Scott, 1998). An example of an ethical issue might be when a health promoter wishes to have an AIDS awareness workshop for students at a local high school. Parents of these students may have a number of issues with holding such a workshop including disputes based in religious or cultural values and traditions. Several approaches to this issue can be considered. First, a parent focus group or survey might be implemented to identify the issues in clear and concrete terms. This might then be followed by an open discussion with a sample of the parents to outline topics the workshop might cover with an aim of gathering parent input and support for doing this workshop. Finally, conducting the workshop for parents first could then help gain parental support to present the workshop for their high school teens.

An ethical *dilemma* is a situation where the health promoter is faced with equally favorable or unfavorable options to a situation and must decide on one of the opposing courses of action (Purtilo, 2005; Scott, 1998). An ethical dilemma also occurs when two or more moral reasons come into contact and the course of action is not obvious (Gabard & Martin, 2003). An example here might be a practitioner caring for a newly diagnosed cancer patient who has been asked by a family member(s) not to disclose the diagnosis to the patient as they do not want this person to be unnecessarily upset and where such stress to the patient might lead to that patient giving up hope of recovery (Searight & Gafford, 2005).

When solving ethical problems, issues, or dilemmas, health practitioners make decisions based on their cultural framework of what they believe is right and wrong. These cultural frameworks originate from the practitioner's personal culture as well as the practitioner's professional culture—beliefs and values learned during professional training and practiced in the work setting (Black & Purnell, 2002; Gard, Cavlak, Sunden, & Razak, 2005; Geddes, Finch, & Graham, 2005). If the practitioner's cultural framework is inherently different from that of the client's, there may be situations where the health practitioner's cultural beliefs and practices are in direct conflict with the client's cultural beliefs and practices (Doswell & Erlen, 1998; Erlen, 1998). Ethical dilemmas occur when the client's views of health and health care delivery conflict with the health practitioner's views (Erlen, 1998). More so, ethical dilemmas are likely to occur when the client's cultural behaviors and practices appear to violate the ethical and moral definitions of human rights and obligations (Donnelly, 2000), such as in the practice of female circumcision or wife beating for some infraction related to the client's culture.

When the health care practices or beliefs of the client clash with those of the practitioner, this dichotomy can lead to cultural imposition or cultural relativism. *Cultural imposition* would occur if the health promoter forces his or her biomedical practices onto the client without any consideration of the client's cultural beliefs and practices (Lattanzi & Purnell, 2006e; Leininger, 1994, 1995). An example would be if a dietician requests an individual to change his or her diet without any regard to cultural dietary preferences or restrictions. Not only can cultural imposition adversely affect patient outcomes, but this practice has also occasionally been the basis for litigation against nurses working in multicultural contexts who have made inadequate nursing judgments (Leininger, 1994, 1995).

Cultural relativism is the premise that cultural beliefs, behaviors, and practices should only be judged within the context of the client's culture. Cultural relativism promotes tolerance of alternative behaviors and practices founded on the assumption that there is no universal determination of right and wrong since value systems are relative to an individual and based on culture (Bandman & Bandman, 1995; Donnelly, 2000). Supporters of cultural relativism state that some practices should be accepted as cultural norms without judgment from outside cultural perspectives, whereas opponents to cultural relativism argue that some cultural practices violate human rights and thus should not be excused or accepted based solely on cultural grounds (Lattanzi & Purnell, 2006e). Thus, cultural relativism places the personal conscience of a health practitioner in a lower priority to the cultural beliefs and practices of the client.

A review of the literature reveals a plethora of bioethical discussions pertaining to topics such as death and dying, patient confidentiality, informed consent, and caring for uninsured or underinsured clients, with a blatant disregard to ethical problems or dilemmas faced during professional transcultural encounters (Iwama, 2003; Sheikh, 2001; Turner, 2003). Yet, it is vital for health promoters to question the ethical basis of health promotion practices aimed at discouraging certain activities and/or encouraging the adoption of others given that the judgment of what practices are right and

what practices are wrong is based within the cultural context of the health practitioner (Bayer, 2003; Coveney, 1998). Even if health promoters practice within the guidelines of their professional code of ethics, conflict can surface if caregivers question or challenge the health care practices of a patient from a different cultural group (Bandman & Bandman, 1995). Ethical issues and dilemmas in practice may only be resolved if the health promoter is engaged in culturally proficient practice.

THE CONTINUUM OF CULTURALLY PROFICIENT PRACTICE IN HEALTH CARE AND HEALTH PROMOTION

The importance of culturally competent practice is increasingly being professed in the health practitioner literature, including public health and health promotion (Burgess, Fu, & van Ryn, 2004; Jenko & Moffitt, 2006; Kreuter, Kukwago, Bucholtz, Clark, & Sanders-Thompson, 2002), medicine (Buchwald et al., 1994; Lavizzo-Mourey & Mackenzie, 1996), nursing (Alpers & Zoucha, 1996; Campinha-Bacote, 1994, 1995, 1999; Campinha-Bacote & Padgett, 1995; Clinton, 1996; Doswell & Erlen, 1998; Jones, Bond, & Mencini, 1998; Kirkham, 1998; Leininger, 1994, 1995; Lister, 1999; Napholz, 1999; Purnell, 2000; Smith, 1998; Talabere, 1996), occupational therapy (Dillard et al., 1992; Yuen & Yau, 1999), and physical therapy (Lattanzi & Purnell, 2006a; Leavitt, 1999a, 1999b; Swisher & Page, 2005). The term *cultural competence* has evolved through a variety of models for providing culturally appropriate health care.

Perhaps one of the earliest terms, *cultural sensitivity*, is defined as having an *awareness* of a client's cultural beliefs and practices to enable the practitioner to respect and value the client's perspectives and be nonjudgmental and inoffensive when working with the client (Clinton, 1996; Purnell & Lattanzi, 2006; Talabere, 1996). Many in the health professions believe that a health practitioner must go beyond providing culturally sensitive care to providing *culturally competent* care (Felder, 1995; Kirkham, 1998; Talabere, 1996), which involves the implementation and integration of cultural knowledge into clinical practice (Clinton, 1996; Smith, 1998; Sue, 1998; Talabere, 1996). Cultural competence is a process of possessing the knowledge to appreciate and respect the cultural differences and similarities within and between cultural groups, acknowledging and incorporating the importance of culture, and working within the cultural context of an individual in an unbiased manner to meet the client's needs (Alpers & Zoucha, 1996; Campinha-Bacote, 1994, 1999; Felder, 1995; Leavitt, 1999a; Lynch, 1998b; St. Clair & McKenry, 1999; Talabere, 1996). A similar ideal, providing *culturally congruent* care, has been defined as acquiring knowledge and an understanding of a patient's cultural orientation, including language and attitudes toward health and illness, to provide safe and effective care (Donnelly, 2000).

The next stage on the culturally appropriate practice continuum is *cultural proficiency*. Cultural proficiency is acknowledging, valuing, responding to, and advocating for individual as well as group differences and involves continually striving to formally and informally increase the awareness level of and knowledge base for culturally proficient practices (Lindsey, Robins, & Terrell, 1999). Culturally proficient practice thus provides culturally competent care while at the same time reaching out into the community to meet their needs through advocacy and action (Andrews & Boyle, 1999; Coveney, 1998; Cross, Bazron, Dennis, & Isaacs, 1989; Lindsey et al., 1999). Thus, culturally proficient practice demands that health promoters act as community advocates, serve as a community resource, lobby for community legislation, and/or become involved in charitable events (Lattanzi & Purnell, 2006b).

Various models can be found throughout the literature with guidelines for how cultural competence can be achieved (Campinha-Bacote, 1995, 1999; Campinha-Bacote & Padgett, 1995; Felder, 1995; Huff & Kline, 1999; Kirkham, 1998; Leavitt, 1999b; Lister, 1999; Purnell, 2000; St. Clair & McKenry, 1999; Talabere, 1996). Based on these frameworks, and noting the need to include several constructs not specifically addressed in these, Kachingwe and Huff have developed a model for the achievement of *culturally proficient and ethical* health care practice regardless of the situation or setting. Inherent in this model are the overarching constructs of ethics and conviction.

KACHINGWE-HUFF MODEL OF CULTURALLY PROFICIENT AND ETHICAL PRACTICE

Culturally proficient practice can be fostered via the incorporation of five components: cultural awareness, cultural knowledge, interpersonal communication skills, cultural collaboration, and cultural experiences (Figure 3.1).

The first step toward providing culturally proficient care is developing cultural awareness. Cultural awareness is the process by which health care providers become sensitive to and reflective of their personal culture as well as their client's culture (Campinha-Bacote, 1994, 1999; Campinha-Bacote & Padgett, 1995; Lynch, 1998b).

Reflecting on personal culture entails that the health practitioner or student be cognizant of his or her own cultural identity and assess how his or her personal beliefs, attitudes, and behaviors affect his or her views of others (Clinton, 1996; Felder, 1995; Huff & Kline, 1999). Health professionals must also realize that they are socialized into the culture of their profession. Initiated during professional training, professional socialization teaches the health profession student a set of beliefs, practices, and rituals inherent in their profession (Purtilo & Haddad, 2002; Spector, 2004).

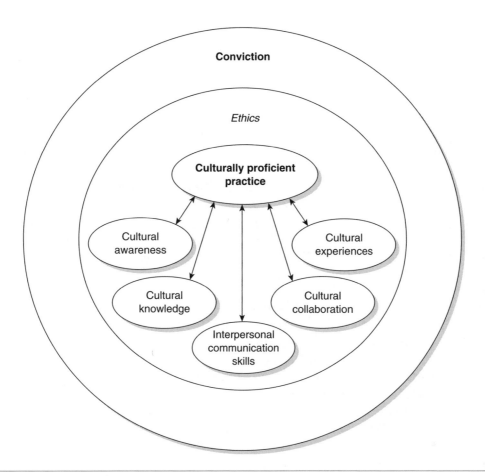

Figure 3.1   Kachingwe-Huff Model of Culturally Proficient and Ethical Practice

Health promoters thus function within the frameworks of their personal culture and their professional culture. Given that individuals are innately ethnocentric, health promoters have a tendency to view their client's health care beliefs and practices from the perspective of their own culture. Ethnocentrism may then lead to distorted perceptions of client behaviors and unfounded judgments and stereotypes of what is appropriate and what is inappropriate behavior (Campinha-Bacote & Padgett, 1995; Dowd, Giger, & Davidhizar, 1998; Felder, 1995; Gordon, 2005; Kirkham, 1998; Leavitt, 1999a; Purnell & Lattanzi, 2006). Huff and Kline (1999) suggest a series of questions health practitioners or students can ask

themselves as a way of getting in touch with their own ethnocentric attitudes.

Consider the last time you saw or interacted with someone you categorized as representing a particular ethnic group. How did you come to categorize that individual as representing a particular ethnic group? How have you come to your knowledge of the specific characteristics you employed to categorize that individual? How accurate do you think these characteristics are with respect to that specific individual? What do you know or not know about that specific individual in terms of his or her cultural heritage, lifestyle, and the like? What more did you seek to learn about that individual? How would you feel knowing that others may be categorizing you in similar ways? (p. 13)

Answering these questions in an honest and open manner may help practitioners better understand how their own ethnocentric attitudes might create problems for their client and themselves in a health care, health education, or other interpersonal encounter.

Cultural awareness also involves having the health promoter reflect on personal attitudes and biases against other cultures. This is particularly important to health practitioners who will be working with culturally diverse clients and/or in ethnically diverse communities (Felder, 1995; Kirkham, 1998; Wells, 2005). Given the current Western paradigm of health care, health promoters must move beyond the perception of culture as a *barrier* to adequate health care and health promotion to the acknowledgment that culture is an integral component of their client's life experience and thus must be embraced to achieve optimal health care and/or health promotion outcomes (Felder, 1995).

The second step toward cultural proficiency is increasing cultural knowledge. Increasing cultural knowledge involves acquiring knowledge of, and understanding of, various cultures to be able to respect and acknowledge the similarities as well as differences between and among cultural groups (Baldonado, 1996; Campinha-Bacote, 1994, 1999; Swisher & Page, 2005). Health promoters can increase cultural knowledge by learning about the cultural beliefs and practices of their clients, including differences in communication, variations in personal space, and differences in perception of time. Yet, it is also important to learn about the physiological variations between people (Dowd et al., 1998). It is virtually impossible to be a "cultural expert" of all cultures since there is a multitude of within-cultural differences. For example, people sharing a common culture may differ in their level of acculturation and thus adherence to cultural beliefs and practices (Leavitt, 1999a). Health professionals

should, however, be encouraged to learn more about specific cultures common among their clients and prevalent in the community they practice (Leavitt, 1999a). This might be done by reading about the different cultures in their community, attending cultural events, visiting these communities to shop and eat, or otherwise interacting with the cultural group(s) outside the confines of the practice setting.

To discuss the general beliefs and practices of cultural groups, one must make generalizations. Making a generalization about a cultural group is a natural approach to managing the overwhelming complexity of culture (MacLachlan, 1997). There is value in being able to generalize about cultural groups in that it provides the health practitioner with a starting point on which to build further inquiry (Purnell & Lattanzi, 2006). However, when cultural generalizations relate more to the motive behind a behavior than to the actual observed behavior, the generalization may be oversimplified—leading to stereotyping. Stereotyping is an oversimplified concept, opinion, or belief about an individual or group of people (Duffy, 2001; Huff & Kline, 1999; Purnell & Lattanzi, 2006). Thus, it is important that when health promoters strive to increase knowledge and respect for culture that they do not label or stereotype cultures, for this may lead to lack of respect and stigmatization (Duffy, 2001; Erlen et al., 1993). Respect for culture entails validating the beliefs and practices of the culture rather than basing interactions on assumptions made about the culture (Erlen, 1998; Erlen et al., 1993; Kreuter et al., 2002).

The third step toward culturally proficient practice is effective *interpersonal communication skills*. Health practitioners must have good communication skills for effective interviewing and for being able to design and effectively implement health education and health promotion programs in their practice and/or community settings. They need to glean pertinent information about a client's beliefs and practices and be able to assess the client's perceptions of his or her health, illness, and treatment (Campinha-Bacote, 1994, 1995, 1999; Campinha-Bacote & Padgett, 1995). Huff and Kline (1999) offer a cultural assessment framework that identifies a variety of potential question areas that can be drawn from to structure a cultural assessment instrument or set of questions for an interview. These can help identify cultural differences that might block or otherwise impede a practitioner's understanding of their culturally diverse client or target community. Conducting a cultural assessment should be the first of a number of assessment processes any health promoter does when they encounter a culturally diverse client or are attempting to develop culturally sensitive and appropriate health education and health promotion programs and services for their community.

Health care practitioners must ask their clients directly about pertinent cultural beliefs and practices, but in an unassuming, approachable, culturally sensitive manner (Buchwald et al., 1994; Campinha-Bacote, 1995). With people for whom English is not their first language, effective communication may involve working with an interpreter (Kirkham, 1998). It is critical, however, to be aware that interpreters must be well trained and should not be a member of the client's family, especially a child of the client (Huff & Kline, 1999; Searight & Gafford, 2005). It is also important to realize any potential discrepancies between the interpreter's ethical code of conduct mandating objectivity and neutrality and the realities of the client-interpreter cultural interaction. If the interpreter and client share similar cultural beliefs and practices, the client will often trust and/or expect advocacy from the interpreter (Brach & Fraserirector, 2000; Kaufert & Putsch, 1997). Conversely, conflicting ethical values systems may lead to cultural and ethical conflict between the client and interpreter (Kaufert & Putsch, 1997).

Effective transcultural communication is vital to ethical practice, as cultural miscommunication

can lead to malpractice claims (Ahmann, 2002). Studies of malpractice claims against physicians found that litigations were most often related to complaints regarding communication (Avery, 1985), while physicians who were never sued were described as concerned, accessible, and willing to communicate (Levinson, 1994).

In addition to effective verbal communication, health promoters must be cognizant of nonverbal communication to have effective interpersonal communication. Professionally inappropriate touch can lead to misinterpretation and misunderstanding of intentions. If a client feels that a practitioner is violating his or her personal space or touching inappropriately, the ethical concern of professionally inappropriate behavior may be raised. On the other hand, professional, appropriate, and respectful touch when performed with the client's consent can be effective in building rapport and trust (Lattanzi & Purnell, 2006c).

The fourth step toward achieving cultural proficiency is *cultural collaboration*. Cultural collaboration involves working as a practitioner-client team and negotiating between the practitioner's beliefs and practices (i.e., the current Western view of medical care) and that of the patient's. The goal of collaboration is to devise a plan of care and to formulate goals that are mutually agreed on by both parties (Felder, 1995). There are instances when traditional or folk health care practices can be harmful if combined with current medical practices. An example would be a herbal remedy that conflicts with, intensifies, or even results in an overdose of prescription medications (Lattanzi & Purnell, 2006d).

Oftentimes traditional or folklore practices can be safely incorporated into the plan of care for the client—leading to better patient compliance and outcomes (Lattanzi & Purnell, 2006d). A study by Sue (1998) examined the outcomes of African American, Asian American, Mexican American, and Caucasian clients receiving counseling in a Los Angeles mental health system to determine if outcomes were affected by providing services within the client's cultural context. When the clients were given culturally appropriate services (using bilingual staff, serving tea instead of coffee), they had lower dropout rates and stayed in the counseling program longer than the clients who received mainstream services. Thus, it can be inferred that working within the cultural context of the client can be beneficial to treatment.

Lack of cooperation between traditional and conventional medicine may lead to conflict (Brach & Fraserirector, 2000). It has been reported that if there are discrepancies between the advice from conventional Western practitioners and traditional healers, the patients will often listen to their traditional healer's advice (Marbella, Harris, Diehr, Ignace, & Ignace, 1998). From an ethical standpoint, it is the client's right to incorporate traditional practices if they "do no harm." Cultural collaboration thus involves working in partnership with traditional forms of medicine and healing, such as inviting traditional healers (e.g., a medicine man) to the hospital to practice traditional healing techniques in conjunction with conventional medical health care practices (Huff & Kline, 1999; Talabere, 1996). Finally, cultural collaboration is also critical for the health promoter who is planning programs and services that reach out into the community. This means connecting with organizations and individuals in the community who represent the targeted population and who can provide insights, suggestions, and support for designing, implementing, and evaluating such programs and services prior to their actually being presented or opened in the community.

The final step toward culturally proficient practice is obtaining cultural experience. This may start by providing health professional students with immersion experiences during their training, and this can take place during service learning activities, internships, and/or clinical affiliations (Hoppes, Bender, & DeGrace, 2005; Reynolds, 2005; Vanderhoff,

2005). Participation in immersion projects, especially international encounters, provides students with the valuable opportunity to obtain direct, firsthand experiences working with, and perhaps living with, culturally diverse clients within their communities (Campinha-Bacote, 1994, 1995; Campinha-Bacote & Padgett, 1995). It is important that immersion experiences incorporate some type of self-reflection exercise to encourage synthesis, understanding, and transformation (Ekelman, Bello-Haas, Bazyk, & Bazyk, 2003; Hoppes et al., 2005).

A study by St. Clair and McKenry (1999) found that nursing students working with culturally diverse patients in community-based practices (i.e., home visits) where they returned to their own homes every day did heighten cultural awareness, but did little to help the students overcome their ethnocentrism. Conversely, when students were *immersed* in another culture (completed a 2- to 3-week experience in Jamaica, Northern Ireland, England, or Ghana), they became aware of their own ethnocentrism, and subsequently, this heightened their ability to provide culturally competent care.

Another study by Jones, Bond, and Mencini (1998) explored a 1-week continuing education immersion experience for health care workers from a Texas hospital who went to a hospital in Mexico. These individuals were immersed in Mexican culture by living with a Mexican family, taking field trips to local hospitals and the traditional herbal stalls, and through one-on-one observational experiences in selected health care settings. The purpose of this experience was for U.S. health care professionals to become familiar with Mexican cultures and the culture of the health care delivery system and increase their proficiency in the Spanish language. Through use of a survey instrument, participants reported that they met the objectives of the experience and gained valuable insights into the Mexican patient perspective.

Returning to the Kachingwe-Huff model of culturally proficient and ethical practice (Figure 3.1), the components of culturally proficient practice, including cultural awareness, cultural knowledge, interpersonal communication skills, cultural collaboration, and cultural experiences, have been discussed. Enveloping culturally proficient practice is ethics. To practice in a culturally proficient manner, there must be an ethical framework by which health practitioners can solve ethical problems, issues, and dilemmas that may be encountered during a transcultural client-practitioner relationship. In addition, there must be a mandate from professional associations for culturally ethical practice. The next logical question then is "What determines whether culturally proficient and ethical practice is indeed being conducted in the health professions?" Although a mandate on cultural ethics from professional associations through the code of ethics is important, this does not *ensure* that culturally proficient and/or ethical practice will occur. Health promoters must also have a personal *conviction* in the centrality of culture for cultural proficiency to be manifested not only in their personal practice but also within the agency or organization(s) for which they work.

CONVICTION TO ACHIEVE CULTURALLY PROFICIENT AND ETHICAL PRACTICE

Conviction is the key component for providing culturally proficient and ethical practice (Figure 3.1). *Conviction* is a belief, held as a truth, so as to become an ideology compelling one to action (Kachingwe, 2000). Conviction related to cultural competence and health promotion is twofold. First and foremost, professions must have a conviction in the importance of, and impact of, client culture on health promotion and health care practices to compel professional associations to explicitly include culture in the code of ethics. Codes stating that "health practitioners must respect the rights and dignity of each client as an individual" *infer* that culture is integral to individual beliefs, behaviors, and actions. If, however, health care professionals are making ethical decisions based on current bioethical principles, they may lack a framework for investigating and resolving ethical conflicts that occur due to the client's cultural reality (Wells, 2005). Conviction from the professional association in the centrality of cultural proficiency should ensure that the practice of cultural ethics is explicitly stated in health professions' code of ethics.

Although we applaud professions that incorporate cultural competence into their ethical standards of practice, mandating ethical practice does not ensure ethical practice. Best practice, community advocacy, and action can only be realized if each health care practitioner or health promoter possesses a *personal conviction* in the importance of culture. Kachingwe (2000, 2003) conducted a grounded theory investigation of diversity and multiculturalism in physical therapy education and concluded that the key component for culturally proficient practice is conviction. Thus, the goals of increasing student and practitioner ethnic diversity within the profession and increasing the multiculturalism content of educational programs can only be obtained if educators and practitioners have a conviction in the importance of these constructs to compel them to act accordingly through recruitment and retention, mentoring, and policy change (Kachingwe, 2000, 2003).

The only way to *ensure* culturally proficient and ethical practice in health promotion and health care is for each health care practitioner to possess a conviction in the fundamentalism of culture. Conviction will lead to a greater awareness and understanding of culture resulting in optimal culturally appropriate client and community outcomes. Health promotion cannot be practiced ethically unless culturally proficient care is central to the philosophy and practice of the profession.

CHAPTER SUMMARY

This chapter sought to discuss the importance of ethics as a major feature of any culturally competent practice. It was noted that codes of ethics for the various health professions must include the domain of culture, as not doing so ignores the importance of cultural differences and cultural responses to health interventions targeting diverse cultural groups. In doing so, a number of ethical problems and dilemmas can surface that can, at the very least, lead to misinformation, feelings of disrespect and distrust, and even to malpractice claims against the health practitioner. A continuum of culturally proficient care was described and discussed and led to a description and presentation of the Kachingwe-Huff model of culturally proficient and ethical practice. It was noted that without a conviction toward culturally proficient practice, the health care professional or health promoter may not be engaged in culturally proficient and ethical practice with the multicultural population groups and clients they serve.

Chapter 4 discusses how important cultural influences have become in contemporary theories explaining the factors that determine health and quality of life. Historically, theories applied in health promotion (and health education) have focused on individual determinants of health. More recently, this focus has expanded to include social and cultural influences. To address health problems effectively, health promotion professionals must be able to examine cultural factors and understand beliefs about health within a context that is relevant to the population of interest. HPDP programs need to be consistent with people's and community's cultural framework, rather than based solely on the Western paradigm within which most health, education, and development programs are planned, implemented, and evaluated. The chapter provides a brief overview of relevant theories of behavior change as they relate to health promotion with multicultural populations or groups.

DISCUSSION QUESTIONS AND ACTIVITIES

1. What are your own personal ethical standards and how did you arrive at these?

2. Under what circumstances or situations are you likely to modify these standards? How do you feel when you do this?

3. If you had to write a set of ethical standards for your professional organization, what would these include?

4. Discuss an ethical problem, issue, or dilemma you have encountered in the health promotion field. How did you resolve it? How might you have resolved it differently within the framework of practicing cultural ethics?

5. Provide some examples of how your program could provide more culturally appropriate services.

6. Take a few moments to consider a time you might have stereotyped someone you did not know. What was the reason for you stereotyping and how did you feel when you did this? When was the last time you were stereotyped? What was the situation and how did this make you feel? What could you have done differently in both situations?

REFERENCES

Ahmann, E. (2002). Developing cultural competence in health care settings. *Pediatric Nursing, 28*, 133–137.

Alpers, R. R., & Zoucha, R. (1996). Comparison of cultural competence and cultural confidence of senior nursing students in a private southern university. *Journal of Cultural Diversity, 3*(1), 9–15.

American Medical Association. (2006). *Principles of medical ethics*. Retrieved March 19, 2006, from www.ama-assn.org/ama/pub/category/2512.html

American Occupational Therapy Association. (2005). *Occupational therapy code of ethics*. Retrieved March 19, 2006, from www.aota.org/general/docs/ethicscode05.pdf

American Physical Therapy Association. (2005). Code of ethics. *Physical Therapy, 85*(1), 88.

American Public Health Association. (2002). *Public health code of ethics.* Retrieved March 19, 2006, from www.apha.org

Andrews, M. M., & Boyle, J. S. (1999). *Transcultural concepts in nursing care* (3rd ed.). Philadelphia: Lippincott.

Avery, J. K. (1985). Lawyers tell what turns some patients litigious. *Medical Malpractice Review, 2,* 35–37.

Bailey, D. M., & Schwartzberg, S. L. (1995). *Ethical and legal dilemmas in occupational therapy.* Philadelphia: F. A. Davis.

Baldonado, A. A. (1996). Transcending the barriers of cultural diversity in health care. *Journal of Cultural Diversity, 3*(1), 20–22.

Bandman, E., & Bandman, B. C. (1995). *Nursing ethics through the life span.* Norwalk, CT: Appleton & Lange.

Bayer, R. (2003). *Ethics and public health: Model curriculum, Module 6.* Retrieved March 15, 2006, from www.asph.org/UserFiles/Module6.pdf

Black, J. D., & Purnell, L. D. (2002). Cultural competence for the physical therapy professional. *Journal of Physical Therapy Education, 16,* 3–10.

Brach, C., & Fraserirector, I. (2000). Can cultural competency reduce racial and ethnic health disparities? A review and conceptual model. *Medical Care Research and Review, 57,* 181–217.

Brown, C. M., & Segal, R. (1996). Ethnic differences in temporal orientation and its implications for hypertension management. *Journal of Health and Social Behavior, 37,* 350–361.

Buchwald, D., Caralis, P. V., Gany, F., Hardt, E. J., Johnson, T. M., Muecke, M. A., et al. (1994). Caring for patients in a multicultural society. *Patient Care, 28*(11), 105–109, 113–114, 116.

Burgess, D. J., Fu, S. S., & van Ryn, M. (2004). Why do providers contribute to disparities and what can be done about it? *Journal of General Internal Medicine, 19*(11), 1154–1159.

Campinha-Bacote, J. (1994). Cultural competence in psychiatric mental health nursing: A conceptual model. *Nursing Clinics of North America, 29*(1), 1–8.

Campinha-Bacote, J. (1995). The quest for cultural competence in nursing care. *Nursing Forum, 30*(4), 19–25.

Campinha-Bacote, J. (1999). A model and instrument for addressing cultural competence in health care. *Journal of Nursing Education, 38*(5), 203–207.

Campinha-Bacote, J., & Padgett, J. J. (1995). Cultural competence: A critical factor in nursing research. *Journal of Cultural Diversity, 2*(1), 31–34.

Carrese, J. A., & Rhodes, L. A. (1995). Western bioethics on the Navajo reservation: Benefit or harm? *Journal of American Medical Association, 274*(10), 826–829.

Clinton, J. F. (1996). Cultural diversity and health care in America: Knowledge fundamental to cultural competence in baccalaureate nursing students. *Journal of Cultural Diversity, 3*(1), 4–8.

Coveney, J. (1998). The government and ethics of health promotion: The importance of Michel Foucault. *Health Education Research, 13*(3), 459–468.

Cross, T. L., Bazron, B. J., Dennis, K. W., & Isaacs, M. R. (1989). *Towards a culturally competent system of care* (Vol. 1). Washington, DC: Georgetown University Press.

Davis, A. J. (1999). Global influence of American nursing: Some ethical issues. *Nursing Ethics: International Journal for Health Care Professionals, 6*(2), 118–125.

Davis, A. J., Aroskar, M. A., Liaschenko, J., & Drought, T. S. (1997). *Ethical dilemmas and nursing practice* (4th ed.). Stanford, CT: Appleton & Lange.

Davis, M. (1991). Thinking like an engineer: The place of a code of ethics in the practice of a profession. *Philosophy and Public Affairs, 20*(2), 150–167.

Dillard, M., Andonia, L., Flores, O., Lai, L., MacRae, A., & Shakir, M. (1992). Culturally competence occupational therapy in a diversely populated mental health setting. *American Journal of Occupational Therapy, 46*(8), 721–726.

Donnelly, P. D. (2000). Ethics and cross-cultural nursing. *Journal of Transcultural Nursing, 11*(2), 119–126.

Doswell, W. M., & Erlen, J. A. (1998). Multicultural issues and ethical concerns in the delivery of nursing care interventions. *Nursing Clinics of North America, 33*(2), 353–361.

Dowd, S. B., Giger, J. N., & Davidhizar, R. (1998). Use of Giger and Davidhizar's transcultural assessment model by health professions. *International Nursing Review, 45*(4), 119–122, 128.

Duffy, M. E. (2001). A critique of cultural education in nursing. *Journal of Advanced Nursing, 36*, 487–495.

Ekelman, B., Bello-Haas, V. D., Bazyk, J., & Bazyk, S. (2003). Developing cultural competence in occupational therapy and physical therapy education: A field immersion approach. *Journal of Allied Health, 32*, 131–137.

Eliason, M. J. (1993). Ethics and transcultural nursing care. *Nursing Outlook, 41*, 225–228.

Elliot, A. C. (2001). Health care ethics: Cultural relativity of autonomy. *Journal of Transcultural Nursing, 12*(4), 326–330.

Erlen, J. A. (1998). Culture, ethics, and respect: The bottom line is understanding. *Orthopaedic Nursing, 17*(6), 79–82.

Erlen, J. A., Lebeda, M., & Tamenne, C. J. (1993). Respect for persons: The patient with AIDS. *Orthopaedic Nursing, 12*(4), 7–10.

Felder, E. (1995). Integrating cultural diversity theoretical concepts into the educational preparation of the advanced practice nurse: The cultural diversity practice model. *Journal of Cultural Diversity, 2*(3), 88–92.

Gabard, D. L., & Martin, M. W. (2003). *Physical therapy ethics.* Philadelphia: F. A. Davis.

Gard, G., Cavlak, U., Sunden, B. T., & Razak, A. (2005). Life-views and ethical viewpoints among physiotherapy students in Sweden and Turkey: A comparative study. *Advances in Physiotherapy, 7*, 20–31.

Geddes, E. L., Finch, E., & Graham, K. (2005). Ethical choices: A moral and legal template for health care practice. *Physiotherapy Canada, 57*, 113–122.

Gordon, S. P. (2005). Making meaning of whiteness: A pedagogical approach for multicultural education. *Journal of Physical Therapy Education, 19*(1), 21–27.

Graham, R. (1981). The role of perception of time in consumer research. *Journal of Consumer Research, 17*, 335–342.

Haddad, A. (2005). Teaching for enduring understanding in ethics. *Journal of Physical Therapy Education, 19*(3), 73–77.

Harris, C. E., Jr., Pritchard, M., & Rabins, M. J. (1995). *Engineering ethics: Concepts and cases.* Belmont, CA: Wadsworth.

Hinman, L. M. (2002). *Basic moral orientations overview.* Retrieved April 11, 2006, from http://ethics.sandiego.edu/presentations/Theory/BasicOrientations/

Hoppes, S., Bender, D., & DeGrace, B. W. (2005). Service learning is a perfect fit for occupational and physical therapy education. *Journal of Allied Health, 34*, 47–50.

Huff, R. M., & Kline, M. V. (1999). *Promoting health in multicultural populations: A handbook for practitioners.* Thousand Oaks, CA: Sage.

Hyun, I. (2002). Waiver of informed consent, cultural sensitivity, and the problem of unjust families and traditions. *Hastings Center Report, 32*(5), 14–22.

Iwama, M. (2003). Toward culturally relevant epistemologies in occupational therapy. *American Journal of Occupational Therapy, 57*(5), 582–588.

Jenko, M., & Moffitt, S. R. (2006). Transcultural nursing principles: An application to hospice care. *Journal of Hospice and Palliative Nursing, 8*(3), 172–180.

Jensen, G. M., & Richert, A. E. (2005). Reflection on the teaching of ethics in physical therapy education: Integrating cases, theory, and learning. *Journal of Physical Therapy Education, 19*(3), 78–84.

Jones, M. E., Bond, M. L., & Mencini, M. E. (1998). Developing a culturally contempt work force: An opportunity for collaboration. *Journal of Professional Nursing, 14*(5), 280–287.

Jonsen, A. R., Seigler, M., & Winslade, W. J. (1992). *Clinical ethics* (3rd ed.). New York: McGraw-Hill.

Kachingwe, A. F. (2000). *Interculturalization and the education of professionals: A grounded theory investigation of diversity, multiculturalism and conviction in the physical therapy profession.* Unpublished dissertation, Northern Illinois University, DeKalb.

Kachingwe, A. F. (2003). A grounded theory investigation of diversity and multiculturalism in the physical therapy profession. *Journal of Physical Therapy Education, 17*(1), 5–17.

Kaufert, J. M., & Putsch, R. W. (1997). Communication through interpreters in healthcare: Ethical dilemmas arising from differences in class, culture, language, and power. *Journal of Clinical Ethics, 8*(1), 71–87.

Kenyon, P. (1999). *What would you do? An ethical case workbook for human service professionals.* Pacific Grove, CA: Brooks/Cole.

Kirkham, S. R. (1998). Nurses' descriptions of caring for culturally diverse clients. *Clinical Nursing Research, 7*(2), 125–146.

Kreuter, M. W., Kukwago, S. N., Bucholtz, D. C., Clark, E. M., & Sanders-Thompson, V. (2002). Achieving cultural appropriateness in health promotion programs: Targeted and tailored approaches. *Health Education & Behavior, 30*(2), 133–146.

La Puma, J. (1990). Clinical ethics, mission, and vision: Practical wisdom in health care. *Hospital and Health Services Administration, 35*(3), 321–326.

Ladd, J. (1995). The quest for a code of professional ethics: An intellectual and moral confusion. In D. G. Johnson (Ed.), *Ethical issues in engineering* (pp. 130–136). Englewood Cliffs, NJ: Prentice Hall.

Lattanzi, J. B., & Purnell, L. D. (2006a). *Developing cultural competence in physical therapy practice.* Philadelphia: F. A. Davis.

Lattanzi, J. B., & Purnell, L. D. (2006b). Establishing a culturally competent practice. In J. B. Lattanzi & L. D. Purnell (Eds.), *Developing cultural competence in physical therapy practice* (pp. 381–394). Philadelphia: F. A. Davis.

Lattanzi, J. B., & Purnell, L. D. (2006c). Exploring communication in cultural context. In J. B. Lattanzi & L. D. Purnell (Eds.), *Developing Cultural competence in physical therapy practice* (pp. 52–68). Philadelphia: F. A. Davis.

Lattanzi, J. B., & Purnell, L. D. (2006d). Exploring cultural healthcare practices and roles of healthcare practitioners. In J. B. Lattanzi & L. D. Purnell (Eds.), *Developing cultural competence in physical therapy practice* (pp. 136–160). Philadelphia: F. A. Davis.

Lattanzi, J. B., & Purnell, L. D. (2006e). Introducing cultural concepts. In J. B. Lattanzi & L. D. Purnell (Eds.), *Developing cultural competence in physical therapy practice* (pp. 3–20). Philadelphia: F. A. Davis.

Lavizzo-Mourey, R., & Mackenzie, E. R. (1996). Cultural competence: Essential measurement of quality for managed care organizations. *Annals of Internal Medicine, 124*(10), 919–921.

Leavitt, R. (1999a). Cultural considerations when treating a diverse patient population. *Orthopaedic Physical Therapy Clinics of North America, 8*(2), 185–201.

Leavitt, R. (1999b). Introduction to cross-cultural rehabilitation. In R. Leavitt (Ed.), *Cross-cultural rehabilitation: An international perspective* (pp. 1–7). London: W. B. Saunders.

Leininger, M. (1994). Transcultural nursing education: A worldwide imperative. *Nursing & Health Care, 15*(5), 254–257.

Leininger, M. (1995). *Transcultural nursing: Concepts, theories, research and practices* (2nd ed.). New York: McGraw-Hill.

Levinson, W. (1994). Physician-patient communication: A key to malpractice prevention. *Journal of American Medical Association, 272*(20), 1619–1620.

Lindsey, R. B., Robins, K. N., & Terrell, R. D. (1999). *Cultural proficiency: A manual for school leaders.* Thousand Oaks, CA: Corwin Press.

Lister, P. (1999). A taxonomy for developing cultural competence. *Nurse Education Today, 19*(4), 313–318.

Ludwick, R., & Silva, M. C. (2000). Nursing around the world: Cultural values and ethical conflict [Electronic version]. *Journal of Issues in Nursing, 5*(3). Retrieved from www.nursingworld.org/ojin/ethicol/ethics_4.htm

Luegenbiehl, H. C. (1983). Codes of ethics and the moral education of engineers. *Business and Professional Ethics Journal, 2*, 41–61.

Lynch, E. W. (1998a). Developing cross-cultural competence. In E. W. Lynch & M. J. Hanson (Eds.), *Developing cross-cultural competence* (pp. 47–86). Baltimore: Brookes.

Lynch, E. W. (1998b). Developing cross-cultural competence. In E. W. Lynch & M. J. Hanson (Eds.), *Developing cross-cultural competence: A guide for working with children and their families* (2nd ed., pp. 47–86). Baltimore: Brookes.

MacLachlan, M. (1997). *Culture and health.* Chichester, UK: Wiley.

Marbella, A. M., Harris, M. C., Diehr, S., Ignace, G., & Ignace, G. (1998). Use of Native American healers among Native American patients in an urban Native American health center. *Archives of Family Medicine, 7*(2), 182–185.

Napholz, L. (1999). A comparison of self-reported cultural competency skills among two groups of nursing students: Implications for nursing education. *Journal of Nursing Education, 38*(2), 81–83.

National Association of Social Workers. (2006). *Code of ethics of the National Association of Social Workers.* Retrieved March 19, 2006, from www.naswdc.org/pubs/code/code.asp

Purnell, L. D. (2000). A description of the Purnell model for cultural competence. *Journal of Transcultural Nursing, 11*(1), 40–46.

Purnell, L. D., & Lattanzi, J. B. (2006). Introducing steps to cultural study and cultural competence. In J. B. Lattanzi & L. D. Purnell (Eds.), *Developing cultural competence in physical therapy practice* (pp. 21–37). Philadelphia: F. A. Davis.

Purtilo, R. (2005). *Ethical dimensions in the health professions* (4th ed.). Boston: Elsevier.

Purtilo, R., & Haddad, A. (2002). *Health professional and patient interaction* (6th ed.). Philadelphia: W. B. Saunders.

Purtilo, R. B., Jensen, G. M., & Royeen, C. B. (2005). *Educating for moral action: A sourcebook in health and rehabilitation ethics.* Philadelphia: F. A. Davis.

Reynolds, P. J. (2005). How service-learning experiences benefit physical therapist students' professional development: A grounded theory story. *Journal of Physical Therapy Education, 19*(1), 41–54.

Scott, R. (1998). *Professional ethics: A guide for rehabilitation professionals.* San Antonio, TX: Mosby.

Searight, H. R., & Gafford, J. (2005). Cultural diversity at the end of life: Issues and guidelines for family physicians. *American Family Physician, 71*(3), 515–522.

Sheikh, A. (2001). Dealing with ethics in a multicultural world. *Western Journal of Medicine, 174,* 87–88.

Shive, S. E., & Marks, R. (2006). The influence of ethical theories in the practice of health education. *Health Promotion Practice, 7*(3), 287–288.

Smith, L. S. (1998). Concept analysis: Cultural competence. *Journal of Cultural Diversity, 5,* 4–10.

Society for Public Health Education. (2006). Code of ethics for the health education profession. Retrieved September 14, 2006, from www.sophe.org/about/ethics.html

Spector, R. E. (2004). *Cultural diversity in health and illness* (6th ed.). Upper Saddle River, NJ: Pearson-Prentice Hall.

St. Clair, A., & McKenry, L. (1999). Preparing culturally competent practitioners. *Journal of Nursing Education, 38*(5), 228–234.

Sue, S. (1998). In search of cultural competence in physiotherapy and counseling. *American Psychologist, 53*(4), 440–448.

Swisher, L. L., & Page, C. G. (2005). *Professionalism in physical therapy: History, practice, and development.* St. Louis, MO: Elsevier-Saunders.

Talabere, L. R. (1996). Meeting the challenge of cultural care in nursing: Diversity, sensitivity, competence, and congruence. *Journal of Cultural Diversity, 3*(2), 53–61.

Turner, L. (2003). Bioethics in a multicultural world: Medicine and morality in pluralistic settings. *Health Care Analysis, 11*(2), 99–117.

U.S. Census Bureau. (1990). *General population and housing characteristics: 1990.* Retrieved May 26, 2006, from http://factfinder.census.gov/

U.S. Census Bureau. (2000a). *Profile of general demographic characteristics: 2000.* Retrieved May 26, 2006, from http://censtats.census.gov/data/US/

U.S. Census Bureau. (2000b). *Projections of the total resident population by 5-year age groups, race, and Hispanic origin with special age categories: Middle series, 2075 to 2100.* Retrieved April 11, 2006, from www.census/gov/population/projections/nation/summary/

Vanderhoff, M. (2005, May). Service learning: The world as a classroom. *PT Magazine,* 34–41.

Wells, S. A. (2005,). An ethic of diversity. In R. B. Purtilo, G. M. Jensen & C. B. Royeen (Eds.), *Educating for moral action: A sourcebook in health and rehabilitation ethics.* Philadelphia: F. A. Davis.

Yuen, H. K., & Yau, M. K. (1999). Cross-cultural awareness and occupational therapy education. *Occupational Therapy International, 6,* 24–34.

4

Models, Theories, and Principles of Health Promotion

Revisiting Their Use With Multicultural Populations

C. JAMES FRANKISH

CHRIS Y. LOVATO

IRAJ POURESLAMI

Chapter Objectives

On completion of this chapter, the health promotion student and practitioner will be able to

- Identify and define the levels of change sought by programs at the health promotion and health education levels

- Define and explain the differences between theory, models, and theoretical frameworks

- Identify and discuss the usefulness of traditional and current health education and health promotion behavior change theories and models and how they can help us understand the determinants of health behaviors when developing interventions that will influence change in multicultural populations

- Define and apply the following principles of health education to multicultural health promotion activities:

  o Principle of educational diagnosis

  o Principle of hierarchy

(Continued)

(Continued)

- o Principle of cumulative learning
- o Principle of participation
- o Principle of situational specificity
- o Principle of multiple methods
- o Principle of individualization
- o Principle of relevance
- o Principle of feedback
- o Principle of reinforcement

Cultural influences have become more prominent in contemporary theories explaining the factors that determine health and quality of life. Historically, theories applied in health promotion (and health education) have focused on individual determinants of health. More recently; this focus has expanded to social and cultural influences (Tang, Beaglehole, & Byrne, 2005). It is clear from experience accumulated over the past two decades that to address health problems effectively, we must examine cultural factors and understand beliefs about health within a context that is relevant to the population of interest.

Cultural sensitivity in health promotion programs refers to planning interventions that are relevant and acceptable within the cultural framework of the population to be reached. Although the role of culture has long been acknowledged in theories that are currently being widely used, culture has not been the central focus. For the health educator, developing a culturally sensitive program demands moving outside the paradigm of the dominant culture.

Since no model or learning theory can explain or predict all aspects of health behaviors, from a cultural and developmental perspective, combining compatible theories and models can help create stronger health education programs for diverse multicultural population groups. Such models must also consider changes across the life span (Campbell & Sherman, 1999).

Based on Airhihenbuwa's (1995) Person, Extended Family, Neighborhood (PEN-3) model, in health promotion and behavior change programs, cultural sensitivity refers to the need to develop programs in ways that are consistent with people's and the community's cultural framework, rather than based on the Western paradigm within which most health, education, and development programs are planned, implemented, and evaluated. Health denotes a process of adaptation. It is the result not of instinct but of an autonomous yet culturally shaped reaction to socially creative reality (Illich, 1976). Each culture creates its own responses to health and disease. This model is appealing in that it incorporates existing models or theories and frameworks of health education and reflects theory and application in cultural studies. There are three primary dimensions of health beliefs and behaviors to consider: health education, educational diagnosis of health behavior, and cultural appropriateness of health behaviors (Frankish, Lovato, & Shannon, 1999).

Cultural influences have become more prominent in contemporary theories explaining the factors that determine health. Historically, theories applied in health promotion focused on individual determinants of health. More recently, this focus has expanded to social and cultural influences. It is clear from experience that to address health problems effectively, we must examine cultural factors and understand beliefs about health within a context that is relevant to the population (Frankish et al., 1999). Health needs of individuals in different age groups differ based on gender, the household environment, and the neighborhood where a person was born and has grown up (Zanchetta & Poureslami, 2006). There is a need for different health education models to assess each individual's attitudinal and behavioral intentions and beliefs. There is no single gold standard model to investigate such diversities in terms of individual cultural background, age group, and gender.

There are many different definitions of theory. In this chapter, the authors address theory from the perspective of the health promotion student and practitioner. The theories are examined based on their utility in helping understand the determinants of health behaviors and develop interventions that will influence change. The chapter provides a brief overview of relevant theories of behavior change as they relate to health promotion with multicultural populations or groups. Information is provided regarding the rationale for the use of theory by health promotion practitioners and policy makers. Next, several important theories are reviewed. This overview leads to the articulation of principles of health education that apply across theoretical perspectives. Finally, some practical concluding comments are made.

RATIONALE FOR USING A THEORETICAL FRAMEWORK

A theoretical framework provides researchers and program developers with a perspective from which to organize knowledge and interpret factors and events. All programs are built on assumptions; however, these may or may not be articulated. Identification and classification of elements of programs or interventions and their linkages (associative, causal; explanatory, predictive; direct, indirect) facilitates informed attempts at identifying and replicating promising parts of interventions and programs and the development of creative potential solutions to unsolved problems.

> By telling us about the what, how, when, and why, theories can inform programs in health education. . . . The what tells us the elements we should consider as the targets for the intervention. . . . The why tells us about the processes by which changes occur in the target variables. The when tells us about the timing and sequencing of our interventions in order to achieve maximum effects. The how tells us the methods or ways we should focus our interventions; it includes the specific means of inducing changes in the explanatory variables. (Glanz, Lewis, & Rimer, 1997, p. 21)

The first step in choosing an appropriate theory is clarifying the purpose of goals of the proposed program or intervention. The explicit goals of the program or intervention provide the marker for identifying classes of theories that may be applicable. Theories are often specific to targets of intervention or units of practice. For example, some theories address change in individual behaviors and others, organizational change. For instance, within the class of behavior change theories, some explain and predict solely volitional behaviors, while others generalize to addictive behaviors.

If a multicultural program needs to incorporate aspects that address an addictive behavior, it should not be based on a theory that addresses only voluntary behaviors (Cheung, 2003; Poureslami & Ayyar, 2002). Likewise, a program that has a goal of behavior maintenance should not be based on a theory that explains only initial behavior change (Huff & Kline, 1999; Hyman & Guruge, 2002). Identifying the target and goals of the program will narrow the field of applicable theories. However, once this guideline has been followed, there are often many theories from which to choose. "The next step is to identify the relevant theories and evaluate the evidence for each of them" (van Ryn & Heaney, 1992).

DISTINGUISHING THEORIES, MODELS, AND FRAMEWORKS

When concepts and constructs are related to each other and purposely combined to form a unit, the resulting entity may be labeled a "framework," a "model," or a "theory." There is considerable controversy regarding the boundaries or limits defining and circumscribing each of these creations. Generally speaking, a framework is a planning tool—for example, the PRECEDE model (see www.lgreen.net/precede.htm for a complete bibliography of PRECEDE applications). It can incorporate theories or models or parts thereof and allows for organization of a large and unspecified number of potentially predictive or explanatory variables. A model is a grouping of a set number of selected variables that, taken together, act as an explanatory or predictive indicator of behavior; the interrelationships between the variables are not definitively specified. A theory is, likewise, "a set number of selected factors or variables; however, the hypothesized relationships among the variables are specified, as well as the circumstances under which the relationships do or do not occur."

An example of a framework used in planning prevention health promotion interventions is the PRECEDE/PROCEED framework (Green & Kreuter, 2005). Using this framework, potentially important variables from a wide conceptual domain may be identified and targeted for

intervention. These categories of variables include those identifying relevant quality of life, health, behavioral, environmental, organizational, and administrative concerns.

An example of a model frequently used in designing health surveys and interventions is the health belief model (HBM) (Rosenstock, 1974). It is composed of four constructs: (1) perceived severity, (2) perceived susceptibility, (3) perceived benefits of action, and (4) perceived barriers to action. The constructs are said to be related multiplicatively, but researchers using the model generally do not combine them in this way.

An example of a theory used in elicitation research and intervention planning is the theory of reasoned action (TRA) (Ajzen & Fishbein, 1980; Madden, Ellen, & Ajzen, 1992). Here the relationships between the variables are explicitly set out in directional and mathematical terms. In much of the literature, the terms *theory* and *model* are used interchangeably and/or without specification. This chapter reflects that pattern of usage so as to reflect the literature as accurately as possible. Others (Davies, 2006; Watt, 2006) have recently linked theories of health promotion to issues including the effectiveness of interventions and the social determinants of health. They correctly note that many health education interventions have been heavily influenced by health behavior—research based on psychological theories and models. These theories focus too much at an individual level. Newer approaches explore the relationship between the social environment and health (see the subsection on social ecology).

VALUES AND THEORIES

Competing contemporary theories of health, the reductionist (purportedly value free) and the relativist (purportedly value based) theories, both rest on an understanding of value as grounded in desiring: a subjective state (Sade, 1995). Sade (1995) notes that both can be classified as subjectivist theories. An alternative set of theories, those resting on an understanding of value as grounded in desirability (or goodness) of an objective goal, can be classified as objectivist theories. Whatever one's theoretical perspective, health promotion practitioners and program planners must be cognizant of their own values while respecting the values of the various cultural communities with whom they work (Smaje, 1996). Frankish, Moulton, Rootman, Cole, and Gray (2006) and Moulton, Frankish, Rootman, Cole, and Gray (2006) recently published two papers on the role of values as a necessary foundation for health promotion. Such values are also manifested in community participation in decision making with respect to health systems and in the definitions of success used for community-based health promotion programs (Frankish, Larsen, Ratner, Wharf-Higgins, & Kwan, 2002; Green & Frankish, 2000; Judd, Frankish, & Moulton, 2001; Trifiletti, Gielen, Sleet, & Hopkins, 2005).

THEORIES AND MODELS OF RELEVANCE

In the field of health behavior, health promotion, and illness prevention, many theories have been developed during the past 5 years. Some have been used to try to understand the determinants of and to maintain and improve health, both by behavioral and by environmental change. These theories can be divided into groups according to the scope of their focus (e.g., intrapersonal, interpersonal, and group levels of interaction, with group-level theories including Organizational Change, Diffusion of Innovation, Community Organization, Media Advocacy, and Social Marketing). Theories can also be organized according to their style of focus—for example, cognitive, behavioral, social, and environmental. DiClemente, Crosby, and Kegler (2002) provide an excellent overview of emerging theories in health promotion practice and research (see also Glanz, Lewis, & Rimer, 1997; Nutbeam & Harris,

1998, 2004). Leviton (1989) discusses five relevant "families" of theories:

1. *Cognitive and decision-making theories*, including the Theory of Risk Communication, the HBM, and the TRA;

2. *Learning theories*, including the Theory Of Operant Conditioning, Social Learning Theory (SLT), and subtheories of self-efficacy, relapse, and self-regulation;

3. *Theories of motivation and emotional arousal*, including theories of fear and fear-arousing communications, helplessness, and coping strategies;

4. *Theories of interpersonal relations*, including social influence, reactance, and group processes; and

5. *Theories of communication and persuasion.*

The theories underlying multicultural health promotion include the HBM (Brunswick & Banaszak-Holl, 1996; Rosenstock, 1974); sick-role behaviors (Kasl & Cobb, 1966); locus of control (Wallston & Wallston, 1978); physician-patient relationships (Haynes, Taylor, & Sackett, 1979); Self-Regulation Theory (Leventhal, Meyer, & Gutmann, 1980); Communications Theory (Garrity, 1980); Attribution, Control, and Decision Theory (Janis & Rodin, 1979); Grounded Theory (Mullens & Reynolds, 1978); Ecologic Theory (Sasao, 1993; Stokols, 1992, 1996); family and systems theories (Becker & Maiman, 1975); communication behavior model of behavior change (Matarazzo, Miller, Weiss, Herd, & Weiss, 1984); SLT (Bandura, 1986, 1989, 1991); Hierarchy of Learning Model (Ray et al., 1973); Self-Control Theory (Kanfer, 1975), Communication-Persuasion Model (McGuire, 1969); Attitude Change Model (Ajzen & Fishbein, 1980); and models of social-problem solving (Goldfried & D'Zurilla, 1969). These theories and others have formed the foundation for the major health education, health promotion, and behavior modification programs (Bruhn, 1983) in North America.

This chapter focuses first on the major (the most prevalent) health education models (and their variants), including the (1) SLT; (2) HBM; (3) TRA/Theory of Planned Behavior (TPB); and (4) Transtheoretical Model, or Stages of Change. These models are primarily focused on the individual and derived from the discipline of psychology. We next contrast these models with four broader, more ecological approaches: (1) the PEN-3 model, (2) social ecology, and (3) the PRECEDE-PROCEED model and community. Finally, we present a list of several less common models of health education/health promotion that have relevance for multicultural populations (see Table 4.1).

Four Prevalent Models for Health Education

Social Learning Theory

The three major constructs in SLT (also called Social Cognitive Theory [SCT] or Social Influence Theory) are (1) behavioral capacity (having the skills necessary for the performance of the desired behavior—for example, active living); (2) efficacy expectations (beliefs regarding one's ability to successfully carry out a course of action or perform a behavior); and (3) outcome expectations (beliefs that the performance of a behavior will have the desired effects or consequences) (van Ryn & Heaney, 1992; see Armitage & Conner, 2000, for a review).

The leading concept in SLT is that of "reciprocal determinism." This means that the interaction among three elements, the person, the person's behavior, and the environment, determine behavior. This approach is highly consistent with the view of living as a dynamic process and experience involving the reciprocal interaction of personal, social, and environmental factors. The person's actions contribute to creating the environment, and the actions

and environment contribute to the person's cognitions or "expectancies." Expectancies are of three types: beliefs about how events are connected, about the consequences of one's own actions (outcome expectations), and about one's competence to perform the behavior needed to influence the outcomes (efficacy expectations). "Incentives" also contribute to behavior: Incentive or reinforcement is the value of a particular outcome to a person. Behavior is regulated by its consequences "but only as those consequences are interpreted and understood by the individual" (Maiman, Becker, & Liptak, 1988). The three important explanatory factors of SLT/SCT can be defined as follows:

> SLT is useful to program development because, in addition to describing the important influences on behavior change, it describes the processes through which these influences can be modified. Thus, behavioral capacity or skill level can be modified through both direct experience or practice and through observing someone else model the desired behavior. Both outcome and efficacy expectations can be modified by four different processes. Performance accomplishments refer to performing the behavior or close approximations of the behavior. Successful performance can increase a person's sense of confidence (self-efficacy) in being able to perform the behavior again. If the behavior leads to a desirable outcome, then that person's outcome expectations become more positive as well. (Bandura, 1986, p. 391)

A second important influence on expectations is observational learning or vicarious experience. Through seeing others who are similar to ourselves behave in certain ways and succeed in bringing about desired effects, people modify their expectations about their own behavior. The third influence, verbal persuasion, refers to attempts to change expectations by providing new or newly motivating information.

Table 4.1   Models of Health Education/Health Promotion With Relevance for Multicultural Populations

Model Theory	Authors and Date	Abstract
Cognitive-Behavioral Model	Decaluwe and Braet (2005)	The findings suggest that the mechanism in the Cognitive-Behavioral Model is operational among obese youngsters.
Social Cognitive Theory (SCT)	Rogers et al. (2004)	SCT is a useful framework for the design of physical activity. Intervention studies should consider the unique barriers and program preferences of patients while focusing on self-efficacy, outcome expectations/expectancies, learning, and reinforcement.
SCT and Stages of Change Theory	Chapman-Novakofski and Karduck (2005)	The study found that a diabetes education program based on the SCT resulted in positive impacts of knowledge, health beliefs, and self-reported behaviors.
SCT	Burke and Stephens (1999)	The study shows that the SCT applied to drinking by college students indicates clear relations between social anxiety and drinking that may be moderated by expectancies and self-efficacy beliefs in socially anxious situations.
Theory of Reasoned Action (TRA)	Bos, Hoogstraten, and Prahl-Andersen (2005)	The study found that the patients' intention to comply during the treatment is influenced by factors outside of the TRA. Therefore, it is recommended that a new model be developed in which factors of the TRA are included.
SCT	Dilorio, Dudley, Soet, Watkins, and Maibach (2000)	The study reveals that the SCT could be used to provide implications for HIV interventions that focus on self-efficacy and are likely to reduce anxiety related to condom use, increase positive perceptions about condoms, and increase the likelihood of adopting condom-use behaviors.
SCT	O'Leary, Goodhart, Jemmott, and Boccher-Lattimore (1992)	SCT analysis demonstrated the need for health educators to develop multifaceted approaches to AIDS prevention, including skill and self-efficacy building, enhancing perceptions of risk, and promoting positive social norms.
Health Belief Model (HBM)	Graham, Liggons, and Hypolite (2002)	Health beliefs were much stronger in determining breast self-examination (BSE) performance than were demographic characteristics. The frequency of BSE was related to an increase in perceived seriousness of cancer, benefits of BSE, and health motivation. Frequency of BSE was inversely related to perceived barriers.

(Continued)

Table 4.1 (Continued)

Model Theory	Authors and Date	Abstract
HBM	Norman and Brain (2005)	The study shows the applicability of the HBM of BSE. The results highlight the importance of focusing on excessive as well as infrequent BSE. Interventions designed to enhance women's confidence in their ability to perform BSE, coupled with reduced worry, may lead to appropriate BSE.
TRA	Milette, Richard, and Martel (2005)	The study shows the applicability of TRA in training nurses' behaviors and cognitive attributes with regard to the prevention of overstimulation of premature infants.
TRA	Trost, Saunders, and Ward (2002)	The study demonstrates that although the combination of TRA and TPB on physical activity may result in an acceptable level, the models accounted for only a small percentage of variance in moderate to vigorous physical activity in youth. The utility of this model's activity interventions appears to be limited.
PRECEDE-PROCEED Model	Trifiletti, Gielen, Sleet, and Hopkins (2005)	Authors looked at the potential of different behavioral/social science theories/models to reduce unintentional injuries. The PRECEDE-PROCEED model was viewed as the most relevant model.
Theory of Planned Behavior (TPB)	White (2004)	Applying TPB, this study found health perceptions, beliefs, and attitudes in African American women with faith-based support as important to engaging in a healthy lifestyle, such as exercise, balanced diets, weight reduction, and stress management.
PRECEDE-PROCEED Model	Daniel and Green (1995)	The study illustrates the use of the PRECEDE-PROCEED model in planning strategies to address behavioral and environmental risks for non-insulin-dependent diabetes mellitus (NIDDM) in a Canadian aboriginal community.
SCT	O'Leary, Goodhart, Jemmott, and Boccher-Lattimore (1992)	The results of this study demonstrate the need for health educators to develop multifaceted approaches to AIDS prevention, including skill and self-efficacy building, enhancing perceptions of risk, and promoting positive social norms.
Behavioral and social science models and theories	Nutbeam and Harris (2004)	This book illustrates the applicability and potential of different behavioral and social science models and theories in the community and population health promotion approach.
Health behavior models	Hollister and Anema (2004)	This study describes health behavior models that have been applied to oral health, presents a critical analysis of the effectiveness of each model in oral health education, and provides examples of the application of models to oral health.

Theory/Model	Citation	Description
PRECEDE-PROCEED Model	Green and Kreuter (1991)	The authors applied the PRECEDE-PROCEED model in an injury prevention study and demonstrated that applying the principles of community organization will not guarantee that public health programs will carry on without some expression of community concern, which is a sign of community validity and interest.
PRECEDE-PROCEED Model	Darrow et al. (2004)	The study applied the PRECEDE-PROCEED model for community planning and health promotion to eliminate local disparities in HIV infection. The results show that the intervention reached the target audience, informed young adults of the risk of HIV infection, and encouraged them to take ownership and action.
TRA	Strader, Beaman, and McSweeney (1992)	The study assessed the TRA to determine if individuals communicate with important social referents and to investigate the effects of communications and the effects of race and gender on communication in relation to condom use. They saw that although talking to a partner does not increase the partner's influence, talking about condoms increased the intention to use them.
TRA	Bos et al. (2005)	The findings suggest that patients' intention to comply during treatment is influenced by factors outside of TRA. It is recommended that a new model be developed in which factors of TRA are included, which can be used specifically for the study of compliance in orthodontics.
TRA	Fisher, Fisher, and Rye (1995)	This study has clear implications for the applicability of TRA for the creation of conceptually based, empirically targeted AIDS prevention interventions.
Behavioral and social science models and theories	U.S. Department of Health and Human Services (2005)	No single theory dominated health education and promotion. Most heath behavior theories can be applied to diverse cultural and ethnic groups, but practitioners must understand the characteristics of target populations (e.g., ethnicity, socioeconomic status, gender, age, worldview [beliefs], and geographical location). Adequately addressing these issues may require more than one theory, and no one theory is suitable for all cases.
SCT	Bandura (1986)	SCT addresses the sociocultural determinants of health as well as the personal determinants. The model focuses on health promotion and disease prevention. The study reveals that SCT works on the demand side by helping people stay healthy through good self-management of health habits.
TPB	DiGirolamo, Thompson, Martorell, Fein, and Grummer-Strawn (2005)	This study supports using the intention construct from TRA to predict initiation of behavior. The theory does not account for experience. The study suggests a need to include experience when predicting behavior.
HBM	Lin, Simoni, and Zemon (2005)	The results suggest that self-efficacy as a target for behavioral change/acculturation may need to be incorporated into HBM.
HBM	Adih and Alexander (1999)	Using the concepts of HBM and Social Learning Theory, the results suggest that HIV prevention programs for youth should emphasize personal vulnerability to AIDS, encourage in youth the self-belief that they can use condoms, and address the problem of overcoming the barriers to use.

Last, people develop their sense of efficacy, in part, from how distressed, anxious, and tense they feel when faced with the need to perform the behavior. Efforts to decrease this emotional arousal may directly enhance efficacy expectations. When there are satisfactory levels of self-efficacy, the motivation to perform a particular behavior can be increased through the expectation that the behavior will lead to a desirable outcome (outcome expectation) and through incentives (rewards). Reward expectations can be influenced by observing others receive rewards (vicarious reward) or by being rewarded oneself (direct reward). Rewards may come from external sources, such as awards, promotions, or recognition, or they may come from internal sources, such as the self-satisfaction a health educator might feel after implementing an effective intervention (van Ryn & Heaney, 1992).

Perceived self-efficacy is defined by Bandura (1986) as "people's judgments of their capabilities to organize and execute courses of action required to attain designated types of performances. It is concerned not with the skills one has but with judgments of what one can do with whatever skills one possesses" (p. 391). It should be noted that self-efficacy refers to beliefs about performing specific actions in specific settings; it cannot refer to global situations or personality traits (Costa, Metter, & McCrae, 1994). Perceived self-efficacy is concerned with people's beliefs that they can exert control over their motivation, behavior, and social environment. People's beliefs about their capabilities affect what they choose to do, how much effort they mobilize, how long they will persevere, and whether they engage in self-debilitating or self-encouraging thought patterns. When lacking a sense of self-efficacy, individuals do not manage situations effectively even though they know what to do and possess the requisite skills. Self-inefficacious thinking creates discrepancies between knowledge and self-protective action.

Numerous studies have been conducted linking perceived self-efficacy to health-promoting and health-impairing behavior (Bandura, 1991). Feelings of self-efficacy derive from four sources: performance attainments, vicarious experience, verbal persuasion, and physiological feedback. For example, Sennott-Miller (1994) found differences in perceived self-efficacy among Hispanics and whites. Perceived self-efficacy and perceived difficulty were related to adoption and maintenance of cancer prevention activities.

As can be seen from the above, self-efficacy is strongly linked to Attribution Theory. Attribution Theory informs us that for change to occur and be maintained it is necessary that the person feel in control of his or her own behavior. High self-efficacy can assist a person undergoing a relapse to see it as temporary. Under conditions of success, stable, global, and internal causal attributions for desirable outcomes should be reinforced. Under conditions of failure, unstable, specific, uncontrollable, and external attributions should be reinforced. SLT and its variants are the most extensively applied of the psychosocial theories.

Self-Efficacy Theory is grounded in the notion that people's ability to cope with a given situation is strongly influenced by their perceived sense of self-efficacy or belief in "their capability to mobilize the motivation, cognitive resources, and courses of action needed to meet the situational demands." Gonzalez, Geoppinger, and Lorig (1990) identified four empirically verified ways to enhance self-efficacy: reinterpretation of signs and symptoms, and mastery of skills, modeling, and persuasion. When judging their capabilities, one source of information that people rely on is information from their physiological state. For example, people may learn to reinterpret the symptoms associated with specific health behaviors—for example, physical effort. Reinterpretation of symptoms may, in some cases, improve an individual's sense of self-efficacy; however, it may also lead to inappropriate maintenance of risky behaviors.

Optimism is closely related to the concept of self-efficacy. Scheier and Carver (1992) reviewed longitudinal and prospective research examining the beneficial effects of optimism on psychological and physical well-being. The article identifies potential mechanisms that produce the beneficial effects of optimism and focuses on how optimism may lead a person to cope more adaptively with stress. Data also suggest that optimists are more likely than pessimists to engage in positive health habits. Similarities are noted between conceptualizing optimism versus pessimism in terms of general expectancies for good versus bad outcomes and approaches that conceptualize optimism versus pessimism in terms of attributional style or self-efficacy. Optimism also varies across cultural groups (Zhang & Schwarzer, 1995).

The most effective way to enhance self-efficacy is through mastery of skills. The acquisition of healthy behavior and skills is facilitated by self-identification of goals, breaking down of tasks into manageable units, and programming for success by sequencing subtasks according to difficulty or ordered objectives. Both the goals and the consequences of health behaviors must be clear, consistent, and doable. Gonzalez et al. (1990) argue that contracting and feedback are such important aspects of health education that 30% of efforts should be directed toward these aspects.

Modeling (Bandura, 1986) is another effective way of enhancing health behaviors. The principle of modeling underlies the development of self-help groups. Modeling can be achieved through mutual aid, the use of lay instructors, and the use of age-appropriate models in educational materials such as videos and pamphlets. The final way to enhance self-efficacy is through the use of persuasion. Although persuasive arguments on the part of health educators are a ubiquitous aspect of education, there is strong evidence that, in and of itself, persuasion is a relatively ineffective strategy. The use of persuasion in multicultural health promotion can be made more effective by delivering such arguments in the context of supportive small-group settings.

People should also be persuaded to make small, incremental behavior changes rather than all-or-nothing efforts.

Various uses of SCT can be found with diverse multicultural groups. Rinderknecht and Smith (2004) reported on a 7-month nutrition intervention for Native American children. They found that overweight children significantly improved their dietary self-efficacy. The intervention was not successful among adolescents. SCT was an effective model from which to explore influential constructs of health behavior.

Reference Group–Based Social Influence Theory

Social influence (normative and informational) can be a significant predisposing factor (direct or indirect) for group members' behavior, in either in health-enhancing or nonenhancing directions. J. Fisher (1988) presents a model showing the effects of social networks and reference groups on AIDS risk and preventive behavior, according to whether the social network's values and norms are of high or low consistency with preventive behaviors. Krohn and Thornberry (1993) provide a network theory model for understanding drug abuse among African American and Hispanic youth.

If preventive behavior is consistent with social norms, the network will be likely to exert social influence and exposure to supportive information facilitative of preventive behavior, and sanctions for lack of it. Likewise, if preventive behavior is inconsistent with a group's norms and values, the group is likely to exert pressure against participation in preventive behavior. Group norms and values can be specific (e.g., against smoking) or general (e.g., in favor of exercise). Groups exert pressure on their members to conform to the status quo (normative social influence) and wield their power by means of sanctions (e.g., rejection or perceived future rejection) for nonconformity. There are a number of factors that may moderate the intensity of the network's response in protecting the status quo: These include the centrality of a value or behavior to the core of a group's assumptive world, the level of trust the group has for the entity that is proposing change, and the network's previous history of remaining intact while being able to integrate previously inconsistent values (J. Fisher, 1988).

In addition to exerting normative influence, groups exert informational influence by being open or closed to information relevant to a particular topic. Group members serve as models for each other; they may provide members exposure to general and specific information, and influence members' perceptions of personal vulnerability to negative outcomes. Various factors may moderate group members' reactions to network-based social influence: These include the size of the network (larger may be more influential), cohesiveness of the reference group (more cohesive being more influential), enmeshment of the individual with the reference group (higher being more influential), nonunanimity of group opinion (lessening pressure to conform), and perception that group opinion is changing (lessening pressure to conform).

Cohesive, homogeneous networks can prove difficult for group members who attempt to initiate new behaviors; reference groups attempt to protect their (status quo) norms and values from assault by both outsiders and insiders. Possible reasons for a network to resist change from within include the fact that change that is inconsistent with a group's values may threaten the perceived veracity of group beliefs, the way a group views itself, the correctness of its behavior, or even the relations between group members (J. Fisher, 1988).

Social influence strategies include the use of slightly older peers to model and influence norms, as well as video representations of respected persons and tangible rewards. Awareness of social pressures and resistance training (identify pressures, examine the motivation behind pressures, respond to pressures, develop skills to resist), also known as psychological inoculation, are applications of social influence theory that are of relevance to multicultural health promotion. Walter, Vaughan, and Cohall (1993) compared models of substance use among urban minority high school students. The socialization model of substance use was much more powerful than either stress/strain or disaffiliation models in explaining the use of alcohol, cigarettes, and marijuana in the past year. However, certain variables derived from the stress/strain and disaffiliation models were important risk factors for the frequent use of these substances. Their findings suggest the need for further elucidation of the social influence process and development, implementation, and evaluation of intensive programs for high-risk youths.

Rinderknecht and Smith (2004) used SCT to improve dietary self-efficacy through a nutrition intervention for Native American adolescents. SCT was an effective model from which to explore constructs of health behavior. This project demonstrated that a nutrition intervention is an effective way to significantly improve dietary self-efficacy among urban Native American children. The lack of intervention effect among adolescents highlights the need for greater comprehension of personal, environmental, and behavioral constraints influencing dietary self-efficacy and behavior.

Health Belief Model

The HBM, a cognitive theoretical model developed during the 1950s, is a set of interrelated variables that, when accurately measured and multiplicatively correlated, suggest why people might be motivated to engage in health-seeking behavior. It was developed by social psychologists influenced by Kurt Lewin. A major contributing construct from Lewin's work was the view that an individual exists in a life space composed of regions positively, negatively, or neutrally valued (valenced).

Illness would be considered a negative event to be avoided or escaped from; people would try to remain in positive or neutral life spaces. (It was later realized that this view was simplistic; some illnesses may have positive payoffs, and addictions that may lead to future illness might provide gratification in the present that seems impossible to resist.) The term *value expectancy* arose from this concept and describes expectations of the future value (potential outcome), having considered perceived benefits and costs, of taking certain actions in relation to future health and well-being.

The psychological orientation of the creators of the HBM caused them to perceive that the inner world of a person determines his or her actions, with environment influencing the situation only in so far as it would influence a person's inner perceptions. Their orientation was ahistorical; they saw the past exerting an influence only as it is represented in present dynamics (Rosenstock, 1974). The HBM is composed of four constructs: (1) perceived personal susceptibility (to a negative health condition), (2) perceived severity of the condition, (3) perceived benefit(s) of taking a particular action against the threat, and (4) perceived barrier(s) to taking that action. A concept labeled "cues to action" was tentatively incorporated into the model during its early years, but it has been dropped as it was found to be too difficult to measure. Derivative models have also been developed (Facione, 1993). There are several review articles on the HBM (see Austin, Ahmad, & McNally, 2002; Gillam, 1991; Hiltabiddle, 1996; Plowden, 1999; Poss, 2001; Risker, 1996; Roden, 2004; Stout, 1997; VanLandingham, Suprasert, Grandjean, & Sittitrai, 1995; Yarbrough & Braden, 2001).

The construct of "self-efficacy" has lately been added to the HBM. Rosenstock, Strecher, and Becker (1988) argue that

> for behavioral change to succeed, people must (as the HBM theorizes) have an incentive to take action, feel threatened by their current behavioral patterns and believe that change of a specific kind will be beneficial by resulting in a valued outcome at acceptable cost, but they must also feel themselves competent (self-efficacious) to implement that change. A growing body of literature supports the importance of self-efficacy in helping to account for initiation and maintenance of behavioral change. (p. 179)

However, recent results with African Americans suggest an inverted causal sequence from what the model assumes: risk behavior leading to or predicting perceptions. Another delineation of the components (of the HBM) hypothesized to be necessary determinants of a decision to take a health-related action is the existence of sufficient motivation (or a health concern) to make health issues salient or relevant. The belief that one is susceptible (vulnerable) to a serious health problem or to the sequelae of that illness or condition is also important. This is often termed perceived threat. The belief that following a particular health recommendation would be beneficial in reducing the perceived threat, and at a subjectively acceptable cost, increases the likelihood of behavior change. Cost refers to perceived barriers that must be overcome to follow a health recommendation; it includes, but is not restricted to, financial outlays (Brunswick & Banaszak-Holl, 1996; Rosenstock et al., 1988).

Different measures from the HBM (perceived susceptibility, perceived severity, self-efficacy, social support, and perceived barriers) have been used to predict the incidence of a variety of safer-sex behaviors among multicultural adolescents (Steers, Elliott, Nemiro, Ditman, & Oskamp, 1996). Perceived susceptibility, self-efficacy, and social support predicted many safer-sex behaviors. Although the HBM predicted more safer-sex behaviors for Euro-American students than for Hispanic American, African American, and Asian American students, the data also indicated few differences in behavior across these ethnic groups.

Yep (1993) also examined the predictive utility of the HBM in relation to prevention of HIV infection among Asian American college students. Three hypotheses proposed a positive relationship between perceived susceptibility, severity, and benefits, and HIV-preventive behavior; and a fourth postulated a negative relationship between perceived barriers to prevention and actual HIV-preventive behaviors. Severity and barriers were significant predictors of adoption of preventive behaviors among Asian Americans. Severity was a significant predictor of becoming more careful about selection of intimate partners, reducing the number of sexual partners, and generally positive changes toward safer sexual behavior. Barriers were predictive of becoming more selective of intimate partners and ensuring that partners are not infected. It appeared that cultural factors, such as beliefs about HIV, illness, prevention, sexuality, and homosexuality, need to be better incorporated into the model to enhance its predictive power.

Consedine, Magai, Horton, Neugut, and Gillespie (2005) examined health beliefs in mammography screening among Caribbean women. Knowledge, perceived personal risk, and beliefs about treatment efficacy were significantly associated with screening behavior. The results suggest that the HBM can be used for interventions tailored to health belief profiles. Similarly, Juniper, Oman, Hamm, & Kerby (2004) reported on relations among constructs in the HBM and the Transtheoretical Model among African American college women. Perceived barriers were significantly higher and perceived severity, cues to action, and self-efficacy were significantly lower in inactive women.

Lin, Simon, and Zemon (2005) examined the HBM, sexual behaviors, and HIV risk among Taiwanese immigrants. Analyses showed that participants who reported a higher number of sexual partners and more frequent sexual intercourse tended to be more educated. The HBM constructs predicted participants' sexual behaviors. Self-efficacy was the strongest predictor. Acculturation moderated the predictive power of the HBM with respect to intercourse frequency. One limitation is that the HBM was not designed to target Asian immigrants.

Neff and Crawford (1998) also used the HBM to evaluate HIV-risk behaviors among Anglo-American, African American, and Mexican American adults. Analyses of community samples indicated different susceptibility-barriers-risk behaviors among males and females. In a similar study, Brunswick and Banaszak-Holl (1996) looked at relations between HIV avoidance practices and components of the HBM, including HIV-related knowledge, attitudes, and perceptions, with African American adults. Perceived vulnerability was a significant negative predictor and, additionally for women, a positive relationship with a generalized sense of personal efficacy.

The HBM is one of the most widely used models in multicultural groups. Topics include health-seeking behavior (Roy, Torrez, & Dale, 2004), breastfeeding patterns (Sharps, El-Mohandes, Nabil El-Khorazaty, Kiely, & Walker, 2003), diabetes (Brown, Becker, Garcia, Barton, & Hanis, 2002), breast cancer (Smiley, McMillan, Johnson, & Ojeda, 2000), HIV behaviors (Neff & Crawford, 1998), and locus of control (Talavera, Elder, & Velasquez, 1997). For example, Graham, Liggot, and Hypolite (2002) examined the relationship between health beliefs and practice of breast self-examination (BSE) in black women. Their results indicated that health beliefs were much stronger in determining BSE performance for a given individual than were demographic characteristics. The frequency of BSE was related to increased perceived seriousness of breast cancer, benefits of BSE, and health motivation. Frequency of BSE was inversely related to perceived barriers.

Theory of Reasoned Action/ Theory of Planned Behavior

The TRA (Ajzen & Fishbein, 1980) is a highly specific theory outlining cognitive and attitudinal determinants of behaviors. Attitudes and subjective norms determine a person's intentions, which are predictive of behaviors; the shorter the time span between "intentions" and "behaviors," the more likely the behaviors will follow the stated intentions. "An overview of research based on the TRA indicates that correlations between behavioral intentions and behaviors are usually between .6 and .9" (Petosa & Jackson, 1991, p. 466). Questions using this theory are very specific; it is often used for elicitation research to determine which variables to target when introducing a program or intervention. Attitudes are composed of two beliefs: (1) to what extent the subject believes a certain behavior will lead to a certain consequence and (2) whether or not the subject values the consequence. Social norms are also measured by using two constructs: (1) the subject's perception of his or her referent group's desires and (2) the subject's predilection to conform to the referent group's desires.

Closely related to the TRA is the TPB (Jemmott, Jemmott, & Hacker, 1992). Jemmott et al. (1992) found that attitudes and subjective norms predicted intentions to use condoms and that, consistent with the TPB, perceived behavioral control added a significant increment. Adolescents' perceptions of their friends' approval of condom use was unrelated to their intentions, but their behavioral beliefs about the effects of condoms on sexual enjoyment, normative beliefs regarding partners' and mothers' approval, and control beliefs regarding technical skill at using condoms were associated with such intentions.

It is also possible to combine one or more theoretical perspectives. Norris and Ford (1995a) used structural equation modeling to evaluate gender and ethnic differences in a theoretical model of condom use. Their sample consisted of urban, low-income African Americans and Hispanics. Their model incorporated concepts from the HBM, TRA, and Construct Accessibility Model. A new theoretical concept, condom predisposition, emerged as a predictor of condom use in all four groups. This concept combines attitude, partner norms, and accessibility of condom-related constructs. These results underscore the importance of investigating gender differences within ethnic groups and the benefits of integrating different theoretical perspectives.

Pawlak, Connell, Brown, Meyer, and Yadrick (2005) examined predictors of multivitamin supplement use among African American female students by using the TPB. Subjective norms had the greatest influence, followed by perceived behavioral control and attitude. Compton and Esterberg (2005) used the TPB to examine associations between three central constructs of the TPB and the length of treatment delay among patients hospitalized for psychosis. There had been no prior research using health behavior theories to study potential predictors of treatment delay or the duration of untreated psychosis.

TPB has been used to study exercise behaviors. Kerner (2005) used the TPB as a framework to assess attitude to activity, expectations of others, perceived control, and intention to engage in activity among middle school students. In a similar manner, Blanchard et al. (2003) examined ethnicity and the TPB in the exercise domain. They concluded that exercise was related to intentions and attitudes and noted that ethnicity and gender need to be considered when dealing with interventions.

Villarruel, Jemmott, Jemmott, and Ronis (2004) used TPB to predict sexual intercourse and condom use intentions among Spanish-dominant Latino youth. The authors concluded that identification of salient beliefs may predict sexual risk and protective behaviors relevant to the design of culturally and linguistically effective interventions. In another study with Latino youth Jemmott, Jemmott, Hines, and Fong (2001) used TPB as a model of intentions for fighting among African American and Latino adolescents. Consistent with the theory, regression analyses revealed that attitudes, subjective norms, and perceived behavioral control predicted intentions for fighting. Their findings suggest that the theory is a useful framework for guiding interventions for adolescents.

This theory has also been used to study a range of health behaviors. Hanson (1997) used the TPB to examine smoking in African American, Puerto Rican, and non-Hispanic white teenage females. Consistent with the theory, analyses showed direct relationships among attitude, subjective norm, perceived behavioral control, and smoking intention for African Americans. Their results suggest that the TPB provides an empirically adequate explanation of cigarette smoking among African American teenage women. Jemmott et al. (1992) predicted intentions to use condoms among African American adolescents with the TPB. Analyses revealed that attitudes and subjective norms predicted intentions to use condoms and that perceived behavioral control added significant explanatory power. More recently, Jemmott, Jemmott, Braverman, and Fong (2005) studied HIV/STD-risk reduction interventions for African American and Latino adolescent girls. Three interventions based on cognitive-behavioral theories and elicitation research were offered. Skills intervention participants reported less unprotected sexual intercourse and fewer sexual partners and were less likely to test positive for STD.

Díaz-Loving and Villagrán-Vázquez (1999) studied Mexican male and female state workers of low socioeconomic status. They answered a survey that included components of the TRA: behavioral beliefs, behavioral attitudes, behavioral intentions, subjective norm, motivation to comply, condom use, and request for condom use. When people referred to occasional partners, personal behavior beliefs and attitudes were more important. When they referred to regular sexual partners, the subjective norm and motivation to comply with the reference groups took precedence. Condom use was better predicted by a model that includes the intentions to use the condom versus a model that has the "goal behavior" of requesting the partner for condom use.

A limitation of the model is that more is needed to produce a behavior change than an expression of intention (Boyle & Holben, 2006, Chap. 15). It has been stated before that the TRA is an accurate description of some behaviors—for some people, in some situations, whereas for other behaviors—and for other people, in other situations—more or less major changes to the TRA should be incorporated (Bos, Hoogstraten, & Prahl-Andersen, 2005).

Transtheoretical (Stages of Change) Model

Another model useful in planning behavioral intervention programs is the Transtheoretical Model (Prochaska & DiClemente, 1983; Prochaska, DiClemente, Velicer, Rossi, & Guadagnoli, 1992). According to this conceptual model, health behaviors change is a gradual, continuous, and dynamic process. People do not move directly from old to new behaviors but progress through a sequence of five discrete stages.

1. *Precontemplative:* Individuals in this stage have no intention to change their behaviors. (They are unaware of the risk, deny the adverse outcome could happen to them, or are aware of the risk but have made a decision not to change behaviors.)

2. *Contemplative:* People in this stage have formed intentions to change but have no specific plans to change in the near future.

3. *Ready for action:* These people have plans to change their behaviors in the immediate future and may have taken some initial action.

4. *Action:* People in this stage have begun changing their behaviors, but the change is relatively recent and may be inconsistent.

5. *Maintenance:* These people have maintained consistent behavioral change for an extended period; the newly acquired behaviors have become a part of their lives.

The model postulates that individuals engaging in a new behavior move through the stages of precontemplation, contemplation, preparation, action, and maintenance. Movement through these stages does not always occur in a linear manner but may also be cyclical as many individuals must make several attempts at behavioral change before their goals are realized. The amount of progress people make as a result of intervention tends to be a function of the stage they are in at the start.

The stages reflect motivational (cognitive, predisposing), social learning (enabling), and relapse prevention (reinforcing) theories and represent a temporal dimension that allows understanding of when particular shifts in attitudes, intentions, and behaviors occur. Another aspect of the Transtheoretical Model is its delineation of processes of change; these reflect how shifts in behaviors occur (Prochaska, DiClemente, & Norcross, 1992) and relate to enabling or skill-related factors.

Change processes involve covert and overt activities and experiences that individuals engage in when they attempt to modify their problem behaviors. Each process is a broad category encompassing multiple techniques, methods, and interventions traditionally associated with different theoretical orientations (Prochaska, DiClemente, & Norcross, 1992).

Change processes identified by the authors of the model include

- Consciousness raising (increasing information about oneself and one's problem)
- Self-reevaluation (assessing how one feels and thinks about oneself with respect to a problem)
- Self-liberation (choosing and committing to act or belief in one's ability to change)
- Counterconditioning (substituting alternatives for problem behaviors
- Stimulus control (avoiding or countering stimuli that elicit problem behaviors)
- Reinforcement management (rewarding oneself or being rewarded for making changes)
- Helping relationships (being open and trusting about problems with someone who cares)
- Dramatic relief (experiencing and expressing feelings about one's problems and solutions)
- Social liberation (increasing alternatives for nonproblem behaviors available in society) (Prochaska, DiClemente, & Norcross, 1992) (derived from a wide range of psychosocial theories)

The Pawtucket Heart Health Project employed stages of change theory in designing a social marketing campaign (IMAGINE ACTION) that was designed to get residents to exercise more frequently. Planners matched the intervention to the different stages of changes (precontemplation, contemplation, preparation, action) with respect to exercise behaviors. The results indicated that most participants moved to a higher stage in the process. For example, two of three individuals in the contemplation of preparation groups became more active.

Below, we provide additional examples of the use of the Stages of Change Model. Ashing-Giwa (1999) examined health behavior change models and their sociocultural relevance for breast cancer screening in African American women. They noted that the model was not designed for and had not been adequately tested with African American women.

They identified sociocultural dimensions that are not accounted for by the model and argued that it is critical that researchers include sociocultural dimensions such as interconnectedness, health socialization, ecological factors, and health care system factors in their intervention models.

Recently, Di Noia, Schinke, Prochaska, and Contento (2006) reported the application of the Transtheoretical Model to fruit and vegetable consumption among economically disadvantaged African American adolescents. Participants in action-maintenance stages evidenced higher pros, self-efficacy, and fruit and vegetable consumption and significantly lower cons than did participants in precontemplation and contemplation-preparation stages. Also, participants in action-maintenance stages used processes of change more frequently than did those in precontemplation-contemplation-preparation stages.

Frenn et al. (2005) explored the determinants of physical activity and low-fat diet among low-income African American and Hispanic middle school students. Exercise and diet behaviors were closely related to social support. They suggest that a school-based approach may be useful to build peer support for physical activity and lower dietary fat. Parish nurse or clinic settings may be most appropriate for building family role models and support. Living in a neighborhood with traditional Hispanic culture and foods appears to have ameliorated the harmful effects of lower income.

This model can also be used to examine gender differences. O'Hea, Wood, and Brantley (2003) used the Transtheoretical Model to explore gender differences across three health behaviors. Evidence suggested that males and females differed in stages of change for smoking and exercise but not dietary fat intake. Gender-specific interventions may be needed to promote certain health behaviors but not others, and self-efficacy and decisional balance may be related differently to stage of change in low-income and ethnic populations.

More Ecological Models

PRECEDE-PROCEED

PRECEDE-PROCEED (Green & Kreuter, 1999) is a conceptual model for planning health education and health promotion programs. It provides program planners with a well-tested means of articulating a program plan and rationale and a means of documenting and using a systematic, step-by-step approach to planning, implementing, and evaluating health promotion activities. The model can be used to guide the planning process of the regional health promotion program; the implementation of specific regional intervention strategies and policies; the selection or development and implementation of educational, organizational, and political strategies for change; the evaluation of change in factors predisposing, enabling, or reinforcing behavioral or environmental factors; and the extrapolation of impact to outcomes measured in terms of the causal factors themselves or in terms of health or quality of life. The model is thus comprehensive enough to encompass the full range of activities, initiatives, and outcomes that programs or policies might attempt to address.

The model grows out of the science and practice of health promotion (Green & Kreuter, 1999). The PRECEDE-PROCEED model has been widely applied in disease prevention and health promotion programs and tested in research and evaluation projects with over 1,000 published applications on a variety of health issues, including AIDS, smoking, cancer, injury prevention, patient education, sex education, and worksite and school health promotion. The model also provided the framework for the construction of Canada's Health Promotion Survey.

Keith (1998) used the PRECEDE model to address diabetes in Native Americans. A PRECEDE-PROCEED description emerged of non-insulin-dependent diabetes mellitus (NIDDM) and influencing factors (including behavioral diagnosis) within the Choctaw Nation. The model also suggested program design, specific objectives, and evaluation procedures. By incorporating cultural values into health education programs for American Indians, the programs should have a better chance to succeed. Recently, Song and Lee (2006) used the PRECEDE model to examine the factors influencing Korean health behavior. They modified the PRECEDE-PROCEED model and found that overall health behaviors were positively related to age, educational level, income level, disease in the family, medical examination, subjective weight, and concern about health. Factors that had negative relations with overall health behavior were sex, subjective health, stress, and degree of physical activity. Quandt, Arcury, Austin, and Cabrera (2001) studied occupational exposure to pesticides in Latino farmworkers. Participatory research within the PRECEDE-PROCEED planning framework was used to design a training program for Mexican farmworkers. Data were gathered and analyzed through individual and group interviews, community forums, an advisory board, and a partnership between academic researchers and a community-based organization. The intervention's dominant features focused on key health behaviors, relevance to local conditions, and issues of control in the workplace.

Chiang, Huang, Yeh, and Lu (2004) evaluated the effectiveness of two different asthma education programs. One was self-management asthma education based on PRECEDE-PROCEED. The other consisted of regular outpatient asthma education. Asthma knowledge, self-efficacy, perceived effectiveness, children's cooperation, and self-management behaviors significantly improved after the self-management asthma education program based on PRECEDE-PROCEED. Except for perceived effectiveness, all variables still had good effectiveness after 6 months of follow-up. The experimental group was better than the control group in knowledge, children's cooperation, and self-management behaviors at the 3-month follow-up, as well as in knowledge and children's cooperation at the 6-month follow-up. In a community coalition, Darrow et al. (2004) adopted the PRECEDE-PROCEED model for community planning and health promotion to eliminate local disparities in HIV disease. The results from computer-assisted telephone surveys showed that awareness of program efforts had increased, recognition of the extent of HIV/AIDS had increased, and participation in HIV prevention efforts had increased significantly.

Satia-Abouta, Patterson, Kristal, Teh, and Tu (2002) examined the influence of diet-related psychosocial constructs on the dietary practices of Chinese in North America. They used an interviewer-administered questionnaire and PRECEDE-PROCEED as a model. Chinese cultural beliefs played an important role in the dietary practices of Chinese living in North America. Traditional health beliefs as well as socioeconomic and environmental factors related to diet should be incorporated into the design and implementation of culturally appropriate health promotion programs for Chinese immigrants.

Social Ecology

The dominant theoretical models used in health education today are based in social psychology. These theories have increasingly acknowledged the role of social and cultural influences in health behavior (Freudenberg et al., 1995) by adopting an "ecological" perspective. Complementary to the population-based approach described above, social ecology involves understanding health problems within the broader context of society (Marsiglia, 2002). It strives to move away from an emphasis limited to individual determinants and toward a broader perspective that considers social, economic, organizational, and political environments as potential points of intervention. By considering both the individual and the context in which he or she lives, the potential for achieving and sustaining meaningful behavioral and environmental changes is maximized (Green, Richard, & Potvin, 1996; Richard, Potvin, Kishchuck, Prlic, & Green, 1996; Perry, Baranowski, & Parcel, 1990).

Stokols (1992) offered a social ecological analysis of health-promotive environments, emphasizing the transactions between individual or collective behavior and the health resources and constraints that exist in specific environmental settings. He argues that health promotion programs often lack a clear theoretical foundation or are based on narrow conceptual models. For example, lifestyle programs typically emphasize individual behavior-change strategies. They neglect environmental underpinning of health and illness. While the behavioral, environmental, and social ecological models each have key strengths and limitations, they are complementary and can be used to derive practical guidelines for designing and evaluating multicultural programs.

Social ecology focuses on contemporary problems of the social and physical environments and their impact(s) on humans. Stokols (1992) identified key assumptions of the social ecology perspective and the core principles of Social Ecological Theory. He also described the development of the ecological paradigm and applied the social ecological perspective to the problem of health promotion. The six underlying principles of social ecology are (1) identify a phenomenon as a social problem; (2) view the problem from multiple levels and methods of analysis; (3) use and apply diverse theoretical perspectives; (4) recognize human-environment interactions as dynamic and active processes; (5) consider the social, historical,

cultural, and institutional contexts of people-environment relations; and (6) understand people's lives in an everyday sense.

Multiple levels of analysis include the macro level, the micro level, and the meso level applied, for example, to individuals, small groups, organizations, neighborhoods, and geographical regions. Multiple methods of analysis include both qualitative and quantitative methods applied in laboratory and naturalistic settings.

The social ecology perspective, according to Stokols (1992), is distinguished by four assumptions: (1) multiple facets of both the physical environment and the social environment are integral to a social ecological analysis; (2) the relative scale and complexity of environments may be characterized in terms of physical and social components, objective or subjective qualities, and scale or immediacy to individuals and groups; (3) the social ecological perspective incorporates multiple levels of analysis and diverse methodologies; and (4) the perspective incorporates concepts from systems theory to take into account both the interdependencies that exist among immediate and more distant environments and the dynamic interrelations between people and their environments. Stokols indicates that a social ecological perspective on health promotion has important implications for theory development and basic research, as well as for the development of public policy, community intervention, and program evaluation.

PEN-3 Model

Whatever theoretical perspective program planners or policy makers may adopt, they need to somehow integrate such theories into some broader frameworks. The most widely applied framework in health promotion and health education is the PRECEDE-PROCEED model of Green and Kreuter (1991), which has nearly 1,000 published applications, many with multicultural groups. More recently, the

PEN-3 model (Airhihenbuwa, 1995) provides a practical approach to ensuring the cultural relevance of a health promotion intervention. Similar frameworks addressing the ecological validity and cultural sensitivity of psychosocial treatments have been offered (Bernal, Bonilla, & Bellido, 1995).

According to a study done by Imamura (2002), cultural competence by the investigators is also essential to complete the steps of the PRECEDE-PROCEED model. Clearly, beliefs about health and disease are deeply rooted in cultural values. Furthermore, understanding reinforcing or enabling factors that contribute to a specific health problem requires a deep understanding of the cultural roots of those factors. No program designed to alter tobacco use in Native American adolescents, for example, will be successful unless grounded in a thorough understanding of the traditional role that tobacco has played in this community since long before the arrival of the Europeans.

Similarly, Abernethy et al. (2005), argued for the use of a broad framework (i.e., the PEN-3 model) to conduct cancer prevention research in the African American community, engage in health promotion in collaboration with churches, and recruit African American men. Together, they argue that a culturally competent approach that incorporates the values of the community is essential.

Erwin, Johnson, Feliciano-Libid, Zamora, and Jandorf (2005) also argued for incorporating cultural constructs in work regarding Latina breast and cervical cancer education programs. Findings were analyzed using the PEN-3 model, and the results demonstrated a mechanism for creating a culturally competent program. Esperanza y Vida defined the key perceptions, enablers, and nurturers in a diverse Latino population. In another PEN-3 study, James (2004) examined food choices, dietary intake, and nutrition-related attitudes among African Americans. The data were analyzed using the PEN-3 model and showed

a general perception that "eating healthfully" meant giving up part of their cultural heritage and trying to conform to the dominant culture. Barriers to eating a healthful diet also included no sense of urgency, the social and cultural symbolism of certain foods, the poor taste of "healthy" foods, the expense of "healthy" foods, and lack of information. Their findings suggest that the PEN-3 model is an appropriate framework for assessing how one's community and culture influence one's dietary habits and highlight the need for programs and materials developed for churches, neighborhood grocery stores, and local restaurants.

In a landmark paper, Airhihenbuwa et al. (2005) reported on the *National Health Educator Competencies Update Project* and argued for training and improved cultural competencies among health educators, service providers, and policy makers. Airhihenbuwa and Obregon (2000) provided a critical assessment of theories/models used in health communication for HIV/AIDS. They argued that flaws in commonly used, "classical" models in health communication are due to contextual differences in locations where these models are applied. These theories and models are being applied in contexts for which they were not designed. Most important, they note that differences in health behaviors are often the function of culture and that culture should be viewed as a strength and not a barrier. In a parallel paper, Airhihenbuwa, Kumanyika, TenHave, and Morssink (2000) found that cultural identity was related to higher socioeconomic status, lower-fat diets, not smoking, current drinking, and higher physical activity. They correctly concluded that there is a need for a greater emphasis on aspects of cultural identity that are positively related to healthy lifestyles as distinct from aspects that might act as barriers.

These approaches challenge professionals to address health issues at the macro level as well as the micro level. It is based on the assumption that any program should be anchored in a participatory approach that involves a dialogue among members of the targeted culture to address cultural sensitivity and appropriateness. The model is appealing in that it incorporates existing models or theories and frameworks of health education and reflects theory and application in cultural studies. There are three primary dimensions of health beliefs and behaviors to consider: health education, educational diagnosis of health behavior, and cultural appropriateness of health behavior. Within each of these dimensions are three categories.

The first dimension, the process of health education, is focused at three levels:

1. *Person:* Health education is committed to the health of all. Individuals should be empowered to make informed health decisions that are appropriate to their roles in their families and communities.

2. *Extended family:* Health education is concerned not only with the immediate nuclear family but also with extended kin.

3. *Neighborhood:* Health education is committed to promoting health and preventing disease in neighborhoods and communities. Involvement of community members and their leaders becomes critical in providing culturally appropriate programs.

The second dimension, the educational diagnosis of health behavior, also has three levels:

1. *Perceptions:* These include knowledge, attitudes, values, and beliefs, within a cultural context, that may facilitate or hinder personal, family, and community motivation to change.

2. *Enablers:* These include cultural, societal, systematic, or structural influences or forces that may enhance or be barriers to change, such as the availability of resources, accessibility, referrals, employers, government officials, skill, and types of services.

3. *Nurturers:* These represent the degree to which health beliefs, attitudes, and actions are influenced and mediated or nurtured by the extended family, kin, friends, peers, and the community.

The third dimension, cultural appropriateness, is the most critical component of the model and is pivotal to the development of a culturally sensitive health education program:

1. *Positive behaviors:* These are behaviors that are based on health beliefs and actions that are known to be beneficial and must be encouraged.

2. *Existential behaviors:* These are cultural beliefs, practices, and/or behaviors that are indigenous to a group and have no harmful health consequences and, thus, need not be targeted for change and should not be blamed for the failure of the program simply because they are not understood.

3. *Negative behaviors:* These are behaviors based on health beliefs and actions that are known to be harmful to one's health.

Abernethy et al. (2005) studied cancer screening of African American men. Key strategies included addressing specific barriers to screening and placing recruitment efforts in a conceptual framework that addressed cultural issues (PEN-3 model). A culturally competent approach that incorporates the values of the community is essential. In a parallel study, Lewis (2005) sought to use a culturally relevant theory to recruit African American men for cancer screening. Lewis applied the PEN-3 model (Airhihenbuwa, 1995) of health education, an educational diagnosis of behavior, and cultural appropriateness to recruit. This study strongly suggests that applying culturally relevant theories to health might change the health behavior patterns of African Americans. We suggest that Abernethy et al. (2005) need to focus more on ways to disseminate their findings to other health professionals targeting health disparities.

Erwin et al. (2005) focused on Latino immigrants at higher risk of death from breast and cervical cancer. Qualitative and quantitative information was obtained through focus groups and questionnaires. Their findings were analyzed using the PEN-3 model, and the results demonstrated the value of creating a culturally competent program by defining the key perceptions, enablers, and nurturers.

James (2004) used the PEN-3 to explore how culture and community influence the nutrition attitudes, food choices, and dietary intake of African Americans and to identify segments of the population and community that should be targeted for education programs. Data were analyzed using the PEN-3 model. Barriers to eating a healthful diet also included no sense of urgency, the social and cultural symbolism of certain foods, the poor taste of "healthy" foods, the expense of "healthy" foods, and lack of information. Segments of the population that potentially could be motivated to make dietary changes included women, men with health problems, young adults, the elderly, and those diagnosed with a severe, life-threatening disease. The PEN-3 model was an appropriate framework for assessing how community and culture influence the dietary habits of African Americans.

Beech and Scarinci (2003) examine the sociocultural factors associated with smoking attitudes and practices among low-income African American young adults. Themes elicited from focus groups were classified according to the PEN-3 model. They included lighting cigarettes for parents as a first experience with cigarettes; perceived stress relief benefits of smoking; use of cigarettes to extend the sensation of marijuana; and protective factors against smoking, such as respect for parental rules.

Community Participation

The concept of community participation is closely tied to population health and the ecological approaches described above. The past decade has seen a clear trend away from intervention approaches that are technology and institution based toward a more people–based approach that involves citizens in a more direct way (Frankish, Kwan, Ratner, Higgins, & Larsen, 2002). This trend places the health education professional in a different role. Rather than being the initiator, developer, implementer, and decision maker, he/she acts more as consultant, advocate, mediator, and supporter.

The basic premise underlying this approach is that communities themselves can act as their own change agents to achieve social and behavioral outcomes. Program planning, implementation, and evaluation require the early involvement and ongoing participation of leaders and community members, thus creating ownership and enhancing program maintenance. Underlying this perspective is an emphasis on the social forces that influence behavior—the idea that behavior is formed and influenced by cultural factors. It is through community participation that these cultural influences are examined and incorporated into the program approach.

Black, Cook, and Murry (2005) looked at the implications of social support for rural, partnered African American women's health functioning. Ecological theory was used to explore the pathways through which intimate relationships influenced health. Women's relationship quality was positively associated with their psychological and physical health functioning. Support from community residents moderated this link, which was strongest for women who felt most connected with their neighbors and for women who believed their neighborhood to have a sense of communal responsibility. Kim (2005) also used a social ecological model to examine disparities in dental care for Hispanic children from low-income families. Initiation of dental care was related to the mothers' beliefs and her social network's beliefs in the value of preventive dental care. Extended clinic hours also increased the likelihood of mothers' return to the dentists. Provider availability, dental insurance, and family income were related to frequency of planned visits.

In a similar way, Adelson (2005) reported on health disparities in aboriginal Canada. She noted that health inequities point to the underlying causes of disparities, many if not most of which sit largely outside of the typically constituted domain of "health." Disparities are directly and indirectly associated with social, economic, cultural, and political inequities, the end result of which is a disproportionate burden of ill health and social suffering on the aboriginal populations. She argues that research and policy must address the contemporary realities of aboriginal health and well-being, including the individual and community-based effects of health disparities and the direct and indirect sources of those disparities.

PRINCIPLES OF HEALTH EDUCATION AS APPLIED TO MULTICULTURAL HEALTH PROMOTION

The foregoing theories of behavior change and health share a number of common elements. These elements can be distilled into several "principles of behavior change and health education"—that is, educational diagnosis, hierarchy, cumulative learning, participation, situational specificity, multiple methods, individualization, relevance, feedback, reinforcement, and facilitation—that can usefully inform the design and evaluation of multicultural health promotion programs. Green and Frankish (1994) provide a review of theories and principles of health education and applied them to asthma prevention.

- *Principle of educational diagnosis:* This principle involves identification of the causes of health behavior in specific cultural groups.
- *Principle of hierarchy:* This states that there is a natural order in the sequence of factors influencing health behavior.

- *Principle of cumulative learning:* This states that experiences must be planned in a sequence that takes into account the person's prior learning experiences and the concurrent incidental learning experiences or opportunities to which people may be exposed.
- *Principle of participation:* This states that changes in health behavior will be greater if people have identified their own need for change and have actively selected a method or approach that they believe will enable them to change.
- *Principle of situational specificity:* This states that there is nothing inherently superior or inferior about any method of intervention but that the effectiveness and efficiency of any multicultural health promotion program will depend on the circumstances and on the characteristics of the person and/or the change agent—that is, peer, teacher.
- *Principle of multiple methods:* This states that comprehensive multicultural health promotion programs should employ different methods or components in consideration of the interaction of person–specific and situation-specific factors.
- *Principle of individualization:* Individualization, or tailoring, of educational interventions applies the principles of participation, situational specificity, and cumulative learning in producing interventions that are both person and situation relevant.
- *Principle of relevance:* This states that the more relevant the contents and methods used are to the person's (learner's) circumstances and interests, the more likely the learning and behavior change process is to be successful.
- *Principle of feedback:* This states that provision of feedback allows the person to adapt both the learning process and the resultant responses to his or her own situation and pace.
- *Principle of reinforcement:* This states that healthy behavior that is rewarded tends to be repeated.
- *Principle of facilitation:* This involves the degree to which an intervention either provides the means for people to take action or reduces the barriers to health behaviors.

Principle of Educational Diagnosis

The first task in changing behavior(s) is to determine its causes. Here, this is referred to as the diagnostic principle of changing behavior (Green, Eriksen, & Schor, 1989). Just as the physician must diagnose an illness before it can be properly treated, so too must a behavior be diagnosed before it can be properly changed. *Properly* in this context refers to interventions that are educational rather than manipulative or coercive. If the causes of unhealthy behaviors can be understood, then health professionals can intervene with the most appropriate combination of health education, training, resource development, support, and rewards to influence the factors that predispose, enable, or reinforce healthy behaviors. An intervention linked to a diagnosed problem and an understanding of the social and cultural context has the greatest chance of success.

Principle of Hierarchy

The second principle of behavior change can be called the hierarchical principle. This principle states that there is a natural order in the sequence of factors influencing health behaviors. Predisposing factors must be dealt with before attempting to influence enabling factors, which must in turn be dealt with before focusing on reinforcing factors. The principle then suggests that the beliefs of people should be addressed prior to intervening in order to provide skills or training and that changes in beliefs and abilities must precede an examination of those factors that serve to reinforce attitudinal or behavioral changes.

Evidence exists that it is inefficient and difficult to attempt to train a person in skills to enable behavior when he or she lacks prior motivation. Unless a belief in the potential efficacy of preventive actions and a sense of competence or ability to engage in such actions exist, there is little point in attempting to train people in preventive or health promotion skills. Similarly, attempts to reinforce or reward active living behavior that is not predisposed or properly enabled are likely to fail (Green et al., 1989).

In reality, the principle of hierarchy is often violated for two reasons. First, a single intervention may address several factors at once. Second, the limited occurrence of opportunities for intervention may demand that predisposing, enabling, and reinforcing factors be dealt with simultaneously (Kippax & Crawford, 1993).

Principle of Cumulative Learning

The principle of cumulative learning is closely related to the principle of hierarchy. To maximally influence health behaviors, learning experiences must be planned in a sequence that takes into account the person's prior learning experiences and the concurrent incidental learning experiences or opportunities to which people may be exposed (Chavez & Oetting, 1995). Behavior responds to the cumulative learning experience of a person, including those experiences that were incidental to or preceded the individual's participation in a health education or behavior change program. It must also be recognized that behavior is strongly influenced by social and cultural determinants of health.

Principle of Participation

The prospects for success in any attempt to change health behavior(s) will be greater if the people have identified their own need for change and have actively selected a method or approach that they believe will enable them to change (Young & Klingle, 1996). No principle of behavior change has greater generalizability than the principle of participation (Green, 1986; Uhl, 1989). In fact, this principle forms the foundation of the definition of health promotion (Green & Kreuter, 1991; World

Health Organization [WHO], 1986). The Ottawa Charter for Health Promotion defined health promotion as "the process of enabling people to increase control over, and to improve their health" (WHO, 1986). Health promotion defined more operationally is "any combination of educational, organizational, economic and environmental supports for actions conducive to health" (Green & Kreuter, 1991).

Howell, Flaim, and Lung (1992) noted that an effective program does not consist of a passive transfer of information. Rather, it involves the participants in an interactive manner, with an emphasis on skills building that is enhanced by effective communication and frequent feedback. They note further that the process requires valid observations, use of good judgment, and appropriate decision making. Participation, in turn, relates to the principle of "ownership"—that is, that people have a sense of responsibility for and control over promoting changes in their behavior and health status. Rifkin, Muller, and Bichmann (1988) note that participation cannot be divorced from equity and that it is crucial that professionals see the benefits of people's participation in order to allocate the necessary time and resources to developing an approach to empowering people.

Principle of Situational Specificity

The principle of situational specificity argues against the notion of the "magic bullet" approach and holds instead that there is nothing inherently superior or inferior about any method of intervention that attempts to achieve change in health behaviors. The effectiveness/efficiency of any multicultural health promotion program will depend on circumstances, characteristics of the people or target audience, and characteristics of the change agent—that is, teacher.

New methods of education or intervention may appear to be superior to "traditional" methods, but this advantage typically fades when the method loses its novelty. Green and

Kreuter (1991) note that the field of health education is strewn with failed approaches. The key to successful intervention appears to lie in the strategic application of a given intervention to the right audience, at the right time, in the right way. Efforts to change people's behavior should rely more on the diagnostic principle and the principle of participation than on the development of "novel" approaches.

Principle of Multiple Methods

Insofar as multiple causes will invariably be found for any given person's behavior, the principle of multiple methods is relevant. This principle suggests that a different method or component of a comprehensive multicultural health promotion program must be provided for each of the different predisposing, enabling, and reinforcing factors. This principle is akin to the multitrait-multimethod matrix approach in personality psychology, which suggests that behavior change results from a complex interaction of person-specific and situation-specific factors.

Principle of Individualization

The individualization, or tailoring, of health promotion interventions applies the principles of participation, situational specificity, and cumulative learning (Rohrbach, Montgomery, & Hansen, 1993). It argues for an interactive approach to learning in which people are actively involved in the learning experience. Programmed instruction, exit interviews in which people's expectations can be clarified or questions answered, and follow-up contact with people after completion of a program are examples of techniques that incorporate this principle. The provision of written or audiovisual materials in combination with personal communication from a health professional may enhance a person's ability to engage in successful health behaviors. The principle of multiple methods suggests that a combination approach may have a greater likelihood of success. However, health professionals must not mistake the simple provision of multiple forms of information for an effective intervention. They should also resist the temptation to substitute the pamphlet approach for more time-consuming, but effective personal interactions with people.

West, Aiken, and Todd (1993) reviewed the strengths and weaknesses of designs and analyses of multicomponent intervention programs. Their analysis is useful in answering questions that assess whether each of the individual components contributes to the outcome, whether the program is optimal, and which processes are the components of the program achieving their effects. Given that *tailoring* suggests the adaptation of learning experiences for each person, such an approach may become impossible in a large-scale program. The difficulties inherent in designing person-specific interventions may lead to the development of simplistic "lowest-common-denominator" approaches to interventions.

Principle of Relevance

Closely, related to the principle of individualization is the principle of relevance. The principle of relevance states that the more relevant the contents and methods used are to the person's (learner's) circumstances and interests, the more likely the learning process is to be successful. The more interested the person is in learning, the more likely it is that information pertaining to specific health behaviors will be retained and that appropriate (self-care) action will be taken. Gregg and Curry (1994) provide evidence to this effect in their study of explanatory models for cancer among African American women and their implications for a cancer-screening program.

Principle of Feedback

Given the principles above, the principle of feedback is crucial in designing health promotion efforts. It ensures that people obtain direct and immediate feedback on their progress and the effects of their health behaviors. The provision of feedback allows individuals to adapt to both the learning process and the behavioral responses within their own situation and at their own pace. When comprehension of a specific regimen is the goal, feedback can take the form of asking questions to determine the amount of information that has been acquired or retained. For long-term regimens, any method that makes progress visible to the person can provide the necessary supportive feedback. The feedback principle is relevant to both program participants and health professionals or caregivers.

Principle of Reinforcement

A fundamental principle of human behavior is that behavior that is rewarded tends to be repeated. Unrewarded behaviors tend to be extinguished or to disappear. Application of the principle of reinforcement involves any activity (other than feedback) that is designed to reward a person for health behavior. Reinforcement may be intrinsic or extrinsic in nature.

Hugo (2000) reported on a grading model for media appropriateness and cultural sensitivity in health education. He noted that many forms of media used in health education have only a limited effect in promoting a healthy lifestyle. One reason is the insufficient attention paid to different sociocultural variables in choosing suitable media for particular audiences in a culturally diverse society. Hugo presents a model based on the interaction between principles of health education, appropriate media and technology, and sociocultural sensitivity. A strong point of this model is its flexibility, because it can be combined with other instruments for formative assessment of different health learning materials.

Principle of Facilitation

This principle is closely tied to the foregoing discussion of enabling factors. Application of this principle includes the development of skills to apply behavioral techniques for self-management. These skills may include avoiding risk behavior, "triggers," or risky environments; devising alter responses to unavoidable triggers; pairing new behaviors with a natural cue; adjusting the active living regimen to suit the people's reality; and learning requisite skills and identifying sources of support to overcome barriers to maintaining healthy behaviors in different environments—that is, home, school, work, outdoors.

THEORETICAL TRENDS INFLUENCING HEALTH PROMOTION

The use of theory in the planning, implementation, and evaluation of multicultural health promotion programs also must be considered within broader contextual trends. Three such trends are the movement toward the so-called population health perspective, the social ecology approach, and the importance of community participation in all aspects of health planning and decision making.

Population Health Promotion

The term *population health* refers to a perspective that suggests that to improve the health of people, action must be taken on a broad range of factors that determine health (Hamilton & Bhatti, 1996). These determinants acknowledge the diversity of the population, on the basis of specific factors including age, sex, economic status, and culture, as leading to differences in health status that cannot be changed by medical care alone. The underlying assumption is that by improving the health of individuals, the health of the entire population will be improved.

There are many similarities between population health, health promotion, public health, and community health, all of which address the health of the larger public. Population health is a more contemporary term that describes an approach based on a synthesis of the available evidence regarding key factors and conditions that determine health status. These factors are identified in *Strategies for Population Health* (Federal, Provincial and Territorial Advisory Committee on Population Health, 1994) as follows:

- *Income and social status:* The relative distribution of wealth is a key factor that determines health status. Social status also affects health by determining the degree of control individuals have over life's circumstances, as well as their capacity to take action.
- *Social support networks:* Support from families, friends, and communities helps people deal with difficult circumstances in their lives and maintain a sense of mastery over the circumstances they encounter.
- *Education:* Education provides people with knowledge and skills for living, enables them to participate in their community, and increases opportunities for employment.
- *Employment and working conditions:* Meaningful employment, economic stability, and a healthy work environment are associated with health.
- *Physical environment:* Air and water quality, housing, and community safety all play a role in determining health.
- *Biology and genetic endowment:* Inherited genetic factors play an important role in determining health.
- *Personal health practices and coping skills:* Personal health practices can play a major role in preventing disease, and coping skills can enable people to be self-reliant, solve problems, and make choices that enhance health.
- *Health child development:* Prenatal and early childhood experiences have a significant effect on later health.
- *Health services:* The availability of preventive and primary care services is important in determining health.

To implement a population health promotion model requires the identification of one of the health determinants identified above, the action strategy to be used (e.g., strengthen community action, build healthy public policy, create supportive environments, develop personal skills, or reorient health services), and the level of action to be taken (e.g., society, a specific sector/system, community, family, individual). By using this approach, program planning can move toward addressing a more comprehensive range of actions-related health.

INTEGRATING THEORY IN HEALTH PROMOTION WITH MULTICULTURAL POPULATIONS

It has been observed by many that practitioners do not seem to use theory and commonly regard it as unrealistic and inapplicable (Hochbaum, Sorenson, & Lorig, 1992). Theory is difficult to apply to the real world because the real world is much more complex than anything we can anticipate. After all, theory is by definition only a reified and hypothetical explanation of the way the world operates. Health promotion theories cannot tell a practitioner specifically how to plan a program or what interventions to use. Theories are merely instruments that guide our thinking as to the most promising approaches to planning intervention strategies (Hochbaum et al., 1992).

It has been acknowledged that while the training of health promotion practitioners emphasizes the use of theory, it is often taught from an academic perspective, which makes application difficult and elusive. In applying theory to a practical situation, D'Onofrio (1992) suggests that health educators should be active consumers who question and analyze the utility of theory by (1) dismantling the myth of theory as the almighty standard, (2) acknowledging the limitations of theory in practice, and (3) exerting leadership by directly identifying and openly discussing the issues confronted in practice. For example, D'Onofrio suggests the following questions as useful issues to consider in making planning decisions:

- What dimensions of the problem does the theory concern?
- How does the theory explain this portion of the problem?
- What additional information does the theory suggest you should gather?
- How accurately does the theoretical explanation coincide with your own understanding of the problem?
- What important aspects of the problem does the theory fail to consider?
- What would an educational program based on the theory be like?
- How effective do you expect the program would be in reducing the problem? Why?
- If the program did result in change, how would the theory explain it?
- If you were guided by theory, what questions would you ask in program evaluation?
- In your own judgment, how helpful is the theory in working with the problem? What are the limitations?

CHAPTER SUMMARY

Taken together, the examined theories have demonstrated relevance to the work of practitioners, program planners, and policy makers who work in multicultural settings. Theories can help us understand the nature of health behaviors. They can explain the dynamics of behavior, the processes for changing behavior, and the effects of external influences on the behavior. Theories can help us identify the most suitable targets for programs, the methods for accomplishing change, and the outcomes for evaluation. Theories and models explain behavior and suggest ways to achieve behavior change (Table 4.2).

Recently, Davies (2006) argued for the use of theory as one tool for evaluating interventions. However, Jones and Donovan (2004) concluded that none of the theories or models included in "standard" theories and models taught in health promotion courses and leading textbooks were used by more than 50% of practitioners. The only models being used by more than one third of the practitioners were PRECEDE–PROCEED

Table 4.2   Examples of Additional Health Education and Health Promotion Models or Theories

Name of Model or Theory	Reference(s)	Multicultural Groups Addressed
AIDS Risk Reduction Model		
Coping Theory	Chavez, Hubbell, McMullin, Martinez, and Mishra (1995); Lazarus and Folkman (1984); Gonzalez, Geoppinger, and Lorig (1990); Negy (1995); Vega, Zimmerman, Gil, Warheit, and Apospori (1993); Wasti and Cortina (2002)	African American mothers, Cuban and Hispanic youth, Anglo-Americans and Mexicans, Turkish and Hispanic American women
Cognitive-Behavioral Theory	Finlayson, Siefert, Ismail, Delva, and Sohn (2005); Mishel et al. (1995); Rosal et al. (2005)	African American children, African American adolescents, African American cancer survivors, Latino diabetes patients
Communication Theory	McGuire (1985); Resnicow, Baranowski, Ahluwalia, and Braithwaite (1999)	
Diffusion of Innovation	Orlandi, Landers, Weston, and Haley (1990); Powe and Adderley-Kelly (2005); Rogers and Storey (1987); Schlundt, Mushi, Larson, and Marrs (2001); Sherrill et al. (2005)	Hispanic communities, African Americans cancer patients
Expectancy Value Theory	Carter, Gayle, and Baker (1990); Gleicher and Petty (1993); Leviton (1989); Kahn, Emans, and Goodman (2001)	
Information Motivation Model	Fisher and Fisher (2002), Kalichman et al. (2006) Aronowitz, Rennells, and Todd (2005)	Afro-American girls, inner-city minority students, AIDS patients

Name of Model or Theory	Reference(s)	Multicultural Groups Addressed
Learned Helplessness Theory	Dancy et al. (2001); Linn, Poku, Cain, Holzapfel, and Crawford (1995); Perilla, Bakeman, and Norris (1994); Tomes, Brown, Semenya, and Simpson (1990); Underwood (1992); Waschbusch, Sellers, LeBlanc, and Kelley (2003); Zimmerman, Ramirez-Valles, and Maton (1999)	Caucasian women, African Americans
Precaution Adoption Model	Weinstein and Sandman (2002)	
Social Marketing Theory	Alden, Tice, and Berthiaume (2006); Brown and Wimberly (2005); Dharod, Perez-Escamilla, Bermudez-Millan, Segura-Perez, and Damio (2004); Levy, Carter, Priloutskaya, and Gallegos (2003); Samuels (1993)	African Americans, Asians and Pacific Islanders, Filipino patients, Latino population, Hispanics
Social Support Theory	Bradley, Schwartz, and Kaslow (2005); Cohen and Wills (1985); Compton, Thompson, and Kaslow (2005); Cortina (2004); Edwards (2006); Ford, Tilley, and McDonald (1998a, 1998b); Gotay and Wilson (1998); Nollen, Catley, Davies, Hall, and Ahluwalia (2005); Schulz et al. (2006); Thomas (2002); Wingate et al. (2005); Wolfe (2004); Thrasher (2004)	African American women, African American men

and the Transtheoretical (Stages of Change) Model. The HBM and other models and theories with similar principles were designed to address health prevention from an individual, linear, and rational perspective. Although these theories and models have proven effective in certain societies for addressing certain diseases, they seem to be inadequate for multicultural groups.

Cultural influences have become more prominent in contemporary theories explaining the factors that determine health. Historically, theories applied in health promotion focused on individual determinants of health. More recently, this focus has expanded to social and cultural influences. It is clear from experience accumulated over the past two decades that to address health problems effectively, we must examine cultural factors and understand beliefs about health within a context that is relevant to the population of interest (Frankish et al., 1999).

According to the literature, the health needs of individuals in different age groups differ based on gender, the household environment, and the neighborhood the person has been born and grown in. There is, therefore, a need for different health education models to assess each individual's attitudinal and behavioral intentions and beliefs. However, as evidenced by the literature, there is no single gold standard model to investigate such diversities in terms of individual cultural background, age group, and gender identity. Cultural sensitivity in health promotion, education, and development programs can be realized only when we centralize the cultural experiences of those who have hitherto been marginalized in the production of knowledge and cultural identity. To be specific, it is counterproductive to target individuals for most health risk reduction efforts without considering the effects of those individuals' cultures, languages, and environments. Educators must use source expertise to manipulate the social, political, and environmental forces that influence health behavior within the context of particular cultures (Airhihenbuwa,

1992). Thus, to locate culture at the core of health education/promotion programs is to require cultural and political understanding of the historicity within the cultural and political context of the present health beliefs and actions of a people. This is a process of cultural empowerment (Airhihenbuwa, 1995).

There are several reasons why it is critical to consider culture and ethnicity when applying theory to a health problem (Reybold, 2006). First, morbidity and mortality rates for different diseases vary by race and ethnicity; second, there are differences in the prevalence of risk behaviors among those groups; and third, the determinants of health behaviors vary across racial and ethnic groups. Based on the evidences, no single theory dominated health education and promotion, nor should it; the problems, behaviors, populations, cultures, and contexts of public health practice are broad and varied. Some theories focus on individuals as the unit of change. Others examine change within families, institutions, communities, or cultures. Adequately addressing an issue may require more than one theory, and no one theory is suitable for all cases (Glanz, Rimer, & Su, 2005). The North American population is growing more culturally and ethnically diverse; an increasing body of research shows that health disparities exist among various ethnic and socioeconomic groups. These findings highlight the important of understanding the cultural backgrounds and life experiences of community members, though research has not yet established when and under what circumstances targeted or tailored health communications are more effective than generic ones. There is also a call for theory to support evidenced-based decision making (Wang, Moss, & Hiller, 2006). Others have noted that much research on health behaviors is theory based. For example, Glanz et al. (1997) found that almost half the articles used some theory or model. The continuing value placed on theory suggests a continuing need for rigorous validation of theories. As stated by Rimer (1997), "theory is not theology." Theory needs questioners more than loyal followers.

Most health behavior theories can be applied to diverse cultural and ethnic groups, but health practitioners must understand the characteristics of target populations (e.g., ethnicity, socioeconomic status, gender, age, and geographical location) to use these theories correctly. Acculturation and education are key factors that should be considered in developing health education messages and interventions that are culturally and educationally appropriate to subpopulations in terms of language and informational content of the message and in terms of psychological factors related to health behavior change (Balcazar, Castro, & Krull, 1995).

Evidence shows that most of the models are not applicable in diverse groups including people of ethno-cultural communities and those of low-income status. Models should place an emphasis on ethno-cultural and vulnerable populations (low socioeconomic status, low health literacy). Issues of literacy and *health literacy* (i.e., a person's ability to access, understand, appraise, and communicate information to make informed decisions regarding his or her health) should be considered (Rootman et al., 2004). Gender-specific issues must also be examined (Shapiro, 2005). In summary, more culturally relevant (competent) and tailored interventions, as well as research that incorporates culturally meaningful concepts with tailored assessment instruments, are needed (Lin et al., 2005; Yeatman & Nove, 2002).

Mulatu and Berry (2001) argue that there will be a growing, diverse worldwide population for whom the health care demands will also be rapidly increasing. As a result, there will also be an increasing demand for multicultural health interventions. They correctly suggest that issues of acceptability, effectiveness, and equity will continue to be key to multicultural health interventions. They discuss several

models that blend ecological and sociocultural processes (e.g., PEN-3 Model; Airhihenbuwa, 1995) in an ecocultural framework (Georgas, van de Vijver, & Berry, 2004), those that target population-level factors and those that aim at individual behavioral and cognitive factors.

In summary, models and theories remain a powerful tool in the planning, implementation, and evaluation of health promotion or health education policy and programs (Bryant, 2002). However, much work remains to be done. The vast majority of existing models have not been adequately validated. Their relevance to multicultural populations needs to be better developed. The movement toward greater emphasis on ecological considerations, culturally appropriate models of evidence and accountability, and increased citizen participation in health education decision making gives hope for a brighter future—in which multicultural groups will be more fully engaged in the design, testing, and application of health education models. This challenge is particularly salient in the "developing" world (Catford, 2005, 2006; Gonzalez-Block, 2004; Haines, Kuruvilla, & Borchert, 2004). Models must also be tools for engendering dialogue, building capacities, and reducing health inequities.

Chapter 5, provides a further dimension of information to the health promotion student and practitioner. The authors Stevens and Cousineau tell us that the relationship between inequality and health is not new. Health differences still persist between racial and ethnic groups, the wealthy and the poor, the insured and the uninsured, and so on. An increasing disparity in health and well-being across these social divisions is seen. The next chapter, then, reviews the current theories and evidence for the creation of health disparities. A model is presented to help the health promotion/disease prevention planner better understand how health disparities are manifested in multicultural populations. Also, some of the major disparities in health and health care by race/ethnicity are explored. The chapter will focus on the role of culture in the production of disparities and considers some of the major programs and interventions that have been designed to address disparities. Finally, the chapter summarizes key steps that health education and promotion professionals can take to further reduce disparities.

DISCUSSION QUESTIONS AND ACTIVITIES

Bringing about behavioral change at the individual, group, and community levels is a complex task, and working with multicultural population groups adds even greater challenges. Different cultural and ethnic groups and their subgroups are at high risk for specific health problems—for example, lung cancer, asthma, breast cancer, heart attack, HIV/AIDS, tuberculosis, accidents and injuries, hypertension, obesity, type 2 diabetes, to identify just a few.

Working in small groups, select a multicultural target group and a health problem.

1. Then, select a change model for developing a program at each level of change—that is, individual, group, community. Explain why you selected that model as relevant to the level and type of change you wish to bring about.

2. For each level of change, identify the desired outcomes of your program; for example, at the community level, you might select the ecological/environmental approach to reduce health risk through changing or adopting new regulations that result in putting fewer community members at risk of a particular disease (such as laws that prevent smoking in the workplace).

3. Share and discuss your small-group work with the rest of the class.

REFERENCES

Abernethy, A. D., Magat, M. M., Houston, T. R., Arnold, H. L., Jr., Bjorck, J. P., & Gorsuch, R. L. (2005). Recruiting African American men for cancer screening studies: Applying a culturally based model. *Health Education & Behavior, 32*(4), 441–451.

Adams, J., & White, M. (2005).Why don't stage-based activity promotion interventions work? *Health Education Research, 20*, 237–243.

Adelson, N. (2005). The embodiment of inequity: Health disparities in aboriginal Canada. *Canadian Journal of Public Health, 96*(Suppl. 2), S45–S61.

Adih, W. K., & Alexander, C. S. (1999). Determinants of condom use to prevent HIV infection among youth in Ghana. *Journal of Adolescent Health, 24*, 63–72.

Airhihenbuwa, C. O. (1992). Health promotion and disease prevention strategies for African-Americans. In R. L. Braithwaite & S. E. Taylor (Eds.), *Health issues in the black community* (pp. 267–280). San Francisco: Jossey-Bass.

Airhihenbuwa, C. O. (1995). *Health and culture: Beyond the Western paradigm.* Thousand Oaks, CA: Sage.

Airhihenbuwa, C. O., Cottrell, R., Adeyanju, M., Auld, M. E., Lysoby, L., & Smith, B. J. (2005). The National Health Educator Competencies Update Project: Celebrating a milestone and recommending next steps to the profession. *Health Education & Behavior 32*(6), 722–724.

Airhihenbuwa, C. O., Kumanyika, S. K., TenHave, T. R., & Morssink, C. B. (2000). Cultural identity and health lifestyles among African Americans: A new direction for health intervention research? *Ethnicity & Disease, 10*(2), 148–164.

Airhihenbuwa, C. O., & Obregon, R. (2000). A critical assessment of theories/models used in health communication for HIV/AIDS. *Journal of Health Communication, 5*(Suppl.), 3.

Ajzen, I., & Fishbein, M. (1980). *Understanding and predicting social change.* Englewood Cliffs, NJ: Prentice Hall.

Alden, D. L., Tice, A., & Berthiaume, J. (2006). Antibiotics and upper respiratory infections: The impact of Asian and Pacific Island ethnicity on knowledge, perceived need, and use. *Ethnicity & Disease, 16*(1), 268–274.

Armitage, C., & Conner, M. (2000). Social cognition models and health behaviour: A structured review. In Methods and models in health psychology [Special issue]. *Psychology & Health, 15*(2), 173–189.

Aronowitz, T., Rennells, R. E., & Todd, E. (2005). Heterosocial behaviors in early adolescent African American girls: The role of mother-daughter relationships. *Journal of Family Nursing, 11*(2), 122–139.

Ashing-Giwa, K. (1999). Health behavior change models and their socio-cultural relevance for breast cancer screening in African American women. *Women & Health, 28*(4), 53–71.

Austin, L. T., Ahmad, F., & McNally, M. J. (2002). Breast and cervical cancer screening in Hispanic women: A literature review using the Health Belief Model. *Women's Health Issues, 12*(3), 122–128.

Balcazar, H., Castro, F, G., & Krull, J. L. (1995). Cancer risk reduction in Mexican American women: The role of acculturation, education, and health risk factors. *Health Education Quarterly, 22*(1), 61–84.

Bandura, A. (1986). *Social foundations of thought and action: A Social Cognitive Theory.* Englewood Cliffs, NJ: Prentice Hall.

Bandura, A. (1989). Perceived self-efficacy in the exercise of control over AIDS infection. In V. M. Mayes, G. W. Albee, & S. F. Schneider (Eds.), *Primary prevention of AIDS: Psychological approaches* (pp. 128–141). London: Sage.

Bandura, A. (1991). Social Cognitive Theory of moral thought and action. In W. Kurtines & J. Gerwitz (Eds.), *Handbook of moral behavior and development* (pp. 45–103). Hillsdale, NJ: Lawrence Erlbaum.

Becker, M., & Maiman, L. (1975). Sociobehavioral determinants of compliance with health and medical recommendations. *Medical Care, 13,* 10–24.

Beech, B. M. & Scarinci, I. C. (2003). Smoking attitudes and practices among low-income African Americans: Qualitative assessment of contributing factors. *American Journal of Health Promotion, 17*(4), 240–248.

Bernal, G., Bonilla, J., & Bellido, C. (1995). Ecological validity and cultural sensitivity for outcome research: Issues for the cultural adaptation and development of psychosocial treatments with Hispanics. *Journal of Abnormal Child Psychology, 23,* 1.

Black, A., Cook, J., & Murry, V. (2005). Ties that bind: Implications of social support for rural, partnered African American women's health functioning. *Women's Health Issues, 15*(5), 216–223.

Blanchard, C. M., Rhodes, R. E., Nehl, E., Fisher, J., Sparling, P., & Courneya, K. S. (2003). Ethnicity and the Theory of Planned Behavior in the exercise domain. *American Journal of Health Behavior, 27*(6), 579–591.

Bos, A., Hoogstraten, J., & Prahl-Andersen, B. (2005). The Theory of Reasoned Action and patient compliance during orthodontic treatment. *Community Dentistry and Oral Epidemiology, 33,* 419–426.

Boyle, M. A., & Holben, D. H. (2006). Designing community nutrition interventions. In *Community nutrition in action: An entrepreneurial approach* (4th ed., pp. 474–495). Belmont, CA: Thomson/Wadsworth.

Bradley, R., Schwartz, A. C., & Kaslow, N. J. (2005). Posttraumatic stress disorder symptoms among low-income, African American women with a history of intimate partner violence and suicidal behaviors: Self-esteem, social support, and religious coping. *Journal of Traumatic Stress, 18*(6), 685–696.

Brown, S. A., Becker, H. A., Garcia, A. A., Barton, S. A., & Hanis, C. L. (2002). Measuring health beliefs in Spanish-speaking Mexican Americans with Type 2 diabetes: Adapting an existing instrument. *Research in Nursing & Health, 25*(2), 145–158.

Brown, S., & Wimberly, Y. (2005). Reducing HIV/AIDS transmission among African-American females: Is the female condom a solution? *Journal of the National Medical Association, 97*(10), 1421–1423.

Bruhn, J. (1983). The application of theory in childhood asthma self-help programs. *Journal of Allergy and Clinical Immunology, 72*(5, Pt 2), 561–578.

Brunswick, A. F., & Banaszak-Holl, J. (1996). HIV risk behavior and the Health Belief Model: An empirical test in an African American community sample. *Journal of Community Psychology, 24*(1), 44–65.

Bryant, T. (2002). Role of knowledge in public health and health promotion policy change. *Health Promotion International, 17*(1), 89–98.

Burke, R., & Stephens, R. S. (1999). Social anxiety and drinking in college students: A Social Cognitive Theory analysis. *Clinical Psychology Review, 19*(5), 513–530.

Campbell, M. K., & Sherman, S. G. (1999). Nutrition behavior: Implementing change in communities. In A. L. Owen, P. L. Splett, & G. M. Owen (Eds.), *Nutrition in the community: The art and science of delivering services* (pp. 172–195). Boston: McGraw-Hill.

Carter, W., Gayle, T., & Baker, S. (1990). Behavioral intervention and the individual. In K. Holmes, P. Mardh, P. Sparling, & P. Wieser (Eds.), *Sexually transmitted diseases* (pp. 1069–1074). New York: McGraw-Hill.

Catford, J. (2005). The Bangkok conference: Steering countries to build national capacity for health promotion. *Health Promotion International, 20*(1), 1–6.

Catford, J. (2006). Creating political will: Moving from the science to the art of health promotion. *Health Promotion International, 21*(1), 1–4.

Chapman-Novakofski, K., & Karduck, J. (2005). Improvement in knowledge, Social Cognitive Theory variables, and movement through stages of change after a community-based diabetes program. *Journal of the American Dietetic Association, 105*(10), 1613–1616.

Chavez, E. L., & Oetting, E. R. (1995). A critical incident model for considering issues in cross-cultural research. Failures in cultural sensitivity. *International Journal of the Addictions, 30*(7), 863–874.

Chavez, L., Hubbell, F., McMullin, J., Martinez, R., & Mishra, S. (1995). Structure and meaning in models of breast/cervical cancer risk factors: A comparison of perceptions among Latinas, Anglo women, and physicians. *Medical Anthropology Quarterly, 9*(1), 40–74.

Cheung, Y. W. (2003). Beyond liver and culture: A review of theories and research in drinking among Chinese in North America. *International Journal of the Addictions, 28*(14), 1497–1513.

Chiang, L. C., Huang, J. L., Yeh, K. W., & Lu, C. M. (2004). Effects of a self-management asthma educational program in Taiwan based on PRECEDE-PROCEED model for parents with asthmatic children. *Journal of Asthma, 41*(2), 205–215.

Cohen, S., & Wills, T. (1985). Stress, social support, and the buffering hypothesis. *Psychological Bulletin, 98*(2), 310–357.

Compton, M. T., & Esterberg, M. L. (2005). Treatment delay in first-episode nonaffective psychosis: A pilot study with African American family members and the Theory of Planned Behavior. *Comprehensive Psychiatry, 46*(4), 291–295.

Compton, M. T., Thompson, N., & Kaslow, N. (2005). Social environment factors associated with suicide attempt among low-income African Americans. *Social Psychiatry and Psychiatric Epidemiology, 40*(3), 175–185.

Consedine, N. S., Magai, C., Horton, D., Neugut, A. I., & Gillespie, M. (2005). Health Belief Model factors in mammography screening: Testing for interactions among subpopulations of Caribbean women. *Ethnicity & Disease, 15*(3), 444–452.

Cortina, L. M. (2004). Hispanic perspectives on sexual harassment and social support. *Personality and Social Psychology Bulletin, 30*(5), 570–584.

Costa, P., Jr., Metter, J., & McCrae, R. (1994). Personality stability and its contribution to successful aging. *Journal of Geriatric Psychiatry, 27*(1), 41–59.

Dancy, B. L., McCreary, L., Daye, M., Wright, J., Simpson, S., & Williams, C. (2001). Empowerment: A view of two low-income African-American communities. *Journal of the National Black Nurses Association, 12*(2), 49–52.

Daniel, M., & Green, L. W. (1995). Application of the PRECEDE-PROCEED planning model in diabetes prevention and control: A case illustration from a Canadian aboriginal community. *Diabetes Spectrum, 8*(2), 74–84.

Darrow, W., Montanea, J., Fernandez, P., Zucker, U., Stephens, D., & Gladwin, H. (2004). Eliminating disparities in HIV disease: Community mobilization to prevent HIV among black and Hispanic young adults. *Ethnicity & Disease, 14*(3), S108–S116.

Davies. K. (2006). What is effective intervention? Using theories of health promotion. *British Journal of Nursing, 15*(5), 252–256.

Decaluwe, V., & Braet, C. (2005). The cognitive behavioural model for eating disorders: A direct evaluation in children and adolescents with obesity. *Eating Behaviors, 6*(3), 211–220.

Dharod, J., Perez-Escamilla, R., Bermudez-Millan, A., Segura-Perez, S., & Damio, G. (2004). Influence of the Fight BAC! food safety campaign on an urban Latino population in Connecticut. *Journal of Nutrition Education and Behavior, 36*(3), 128–132.

Díaz-Loving, R., & Villagrán–Vázquez, G. (1999). The Theory of Reasoned Action applied to condom use and request of condom use in Mexican government workers. *Applied Psychology 48*(2), 139–151.

DiClemente, R., Crosby, R., & Kegler, M. (2002). *Emerging theories in health promotion practice and research: Strategies for improving public health.* New York: Jossey-Bass.

DiGirolamo, A., Thompson, N., Martorell, R., Fein, S., & Grummer-Strawn, L. (2005). Intention or experience? Predictors of continued breastfeeding. *Health Education & Behavior, 32*(2), 208–226.

DiIorio, C., Dudley, W. N., Soet, J., Watkins, J., & Maibach, E. (2000). A social cognitive-based model for condom use among college students. *Nursing Research, 49*(4), 208–214.

Di Noia, J., Schinke, S., Prochaska, J., & Contento, I. R. (2006). Application of transtheoretical model to fruit and vegetable consumption among economically disadvantaged African-American adolescents. *American Journal of Health Promotion, 20*(5), 342–348.

D'Onofrio, C. (1992). Theory and the empowerment of health education practitioners. *Health Education Quarterly, 19*(3), 385–403.

Edwards, L. (2006). Perceived social support and HIV/AIDS medication adherence among African American women. *Qualitative Health Research, 16*(5), 679–691.

Erwin, D. O., Johnson, V. A., Feliciano-Libid, L., Zamora, D., & Jandorf, L. (2005). Incorporating cultural constructs and demographic diversity in the research and development of a Latina breast and cervical cancer education program. *Journal of Cancer Education, 20*(1), 39–44.

Facione, N. (1993). The Triandis model for the study of health and illness behavior: A social behavior theory with sensitivity to diversity. *Advances in Nursing Science, 15*(3), 49–58.

Federal, Provincial and Territorial Advisory Committee on Population Health. (1994). *Strategies for population health: Investing in the health of Canadians.* Retrieved from www.hc-sc.gc.ca/hppb/phdd/resources/

Finlayson, T., Siefert, K., Ismail, A., Delva, J., & Sohn, W. (2005). Reliability and validity of brief measures of oral health-related knowledge, fatalism, and self-efficacy in mothers of African American children. *Pediatric Dentistry 27*(5), 422–428.

Fisher, J. D. (1988). Possible effects of reference group-based social influence on AIDS-risk behavior and AIDS-prevention. *American Psychologist, 43*(11), 914–920.

Fisher, J. D., & Fisher, W. A. (2002). The information-motivation-behavioral skills model. In R. DiClemente, R. Crosby, & R. Kegler (Eds.), *Emerging promotion research and practice* (pp. 40–70). San Francisco: Jossey-Bass.

Fisher, W. A., Fisher, J. D., & Rye, B. J. (1995). Understanding and promoting AIDS-preventive behavior: Insights from the Theory of Reasoned Action. *Health Psychology, 14*(3), 255–264.

Ford, M. E., Tilley, B. C., & McDonald, P. E. (1998a). Social support among African-American adults with diabetes. Part 1: Theoretical framework. *Journal of the National Medical Association, 90*(6), 361–365.

Ford, M. E., Tilley, B. C., & McDonald, P. E. (1998b). Social support among African-American adults with diabetes, Part 2: A review. *Journal of the National Medical Association, 90*(7), 425–432.

Frankish, C. J., Kwan, B., Ratner, P. A., Higgins, J. W., & Larsen, C. (2002). Challenges of citizen participation in regional health authorities. *Social Science & Medicine, 54*(10), 1471–1480.

Frankish, C. J., Larsen, C., Ratner, P., Wharf-Higgins, J., & Kwan, B. (2002). Social and political factors influencing the functioning of regional health boards in British Columbia (Canada). *Health Policy, 61*(2), 125–151.

Frankish, C. J., Lovato, C. Y., & Shannon, W. J. (1999). Models, theories, and principles of health promotion with multicultural populations. In *Promoting health in multicultural populations* (pp. 41–99). Thousand Oaks, CA: Sage.

Frankish, J., Moulton, G., Rootman, I., Cole, C., & Gray, D. (2006). Setting a foundation:

Values and structures as a foundation for health promotion in primary health care. *Primary Health Care Research & Development,* 7, 172–182.

Frenn, M., Malin, S., Villarruel, A., Slaikeu, K., McCarthy, S., Freeman, J., et al. (2005). Determinants of physical activity and low-fat diet among low income African American and Hispanic students. *Public Health Nursing,* 22(2), 89–97.

Freudenberg, N., Eng, E., Flay, B., Parcel, G., Rogers, T., & Wallerstein, N. (1995). Strengthening individual and community capacity to prevent disease and promote health: In search of relevant theories and principles. *Health Education Quarterly,* 22(3), 290–306.

Garrity, T. (1980, October). Medical compliance and the patient-provider relationship. In R. Haynes (Ed.), *Patient compliance to antihypertensive medications.* Washington, DC: National Institutes of Health.

Georgas, J., van de Vijver, F., & Berry, J. (2004). The ecocultural framework, ecosocial indices, and psychological variables in cross-cultural research. *Journal of Cross-Cultural Psychology,* 35(1), 74–96.

Gillam, S. J. (1991). Understanding the uptake of cervical cancer screening: The contribution of the Health Belief Model. *British Journal of General Practice,* 41(353), 510–513.

Glanz, K., Lewis, F. M., & Rimer, B. K. (Eds.). (1997). *Health behavior and health education: Theory, research, and practice* (2nd ed.). San Francisco: Jossey-Bass.

Glanz, K., Rimer, B. K., & Su, S. M. (2005). *Theory at a glance: A guide for health promotion practice.* New York: United States National Cancer Institute.

Gleicher, F., & Petty, R. (1993). Expectations of reassurance influence the nature of fear stimulated attitude change. *Journal of Experimental Social Psychology,* 28(1), 86–100.

Goldfried, M., & D'Zurilla, T. (1969). A behavior analytic model for assessing competence. In L. Spielberger (Ed.), *Current topics in clinical and community psychology* (pp. 151–196). New York: Academic Press.

Gonzalez, V., Geoppinger, J., & Lorig, K. (1990). Four psychosocial theories and their application to patient education and clinical practice. *Arthritis Care and Research,* 3(3), 132–143.

Gonzalez-Block, M. A. (2004). Health policy and systems research agendas in developing countries. *Health Research Policy and Systems,* 2(6), 1–12.

Gotay, C., & Wilson, M. (1998). Use of quality-of-life outcome assessments in current cancer clinical trials. *Evaluation and the Health Health Professions,* 21(2), 157–178.

Graham, M. E., Liggons, Y., & Hypolite, M. (2002). Health beliefs and self breast examination in black women. *Journal of Cultural Diversity,* 9(2), 49–54.

Green, L. W. (1986). The Theory of Participation: A qualitative analysis of its expression in national and international policies. *Advances in Health Education and Promotion,* 1(A), 211–236.

Green, L. W., Eriksen, M. P., & Schor, E. L. (1989). Preventive practices by physicians: Behavioral determinants and potential interventions. *American Journal of Preventive Medicine,* 4(Suppl. 4), 101–107.

Green, L. W., & Frankish, C. J. (1994). Theories and principles of health education applied to asthma. *Chest,* 106(4 Suppl.), 219S–230S.

Green, L. W., & Frankish, C. J. (2000). Health promotion, health education and disease prevention. In C. Koop, C. Pearson, & R. Schwarz (Eds.), *Critical issues in global health* (pp. 321–330). New York: Viking.

Green, L. W., & Kreuter, M. W. (1991). *Health promotion planning: An educational and environmental approach* (2nd ed.). Palo Alto, CA: Mayfield.

Green, L. W., & Kreuter, M. W. (1999). *Health promotion planning: An educational and environmental approach* (3rd ed.). Mountain View, CA: Mayfield.

Green, L. W., & Kreuter, M. W. (2005). *Health program planning: An educational and ecological approach* (4th ed.). New York: McGraw-Hill.

Green, L. W., Richard, L., & Potvin, L. (1996). Ecological foundations of health promotion. *American Journal of Health Promotion,* 10(4), 270–281.

Gregg, J., & Curry, R. H. (1994). Explanatory models for cancer among African-American women at two Atlanta neighborhood health centers: The implications for a cancer screening program. *Social Science & Medicine, 39*(4), 519–526.

Haines, A., Kuruvilla, S., & Borchert, M. (2004). Bridging the implementation gap between knowledge and action for health. *Bulletin of the World Health Organization, 82*(10), 724–732.

Hamilton, N., & Bhatti, T. (1996). *Population health promotion: An integrated model of population health and health promotion*. Toronto, Ontario: Health Canada, Health Promotion Development Division.

Hanson, M. J. (1997). The Theory of Planned Behavior applied to cigarette smoking in African-American, Puerto Rican, and non-Hispanic white teenage females. *Nursing Research, 46*(3), 155–162.

Haynes, R., Taylor, D., & Sackett, D. (1979). *Compliance in health care*. Baltimore, MD: Johns Hopkins University Press.

Hiltabiddle, S. J. (1996). Adolescent condom use, the Health Belief Model, and the prevention of sexually transmitted disease. *Journal of Obstetric, Gynecologic, and Neonatal Nursing, 25*(1), 61–66.

Hochbaum, G., Sorenson, J., & Lorig, K. (1992). Theory in health education practice. *Health Education Quarterly, 19*(3) 295–313.

Hollister, C., & Anema, M. (2004). Health behavior models and oral health. *Journal of Dental Hygiene, 3,* 6.

Howell, J., Flaim, T., & Lung, C. (1992). Patient education. *Pediatric Clinics of North America, 39*(6), 1343–1361.

Huff, R. M., & Kline, M. V. (1999). *Promoting health in multicultural populations: A handbook for practitioners*. Thousand Oaks: Sage.

Hugo, J. (2000). A grading model for media appropriateness and cultural sensitivity in health education. *Journal of Audiovisual Media in Medicine, 23*(3), 103–109.

Hyman, I., & Guruge, S. (2002). A review of theory and health promotion strategies for new immigrant women. *Canadian Journal of Public Health, 93*(3), 183–187.

Illich, I. (1976). *Medical nemesis: The expropriation of health*. New York: Pantheon.

Imamura, E. (2002). Amy's chat room: Health promotion programmes for community dwelling elderly adults. *International Journal of Nursing Practice, 8*(1), 61.

James, D. (2004). Factors influencing food choices, dietary intake, and nutrition-related attitudes among African Americans: Application of a culturally sensitive model. *Ethnicity & Health, 9*(4), 349–367.

Janis, I., & Rodin, J. (1979). Attribution, control and decision-making. In G. Stone (Ed.), *Health psychology* (pp. 487–521). San Francisco: Jossey-Bass.

Jemmott, J. B., III, Jemmott, L. S., Braverman, P. K., & Fong, G. T. (2005). HIV/STD risk reduction interventions for African American and Latino adolescent girls at an adolescent clinic: A randomized controlled trial. *Archives of Pediatrics & Adolescent Medicine, 159*(5), 440–449.

Jemmott, J. B., III, Jemmott, L. S., & Hacker, C. I. (1992). Predicting intentions to use condoms among African-American adolescents: The Theory of Planned Behavior as a model of HIV risk-associated behavior. *Ethnicity & Disease, 2*(4), 371–380.

Jemmott, J. B., III, Jemmott, L. S., Hines, P. M., & Fong, G. T. (2001). The Theory of Planned Behavior as a model of intentions for fighting among African American and Latino adolescents. *Maternal and Child Health Journal, 5*(4), 253–263.

Jones, S., & Donovan, R. (2004). Does theory inform practice in health promotion in Australia? *Health Education Research, 19*(1), 1–14.

Judd, J., Frankish, J., & Moulton, G. (2001). A unifying approach to setting standards in the evaluation of community-based health promotion programs. *Health Promotion International, 16*(4), 367–380.

Juniper, K., Oman, R., Hamm, R., & Kerby, D. (2004). The relationships among constructs in the Health Belief Model and Transtheoretical Model among African-American college women for physical activity. *American Journal of Health Promotion, 18*(5), 354–357.

Kahn, J, A., Emans, S. J., & Goodman, E. (2001). Measurement of young women's attitudes about communication with providers regarding Papanicolaou smears. *Journal of Adolescent Health, 29*(5), 344–351.

Kalichman, S., Simbayi, L., Cain, D., Jooste, S., Skinner, D., & Cherry, C. (2006). Generalizing a model of health behaviour change and AIDS stigma for use with sexually transmitted infection clinic patients in Cape Town, South Africa. Research Support. NIH, *Extramural AIDS Care, 18*(3):178–182.

Kanfer, F. (1975). Self-management methods. In F. Kanfer & A. Goldstein (Eds.), *Helping people change* (pp. 334–389). New York: Pergamon Press.

Kasl, S., & Cobb, S. (1966). Health behavior, illness behavior and sick-role behavior. *Archives of Environmental Health, 12,* 246–250.

Keith, S. (1998). Using PRECEDE/PROCEED to address diabetes within the Choctaw nation of Oklahoma. *American Journal of Health Behavior, 22*(5), 358–359.

Kerner, M. S. (2005). Development of measures from the Theory of Planned Behavior applied to leisure-time physical activity. *Perceptual and Motor Skills, 100*(3, P. 1), 851–858.

Kim, Y. O. (2005). Reducing disparities in dental care for low-income Hispanic children. *Journal of Health Care for the Poor and Underserved, 16*(3), 431–443.

Kippax, S., & Crawford, J. (1993). Flaws in the Theory of Reasoned Action. In D. J. Terry, C. Gallois, & M. McCamish (Eds.), *The Theory of Reasoned Action: Its application to AIDS-preventive behavior* (pp. 253–269). New York: Pergamon Press.

Krohn, M., & Thornberry, T. (1993). Network theory: A model for understanding drug abuse among African-American and Hispanic youth. *NIDA Research Monograph, 130,* 102–128.

Lazarus, R., & Folkman, S. (1984). *Stress, appraisal and coping.* New York: Springer.

Leventhal, H., Meyer, D., & Gutmann, M. (1980, October). The role of theory in the study of compliance. In R. Haynes (Ed.), *Patient compliance to antihypertensive medications.* Washington, DC: National Institutes of Health.

Leviton, L. (1989). Can organizations benefit from worksite health promotion? *Health Services Research, 24*(2), 159–189.

Levy, C., Carter, S., Priloutskaya, G., & Gallegos, G. (2003). Critical elements in the design of culturally appropriate interventions intended to reduce health disparities: Immunization rates among Hispanic seniors in New Mexico. *Journal of Health and Human Services Administration, 26*(2), 199–238.

Lewis, R. (2005). Using a culturally relevant theory to recruit African American men for prostate cancer screening. *Health Education & Behavior, 32*(4), 452–454.

Lin, P., Simoni, J. M., & Zemon, V. (2005). The Health Belief Model, sexual behaviors, and HIV risk among Taiwanese immigrants. *AIDS Education and Prevention, 17*(5), 469–483.

Linn, J. G., Poku, K. A. Cain, V. A., Holzapfel, K. M., & Crawford, D. F. (1995). Psychosocial outcomes of HIV illness in male and female African American clients. *Social Work in Health Care, 21*(3), 43–47.

Madden, M. J., Ellen, P. S., & Ajzen, I. (1992). A comparison of the Theory of Planned Behavior and the Theory of Reasoned Action. *Personality and Social Psychology Bulletin, 18*(1), 3–9.

Maiman, L., Becker, M., & Liptak, G. (1988). Improving pediatrician's compliance enhancing practices, *American Journal of Disorders in Childhood, 142,* 773–779.

Marsiglia, F. (2002). Ties that protect: An ecological perspective on Latino/a urban pre-adolescent drug use. In D. de Anda (Ed.), *Social work with multicultural youth* (pp. 191–220). Binghamton, NY: Haworth.

Matarazzo, J., Miller, N., Weiss, S., Herd, J., & Weiss, S. (1984). *Behavioral health: A handbook of health enhancement and disease prevention.* New York: Wiley.

McGuire, W. J. (1969). Attitudes and attitude change. In G. Lindzey & E. Aronson (Eds.), *Handbook of social psychology* (Vol. 2). Reading, MA: Addison-Wesley.

McGuire, W. J. (1985). Attitudes and attitude change. In G. Lindzey & E. Aronson (Eds.), *Handbook of social psychology* (Vol. 2, 3rd ed., pp. 233–346). New York: Random House.

Milette, I. H., Richard, L., & Martel, M. J. (2005). Evaluation of a developmental care training programme for neonatal nurses. *Journal of Child Health Care, 9*(2), 94–109.

Mishel, M. H., Germino, B. B., Gil, K. M., Belyea, M., Laney, I. C., Stewart, J., et al. (2005). Benefits from an uncertainty management intervention for African-American and Caucasian older long-term breast cancer survivors. *Psycho-Oncology, 14*(11), 962–978.

Moulton, G., Frankish, J., Rootman, I., Cole, C., & Gray, D. (2006). Building on a foundation: Strategies, processes and outcomes of health promotion in primary health care settings. *Primary Health Care Research & Development, 7,* 269–277.

Mulatu, M., & Berry, J. (2001). Cultivating health through multiculturalism. In M. MacLachlan (Ed.), *Cultivating health: Cultural perspectives on promoting health* (pp. 15–35). New York: Wiley.

Mullens, P., & Reynolds, R. (1978). Potential for grounded theory in health education research. *Health Education Research, 6,* 280–285.

Neff, J. A., & Crawford, S. L. (1998). The Health Belief Model and HIV risk behaviors: A causal model analysis among Anglos, African-Americans and Mexican-Americans. *Ethnicity & Health, 3*(4), 283–299.

Negy, C. (1995). Coping and culture: A research note on Diaz-Guerrero's theory. *Psychological Reports, 76*(2), 680–682.

Nollen, N. L., Catley, D., Davies, G., Hall, M., & Ahluwalia, J. S. (2005). Religiosity, social support, and smoking cessation among urban African American smokers. *Addictive Behaviors, 30*(6), 1225–1229.

Norman, P., & Brain, K. (2005). An application of an extended Health Belief Model to the prediction of breast self-examination among women with a family history of breast cancer. *British Journal of Health Psychology, 10*(1), 1–16.

Norris, A. E., & Ford, K. (1995a). Condom use by low-income African American and Hispanic youth with a well-known partner: Integrating the Health Belief Model, Theory of Reasoned Action, and the Construct Accessibility Model. *Journal of Applied Social Psychology, 25*(20), 1801–1830.

Nutbeam, D., & Harris, E. (1998). *Theory in a nutshell: A practitioner's guide to commonly used theories and models in health promotion.* Sydney, Australia: National Center for Health Promotion.

Nutbeam, D., & Harris, E. (2004). *Theory in a nutshell: A practical guide to health promotion theories* (2nd ed.). Sydney, Australia: McGraw-Hill.

O'Hea, E. L., Wood, K. B., & Brantley, P. J. (2003). The Transtheoretical Model: Gender differences across 3 health behaviors. *American Journal of Health Behavior, 27*(6), 645–656.

O'Leary, A., Goodhart, F., Jemmott, L. S., & Boccher-Lattimore, D. (1992). Predictors of safer sex on the college campus: A Social Cognitive Theory analysis. *Journal of American College Health, 40*(6), 254–263.

Orlandi, M., Landers, C., Weston, R., & Haley, N. (1990). Diffusion of health promotion innovation. In K. Glanz, F. M. Lewis, & B. Rimer (Eds.), *Health Behavior and Health Education: Theory, Research and Practice* (pp. 288–313). San Francisco: Jossey-Bass.

Pawlak, R., Connell, C., Brown, D., Meyer, M. K., & Yadrick, K. (2005). Predictors of multivitamin supplement use among African-American female students: A prospective study utilizing the Theory of Planned Behavior. *Ethnicity & Disease, 15*(4), 540–547.

Perilla, J., Bakeman, R., & Norris, F. (1994). Culture and domestic violence in Latinas. *Violence and Victims, 9*(4), 325–339.

Perry, C. L., Baranowski, T., & Parcel, G. S. (1990). How individuals, environments, and health behavior interact: Social Learning Theory. In K. Glanz, F. M. Lewis, & B. K. Rimer (Eds.), *Health behavior and health education* (p. 161). San Fransisco: Jossey-Bass.

Petosa, R., & Jackson, K. (1991). Using the Health Belief Model to predict safer sex intentions among adolescents. *Health Education Quarterly, 18*(4), 463–476.

Plowden, K. (1999). Using Health Belief Model in understanding prostate cancer in African American men. *ABNF Journal, 10*(1), 4–8.

Poss, J. (2001). Developing a new model for cross-cultural research: Synthesizing the Health Belief Model and the Theory of Reasoned Action. *Advances in Nursing Science, 23*(4), 1–15.

Poureslami, I. M., & Ayyar, S. (2002). *Health promotion in disadvantaged communities.* Health Promotion NGO Press: Tehran, Iran.

Powe, B., & Adderley-Kelly, B. (2005). Colorectal cancer in African-Americans: Addressing the need for further research and research utilization. *Journal of National Black Nurses Association, 16*(1), 48–54.

Prochaska, J. O., & DiClemente, C. C. (1983). Stages and processes of self-change of smoking: Toward an integrated model of change.

Journal of Consulting and Clinical Psychology, *51,* 390.

Prochaska, J. O., DiClemente, C. C., & Norcross, J. C. (1992). In search of how people change: Applications to addictive behaviors. *American Psychologist, 47*(9), 1102–1114.

Prochaska, J. O., DiClemente, C. C, Velicer, W. F., Rossi, J. S., & Guadagnoli, E. (1992). *Patterns of change in smoking cessation: Between variable comparisons.* Manuscript submitted for publication.

Quandt, S. A., Arcury, T. A., Austin, C. K., & Cabrera, L. F. (2001). Preventing occupational exposure to pesticides: Using participatory research with Latino farmworkers to develop an intervention. *Journal of Immigrant Health, 3*(2), 85–96.

Ray, M., Sawyer, A., Rothschild, M., Heeler, R., Strong, E., & Reed, J. (1973). Marketing communication and the hierarchy of effects. In P. Clarke (Ed.), *New models for mass communication research* (pp. 147–176). Beverly Hills, CA: Sage.

Resnicow, K., Baranowski, T., Ahluwalia, J. S., & Braithwaite, R. (1999). Cultural sensitivity in public health: Defined and demystified. *Ethnicity & Disease, 9*(1), 10–21.

Reybold, L. (2006). A critical perspective of health empowerment: The breakdown of theory to practice in one Hispanic subculture. *Family & Community Health, 29*(2), 153–157.

Richard, L., Potvin, L., Kishchuk, N., Prlic, H., & Green, L. W. (1996). Assessment of the integration of the ecological approach in health promotion programs. *American Journal of Health Promotion, 10*(4), 318–328.

Rifkin, S. B., Muller, F., & Bichmann, W. (1988). Primary health care: On measuring participation. *Social Science & Medicine, 26*(9), 931–940.

Rimer, B. K. (1997). Perspectives on intrapersonal theories of health behavior. In K. Glanz, F. M. Lewis, & B. K. Rimer (Eds.), *Health behavior and health education: Theory, research and practice* (2nd ed., pp. 139–147). San Francisco: Jossey-Bass.

Rinderknecht, K., & Smith, C. (2004). Social Cognitive Theory in an after-school nutrition intervention for urban Native American youth. *Journal of Nutrition Education and Behavior, 36*(6), 298–304.

Risker, D. (1996). The Health Belief Model and consumer information searches: Toward an integrated model. *Health Marketing Quarterly, 13*(3), 13–26.

Roden, J. (2004). Revisiting the Health Belief Model: Nurses applying it to young families and their health promotion needs. *Nursing & Health Sciences, 6*(1), 1–10.

Rogers, E., & Storey, D. (1987). Communication campaigns. In C. Berger & S. Chaffee (Eds.), *Handbook of communication science* (pp. 817–846). Newbury Park, CA: Sage.

Rogers, L., Matevey, C., Hopkins-Price, P., Shah, P., Dunnington, G., & Courneya, K. (2004). Exploring Social Cognitive Theory constructs for promoting exercise among breast cancer patients. *Cancer Nursing, 27*(6), 462–473.

Rohrbach, L., Montgomery, S. B., & Hansen, W. B. (1993). *The importance of theory to tailor prevention messages to subgroups in an STD clinic population.* Paper presented at the IV International Conference on AIDS (Abstr. PO-D14–3844), Berlin, Germany.

Rootman, I. R., Gordon-El-Bihbety, D., Frankish, C., Hemming, H., Kaszap, M. Langille, L., et al. (2004, November 2). Toward an agenda for literacy and health research in Canada. *Literacies* (2), 38–41.

Rosal, M. C., Olendzki, B., Reed, G. W., Gumieniak, O., Scavron, J., & Ockene, I. (2005). Diabetes self-management among low-income Spanish-speaking patients: A pilot study. *Annals of Behavioral Medicine, 29*(3), 225–235.

Rosenstock, I. (1974). Historical origins of the Health Belief Model. Health Education Monographs, 2, 328–343.

Rosenstock, I., Strecher, V., & Becker, M. (1988). Social Learning Theory and the Health Belief Model. *Health Education Quarterly, 5*(2), 175–183.

Roy, L. C., Torrez, D., & Dale, J. C. (2004). Ethnicity, traditional health beliefs, and health-seeking behavior: Guardians' attitudes regarding their children's medical treatment. *Journal of Pediatric Health Care, 18*(1), 22–29.

Sade, R. (1995). A theory of health and disease: The objectivist-subjectivist dichotomy. *Journal of Medicine and Philosophy, 20*(5), 513–525.

Samuels, S. (1993). Project LEAN: A national campaign to reduce dietary fat consumption.

American Journal of Health Promotion, 4(6), 435–440.

Sasao, T. (1993). Toward a culturally anchored ecological framework of research in ethnic-cultural communities. *American Journal of Community Psychology, 21*(6), 705–727.

Satia-Abouta, J., Patterson, R. E., Kristal, A. R., Teh, C., & Tu, S.-P. (2002). Psychosocial predictors of diet and acculturation in Chinese American and Chinese Canadian women. *Ethnicity & Health, 7*(1), 21–39.

Scheier, M., & Carver, C. (1992). Effects of optimism on psychological and physical well-being: Theoretical overview and empirical update. *Cognitive Therapy and Research, 16*(2), 201–228.

Schlundt, D., Mushi, C., Larson, C., & Marrs, M. (2001). Use of innovative technologies in the evaluation of Nashville's REACH 2010 community action plan. *Journal of Ambulatory Care Management, 24*(3), 51–60.

Schulz, A., Israel, B., Zenk, S., Parker, E., Lichtenstein, R., Shellman-Weir, S., et al. (2006). Psychosocial stress and social support as mediators of relationships between income, length of residence and depressive symptoms among African American women on Detroit's Eastside. *Social Science & Medicine, 62*(2), 510–22.

Sennott-Miller, L. (1994). Using theory to plan appropriate interventions: Cancer prevention for older Hispanic and non-Hispanic white women. *Journal of Advanced Nursing, 20*(5), 809–814.

Shapiro, E. R. (2005). Because words are not enough: Latina re-visionings of transnational collaborations using health promotion for gender justice and social change. *NWSA Journal, 17*(1), 141–171.

Sharps, P. W., El-Mohandes, A. A., Nabil El-Khorazaty, M., Kiely, M., & Walker, T. (2003). Health beliefs and parenting attitudes influence breastfeeding patterns among low-income African-American women. *Journal of Perinatology, 23*(5), 414–419.

Sherrill, W. W., Crew, L., Mayo, R. M., Mayo, W. F., Rogers, B. L., & Haynes, D. F. (2005). Educational and health services innovation to improve care for rural Hispanic communities in the U.S. *Education for Health, 18*(3), 356–367.

Smaje, C. (1996). Ethnic patterning of health: New directions for theory and research. *Sociology of Health & Illness, 18*(2), 139–171.

Smiley, M. R., McMillan, S. C., Johnson, S., & Ojeda, M. (2000). Comparison of Florida Hispanic and non-Hispanic Caucasian women in their health beliefs related to breast cancer and health locus of control. *Oncology Nursing Forum, 27*(6), 975–984.

Song, Y. L., & Lee, K. S. (2006). The factors influencing Korean health behavior. *Daehan Ganho Haghoeji, 36*(2), 330–334.

Steers, W. N., Elliott, E., Nemiro, J., Ditman, D., & Oskamp, S. (1996). Health beliefs as predictors of HIV-preventive behavior and ethnic differences in prediction. *Journal of Social Psychology, 136*(1), 99–110.

St. Lawrence, J. S., Brasfield, T. L., Jefferson, K. W., Alleyne, E., O'Bannon, R. E., III, & Shirley, A. (1995). Cognitive-behavioral intervention to reduce African American adolescents' risk for HIV infection. *Journal of Consulting and Clinical Psychology, 63*(2), 221–237.

Stokols, D. (1992). Establishing and maintaining healthy environments. Toward a social ecology of health promotion. *American Psychologist, 47*(1), 6–22.

Stokols, D. (1996). Translating Social Ecological Theory into guidelines for community health promotion. *American Journal of Health Promotion, 10*(4), 282–298.

Stout, A. (1997). Prenatal care for low-income women and the Health Belief Model: A new beginning. *Journal of Community Health Nursing, 14*(3), 169–180.

Strader, M. K., Beaman, M. L., & McSweeney, M. (1992). Effects of communication with important social referents on beliefs and intentions to use condoms. *Journal of Advanced Nursing, 17*(6), 699–703.

Talavera, G. A., Elder, J. P., & Velasquez, R. J. (1997). Latino health beliefs and locus of control: Implications for primary care and public health practitioners. *American Journal of Preventive Medicine, 13*(6), 408–410.

Tang, K. C., Beaglehole, R., & Byrne, D. O. (2005). Policy and partnership for health promotion: Addressing the determinants of health. *Bulletin of the World Health Organization, 83*(12), 884.

Thomas, C. J. (2002). The context of religiosity, social support and health locus of control: Implications for the health-related quality of life of African-American hemodialysis patients. *Journal of Health & Social Policy, 16*(1–2), 43–54.

Tomes, E. K., Brown, A., Semenya, K., & Simpson, J. (1990). Depression in black women of low socioeconomic status: Psychosocial factors and nursing diagnosis. *Journal of National Black Nurses Association, 4*(2), 37–46.

Thrasher, J. (2004). Behavior-specific social support for healthy behaviors among African American church members: Applying optimal matching theory. *Health Education & Behavior, 31*(2), 193–205.

Trifiletti, L. B., Gielen, A. C., Sleet, D. A., & Hopkins, K. (2005). Behavioral and social sciences theories and models: Are they used in unintentional injury prevention research? *Health Education Research, 20*(3), 298–307.

Trost, S. G., Saunders, R., & Ward, D. S. (2002). Determinants of physical activity in middle school children. *American Journal of Health Behavior, 26*(2), 95–102.

Uhl, J. (1989). International networking: Coordinating health promotion strategies with multiple interventions. *Annals of Academy of Medicine, 18*(3), 280–285.

Underwood, S. (1992). Cancer risk reduction and early detection behaviors among black men: Focus on learned helplessness. *Journal of Community Health Nursing, 9*(1), 21–31.

U.S. Department of Health and Human Services, National Institutes of Health, Office of Behavioral and Social Sciences Research. (2005). *The contributions of behavioral and social sciences research to improving the health of the nation: A prospectus for the future.* Washington, DC: Author.

VanLandingham, M. J., Suprasert, S., Grandjean, N., & Sittitrai, W. (1995). Two views of risky sexual practices among Northern Thai males: The Health Belief Model and the Theory of Reasoned Action. *Journal of Health and Social Behavior, 36*, 195–212.

van Ryn, M., & Heaney, C. (1992). What's the use of theory? *Health Education Quarterly, 19*(3), 315–330.

Vega, W. A., Zimmerman, R., Gil, A., Warheit, G. J., & Apospori, E. (1993). Acculturation Strain Theory: Its application in explaining drug use behavior among Cuban and other Hispanic youth. *NIDA Research Monograph, 130*, 144–166.

Villarruel, A. M., Jemmott, J. B., III, Jemmott, L. S., & Ronis, D. L. (2004). Predictors of sexual intercourse and condom use intentions among Spanish-dominant Latino youth: A test of the Planned Behavior Theory. *Nursing Research, 53*(3), 172–181.

Wallston, B., & Wallston, K. (1978). Locus of control and health. *Health Education Monographs, 6*, 107–115.

Walter, H. J., Vaughan, R. D., & Cohall, A. T. (1993). Comparison of three theoretical models of substance use among urban minority high school students. *Journal of the American Academy of Child and Adolescent Psychiatry, 32*(5), 975–981.

Wang, S., Moss, J. R., & Hiller, J. E. (2006). Applicability and transferability of interventions in evidence-based public health. *Health Promotion International, 21*(1), 76–83.

Waschbusch, D. A., Sellers, D. P., LeBlanc, M., & Kelley, M. L. (2003). Helpless attributions and depression in adolescents: The roles of anxiety, event valence, and demographics. *Journal of Adolescence, 26*(2), 169–183.

Wasti, S., & Cortina, L. (2002). Coping in context: Sociocultural determinants of responses to sexual harassment. *Journal of Personality and Social Psychology, 83*(2), 394–405.

Watt, R. (2006). Emerging theories into the social determinants of health: Implications for oral health promotion. *Community Dentistry and Oral Epidemiology, 30*(4), 241–247.

West, S. G., Aiken, L. S., & Todd, M. (1993). Probing the effects of individual components in multiple component prevention programs. In T. A. Revenson (Ed.), *Ecological research to promote social change.* New York: Kluwer.

Weinstein, N. D., & Sandman, P. M. (2002). Reducing the risks of exposure to radon gas: An application of the precaution adoption process model. In D. R. Rutter & L. Quine (Eds.), *Changing health behavior: Intervention and research with social cognition models* (pp. 66–86). Buckingham, UK: Open University Press.

Wingate, L., Bobadilla, L., Burns, A., Cukrowicz, K., Hernandez, A., Ketterman, R., et al. (2005). Suicidality in African American men: The roles of southern residence, religiosity, and social support. *Suicide & Life-Threatening Behavior, 35*(6), 615–629.

Wolfe, W. (2004). A review: Maximizing social support—a neglected strategy for improving weight management with African-American women. *Ethnicity & Disease, 14*(2), 212–218.

World Health Organization. (1986, November 21). *The Ottawa charter for health promotion,* 3–5. Presented at the first international conference on health promotion, Ottawa, Ontario, Canada.

Yarbrough, S. S., & Braden, C. (2001). Utility of Health Belief Model as a guide for explaining or predicting breast cancer screening behaviors. *Journal of Advanced Nursing, 33*(5), 677–688.

Yeatman, H. R., & Nove, T. (2002). Reorienting health services with capacity building: A case study of the core skills in health promotion project. *Health Promotion International, 17*(4), 341–350.

Yep, G. (1993). HIV prevention among Asian-American college students: Does the Health Belief Model work? *Journal of American College Health, 41*(5), 199–205.

Young, M., & Klingle, R. S. (1996). Silent partners in medical care: a cross-cultural study of patient participation. *Health Communication, 8*(1), 29–53.

Zanchetta, S. Z., & Poureslami, I. M. (2006). Health literacy within the reality of immigrants' culture and language. *Canadian Journal of Public Health, 97*(Suppl. 2), S26–S30.

Zhang, J. X., & Schwarzer, R. (1995). Measuring optimistic self-beliefs: a Chinese adaptation of the general self-efficacy scale. *Psychologia, 38*(3), 174–181.

Zimmerman, M. A., Ramirez-Valles, J., & Maton, K. (1999). Resilience among urban African American male adolescents: A study of the protective effects of sociopolitical control on their mental health. *American Journal of Community Psychology, 27*(6), 733–751.

5

Health Disparities in Multicultural Populations

An Overview

GREGORY D. STEVENS

MICHAEL R. COUSINEAU

Chapter Objectives

On completion of this chapter, the health promotion student and practitioner should be able to

- Understand and describe the extent of health and health care disparities across racial and ethnic groups in the United States

- Define, understand, and discuss some of the major risk factors for health and health care disparities and why they are associated with poorer outcomes among some multicultural populations

- Understand and explain at least five steps for applying information about the causes of health disparities to develop or improve multicultural-related interventions for resolving disparities in health and health care

HEALTH INEQUALITY IN THE UNITED STATES

The United States has experienced and, at times, promulgated a long history of **inequality** among its citizens. From civil rights violations and suffrage restrictions that only started to resolve in the past 60 years, to increasing income gaps between the poor and rich through the early 21st century, inequality continues to pervade many aspects of modern life, including education, employment, housing, and other necessities of life. Most deeply affected have been groups delineated by race or ethnicity, socioeconomic status (SES), immigration status, culture and language, and sexual orientation (Shi & Stevens, 2005).

Perhaps the most persistent manifestation of inequality has been an ongoing and, in some cases, increasing disparity in health and well-being across these social divisions. The relationship between inequality and health is not new. Later than their colleagues in Europe, researchers in the United States began documenting the extent to which those who are impoverished were less healthy than more affluent members of society. These findings have been replicated so frequently that today, we rarely raise an eyebrow when we see health differences that persist between racial and ethnic groups, the wealthy and the poor, the insured and the uninsured, and many other social divisions. But perhaps it *should* be much more surprising news, considering that most present day health disparities are *not* caused by a lack of sanitation, poor drinking water, or famine that claimed so many lives of the underprivileged in the initial years after the country's formation.

Things, in fact, have changed dramatically. The causes of health disparities now are not always obvious and are infrequently tied to characteristics of the health care system; rather, they are rooted in the social context surrounding modern life. Public health and the medical professions are beginning to acknowledge the impact, for example, that personal social position and **social class**, racism and discrimination, social networks, and other relational community factors have on the health of populations. Some of this recent knowledge is being applied to design interventions to address disparities in multicultural populations, but most efforts are still very much in their infancy (Cooper, Hill, & Powe, 2002).

The purpose of this chapter is to review the current theories and evidence for the creation of health disparities, discuss a model to better understand how health disparities are manifested in multicultural populations, and explore some of the major disparities in health and health care by race/ethnicity. The chapter focuses on the role of culture in the production of disparities and considers some of the major programs and interventions that have been designed to address disparities. Finally, the chapter summarizes key steps that health education and promotion professionals can take to further reduce disparities.

WHAT ARE HEALTH DISPARITIES?

The term **health disparities** refers to distinct patterns of differences in health status and well-being across population groups. Use of the term *disparities* today most often implies differences across racial/ethnic groups, but the term has also been extended to differences in health across income, education, cultures, and gender groups. The term is regularly used interchangeably with the term *health inequalities*; and application of the term to health care (i.e., health care disparities) refers to patterns of differences in health care access, quality, utilization of health services, satisfaction, or outcomes.

Why Should Health Promotion Professionals Focus on Disparities?

There are several overarching reasons that health professionals should focus on reducing health disparities. First, the United States was founded on the principle of equality and freedom. Where this equality has been infringed (e.g., slavery, segregation, and other civil riots violations), policy changes have eventually occurred to begin correcting these infringements. Personal health, however, has remained conspicuously absent from the list of advocated civil rights. Its absence reflects a lack of consensus regarding the extent to which health is considered a right protected by the Constitution. In a broader view, its absence might rightly be considered a national failure since most other developed nations have recognized health as a human right for decades, evidenced in part by their assurances of universal access to health services.

Second, the health of the overall U.S. population lags behind that of many other developed countries. For example, average life expectancy in the United States (about 76.4 years) remains up to 5 years less than in about 25 other developed countries. Infant mortality in the United States also remains substantially higher compared with more than 40 other developed countries (e.g., a rate of 6.9 deaths per 1,000 births in the United States vs. just 2.8 deaths per 1,000 births in Sweden) (National Center for Health Statistics, 2005). Because such health disparities affect a large proportion of the U.S. population, improvements in the U.S. health and well-being that rivals other countries cannot likely be attained without attention to resolving the health disparities experienced by the most **vulnerable populations** (e.g., the poor, racial/ethnic minorities, the uninsured).

Third, the number of vulnerable individuals is rapidly increasing in the United States. As an example, the poverty rate, having reached its most recent low point at 11.3% of the population in 2000, has been increasing in the past 4 years, reaching 12.7% in 2004, equating to about 37 million individuals. Similarly, the proportion of individuals lacking health insurance coverage has increased significantly since 1990, reaching 15.7% of the population or about 45.8 million individuals in 2004 (DeNavas-Walt, Proctor, & Lee, 2005). With increases in the prevalence of these vulnerable populations, health disparities will become an issue affecting more of the mainstream and thus require greater policy attention of the United States.

UNDERSTANDING THE OCCURRENCE OF HEALTH DISPARITIES

Perhaps what is most relevant to health promotion professionals is that while advances in health promotion strategies have contributed to improvements in population health, these gains in health have not necessarily benefited population groups equally. For example, despite overall declines in smoking rates during pregnancy, American Indians/Native Americans remain more likely to smoke during pregnancy than other racial or ethnic groups (19.7% vs. 15.0% of whites, 8.7% of African Americans, and 3.0% of Latinos) (National Center for Health Statistics, 2006). Reducing the rate of smoking during pregnancy might be achieved through health education efforts that are aimed at American Indians/Native Americans. But such efforts are likely to be more effective if they were tailored to address the deeper reasons behind the disparities.

To understand the underlying causes of disparities, we explore and summarize the range of risk factors that commonly contribute to health disparities among racial/ethnic minority groups and then examine the mechanisms by which these risk factors may lead to health problems. To summarize these relationships, we highlight the general model of vulnerability developed by Shi and Stevens (2005) that is useful in categorizing the range of community- and individual-level risk factors that influence poor health (Shi & Stevens, 2005). To help make the concepts in the model clearer, we provide an example of the range of risk factors that influence cardiovascular disease, a health problem commonly addressed by many health promotion professionals.

The General Model of Vulnerability

Many models have been developed to explain the roles of various risk factors in predicting disease. Shi and Stevens (2005) have developed a general model to highlight the contributions of a very broad range of risk factors to poor health. Figure 5.1 shows this general model, which notes the combined contributions of community and individual risk factors to *vulnerability* that reflects the sum of independent risk factors. This combined level of

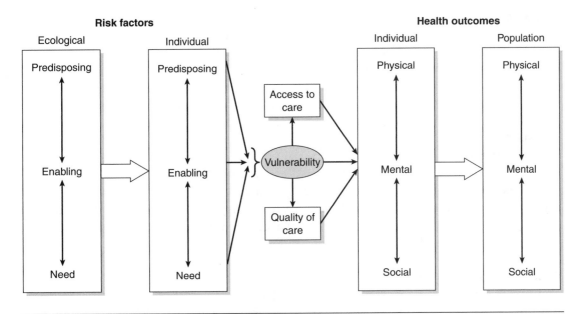

Figure 5.1   The General Model of Vulnerability

SOURCE: The General Model of Vulnerability from *Vulnerable Populations in the United States* (p. 336) by L. Shi and G. D. Stevens, 2005, San Francisco: Jossey-Bass.

risk, in turn, contributes to poor health outcomes at the individual and ultimately community or population levels. Access to medical care and the quality of care received play intermediary roles by helping prevent health problems and treat health problems that have already occurred (Shi & Stevens, 2005).

The model organizes risk factors according to *predisposing, enabling,* and *need* categories that have been previously developed by Andersen (1995). The risk factors that fall into each category can occur at both the individual and community levels. *Predisposing* risk factors are those factors that predispose an individual to poor health, including individual factors such as age, gender, race/ethnicity, and culture; and community factors such as rural or urban geographic setting, the physical environment, and even the social or cultural norms of a community. *Enabling* risk factors are those factors that socially or even materially enhance the ability of individuals to improve their health, including individual factors such as income, education, and

health insurance, and community factors such as the availability of well-paying jobs, excellent schools, and availability of health services. *Need* risk factors are the existing health problems that may contribute to overall poor health or the ability to address other health issues, including individual factors such as personal mental health issues, disabilities, and disease rates, and community factors such as rates of transmissible diseases in the community, the availability of illegal drugs, and even the presence of liquor stores that contribute to population rates of drug and alcohol abuse.

Application of the Model to Cardiovascular Disease

Cardiovascular disease occurs at higher rates among vulnerable populations. As an example, we will apply the model to the well-known finding that African American men are more likely than other racial/ethnic groups to report having hypertension, a major contributor to cardiovascular disease. In 2003, nearly one in three African American adults (~32%) reported that they had hypertension compared with 20% of whites, 19% of Latinos, and just 16% of Asian Americans (National Center for Health Statistics, 2006). Researchers have studied and documented a wide array of both predisposing and enabling risk factors that contribute to this disparity by their differences in distribution across racial/ethnic groups.

Predisposing risk factors for cardiovascular disease include race/ethnicity, which may indeed reflect some genetic differences in the predisposition for hypertension among African Americans (Brandon et al., 2003). Predisposing risk factors are also present at the community or environment level. African Americans are more likely than whites, Asian Americans, or Latinos to live in inner-city areas that have higher levels of pollution, greater crowding and more congested thoroughfares, few parks and recreation areas (leading to fewer opportunities for regular exercise), and fewer comprehensive grocery stores (Diez Roux, 2003; Diez Roux et al., 2001; Schulz & Northridge, 2004; Schulz, Williams, Israel, & Lempert, 2002), leaving families with few choices other than to shop at convenience or liquor stores where junk food, alcohol, and cigarettes reigns supreme.

Employment in lower wage or blue-collar professions—leading to higher levels of stress due to lack of job control, inflexible work environments, etc.—may also contribute to some of the disparity, since African Americans are more likely than other groups (except Latinos) to be employed at these levels (Bosma et al., 1997; Bosma, Stansfeld, & Marmot, 1998; Marmot, Bosma, Hemingway, Brunner, & Stansfeld, 1997). Another potential community predisposing risk factor for hypertension is the long-term social relegation of African Americans in the United States due to both overt and subtle prejudices, stereotyping, and racism (LaVeist, Diala, & Jarrett, 2000). Studies have shown that African American adults who experience higher levels of perceived

discrimination are also more likely to report having hypertension and other risk factors for cardiovascular disease (Cozier et al., 2006; Davis, Liu, Quarells & Din-Dzietham, 2005; Din-Dzietham, Nembhardt, Collins, & Davis, 2004). The causal effect of this is not fully known, but it is theorized, in part, to be a form of long-term chronic stress (Thompson, 2002).

Enabling risk factors for hypertension include individual risk factors such as the lack of income that affords individuals the ability to buy hypertension-protective goods, and services such as healthy foods, participation in organized recreational activities, and even regular leisure time or time off from work. Lack of insurance coverage is another risk factor that is associated with hypertension, since without insurance, individuals do not have regular access to health services that could protect against or resolve hypertension (e.g., screening, nutrition counseling, regular monitoring, and specialist care) (Lurie, Ward, Shapiro, & Brook, 1984; Lurie et al., 1986). African Americans are more likely than whites to be both low-income earners and uninsured (DeNavas-Walt et al., 2005).

These enabling risk factors exist at community level as well. Lower-income communities frequently have fewer well-paying job opportunities, since businesses and larger established companies may avoid or leave these areas in search of areas where the purchasing power is higher and where more skilled employees can be found. Schools in lower-income communities are often not well staffed and greatly underfunded since the main source of financing for education often comes from local tax revenues. Similarly, health care providers are rarely attracted to practice in these communities because most of the residents will be uninsured or covered by health insurance programs for the poor such as Medicaid that reimburse providers much less than private insurance. African Americans are more likely than whites to live in these communities, creating further difficulties with preventing and treating hypertension.

Taken together, these predisposing and enabling risk factors combine to affect the likelihood that African Americans will have hypertension. So combined, African Americans have a slight genetic predisposition for hypertension, are more likely to live where stressors are higher and the opportunities for health promotion are fewer, and are less likely to have access to health care to prevent and treat hypertension. The greater presence of risk factors experienced by African Americans thus likely contributes to the presence of this health disparity.

HEALTH DISPARITIES IN MULTICULTURAL POPULATIONS

There is a vast literature demonstrating health disparities among racial and ethnic minority populations in the United States (U.S. Department of Health and Human Services, 2000). Compared with whites, racial/ethnic minorities experience higher rates of mortality and shorter life expectancy, greater prevalence of chronic illness such as diabetes and asthma, more frequent risk behaviors such as not engaging in regular exercise, and generally poorer health status (National Center for Health Statistics, 2006). The story is not entirely simple, however, in that not all minority groups experience the same deficits, and depending on the condition, some groups have better health than whites. In fact, even greater variations in health can sometimes be found between specific subgroups of a racial/ethnic category than among the simplistic classifications of Asian American, African American, Latino, and whites.

A good example of this greater complexity is with national infant mortality rates. African Americans have a distinctly high rate of infant mortality (~13 deaths per 1,000 live births), a rate that is more than double that of whites (see Figure 5.2). American Indians/Alaska Natives also have high rates of infant mortality (~9 deaths per 1,000 live births), but Latinos and Asian Americans as a whole have equal or slightly lower rates of infant mortality than

whites (~5 deaths per 1,000 live births each). When the mortality rate is examined according to specific Latino and Asian American ethnic subgroups, however, we see that there is much greater variation in risk. Hawaiians, for example, are at higher risk compared with those who are of Chinese background. (~9 deaths vs. ~3 deaths per 1,000 live births), providing greater insight for health professionals making decisions about targeting or tailoring interventions to prevent infant mortality.

One of the most commonly monitored and reported measures of health is self-reported general health status. Using the simple self-rating of one's own general health via the scale, "excellent, very good, good, fair, or poor," a lot can be learned about both current morbidity and future mortality (Franks, Gold, & Fiscella, 2003; McGee, Liao, Cao, & Cooper, 1999). For example, individuals who report having fair or poor health status have at least twice the risk of mortality than individuals who report having excellent, very good, or good health status. Thus, while the reports are entirely subjective for an individual, differences between the groups over time can be used to track changes in mortality risk.

National reports of self-reported general health status by race/ethnicity reflect the current level of health and future mortality of these groups (see Figure 5.3). Although the percentage of individuals reporting fair or poor health status has declined for the most part since the early 1990s, there were striking racial/ethnic differences in health status in 2003, which are the most recent data available. That year, Asian Americans and whites were the least likely to report having fair or poor health (~8% each) compared with approximately 14% of Latinos, 15% of African Americans, and 16% of American Indians/Native Americans.

Overweight and obesity are considered among the latest health challenges to individuals in the United States because they are risk factors for many other problems, including diabetes, hypertension, and heart disease. Overweight is defined as having a body mass

FOUNDATIONS

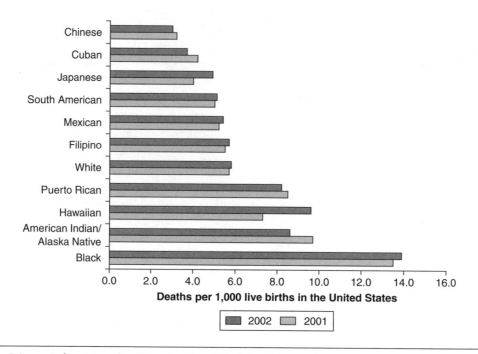

Figure 5.2   Infant Mortality Rates by Race/Ethnicity, 2001 and 2002

SOURCE: Data from *Health, United States 2005*, by the National Center of Health Statistics, 2006, Hyattsville, MD: Centers for Disease Control.

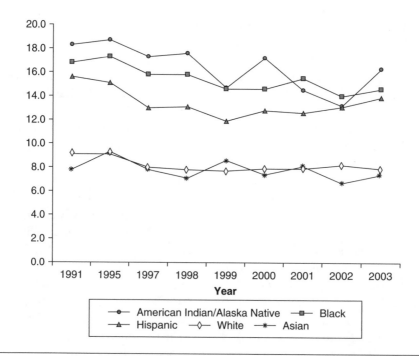

Figure 5.3   Adult Self-Reported Fair/Poor Health Status by Race/Ethnicity, 1991 to 2003

SOURCE: Data from *Health, United States 2005*, by the National Center of Health Statistics, 2006, Hyattsville, MD: Centers for Disease Control.

index (BMI) of 25 or greater (a measure based on the ratio of weight to height), and obesity is defined as having a BMI of 30 or greater (National Center for Chronic Disease Prevention and Health Promotion, 2006). There have been major increases in the past two decades in the proportion of adults in the United States who are overweight or obese with population prevalence increases for most racial/ethnic groups ranging from 5% to 10%. This has prompted many of the major government health authorities to prioritize the prevention and treatment of overweight and obesity.

In 2003, Latino and African American men were slightly more likely than white and much more likely than Asian American men to be overweight and obese (see Figure 5.4). Of particular note, less than 10% of Asian American men were obese compared with 15% to 20% of whites, Latinos, and African

Americans, and about 30% of American Indians/Alaska Natives. Disparities in overweight and obesity were much greater among women, with only 22% of Asian American women and 42% of white women found to be overweight or obese compared with about 60% or more of Latino, African American, and American Indian/Alaska Natives. Even more striking is the prevalence of obesity among Latino, African American, and American Indian and Alaska Native women, which is well over twice that of white and Asian American women.

HEALTH CARE DISPARITIES IN MULTICULTURAL POPULATIONS

As with the health disparities we just reviewed, similar racial/ethnic disparities exist in access to and quality of health care services (Agency

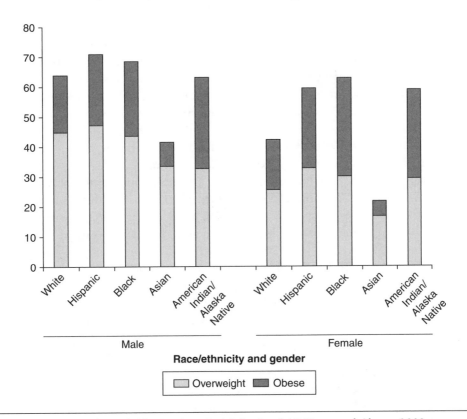

Figure 5.4 Overweight and Obesity Among Adults Aged 18 Years and Above, 2003

SOURCE: Holtby, S., Zahnd, E., Lord, N., McCain, C., Chia, Y. J., & Kurata, J. H. (2006). *Health of California's adults, adolescents and children: Findings from CHIS 2003 and CHIS 2001.* Los Angeles, CA: UCLA Center for Health Policy Research, Table 13, p. 22.

for Healthcare Quality Research, 2003; Smedley, Stith, & Nelson, 2002; Stevens & Shi, 2003). That the disparities in health care follow a similar pattern illustrates an important concept in the public health and medical fields known as the **inverse care law** that aptly describes the phenomenon whereby individuals with the greatest health needs are often the least likely to obtain needed health care services (Hart, 1971). This pattern is, not surprisingly, cyclical such that without access to needed health services, health problems will continue to go untreated, and the risk for greater morbidity and mortality increases.

It is also important to note that costs to society increase as the health care delivery system eventually must respond to this higher level of acuteness and need by caring for patients in emergency or hospital settings. For example, a child with asthma who cannot access to **primary health care** (say, because of no insurance coverage) is much more likely to be treated for an acute asthmatic episode or attack in an emergency room (which, by law, cannot deny uninsured patients). This emergency care is more costly than if primary care had been provided in a clinic or health care provider's office.

One of the most fundamental measures of access to health care is whether or not a person has health insurance coverage. Without health insurance, individuals have been shown to avoid visiting a health care professional even when they experience problems that should receive medical attention (Newacheck, Stoddard, Hughes, & Pearl, 1998; Shi, 2000; Zuvekas & Weinick, 1999). Although a person can obtain health care without health insurance either by paying out-of-pocket or visiting the emergency department of a public hospital, this can place a heavy financial burden on families and rarely results in the receipt of high-quality health (i.e., hospital emergency departments are not designed to deliver primary care).

In 2003, roughly 16.5% of the total population of the United States did not have health insurance coverage, reflecting more than 41.6 million individuals (DeNavas-Walt et al., 2005). The increase in the number of the uninsured reflects a steady decline in employer-sponsored health insurance coverage for the employees and/or their dependents. The number of the uninsured would have been higher were it not for public health insurance programs such as Medicaid and the State Children's Health Insurance programs (SCHIP). In 2003, Medicaid covered an estimated 12.3% of the population below the age of 65 years (or 30.9 million people), both Medicaid and SCHIP provide coverage for about 22% of all children (Anonymous, 2006).

There are major disparities across racial/ethnic groups in the insurance coverage rates (see Figure 5.5). This reflects differences in employment, income, family structure, and other factors that affect the ability to obtain coverage. Whites are the least likely to be uninsured (12%), while Latinos are the most likely (37%). Almost 30% of those of Cuban descent, 35% of American Indians and Alaska Natives, and nearly 38% of those of Mexican descent are uninsured. Conversely, whites are the least likely to be covered by Medicaid (the rest by employer-based insurance) compared with 23% of those of Mexican descent, 24% of African Americans, and more than 30% of Puerto Ricans.

The second most commonly reported measure of access to health care is whether a person has a regular source of care that he or she can go to for the majority of their health care needs. This can be a person's own doctor, nurse practitioner, or other type of provider that a person normally sees when faced with a health problem. This measure is important because having a regular provider is strongly associated with fewer delays in receiving care, fewer hospital and emergency department visits, and much greater use of preventive care (Hayward, Bernard, Freeman, & Corey, 1991; Lambrew, DeFriese, Carey, Ricketts, & Biddle, 1996; Ryan, Riley, Kang, & Starfield, 2000; Sox, Swartz, Burstin, & Brennan, 1998). These differences in having a regular

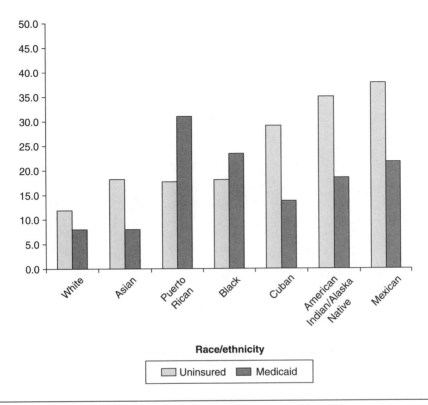

Figure 5.5   Uninsured and Medicaid Insurance Coverage Rates by Race/Ethnicity, 2003

SOURCE: National Center for Health Statistics. (2006). *Health, United States, 2005 with chartbook on trends in the health of Americans.* Tables 133 (p. 382) and 134 (p. 384). Hyattsville, MD: National Center for Health Statistics.

NOTE: Among persons below 65 years of age.

source of care also have implications for the overall costs of health care.

In California, which has perhaps the greatest racial/ethnic diversity in the United States, there have been increases in the proportion of individuals with a regular source of care between 2001 and 2003 (see Figure 5.6). In 2003, however, there remained substantial disparities in having a regular source of care across racial and ethnic groups. About one quarter of Koreans (27%) and Latinos (24%) reported not having a regular source of care, more than twice that of whites (12%), African Americans (10%), and Filipinos (7%).

Racial/ethnic disparities also exist in the types and amount of health services that are received. Receipt of preventive care is often used as an indicator of the overall level of comprehensiveness of care that is received because these services are usually delivered during

checkups where a broader array of services can be provided as opposed to acute care visits where visits often focus on remedying a single problem (Starfield, 1998). Two preventive care services that have a substantive evidence base of effectiveness and are common topics for health promotion professionals are the receipt of a Pap test and receipt of a mammogram among women of particular age groups.

African American women fare well in this regard, despite the fact that they are less likely than whites to be insured and slightly less likely to have a regular source of care. Receipt of a Pap test in the past 3 years and mammogram in the past 2 years was nearly equal between African American and white women, with rates of these services for both groups at about 90% and 78%, respectively (see Figure 5.7). Latino women fare equally well with regard to receipt of a Pap test, but

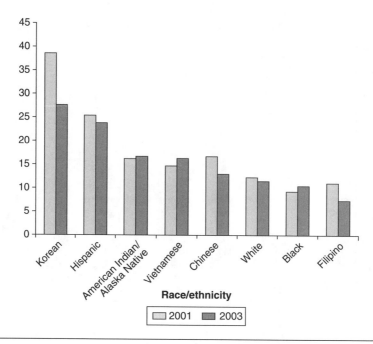

Figure 5.6   No Regular Source of Health Care Among Adults Aged 18 to 65 Years, 2001 to 2003

SOURCE: *California Health Interview Survey,* CHIS 2005 Adult Public Use File, Release 1. Los Angeles, CA: UCLA Center for Health Policy Research, January.

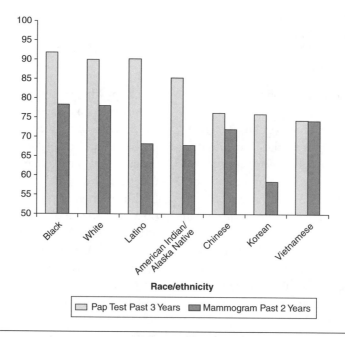

Figure 5.7   Preventive Cancer Screening Rates Among Women, 2003

SOURCE: Holtby, S., Zahnd, E., Lord, N., McCain, C., Chia, Y. J., & Kurata, J. H.(2006). *Health of California's adults, adolescents and children: Findings from CHIS 2003 and CHIS 2001.* Los Angeles, CA: UCLA Center for Health Policy Research, Table 14 (Pap Test, p. 23) and Table 15 (Mammograms, p. 24).

NOTE: Pap test was assessed for women aged 25 to 65 years and mammogram for women aged 40 to 65 years.

are much less likely to report having a mammogram (68%).

Asian American ethnic groups are much less likely to report receiving either service, with Vietnamese women reporting the lowest rate of Pap test (74%) and Korean women reporting the lowest rate of receiving a mammogram. While Asian American women are indeed less likely than others to experience breast and cervical cancer, this does not provide a sufficient rationale for not seeking screening or physicians not offering these tests. The reasons for women not seeking these services may have much to do with culture, which is the focus of the following section.

In addition to the health care disparities we have reviewed, there are very likely to be racial/ethnic disparities in the receipt of health education and promotion. While there is little or no direct evidence reported so far in the literature, there is good reason to think that such disparities may exist. First, health education often occurs in health care settings and during medical visits, where, for example, health information pamphlets or brochures are distributed and many health care providers deliver preventive health counseling and referrals. Since racial/ethnic minorities, low SES individuals, and the uninsured all have reduced access to health services (Hargraves, Cunningham, & Hughes, 2001; Weinick & Krauss, 2000; Weinick, Zuvekas, & Cohen, 2000), they are therefore less likely to have access to these programs or receive important health education.

Second, many of the health education and promotion materials and health counseling services are still available in a limited number of languages (Morales, Elliott, Weech-Maldonado, & Hays, 2006). Only recently, rules and regulations have been implemented to require that health plans and health care providers offer information and materials in **threshold languages** or, rather, languages common in a geographic area or provider service network. No federal law currently mandates that health care facilities provide medical interpreters to patients who need them. The U.S. Department of Health and Human Services only requires that health care sites receiving federal funds make an effort to provide interpreters for patients. Consequently, trained medical interpreters are not available to many patients who need them. Moreover, many health care providers may be reluctant to offer health promotion counseling in cases in which an interpreter is needed (Green et al., 2005). Without informational materials and education commonly available in multiple languages, certain racial/ethnic minorities may be less likely to receive these services.

At the same time, not all health education materials and counseling services are designed to reflect the diversity in cultures, making some health education resources unacceptable and even inappropriate to some groups while effective for others. Tailoring materials and counseling approaches to accommodate the unique cultural bounds is likely to enhance their effectiveness in achieving health goals. *Features of a health promotion strategy must take into account perceptions of health and disease that are determined in part by an individual's culture.* They should also use terminology that is common to a particular population (and free of medical jargon) and unambiguous to improve uptake and incorporation of health education information (Rothschild, 2005). Such tailoring is not commonplace due, in part, to a lack of information about how best to best tailor materials or counseling.

Third, health education and promotion materials are increasingly being developed and delivered using the Internet and other forms of electronic communication. While this presents new and innovative opportunities for disseminating health messages, lower SES individuals and families have less access to the Internet and electronic communications than middle- or upper-income families (Chang et al., 2004; Haughton, Kreuter, Hall, Holt, & Wheetley,

2005; Jackson et al., 2005). These families are therefore less likely to receive exposure to electronic forms of health education and promotion messages and materials. This could further widen disparities in the receipt of health education. Efforts to expand health education could focus on crossing what is increasingly known as the digital divide between the social classes.

Because of the likelihood of disparities in the receipt of health education and the dearth of information actually documenting these disparities, there is a great need for a focused research agenda to study and reveal these potential disparities. Even without this evidence available, based on information about poorer access to care, language barriers, and the digital divide, there may be sufficient reason to enhance health education efforts among racial/ethnic minorities and other vulnerable populations. In addition to the creation of these interventions, there is a need to document and evaluate existing health education programs that focus on addressing disparities in health education and promotion.

THE ROLE OF CULTURE IN HEALTH AND HEALTH CARE DISPARITIES

Culture has been defined in the medical field as the "integrated patterns of human behavior including thoughts, communications, actions, beliefs, values, and institutions of racial, ethnic, religious, or social groups" (Kleinman, Eisenberg, & Good, 1978). Culture is a broad and often referenced term, which has been widely accepted as a factor associated with health, health behaviors, and experiences with the health care system. As American society becomes even more diverse, the notion of culture's role in health and health care is attracting more attention in both public health practice and research (Brach & Fraser, 2000). For example, while the terms *cultural sensitivity* and *cultural competence* have become commonplace in the fields of public health and medicine, both still lack operational definitions

and measures to assess their performance, and explanatory models still do not do a sufficient job of explaining the link of culture with health and health care (Gregg & Saha, 2006).

In many cases, culture is conflated with race/ethnicity or simplified to only reflect language spoken by the group. While these are important aspects of culture, other components of a person's cultural background may affect perceptions of illness or help-seeking behavior (Betancourt, Green, Carrillo, & Ananeh-Firempong, 2003). These include beliefs about health problems or health care providers, values, preferences, and the acceptability of behaviors that are likely associated with health and health care seeking. But even this attempt to list all the attributes of culture fails to fully reflect that culture is dynamic, complex, and adaptive to larger social, political, and environmental forces. Thus, to say that all members of a particular cultural group are a particular way (even if many members share this characteristic) without taking into account the actual context and experience of the individuals that make up the cultural group, risks stereotyping, prejudice, and potentially discrimination.

That said, there is evidence that many different cultural characteristics influence the health and health care experiences of a particular group (Betancourt, Green, Carrillo, & Park, 2005). These cultural factors may influence health and health care directly (e.g., culturally based dietary practices influencing overweight rates) or indirectly by affecting health decisions, behaviors, health care and social service seeking and even the receptiveness to and/or adoption of health promotion messages and programs. For example, it is widely known that when individuals of Japanese descent immigrated to the United States after World War II, they substituted American diets that had higher saturated fats for the more traditional Japanese nutritional practices. There was a corresponding increase in rates of diabetes and heart disease in these individuals compared with those who maintained more traditional diets (Egusa et al., 2002; Huang et al., 1996; Nakanishi et al., 2004; Watanabe et al., 2003).

Differences in culture manifest themselves in how people recognize and describe health symptoms and needs. This in turn affects thresholds for the seeking of health care services as well as preferences for where and from whom health services are sought. Culture also affects the ability of a patient to communicate comfortably and openly with health care providers and their acceptance of and adherence to prescribed therapies and treatments (Park et al., 2005). These cultural differences and their role in the health care system have been catalogued in a growing literature reviewed in the 2002 Institute of Medicine report *Unequal Treatment: Confronting Racial and Ethnic Disparities in Health Care* (Smedley et al., 2002). This text describes a substantial disconnect in the cultures of health care professionals and their patients that may contribute to less use of health care services, poorer quality of care and satisfaction, and perhaps poorer health.

Because of the cultural disconnect between health care providers and patients, there has been much recent discussion around matching patients and health care providers according to their race/ethnicity to reduce disparities in quality. While there is extensive debate on the value of such a practice—with some studies showing improvements in satisfaction and quality of care (King, Wong, Shapiro, Landon, & Cunningham, 2004; LaVeist & Nuru-Jeter, 2002; LaVeist, Nuru-Jeter, & Jones, 2003; Saha, Komaromy, Koepsell, & Bindman, 1999) and others showing no effect or even an opposite effect (Stevens, Mistry, Zuckerman, & Halfon, 2005; Stevens, Shi, & Cooper, 2003), particularly for pediatric care—there may be great difficulty in doing so. While nonwhite physicians are more likely to care for nonwhite patients (Saha, Taggart, Komaromy, & Bindman, 2000; Xu et al., 1997), nonwhite physicians still account for less than 10% of the nation's health care work force (and less than 15% of medical graduates), despite nonwhites accounting for more than 25% of the national population (Cooper & Powe, 2004). Even without a final consensus on the impact of patient-provider matching on access, quality, and outcomes, increasing the number of underrepresented minority health care providers is an important policy goal based on the principle of equity alone.

In the health professions, aligning the public health and medical approaches used to reach and communicate with particular cultural groups may enhance the delivery of care and improve the adoption of both health education and health care treatments (Brach & Fraser, 2002; Brach, Fraser, & Paez, 2005; Schouten & Meeuwesen, 2006). We present one major health disparity according to culture—overweight and obesity. Exactly how health care and health promotion services can be tailored and refined to address such a disparity across cultures is the focus of many of the other chapters of this book.

Previously, we indicated that culture is not necessarily stable over time. One concept that captures part of this change in culture is **acculturation**, which describes the degree to which a particular racial/ethnic group has integrated into the culture of the majority racial/ethnic group. While there are more descriptive and accurate measures of acculturation involving individual ratings of biculturalism and traditionalism, nationally representative data that are available on acculturation are generally based on two major measures: birthplace (U.S. born vs. foreign born) and number of years living in the United States. Neither of the measures is a perfect representation of acculturation but gives some rough indication of the potential level of acculturation and does reveal interesting data.

Figure 5.8 shows differences in rates of obesity among adults according to the two measures

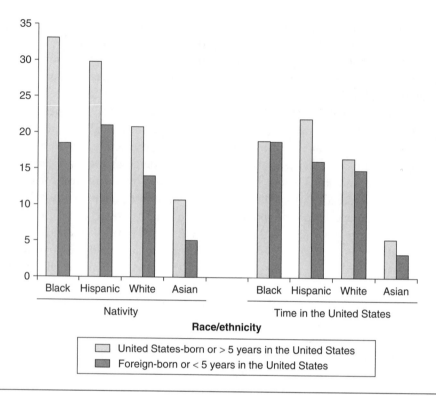

Figure 5.8   Measures of Acculturation and Rates of Obesity by Race/Ethnicity

SOURCE: *California Health Interview Survey*, CHIS 2005 Adult Public Use File, Release 1, Los Angeles, CA: UCLA Center for Health Policy Research, January 2007.

of acculturation. According to the nativity measure of acculturation, those who were born in the United States were much more likely than those born in a foreign country to have a BMI of 30 or more (i.e., be clinically obese). This difference was most apparent among African Americans and Latinos; for example, nearly 34% of U.S.-born African Americans were obese compared with just 18% of foreign-born African Americans. Smaller differences of about 6% to 8% were found for whites and Asian Americans. The differences in obesity rates according to the second measure of acculturation were substantially reduced for most racial/ethnic groups. African Americans had almost identical obesity rates regardless of whether they had lived in the United States less than 5 years or more, and rates of obesity were just slightly higher among whites and Asian Americans who had

resided in the United States for more than 5 years. Among Latinos, however, rates were about 8% higher in the more acculturated group (22% vs. 16%).

As with the individuals of Japanese descent who immigrated to the United States, these differences in obesity according to acculturation suggest that at least one factor that is correlated with obesity may vary according to culture (e.g., dietary habits may have switched from more traditional homemade foods to low-cost fast foods in the United States). Another possible explanation is that cultural physical activity patterns may have changed substantially (e.g., from walking to complete everyday errands, to relying instead on the automobile for these errands in the United States). These differences, while not entirely the sole domain of culture, are either supported or unsupported by community culture in which the family lives. For example, if the norm in the community is to drive around town to complete errands, healthier walking may be discouraged because of concerns about what it may convey about financial status, etc.

Why the rather dramatic differences are present in the measure of obesity between the two measures of acculturation is not entirely clear. Perhaps, the first measure shows a greater difference in culture since the native cultural contexts of the individuals are very different. There are no doubt major differences in inclination towards traditional culture between first- and second-generation residents of the United States. Once in the United States, however, it is possible that there are somewhat fewer differences in culture according to the length of time, or perhaps the cutoff of 5 years (while commonly used) is not long enough to show major differences in level of acculturation.

RESOLVING HEALTH AND HEALTH CARE DISPARITIES

We have shown that there is an extensive range of health disparities in the United States, and thus there is a clear need for a broad range of policy and programmatic interventions to reduce and ultimately resolve these disparities in health and health care. Health education and promotion professionals are in a particularly good position to assist with this aim, given the emphasis on health behavior change that may help promote reduced risk behaviors and increased health-promoting behaviors (Kreuter & McClure, 2004; Perloff, 2006; Schneider, 2006). But health educators must better tailor messages, materials, and communication approaches to be more applicable, and better accepted, adopted, and incorporated.

There are many health programs and interventions that have been developed to address health disparities. One major example is the Racial and Ethnic Approaches to Community Health (REACH) program launched by the U.S. Centers for Disease Control in 1999 and designed to support many community-based interventions to address the broad range of social, environmental, and behavioral determinants of health disparities. While many different programs were funded under the REACH initiative, one example of a successful program is the Cambodian Community Health program in Massachusetts that aimed to improve prevention and management of diabetes and heart disease among Cambodian refugees.

Other programs have been developed to address reduced disparities in access to care among the lower-income families and the uninsured. For example, the national Public Housing Primary Care Program was created by the Bureau of Primary Health Care in the U.S. Department of Health and Human Services in 1996 to locate free or low-cost health centers or individual health care providers within or nearby public housing centers to deliver services to the residents of these facilities. These programs are designed to reduce the financial barriers to care that individuals and families experience, including reducing the costs that are associated with traveling to receive medical care. There are more than 30 of these programs that serve more than 70,000 clients annually (www.bphc .hrsa.gov).

But public policies to reduce financial barriers to care go back more than 40 years when the U.S. Congress extended publicly financed health insurance to both the elderly and the poor. Medicaid, for example, provides free health insurance coverage to individuals living in poverty in the United States. The program is a joint federal and state venture, and it covers more than 11% of the people in the United States, including about one out of every four children in the country (Iglehart, 1999). Enrollment in the program varies quite a bit by race/ethnicity, with African Americans (23%) and Latinos (20%) more than twice as likely to be enrolled in the program than whites (8%) or Asian Americans (10%). Because Medicaid occupies a substantial proportion of federal and state budgets, it is continually threatened by state and federal budget deficits.

These and other programs reflect progress in the United States to address health and health care disparities. But they tend to focus on just a single major risk factor (e.g., targeting race/ethnicity, income level, insurance). These programs tend to be housed and funded by a wide variety of organizations and/or departments within various levels of government, and many compete with each other for funding. Thus, the programs tend to represent a rather fragmented system or strategy for reducing health disparities. A more comprehensive approach whereby several interventions working in concert address multiple risk factors for a given health disparity may produce a more coordinated and effective approach (Shi & Stevens, 2005).

Consider again, for example, the issue of infant mortality. Common sense tells us that many of the risk factors for infant mortality co-occur within the same populations. For example, we know that African Americans are more likely to live in poverty, less likely to be highly educated, and more likely to be uninsured, all of which are risk factors for higher infant mortality (Lane et al., 2001; Macinko, Shi, & Starfield, 2004; Shi et al., 2004). Rather than approaching these individually, a coordinated set of health interventions could be designed to target multiple risk factors contributing to infant mortality. As an example, the REACH program could fund efforts within the public housing primary care program to increase the utilization of prenatal care services by reducing language, transportation, and other barriers to seeking care (i.e., addressing the three major risk factors for inadequate primary care utilization). The same interventions could additionally focus on reducing behavioral risk factors, including smoking cessation or drug and alcohol prevention. The potential of such a coordinated initiative to reduce this disparity may be greater than either strategy alone.

Community health centers (CHCs) are one program that is purposefully designed to address multiple risk factors for many health and health care disparities. The CHCs are a widespread program that has long served an important safety-net primary health care delivery role for vulnerable populations in the United States (Dievler & Giovannini, 1998; Lefkowitz & Todd, 1999; Proser, 2005; Zuvekas, 1990). Started in the mid-1960s, the CHCs provide primary care services at very low or no cost to people living in federally designated underserved areas. In 2008, there were 1200 health centers across the United States that served more than 15 million individuals. The program is operated by the Bureau of Primary Health Care in the U.S. Health Resources and Services Administration (Bureau of Primary Health Care, 2008).

In addition to providing primary care services to vulnerable populations, CHCs offer a wide array of enabling services such as case management, health education and promotion, assistance with transportation and language translation, child care, and parenting classes. This one-stop shop for services, and strategic location in underserved areas, makes the CHCs a potentially very important resource for reducing national disparities in access to health care and health (Politzer, Schempf, Starfield, & Shi, 2003). By addressing multiple risk factors for poor health care access and health status, including targeting health education and promotion efforts to vulnerable populations, the CHCs are exemplary models of how programs and interventions can be comprehensively designed.

Recognizing the potential of the CHCs to improve primary care access for vulnerable populations and potentially national levels of health, the U.S. Congress passed the Health Care Safety Net Amendments of 2002, which is an initiative to enhance primary care access for an additional 6.1 million underserved individuals in 1,200 communities in the United

States by creating new CHC access points and expanding the existing facilities. At the same time, however, the U.S. Congress passed substantial funding cuts to the Medicaid program that will likely place greater stresses on the capacity and stability of the CHCs.

More programs could be designed to concomitantly address a wider range of risk factors for a given disparity, but this would require significant changes in the leadership, organization, and financing of health programs and interventions in this country. While there is no defined course for invigorating new efforts to address health disparities, there are five principles that may help guide public health and health promotion practitioners through this process. These principles were first described by Shi and Stevens (2005) and are summarized here.

• *Preparation.* There is still a false belief in this country among a majority of the population that health disparities do not exist and that health care in the United States is better than the rest of the world. This belief needs correction to reflect reality by enhancing public awareness of the issue through new and available data and research, communicating the severity and breadth of health disparities, and demonstrating their growing relevance to the general population.

• *Design.* Interventions and programs should build on existing knowledge of the risk factors for health disparities, address the range of risk factors that contribute to health disparities in a more comprehensive way, and unite and coordinate efforts across programs to strengthen the effectiveness of any interventions that are developed. In addition to improved efficiency and effectiveness, coordinating efforts leads to less competition among programs and greater sustainability. For example, programs that address a broad range of issues are appealing to a greater number of funders and can make use of a broader range of government funds.

• *Implementation.* Implementing interventions requires effective strategies for conveying messages to the public about the new interventions, setting measurable goals and objectives to measure the progress of the program and its impacts on the target population, and building on prior programs that have been successful to demonstrate continuous improvement. Any new initiative is likely to be taken more seriously and better adopted if it builds on the prior successes that have established its credibility.

• *Evaluation.* After implementation, programs or interventions should be thoroughly monitored, evaluated, and continually improved. This should be built into the funding of the program such that quality improvement is a regular and ongoing activity within a program. Policies should also be developed to include a longer-term perspective. Many programs are now designed with 2- or 3-year trial periods, when direct impacts on the health of the population are not feasible in the short term. Assuming that such programs have the potential to reduce health disparities over the longer term, some room should be granted for the demonstration of achieving key milestones over a longer period of time.

Taking these major steps to reduce health disparities remains a major challenge in the United States. For health education and promotion professionals, the challenge is the same: focusing increased attention on reducing health and health care disparities, understanding the major risk factors for the disparities, redesigning health and health care interventions more comprehensively and simultaneously address these risk factors, and persevering the course and engaging in quality improvement to see short- and longer-term successes. Using this overview of health disparities among multicultural populations, and the other chapters of this book as a guide, practitioners and students of health education and promotion will be well prepared to reduce health disparities, and it is hoped that it will ultimately improve the overall health of the U.S. population.

CHAPTER SUMMARY

The United States has experienced and, at times, promulgated a long history of inequality among its citizens. Perhaps the most persistent manifestation of inequality has been an ongoing and, in some cases, increasing disparity in health and well-being across these social divisions. The causes of health disparities are now not always obvious and are infrequently tied to the characteristics of the health care system, but rather they are rooted in the social context surrounding modern life. Because of this, making major inroads into resolving disparities remains a major challenge for the United States. Among health education and promotion professionals, increased efforts should be made to focus attention on reducing disparities, understand the major roots and causes of disparities, redesign interventions to comprehensively and simultaneously address these risk factors, and persevere the course and engage in quality improvement activities to see short- and longer-term successes.

The next chapter stresses that health promotion student, practitioner, and participants from the target community must be able to accurately identify and assess the roles and relationships of cultural differences, health beliefs and practices in the context of social conditions, such as rural/urban, social class, country of origin, language, generational aspects, and historical experiences with the wider society. The importance of cultural assessment must not be underestimated in the planning processes. Chapter 6 presents the Cultural Assessment Framework (CAF) developed by the authors to provide practitioners with an assessment approach and a framework for better understanding the similarities and differences between the mainstream culture and the specific cultural or ethnic group targeted for intervention. The Framework has value in the clinical setting, but can be a much more powerful tool for health promotion and disease prevention (HPDP) program-planning activities. That is, it provides guidelines that have application to the small group, community, and organizational levels of assessment and provides the practitioner with major suggestions pertinent to identifying important demographics, epidemiological factors, cosmology, general and specific cultural characteristics, general and specific health beliefs and practices, environmental and biocultural factors, and organizational variables. The following chapter will underscore that identification and the understanding of all these variables are critical in HPDP planning.

DISCUSSION QUESTIONS AND ACTIVITIES

1. What are three major reasons for targeting and tailoring health education and promotion efforts to address health disparities among vulnerable populations?

2. What is "culture," and how might culture be causally related to disparities in health or receipt of health care?

3. What reasons exist to believe that there may be substantial racial/ethnic disparities in the receipt of health education and promotion?

4. Identify a public health problem where there are known racial/ethnic disparities. Identify three major risk factors for this problem, explain their relationship with health, and develop a single intervention to reduce the disparity in the public health problem by addressing each of the three risk factors.

GLOSSARY TERMS AND DEFINITIONS

Acculturation—Describes the degree to which a particular racial/ethnic, religious, or other group has integrated into the culture of the majority group.

Health disparities—Distinct patterns of differences in health status and well-being across population groups.

Inequality—Lack of equality in health or health care across population groups.

Inverse care law—Describes the phenomenon whereby individuals with the greatest health needs are often the least likely to obtain needed health care services.

Primary health care—Ideally, the initial point of contact for the receipt of health care, whereby clinicians provide integrated, accessible health services that is able to address the majority of personal health care needs. Typical primary health care providers include family physicians, general practitioners or internists, and pediatricians, although each of these may also practice specialized care to some extent.

Social class—A broad group delineation in society having common economic, cultural, or political status. Health has been shown to vary according to one's social class.

Threshold languages—Languages common enough in a geographic area or provider service network such that a health plan or health care provider (sometimes by law) must offer interpreter services.

Vulnerable populations—Groups that are at risk for poor health status and well-being and also often at risk for poor health care access, quality, and outcomes.

REFERENCES

Agency for Healthcare Quality Research. (2003). *National healthcare disparities report.* Rockville, MD: U.S. Department of Health and Human Services, Agency for Healthcare Quality Research.

Andersen, R. M. (1995). Revisiting the behavioral model and access to medical care: Does it matter? *Journal of Health and Social Behavior, 36,* 1–10.

Anonymous. (2006). *Covering the uninsured: Growing need, strained resources.* Washington, DC: Kaiser Commission on Medicaid and the Uninsured.

Betancourt, J. R., Green, A. R., Carrillo, J. E., & Ananeh-Firempong, O., II. (2003). Defining cultural competence: A practical framework for addressing racial/ethnic disparities in health and health care. *Public Health Report, 118,* 293–302.

Betancourt, J. R., Green, A. R., Carrillo, J. E., & Park, E. R. (2005). Cultural competence and health care disparities: Key perspectives and trends. *Health Affairs (Project Hope), 24,* 499–505.

Bosma, H., Marmot, M. G., Hemingway, H., Nicholson, A. C., Brunner, E., & Stansfeld, S. A. (1997). Low job control and risk of coronary heart disease in Whitehall II (prospective cohort) study. *British Medical Journal, 314,* 558–565.

Bosma, H., Stansfeld, S. A., & Marmot, M. G. (1998). Job control, personal characteristics, and heart disease. *Journal of Occupational Health Psychology, 3,* 402–409.

Brach, C., & Fraser, I. (2000). Can cultural competency reduce racial and ethnic health disparities? A review and conceptual model. *Medical Care Research and Review, 57*(Suppl. 1), 181–217.

Brach, C., & Fraser, I. (2002). Reducing disparities through culturally competent health care: An analysis of the business case. *Quality Management in Health Care, 10,* 15–28.

Brach, C., Fraser, I., & Paez, K. (2005). Crossing the language chasm. *Health Affairs (Project Hope), 24,* 424–434.

Brandon, D. T., Whitfield, K. E., Sollers, J. J., III, Wiggins, S. A., West, S. G., Vogler, G. P., et al. (2003). Genetic and environmental influences on blood pressure and pulse pressure among adult African Americans. *Ethnicity & Disease, 13,* 193–199.

Bureau of Primary Health Care (2008). *Primary health care: The health center program.* Health Resources and Services Administration, Washington, DC: Author. Retrieved March 16, 2008, from, http://bphc.hrsa.gov/

Chang, B. L., Bakken, S., Brown, S. S., Houston, T. K., Kreps, G. L., Kukafka, R., et al. (2004). Bridging the digital divide: Reaching vulnerable populations. *Journal of the American Medical Informatics Association, 11,* 448–457.

Cooper, L., Hill, M., & Powe, N. (2002). Designing and evaluating interventions to eliminate racial and ethnic disparities in health care. *Journal of General Internal Medicine, 17,* 477–486.

Cooper, L. A., & Powe, N. (2004). *Disparities in patient experiences, health care processes, and outcomes: The role of patient-provider racial/ethnic, and language concordance.* New York: Commonwealth Fund.

Cozier, Y., Palmer, J. R., Horton, N. J., Fredman, L., Wise, L. A., & Rosenberg, L. (2006). Racial discrimination and the incidence of hypertension in US black women. *Annals of Epidemiology, 16,* 681–687.

Davis, S. K., Liu, Y., Quarells, R. C., & Din-Dzietharn, R. (2005). Stress-related racial discrimination and hypertension likelihood in a population-based sample of African Americans: The Metro Atlanta Heart Disease Study. *Ethnicity & Disease, 15,* 585–593.

DeNavas-Walt, C., Proctor, B., & Lee, C. (2005). *Income, poverty, and health insurance in the United States: 2004.* Washington, DC: U.S. Census Bureau.

Dievler, A., & Giovannini, T. (1998). Community health centers: Promise and performance. *Medical Care Research and Review, 55,* 405–431.

Diez Roux, A. V. (2003). Residential environments and cardiovascular risk. *Journal of Urban Health, 80,* 569–589.

Diez Roux, A. V., Merkin, S. S., Arnett, D., Chambless, L., Massing, M., Nieto, F. J., et al. (2001). Neighborhood of residence and incidence of coronary heart disease. *New England Journal of Medicine, 345,* 99–106.

Din-Dzietham, R., Nembhard, W. N., Collins, R., & Davis, S. K. (2004). Perceived stress following race-based discrimination at work is associated with hypertension in African-Americans. The Metro Atlanta Heart Disease Study, 1999–2001. *Social Science & Medicine, 58,* 449–461.

Egusa, G., Watanabe, H., Ohshita, K., Fujikawa, R., Yamane, K., Okubo, M., et al. (2002). Influence of the extent of westernization of lifestyle on the progression of preclinical atherosclerosis in Japanese subjects. *Journal of Atherosclerosis Thrombosis, 9,* 299–304.

Franks, P., Gold, M. R., & Fiscella, K. (2003). Sociodemographics, self-rated health, and mortality in the US. *Social Science & Medicine, 56,* 2505–2514.

Green, A. R., Ngo-Metzger, Q., Legedza, A. T., Massagli, M. P., Phillips, R. S., & Iezzoni, L. I. (2005). Interpreter services, language concordance, and health care quality: Experiences of Asian Americans with limited English proficiency. *Journal of General Internal Medicine, 20,* 1050–1056.

Gregg, J., & Saha, S. (2006). Losing culture on the way to competence: The use and misuse of culture in medical education. *Academic Medicine, 81,* 542–547.

Hargraves, J. L., Cunningham, P. J., & Hughes, R. G. (2001). Racial and ethnic differences in access to medical care in managed care plans. *Health Services Research, 36,* 853–868.

Hart, J. T. (1971). The inverse care law. *Lancet, 1,* 405–412.

Haughton, L. T., Kreuter, M., Hall, J., Holt, C. L., & Wheetley, E. (2005). Digital divide and stability of access in African American women visiting urban public health centers. *Journal of Health Care for the Poor and Underserved, 16,* 362–374.

Hayward, R. A., Bernard, A. M., Freeman, H. E., & Corey, C. R. (1991). Regular source of ambulatory care and access to health services. *American Journal of Public Health, 81,* 434–438.

Huang, B., Rodriguez, B. L., Burchfiel, C. M., Chyou, P. H., Curb, J. D., & Yano, K. (1996). Acculturation and prevalence of diabetes among Japanese-American men in Hawaii. *American Journal of Epidemiology, 144,* 674–681.

Iglehart, J. (1999). The American health care system: Medicaid. *New England Journal of Medicine, 340,* 403–408.

Jackson, C. L., Batts-Turner, M. L., Falb, M. D., Yeh, H. C., Brancati, F. L., & Gary, T. L. (2005). Computer and Internet use among urban African Americans with type 2 diabetes. *Journal of Urban Health, 82,* 575–583.

King, W. D., Wong, M. D., Shapiro, M. F., Landon, B. E., & Cunningham, W. E. (2004). Does racial concordance between HIV-positive patients and their physicians affect the time to receipt of protease inhibitors? *Journal of General Internal Medicine, 19,* 1146–1153.

Kleinman, A., Eisenberg, L., & Good, B. (1978). Culture, illness, and care: Clinical lessons from anthropologic and cross-cultural research. *Annals of Internal Medicine, 88,* 251–258.

Kreuter, M. W., & McClure, S. M. (2004). The role of culture in health communication. *Annual Review of Public Health, 25,* 439–455.

Lambrew, J. M., DeFriese, G. H., Carey, T. S., Ricketts, T. C., & Biddle, A. K. (1996). The effects of having a regular doctor on access to primary care. *Medical Care, 34,* 138–151.

Lane, S. D., Cibula, D. A., Milano, L. P., Shaw, M., Bourgeois, B., Schweitzer, F., et al. (2001). Racial and ethnic disparities in infant mortality: Risk in social context. *Journal of Public Health Management and Practice, 7,* 30–46.

LaVeist, T. A., Diala, C., & Jarrett, N. (2000). Social status and perceived discrimination: Who experiences discrimination in the health care system, how and why? In C. Hogue, M. A. Hargraves, & K. Collins (Eds.), *Minority health in America: Findings and policy implications from the Commonwealth Fund Minority Health Survey* (pp. 194–208). Baltimore: Johns Hopkins University Press.

LaVeist, T. A., & Nuru-Jeter, A. (2002). Is doctor-patient race concordance associated with greater satisfaction with care? *Journal of Health and Social Behavior, 43,* 296–306.

LaVeist, T. A., Nuru-Jeter, A., & Jones, K. E. (2003). The association of doctor-patient race concordance with health services utilization. *Journal of Public Health Policy, 24,* 312–323.

Lefkowitz, B., & Todd, J. (1999). An overview: Health centers at the crossroads. *Journal of Ambulatory Care Management, 22,* 1–12.

Lurie, N., Ward, N. B., Shapiro, M. F., & Brook, R. H. (1984). Termination from Medi-Cal—does it affect health? *New England Journal of Medicine, 311,* 480–484.

Lurie, N., Ward, N. B., Shapiro, M. F., Gallego, C., Vaghaiwalla, R., & Brook, R. H. (1986). Termination of Medi-Cal benefits: A follow-up study one year later. *New England Journal of Medicine, 314,* 1266–1268.

Macinko, J. A., Shi, L., & Starfield, B. (2004). Wage inequality, the health system, and infant mortality in wealthy industrialized countries, 1970–1996. *Social Science & Medicine, 58,* 279–292.

Marmot, M. G., Bosma, H., Hemingway, H., Brunner, E., & Stansfeld, S. (1997). Contribution of job control and other risk factors to social variations in coronary heart disease incidence. *Lancet, 350,* 235–239.

McGee, D. L., Liao, Y., Cao, G., & Cooper, R. S. (1999). Self-reported health status and mortality in a multiethnic US cohort. *American Journal of Epidemiology, 149,* 41–46.

Morales, L. S., Elliott, M., Weech-Maldonado, R., & Hays, R. D. (2006). The impact of interpreters on parents' experiences with ambulatory care for their children. *Medical Care Research and Review, 63,* 110–128.

Nakanishi, S., Okubo, M., Yoneda, M., Jitsuiki, K., Yamane, K., & Kohno, N. (2004). A comparison between Japanese-Americans living in Hawaii and Los Angeles and native Japanese: The impact of lifestyle westernization on diabetes mellitus. *Biomedicine & Pharmacotherapy, 58,* 571–577.

National Center for Chronic Disease Prevention and Health Promotion. (2006). *Defining overweight and obesity.* Hyattsville, MD: Centers for Disease Control.

National Center for Health Statistics. (2005). *Health, United States 2004.* Hyattsville, MD: Centers for Disease Control.

National Center for Health Statistics. (2006). *Health, United States 2005.* Hyattsville, MD: Centers for Disease Control.

Newacheck, P. W., Stoddard, J. J., Hughes, D. C., & Pearl, M. (1998). Health insurance and access to primary care for children. *New England Journal of Medicine, 338,* 513–519.

Park, E. R., Betancourt, J. R., Kim, M. K., Maina, A. W., Blumenthal, D., & Weissman, J. S. (2005). Mixed messages: Residents' experiences learning cross-cultural care. *Academic Medicine, 80,* 874–880.

Perloff, R. M. (2006). Introduction: Communication and Health Care Disparities. *The American Behavioral Scientist, 49,* 755–759.

Politzer, R. M., Schempf, A. H., Starfield, B., & Shi, L. (2003). The future role of health centers in improving national health. *Journal of Public Health Policy, 24,* 296–306.

Proser, M. (2005). Deserving the spotlight: Health centers provide high-quality and cost-effective care. *Journal of Ambulatory Care Management, 28,* 321–330.

Rothschild, B. (2005). Health literacy: What the issue is, what is happening, and what can be done. *Health Promotion Practice, 6,* 8–11.

Ryan, S., Riley, A., Kang, M., & Starfield, B. (2000). The effects of regular source of care and health need on medical care use among rural adolescents. *Archives of Pediatrics & Adolescent Medicine, 155,* 184–190.

Saha, S., Komaromy, M., Koepsell, T., & Bindman, A. (1999). Patient-physician racial concordance and the perceived quality and use of health care. *Archives of Internal Medicine, 159,* 997–1004.

Saha, S., Taggart, S. H., Komaromy, M., & Bindman, A. B. (2000). Do patients choose physicians of their own race? *Health Affairs (Project Hope), 19,* 76–83.

Schneider, T. R. (2006). Getting the biggest bang for your health education buck: Message framing and reducing health disparities. *The American Behavioral Scientist, 49,* 812–822.

Schouten, B. C., & Meeuwesen, L. (2006). Cultural differences in medical communication: A review of the literature. *Patient Education and Counseling, 64,* 21–34.

Schulz, A., & Northridge, M. E. (2004). Social determinants of health: Implications for environmental health promotion. *Health Education & Behavior, 31,* 455–471.

Schulz, A. J., Williams, D. R., Israel, B. A., & Lempert, L. B. (2002). Racial and spatial relations as fundamental determinants of health in Detroit. *Milbank Quarterly, 80*(iv), 677–707.

Shi, L. (2000). Type of health insurance and the quality of primary care experience. *American Journal of Public Health, 90,* 1848–1855.

Shi, L., Macinko, J., Starfield, B., Xu, J., Regan, J., Politzer, R., et al. (2004). Primary care, infant mortality, and low birth weight in the states of the USA. *Journal of Epidemiology and Community Health, 58,* 374–380.

Shi, L., & Stevens, G. D. (2005). *Vulnerable populations in the United States.* San Francisco: Jossey-Bass.

Smedley, B., Stith, A., & Nelson, A. (Eds.). (2002). *Unequal treatment: Confronting racial and ethnic disparities in health care.* Washington, DC: National Academy Press.

Sox, C. M., Swartz, K., Burstin, H. R., & Brennan, T. A. (1998). Insurance or a regular physician: Which is the most powerful predictor of health care? *American Journal of Public Health, 88,* 364–370.

Starfield, B. (1998). *Primary care: Balancing health needs, services, and technology.* New York: Oxford University Press.

Stevens, G. D., Mistry, R., Zuckerman, B., & Halfon, N. (2005). The parent-provider relationship: Does race/ethnicity concordance or discordance influence parent reports of the receipt of high quality basic pediatric preventive services? *Journal of Urban Health, 82,* 560–574.

Stevens, G. D., & Shi, L. (2003). Racial and ethnic disparities in the primary care experiences of children: A review of the literature. *Medical Care Research and Review, 60,* 3–30.

Stevens, G. D., Shi, L., & Cooper, L. A. (2003). Patient-provider racial and ethnic concordance and parent reports of the primary care experiences of children. *Annals of Family Medicine, 1,* 105–112.

Thompson, V. L. (2002). Racism: Perceptions of distress among African Americans. *Community Mental Health Journal, 38,* 111–118.

U.S. Department of Health and Human Services. (2000). *Healthy people 2010: Understanding and improving health.* Washington, DC: Government Printing Office.

Watanabe, H., Yamane, K., Fujikawa, R., Okubo, M., Egusa, G., & Kohno, N. (2003). Westernization of lifestyle markedly increases carotid intima-media wall thickness (IMT) in Japanese people. *Atherosclerosis, 166,* 67–72.

Weinick, R., & Krauss, N. (2000). Racial and ethnic differences in children's access to care. *American Journal of Public Health, 90,* 1771–1774.

Weinick, R. M., Zuvekas, S. H., & Cohen, J. W. (2000). Racial and ethnic differences in access to and use of health care services, 1977 to 1996. *Medical Care Research and Review, 57*(Suppl. 1), 36–54.

Xu, G., Fields, S. K., Laine, C., Veloski, J. J., Barzansky, B., & Martini, C. J. (1997). The relationship between the race/ethnicity of generalist physicians and their care for underserved populations. *American Journal of Public Health, 87,* 817–822.

Zuvekas, A. (1990). Community and migrant health centers: An overview. *Journal of Ambulatory Care Management, 13,* 1–12.

Zuvekas, S. H., & Weinick, R. M. (1999). Changes in access to care, 1977–1996: The role of health insurance. *Health Services Research, 34,* 271–279.

6

The Cultural Assessment Framework

ROBERT M. HUFF

MICHAEL V. KLINE

Chapter Objectives

On completion of this chapter, the health promotion student and practitioner will be able to

- Discuss the value of including cultural assessment in any HPDP planning and intervention project
- Identify and discuss the five major components of the Cultural Assessment Framework
- Develop a basic cultural assessment survey instrument for a target group of his or her choice

There are many important factors to be considered in planning health promotion programs across cultural groups. This book seeks to highlight and discuss some of the major issues, barriers, and potentialities of multicultural health promotion within five particular population groups and their many and diverse subgroups. Throughout the text, it will be stressed that practitioners need to gain knowledge that can be used to tailor health promotion programming that is appropriate to each group's needs. In addition, the practitioner and participants from the target community must be able to accurately assess cultural differences, beliefs, and practices in the context of social conditions, such as rural-urban, social class, country of origin, language, generational aspects, and historical experiences with the wider society.

For the health promotion student and practitioner, this chapter emphasizes that owing to the scope and complexity of the planning process, they will need to operate from some rational Cultural Assessment Framework (CAF) or model rather than solely on the basis of pragmatic or expediency considerations. The cultural assessment model, presented in this chapter, provides an organizing framework that encourages a more systematic approach to the planning situation, the cultural characteristics of the target group, setting, and health problem. The importance of cultural assessment should never be underestimated.

Pasick, D'Onofrio, and Otero-Sabogal (1996) discuss the interactions among culture, health behavior, and health promotion and present a framework for *cultural tailoring* in the development of interventions for diverse cultural and/or ethnic groups. They distinguish between *targeting* of interventions for specific subgroups of the population to ensure exposure of the target group to the intervention and *cultural tailoring*, which is the development of interventions, strategies, messages, and materials that reflect specific cultural characteristics of the population group targeted for intervention. Pasick et al. observe that cultural tailoring provides a way to focus more directly on the specific cultural factors including the values, beliefs, and traditions of a particular group that influence behavior related to health and disease. Their framework for cultural tailoring intersects five major components of program planning and implementation. It emphasizes that more cultural tailoring is required at the levels of the behavioral theory being considered for conceptualization of interventions, the intervention design itself, and the implementation plan than at the levels of problem identification and objective setting. Pasick et al. hope that their framework will move researchers and planners to examine old assumptions and to systematically assess the amount of cultural tailoring needed for each phase of the program planning process. Unfortunately, this is not always the case as time, resources, interests, ethnocentric bias, and other related factors can act to mediate

the types and amount of formative needs assessment data that is collected prior to the development of specific intervention strategies. However, awareness of such frameworks can serve to encourage the planners or health promoter to conduct a thorough assessment of the cultural or ethnic population group targeted for intervention with respect to the values, beliefs, attitudes, and traditions directly and indirectly related to the health problem being addressed. It should be noted that the planner also needs to assess the organizational factors that may effect or be affected by cultural differences among the multicultural populations they may serve.

The CAF, developed by the authors and presented in Figures 6.1 through 6.5, provides practitioners with an assessment approach and a framework for better understanding the similarities and differences between the mainstream culture and the specific cultural or ethnic group targeted for intervention. The framework presented in this chapter evolved out of a variety of planning and cultural assessment models (Andrews & Boyle, 1995; Brownlee, 1978; Clark, 1978; Green & Kreuter, 2005; Leininger, 1995; Lipson & Steiger, 1996; Orque, Bloch, & Ahumada Monrroy, 1983; Purnell & Paulanka, 2003; Spector, 2004; Tripp-Reimer, Brink, & Saunders, 1984) that seek to provide guidelines for the identification of the major areas that should be considered when assessing individual patients in the clinical setting. The framework, while having value in the clinical setting, is a much more powerful tool for health promotion/ disease prevention (HPDP) program planning activities. These guidelines also have application to the small group, community, and organizational levels of assessment and provide the practitioner with major suggestions pertinent to identifying important demographics, epidemiological factors, cosmology, general and specific cultural characteristics, general and specific health beliefs and practices, environmental and biocultural factors, and organizational variables. To some degree, assessment of these factors should be part of any basic formative evaluation process conducted to determine baseline characteristics of a population being targeted for a HPDP program. These are not, however, always made explicit or included in any kind of comprehensive way during the assessment process. There is a need to formally include a cultural assessment as a routine component of any needs assessment process that includes a multicultural population within the target group to be addressed by a program plan.

THE CULTURAL ASSESSMENT FRAMEWORK

The CAF incorporates five primary levels of assessment that should be considered when planning a program for any multicultural population group. Because all planning models include some form of early or formative evaluation to assess demographic, epidemiological, social, and behavioral characteristics of target populations to be served by a HPDP program, the CAF has been organized to overlay and enhance this early assessment process. That is, the categories and associated subcategories of assessment within the framework suggest areas of needed inquiry that are culture specific and should be included in assessment tools such as surveys, focus groups, or other formative evaluation processes. The framework, like similar models, involves asking and answering a planned range of questions at each stage of the assessment process. It assumes, at the outset, that the health promoter or planner has begun to acquire an increased level of cultural competence with respect to the target population with which he or she will be working (e.g., history, culture, language, migration patterns). Interestingly, Andrews and Boyle (1995) suggest that biocultural variations such as the distinctive anatomical and physiological characteristics of the ethnic or cultural group also might be important

to the assessment process, although this has not been included as a distinct category in the CAF. Rather, questions associated with this area of assessment can be included as part of the general and specific cultural or ethnic group characteristics within the CAF.

The CAF can be applied to address HPDP questions that target individual or family activities in clinical settings as well as those targeted to small group, community, or higher levels of health behavior intervention. The five major levels of assessment for the CAF are as follows:

1. Culture or ethnic group-specific demographic characteristics

2. Culture or ethnic group-specific epidemiological and environmental influences

3. General and specific cultural or ethnic group characteristics

4. General and specific health care beliefs and practices

5. Western health care organization and service delivery variables

The CAF is further divided into a number of subcategories with associated assessment questions to provide a more in-depth review of the factors that should be considered when planning HPDP programs and services for multicultural groups. Each of the primary components and subcomponents of the CAF is presented in what follows, with examples where appropriate to highlight the value and importance of each of the assessment levels in the framework.

CULTURE OR ETHNIC GROUP DEMOGRAPHIC CHARACTERISTICS

The most basic assessment need in most planning models is to determine as accurately as possible what the demographic characteristics of the intended target audience are (Kline, Chapter 7, this volume). In this first level, we are concerned with characteristics related to age, gender, area of residence, education and literacy, religion, language, housing, income, occupation, and related items. The assumption here is that the more we know about these factors, the better we will be at targeting programs that consider these characteristics and issues in the program planning, intervention design, implementation, and evaluation processes. These same issues from a cultural or ethnic group-specific perspective also must be included, as seen in Table 6.1.

As can be seen in this component of the CAF, age and gender factors, social class and social status, education and literacy, language and dialect, religious preferences and practices, income and occupation, patterns of residence and living conditions, and acculturation and assimilation also should be included with any other demographic factors being explored by the health planner.

Age

Age and gender factors need to be considered where there are cultural rules governing issues such as making decisions for the family regarding health care-related matters, food preparation practices, and other age-related culturally specified behaviors. For example, among Samoans, an interaction with a non-Samoan health care provider might involve an elder or the most educated family member to act as the family spokesperson (Ishida,

Table 6.1   Cultural Assessment Framework: Culture-Specific Demographic Characteristics

Assessment Area	Assessment Questions
Age and gender characteristics	☐ What are the age and gender distributions of the cultural or ethnic group? ☐ What are the cultural or ethnic rules governing behaviors related to age? ☐ What are the cultural or ethnic gender rules governing social and other types of interpersonal interactions within and outside family (e.g., how are different genders perceived and treated)? What roles do men and women have with respect to decision making, child rearing and household management, health and disease, medical encounters with Western health care providers, and so on?
Social class and status	☐ What social class and status distinctions exist within the cultural or ethnic group? ☐ What are the rules governing social class and status within the cultural or ethnic group? ☐ How do these distinctions affect matters of health, illness, and disease? ☐ What specific impact does social class and status have on health-promoting or health care-seeking behaviors?
Education and literacy	☐ What is the distribution of formal educational attainment across the cultural or ethnic group? ☐ What are the general attitudes toward formal education? ☐ What percentage of the cultural or ethnic group can understand, read, and write English? ☐ What percentage of the cultural or ethnic group understands, reads, and writes the language or dialect of the culture of origin? ☐ How does the cultural or ethnic group learn best?

Assessment Area	Assessment Questions
Language and dialect	☐ What is the primary language of the cultural or ethnic group? ☐ What dialect differences exist within the cultural or ethnic group? ☐ What language is spoken most often in the home? ☐ What are the language preferences with respect to entertainment, education, and information seeking? ☐ What words are commonly used by the cultural or ethnic group to describe health, illness, and disease processes? ☐ How does the cultural or ethnic group learn best?
Religious preferences	☐ What is the primary religious orientation of the cultural or ethnic group? ☐ What variations in religious preferences exist across the cultural or ethnic group? ☐ What religious rules govern health and disease practices? ☐ What are the primary religious holidays and celebrations of the cultural or ethnic group? ☐ What role(s) has the culture's religious leaders played with respect to health and disease, community health action, and so on? ☐ Are leaders currently involved in health promotion and disease prevention activities?
Occupation and income	☐ What are the traditional occupations of the cultural or ethnic group? ☐ How have these occupations been affected by migration into the United States? ☐ How do traditional occupations and changes in these affect health and disease within the cultural or ethnic group?
Patterns of residence and living conditions	☐ What is the typical family size within the cultural or ethnic group? ☐ In general, how many families occupy a single-family dwelling? ☐ What are the typical physical conditions of housing within the community where the cultural or ethnic group resides? ☐ What hygiene and/or environmental health issues or problems related to residence patterns and living conditions affect real or potential health and disease issues?
Acculturation and assimilation	☐ In general, how long has the cultural or ethnic group resided in the United States? ☐ What is the distribution of first, second, third, and later generations in the cultural or ethnic group? ☐ Is the community in which the cultural or ethnic group resides an open or more insular community? ☐ What percentage of the target population works outside the community? ☐ How often and with whom does the target population socialize outside the interpersonal and physical boundaries of the community? ☐ What percentages of the target population are traditional, marginal, bicultural, and fully acculturated and assimilated into the mainstream culture?

Toomata-Mayer, & Mayer, 1996). Galanti (1991) cites a case in which the paternal grandmother and several older aunts intervened to keep the parents of a sick child from seeing the child until his condition was stabilized in the hospital. This was because they viewed these parents as babies who would not be able to make appropriate decisions regarding the care of their own child. Lynch and Hanson (1992) note that age plays a role in cultural development and observes that by 5 years of age, children have an understanding of their culture of origin. They also recognize that children are much quicker to learn new cultural patterns than are their parents. Thus, beyond the usual reasons for looking at age in a demographic profile, it is important to understand that decision making based on deference to elders who have lived the longest and have more experience with worldly matters may play a major role in how families perceive and use preventive or curative health services. In addition, it is important to determine how the elderly are cared for, what expectations there are for them with respect to self-care, exercise, and other health promotion activities. HPDP activities might need to be targeted to or involve the older members of the community in planning and implementation efforts.

Gender

Like age, gender rules within a cultural or ethnic group also need to be assessed (Friedman, Bowden, & Jones, 2003; Leddy, 2003). Many cultures have very specific rules and traditional roles prescribed for men and women. For example, among traditional Vietnamese, men are the decision makers and support for the family. Women are expected to prepare all meals, whether they work or not, and to do most of the household chores. Where these roles shift, traditional family relationships are often strained (Farrales, 1996). Gender issues governing modesty, purity, and virginity are also important as many cultural groups highly value and protect these virtues

among their women (Spector, 2004). Programs that may require examinations of female patients or participants (e.g., breast examinations, Pap smears) from a male doctor or other health care worker might be frowned on or avoided altogether by these population groups (Lipson, 1996). Mo (1992), reporting on a study conducted among Chinese women in San Francisco, observes that cultural values with respect to modesty and sexuality contributed to less utilization of breast health services by that group. In addition, she notes that a lack of female physicians and educational materials written in English instead of Chinese were also important barriers. Likewise, the promotion of birth control methods and sexually transmitted disease prevention also might be considered an affront to a cultural group whose religious practices forbid the use of birth control, premarital sex, and the like.

Social Class and Social Status

Social class and status also may be important considerations in a cultural assessment because there are cultural groups where these factors might serve to help or hinder a HPDP program (Leddy, 2003; Lipson, 1996). Ishida et al. (1996) note that among Samoans, persons perceived as being in positions of authority (e.g., elders, family chief, clergy) are given great respect and deference. As a result of their status, these individuals may be able to influence health promoting behaviors if they are involved in the planning and execution of HPDP programs. Helman (2000) notes that symptoms of illness or disease may also be influenced by one's socioeconomic status and cites an example of backache, which was interpreted by members of the highest socioeconomic class as an abnormal symptom, whereas members of the lower socioeconomic class interpreted it as a normal and inevitable part of living. Social class also can play an important role in health care access because, again, those in the lower socioeconomic ranks might be less inclined or able to access HPDP services if those services interfere with or call for them to leave their jobs. The HPDP program planner will need to consider these factors when they plan for how and when to deliver HPDP services to their target groups.

Literacy

Education and literacy should be considered as major points of interest to the practitioner (Doak, Doak, & Root, 1996; Friedman et al., 2003; Rudd, Renzulli, Pereira, & Daltroy, 2005). Each can play a significant role in whether and how well a HPDP program may be used. That is, how a particular individual or cultural group perceives HPDP might well determine whether target group members avail themselves of the program. If the target group does not have a concept for HPDP, then group members might be much less inclined to accept or even acknowledge the program in their community. Literacy also will be an important factor because many HPDP programs rely on written educational materials and advertising to reinforce concepts and skills they teach and to reach the target audiences with their health promoting messages. Furthermore, Western concepts and examples included within these materials may be completely foreign or counter to the target group's worldview and understanding of health and disease principles and practices.

Language

Although closely related to education and literacy, language or dialect is also an important assessment consideration. That is, what is the preferred language and dialect of the target population? Can they read this language or dialect if it is presented to them in a written format? Can they speak and read English? Obviously, program materials need to be developed in the preferred language or dialect of the target group and to be back-translated to ensure their accuracy. Materials developed that fail to include dialect differences might result in confusion or indifference on the part of the target group for which they were designed. For example, using Spanish language materials that have been written in the highest Castillian dialect might not be understood by someone living in a barrio with little education or reading ability. Thus, a program will need to consider how their target group learns best and how best to reach them with information about programs in their community. Perhaps an oral approach will have greater impact than will written materials, and perhaps pictures should be considered over words (Comings & Kirsch, 2005; Doak et al., 1996; Roter, 2005).

Religion

As discussed in numerous places throughout this book, religion and religious preferences are extremely important factors in the lives of many multicultural groups. Knowing how religious views and practices affect the daily lives of target group members, including variables such as food practices and taboos; religious observances; dress; views regarding marriage, family, and sexuality, might well determine how the program is targeted, what can be included with respect to program content, and even on what day(s) a program might be presented. Furthermore, an understanding of how health and disease issues are addressed and taught within the religious cosmology will aid the planner in defining interventions that are more acceptable to the religious hierarchy and the target population itself. It might be possible, as noted earlier, to involve the clergy, priests, and other religious leaders in the planning and implementation of the HPDP program.

Occupation and Income

Occupation and income might appear less important than other cultural factors, but they are relevant in that both are connected to socioeconomic factors as well as epidemiological factors that might be contributing to accidents, illness, and/or disease. For example, occupations that involve high risk, such as the fishing industry, might place certain population groups in greater jeopardy than they do other groups. A personal observation of a Vietnamese fisherman on the West Coast demonstrated to one of the authors (Huff) that attention to the safety of their boats and crew often is a much lower priority than is making the catch and supporting their families. In addition, money to properly outfit their boats is scarce, so this often is a neglected safety factor in their daily occupation. For those population groups in the lower socioeconomic classes, making a living each day often will take priority over matters of health. That is, taking time out to exercise, eat properly, manage their stress, or to visit a physician when they are not feeling well might not be in their concept of what it takes to survive. Finding ways to incorporate issues of income and occupation might well be one of the more challenging aspects facing the HPDP program planner.

Residence

Closely related to income and occupation are the patterns of residence and the living conditions of the target population. Is the target population living in substandard housing, the inner city, or a rural community? How difficult is it for them to access health services? What perceptions do they have concerning their living conditions with respect to health and disease? For example, are the crime rates excessive, and do they contribute to mental stress within the community? How difficult is it to bring HPDP programs into the community? What options do the target group members have for changing their living conditions? How many people, on average, occupy a single family unit? Are they living as they always have and want to live? As previous experience working in an inner city attested to one of the authors (Huff), the priorities of the target population were not always in line with those of the agencies providing health services to the

community. Understanding these factors may help the health planner to develop a more realistic outlook on what is possible and appropriate given the circumstances with which he or she is working.

Acculturation and Assimilation

Acculturation and assimilation are factors that cross all the levels of the CAF, and both have been covered in some depth by many of the chapters in this book. As noted in Chapter 1, populations immigrating to any new country where the values, beliefs, and ways of life are different from those of their old countries will be required, to some degree, to take on some of the characteristics of the dominant culture if they are to successfully assimilate. As is well known, however, this does not always occur, and the reality is that there will be an acculturation continuum ranging from those who remain completely traditional to those who take on all the characteristics of the mainstream culture in which they live. Assessment of this process can help the health promoter to determine how best to target his or her program or service to accommodate the values, beliefs, attitudes, and health practices of those whom the health promoter will be serving. That is, for a target group that might be primarily composed of first- and second-generation immigrants, their perceptions of health, disease, and Western health care practices may be sharply divergent. Programs or services that fail to take these differences into consideration might find target population participation to be low or even nonexistent. There are a number of acculturation scales that have been developed and tested and the reader is encouraged to look at those described and/or referenced elsewhere in this book.

CULTURE-SPECIFIC EPIDEMIOLOGICAL AND ENVIRONMENTAL INFLUENCES

Environmental and epidemiological factors are generally included in all assessment models, but there is a need for the practitioner to look at these factors in a more focused manner than in the general way these factors normally are considered in an assessment. That is, when morbidity and mortality data are aggregated into larger categories of analysis, specific health issues of many subpopulation groups can be masked (e.g., Asian or Pacific Islander). In the same way, we may also overlook specific environmental factors, such as lead-based paints in older homes, other home hazards (e.g., tubs, stairs, and pools), agricultural hazards, alcohol and tobacco advertising, and other associated influences affecting the target group. Table 6.2 identifies some of the most obvious questions that should be considered in the epidemiological and environmental needs assessment.

There are a number of questions that seem worthwhile to explore within this component

Table 6.2   Cultural Assessment Framework: Culture-Specific Epidemiological and Environmental Influences

Assessment Area	Assessment Questions
Morbidity, mortality, and disability rates	☐ What are the leading causes of morbidity in the cultural or ethnic group by age, gender, income, and occupation? ☐ What are the leading causes of mortality in the cultural or ethnic group by age, gender, income, and occupation? ☐ What are the leading causes of disability in the cultural or ethnic group by age, gender, income, and occupation? ☐ What are the immunization rates and levels within the target population? ☐ To what specific illnesses or diseases is the cultural or ethnic group most susceptible? ☐ What specific culturally sanctioned behaviors (e.g., smoking, alcohol, or other substance use or abuse; violence) may be contributing to the morbidity and mortality rates within the cultural or ethnic group? ☐ How do perceptions of quality of life, worldview, and religion influence responses to illness and disease, disease prevention practices, and use of Western health care screening and disease prevention programs and treatment services?
Environmental influences	☐ What types of environmental health hazards can typically be found within the community in which the cultural or ethnic group resides (e.g., toxins, chemicals)? ☐ What types of potentially health-damaging advertising (e.g., billboards, signs) can be found within the target community and in what concentrations? ☐ How does the community react to these types of advertising? ☐ What is the distribution of stores that sell alcoholic products in the community? ☐ How many and what types of westernized fast food restaurants exist in the community, and how frequently are they used by the community? ☐ What is the general appearance of the community (e.g., clean and safe looking, graffiti strewn, dirty and run down)? ☐ What types of people are most often seen on the streets of the community during the day, evening, and night?

of the CAF and that can be used to provide a truer picture of the extent of morbidity and mortality rates for the specific cultural or ethnic group being targeted. Admittedly, this is a difficult challenge and may require a significant effort on the part of the health promoter to discover this data. But if the health promoter does not do so, then he or she might miss something very important and target the program efforts inappropriately. The activities required for obtaining data about culturally sanctioned behaviors of a target group also may be challenging but might ultimately prove to be quite enlightening. For example, smoking is a socially sanctioned behavior among many Third World population groups, and one could expect to encounter resistance to smoking cessation programs without some serious preliminary work aimed at reframing how this population group perceives and uses tobacco products. Food preferences, which might include the use of lard or other high-cholesterol foods, could be playing a significant role in the development of chronic disease. Religious preferences and practices may also present a problem where programs aimed at reducing sexually transmitted diseases are a concern. Finally, other cultural factors, such as a strong value for modesty or a lack of a concept of germ theory, might well be contributing factors to the morbidity and mortality issues in the cultural or ethnic group of concern.

GENERAL AND SPECIFIC CULTURAL CHARACTERISTICS

This book has continually advocated the need for the health promoter to become more culturally competent and sensitive to the target group with which he or she is working. This concern is reflected in the third component of the CAF (Table 6.3).

Table 6.3   Cultural Assessment Framework: General and Specific Cultural Characteristics

Assessment Area	Assessment Questions
Cultural or ethnic identity	☐ How does the target population identify itself with respect to culture or ethnic derivation? ☐ What subgroups, if any, exist within the broader cultural or ethnic group? ☐ What specific customs and practices govern identification and/or participation in these specific subgroups?
Cosmology	☐ How does the cultural or ethnic group view the world with respect to natural, supernatural, and metaphysical forces? ☐ How does the cultural or ethnic group perceive and relate to the mainstream culture in which it is located? ☐ How does the cosmology of the cultural or ethnic group affect perceptions of health, disease prevention, illness, death, and dying practices? ☐ How does the cultural or ethnic group's cosmology parallel, merge, or conflict with that of the mainstream culture?
Time orientation	☐ What is the general time orientation of the cultural or ethnic group (e.g., past, present, future)? ☐ How does the cultural or ethnic group perceive and use time on a daily basis? ☐ How does time orientation affect disease prevention, illness, and treatment-seeking behaviors?

Assessment Area	Assessment Questions
Perceptions of self	☐ How is the concept of "self" perceived and described by the cultural or ethnic group? ☐ How is individual motivation and determination viewed by the cultural or ethnic group? ☐ What impact, if any, do perceptions of self have with respect to disease prevention, illness, treatment seeking, dying, and death practices
Perceptions of community	☐ How is the concept of community defined by the cultural or ethnic group? ☐ How are community gatekeepers defined, described, or identified by the cultural or ethnic group? ☐ How are outsiders perceived by the cultural or ethnic group (e.g., Western politicians, medical providers, and educators)? ☐ Who, outside of the target population, has entry to the community gatekeepers? ☐ How are mainstream laws, rules, social customs, values, and practices perceived by the cultural or ethnic group? ☐ To what degree are the mainstream laws, rules, social customs, values, and practices observed by the cultural or ethnic group?
Social norms, values, and customs	☐ What are the traditional and expected norms, values, and customs related to family and family dynamics (e.g., interpersonal interactions, gender and age roles, decision making and family leadership, dress, food preferences and preparation, child rearing, religious observances, rules and taboos, marriage, sexuality, health and disease practices)? ☐ How has acculturation and assimilation into the mainstream culture been affected by traditional norms, values, and customs of the family and culture? ☐ What are the traditional and expected norms, values, and customs governing interactions between and among families, community institutions, and the outside world (e.g., the mainstream culture or other cultural or ethnic groups in proximity to the cultural or ethnic group in question)? ☐ How do traditional norms, values, and customs merge with, parallel, or conflict with those of the mainstream culture?
Communication patterns	☐ What are the usual and customary communication patterns and practices within the cultural or ethnic group (e.g., the verbal and nonverbal forms of greeting, talking, social interchange, idioms, communication with outsiders)? ☐ How does the cultural or ethnic group communicate or expect to be communicated with where matters of health care and health education with folk or traditional healers and Western medical providers are concerned (e.g., the rules of communication and dialogue)? ☐ How do the traditional forms of communication in the cultural or ethnic group merge with, parallel, or conflict with those of the mainstream culture?

This level of assessment is concerned with a more anthropological evaluation of the cultural or ethnic group under consideration. Of concern are the cosmology; time orientation; perceptions of self and community; social norms, values, and customs; and communication patterns. A thorough cultural assessment must begin with establishing how the group identifies itself with respect to a specific cultural or ethnic tradition. This also will provide a reference point from which to begin this investigation of the group to be targeted for intervention. It also can help ensure that the health promoter is using the correct descriptor when talking about or to the cultural group and can help identify diversity within the culture being studied. As Seidel, Ball, Dains, and Benedict (1995) observe, within the cultural group there will generally be a variety of populations and subgroups, each of which will manifest a number of shared traits that distinguish its members from the mainstream culture.

Cosmology

The cosmology of the cultural or ethnic group is also important to understand because these beliefs can affect behaviors and health practices. For example, some cultural groups, such as the Hmong from Southeast Asia, are highly oriented to the concept of fate, believing that one's life is preordained. Thus, seeking to change what is already established would likely meet with resistance or outright indifference. Certainly, a major question with respect to cosmology would be concerned with whether the cosmology of the group parallels or conflicts with Western beliefs and practices. For the health promoter, understanding these similarities and differences can be helpful in planning programs reflecting, respecting, and working within and between the differing worldviews.

Time Orientation

Time also is an important issue because different cultural groups view and incorporate

time-specific activities into their worldviews. Seidel et al. (1995) and others (Lipson, 1996; Spector, 2004) comment that a present-centered culture (e.g., Hispanic) tends to take each day as it comes and may see the future as unpredictable, whereas a past-oriented worldview (e.g., East Asian) will seek to hold on to traditions that were significant in the past, and a future-oriented group (e.g., dominant American) will likely look to a "better future," thus placing a high value on change. The issue here, then, is about the potential for bringing about change and what the health promoter might need to consider when planning for health or other social change in the target group.

Perceptions of Self

Perceptions of self and one's relationship to their community is another important consideration when working with traditional cultural or ethnic groups. That is, in some cultures, such as the dominant American culture, individualism and self-determination are highly valued traits, whereas in other cultural groups these might be frowned on and even discouraged. For example, among traditional Native American, East Asian, and Hispanic populations, group goals take precedence over those of the individual. Thus, efforts to create change in these cultures might need to give consideration to how change interventions can be brought into alignment with group goals so that these interventions can be accepted, adopted, and promoted by the group to its individual members.

Norms, Values, and Customs

Social norms, values, and customs comprise the next level of assessment. A *cultural norm* is a standard of behavior that is expected by all who represent a cultural or ethnic group. A *value* is a standard that prescribes the relative worth, utility or importance of a particular belief, custom, or behavior. A *custom* can be defined as a learned and patterned response to a given situation or occasion and may be reflected in dress, language, communications, religion, and other aspects of the cultural or social group. Questions aimed at identifying these aspects of a population group are important because if differences in values, norms, and practices between cultural groups are not identified, then misunderstanding and conflict probably will result. Thus, looking at issues such as who makes the decisions in the family, what the gender roles are, expected marriage and family practices, food preferences and preparation practices, and other family and social dynamics components of the culture or ethnic group is extremely important. Where these are in conflict with or different from the mainstream culture's views, efforts to work within these frames of reference will be necessary for the health promoter.

Communication Patterns

Like other components of the cultural characteristics assessment, communication patterns should be of great interest to the health planner. This is especially important in the clinical setting where direct contact with a client or patient will necessitate understanding issues such as the rules of greeting, speaking, presenting information, touching, eye contact, and other verbal and nonverbal behaviors. As Brislin and Yoshida (1994) observe, the typical Western medical model is very directive and aimed at getting to the heart of the matter as quickly as possible. This also is reflected in how patient, community, and worksite health promotion activities are carried out, that is, getting directly to what the issue is and how best to treat or prevent it with little thought to how these messages will be received, perceived, or acted on. Taking the time to discover how best to address, teach, and work with different cultural groups can make the difference in how HPDP messages and programs are received (Friedman et al., 2003; Spector, 2004). Fredericks and Hodge (1999) discuss the value of "talking circles" as a way to educate Native American women

about cancer prevention using Native American stories and myths as the entry point for HPDP activities. At a related level, assessing how a given cultural or ethnic group generally acquires health information and what media approaches are the most effective for reaching group members can be extremely valuable to the health promoter or planner. Ramirez, Cousins, Santos, and Supic (1986) devised a simple scale for assessing media and language preferences among Mexican Americans, and similar assessment questions have been incorporated into other acculturation measurement scales (Castro, Cota, Vega, & Valdez, 1997; Marin & Gamba, 1996).

GENERAL AND SPECIFIC HEALTH BELIEFS AND PRACTICES

Huff and Yasharpour (Chapter 2, this volume) discuss traditional health beliefs and practices that health promoters should be aware of as they design HPDP interventions for multicultural population groups. Table 6.4 identifies four major assessment areas with associated questions that should be considered when assessing any diverse cultural or ethnic group.

Explanatory Model

This level of assessment begins with a consideration of the explanatory model(s) that is used by the target group to explain and make sense of health and disease issues. As we have seen in the other chapters of this book, significant differences between the cultural or ethnic group and the Western biomedical model can lead to differences of opinion, lack of adherence to prescribed treatment methods, and lack of involvement in health promotion efforts. Response to illness episodes is another area to be explored as many multicultural groups begin illness interventions by seeking the assistance of a traditional healer or by using traditional medicines that have been acquired in the community, handed down through the family, or suggested by close

Table 6.4   Cultural Assessment Framework: General and Specific Health Beliefs and Practices

Assessment Area	Assessment Questions
Explanatory model(s)	☐ What are the traditional explanations used by the cultural or ethnic group to describe and make sense of health, illness, disease, and death?
	☐ How do these explanations merge with, parallel, or conflict with Western explanatory models?
	☐ Does the cultural or ethnic group recognize and practice health-promoting behaviors? If so, then what specific health-promoting behaviors are practiced?
Response to illness	☐ What are the usual or traditional responses to a communicable, chronic, or additive illness episode?
	☐ Who makes the decision(s) within the family regarding health care and treatment seeking for sick family members?
	☐ What types of traditional healing methods and healers are routinely consulted, and under what conditions are they consulted?
	☐ What negative consequences, if any, are perceived by the cultural or ethnic group related to the use of traditional healing methods?
	☐ How are episodes of communicable, chronic, addictive, or mental illness perceived and treated within the family?
	☐ What is the usual response to illness when traditional treatment approaches fail?
	☐ In general, who does the cultural or ethnic group consult with or listen to when health-related information is being sought or presented, how do group members like this information to be given?
Western health care and health promotion use	☐ What are the cultural or ethnic group's perceptions of Western health care practices and services?
	☐ In what ways, and under what conditions, does the cultural or ethnic group currently use Western health care services?
	☐ What are the traditional cultural rules governing interaction with a Western health care provider, health educator, or health care professional in the clinical or community setting?
	☐ What are the cultural or ethnic group's perceptions about change and change processes with respect to health behavior change recommendations from Western health providers?
	☐ How are traditional health beliefs and practices mediated by acculturation and assimilation into mainstream society?
	☐ What seem to be the major barriers to the target population's use of Western health care services
	☐ How have past efforts to reach the cultural or ethnic group with Western health care and/or screening and educational services been received? What worked, what did not work, and why?
Health behavior practices	☐ What specific predisposing, enabling, and reinforcing factors are acting to maintain the health issue or problem to be addressed by the program?
	☐ What specific predisposing, enabling, and reinforcing factors will need to be put in place to help promote the health changes being recommended to the cultural or ethnic group?
	☐ What specific cultural or ethnic group factors may act to block the effectiveness of the health promotion program to achieve its objectives?

friends of the family. As noted elsewhere in this book, these traditional health practices are often used in conjunction with Western medical treatments, so determining what traditional measures have been or are likely to be taken can aid the health promoter in determining what interventions or combination of interventions will have the greatest likelihood of acceptance by the target group.

Perceptions

The perceptions of the target group with respect to the Western health care system also may come into play in both the clinical and health promotion setting. For example, if target group members perceive the Western health care facility as a "death house" where family or friends go in alive and come out dead or as a place that shows little respect for or understanding of their traditional health beliefs and practices, then they will be more likely to avoid contact with these facilities except under the most dire circumstances. In addition to these variables, there may be other factors governing the target population's interest or ability to access HPDP services, including barriers such as transportation, distance, hours of availability of the program or service, language, and other related factors. Perceptions of change also may play a role in the target group's interest in or motivation to access HPDP program or service. As noted in the earlier discussion of cosmology, time, and perceptions of self, for some traditional cultural groups the idea of change is foreign and the probability of resistance is quite high unless attention is paid to cultivating the value of a change and how it can be woven into the fabric of the target group's belief system.

Health Behavior Factors

The identification and role of predisposing, enabling, and reinforcing factors that are contributing to the health problem or issue or

that will be brought into play to intervene and promote change is also an important assessment activity (Green & Kreuter, 2005). Here, the focus is on the specific health beliefs and practices that cut across the culture and are supported by other variables within the cultural milieu. For example, there may be specific food preferences and practices such as the use of high-fat foods, little use of fruits and vegetables, or high use of alcohol or tobacco products that might be contributing to the problem. Environmental conditions, including sanitation beliefs and practices or other factors, might also be acting to reinforce the issue or problem. An accurate assessment and educational-behavioral diagnosis is critical to understanding the problem and designing the most appropriate interventions.

WESTERN HEALTH CARE ORGANIZATION AND ASSESSMENT

The final area of the CAF is concerned with the actual organization and staff who are providing the services to the multicultural group. Although one could make the argument that this area is a separate assessment unto itself, the authors would argue that the way in which the health promotion organization perceives the target group, how they prepare to deliver culturally competent services, and how the actual organizational facility is organized both physically and in its mission, conviction to deliver culturally competent services, and policy documents plays as great a role in the assessment process as does looking at those for whom the services are targeted. Table 6.5 presents the organizational assessment areas and associated questions for the reader's consideration.

Cultural Competency and Sensitivity

The first of these areas addresses cultural competence and sensitivity, which was discussed in some detail in Chapter 1. Of concern here are the agency's management and staff perceptions,

Table 6.5   Cultural Assessment Framework: Western Health Care Organization and Service
               Delivery

Assessment Area	Assessment Questions
Cultural competence and sensitivity	☐ How well prepared are the staff and management of the agency to provide culturally competent services to the targeted cultural or ethnic group? ☐ How sensitive are agency staff and management to the cultural nuances and needs of the targeted cultural or ethnic group? ☐ How well prepared are the health promotion staff and management to provide culturally competent health promotion services to the targeted cultural or ethnic group? ☐ How sensitive are the health promotion staff and management to the cultural nuances and needs of the targeted cultural or ethnic group? ☐ How much training have all agency staff and management had in cultural competence and sensitivity to multicultural populations being served by them? ☐ What additional training in cultural competence and sensitivity is needed by all agency staff and management? ☐ How well prepared is the agency to deliver training to staff and management in the areas of cultural competence and sensitivity?
Organizational policy and mission	☐ What written policy and/or mission statements exist pertaining to the provision of culturally competent and sensitive health care and health promotion services? ☐ If policy or mission statement exist, then how well do agency staff and management adhere to these? ☐ If no specific policy or mission statement exist, then how might these be developed and implemented in the agency?
Facilities and program preparation	☐ How well organized is the agency's facility with respect to signs, directions, bilingual or bicultural staff, translators, and written materials specific to the multicultural populations to be served by the agency? ☐ How well prepared is the program with respect to signs, directions, bilingual or bicultural staff, translators, and written program and educational materials specific to the multicultural populations to be served? ☐ What additional preparation will be needed to bring the agency or program online, and who will facilitate that process?
Evaluation of culturally competent services	☐ What evaluation processes currently are in place to monitor the delivery and efficacy of the culturally competent and sensitive program or service being provided to the targeted multicultural population group? ☐ What additional evaluation processes are needed to monitor delivery and efficacy of this program or service, and who will develop these processes? ☐ What staff training is needed to implement evaluation and monitoring of the program or service to be provided? ☐ When will monitoring and evaluation processes be carried out, and who will carry them out? ☐ How will monitoring and evaluation results be used to improve program or service delivery, and at what points will this take place?

interest, motivation, and conviction at every level to understand, respect, and interact appropriately with the target group. As noted in Chapter 1, a failure to take the steps to begin developing cultural competence within the agency is likely to contribute to interpersonal and communication problems between and among the agency's staff and those they are serving. A number of models have been proposed for how to begin developing cultural competence and sensitivity (Bell & Evans, 1981; Borkan & Neher, 1991; Campinha-Bacote, 1994; Lipson, 1996; Office of Minority Health, 2001). However, the first need is to determine through the assessment process, where agency management and staff are in terms of cultural competence and sensitivity. This can set the scene for in-service and continuing education programming to help better prepare the agency to deliver culturally competent and sensitive care.

Organizational Policy and Mission

An agency's policy and mission statements can provide the impetus for moving its management and staff toward higher levels of culturally competent care and programming. Thus, an examination of current policy and mission statements should be undertaken to ensure they incorporate a cultural competence philosophy that all can follow. If these features already exist in the policy and mission statements, then an assessment as to how well they are followed would be worthwhile with variables such as direct observation of staff and management interaction among and between themselves; observation of interactions in the clinic, waiting area, educational area and other areas where the target group and facility staff interact; and observation of materials being given to the target group to determine how they are received, perceived, read, and understood as well as whether they are written in a language the target group can read and at the appropriate grade or reading level. This assessment would also apply to signs within and around the facility and in other locales where services including health promotion programming may be offered.

Performance Evaluation

Perhaps the most critical aspect of the agency's preparation and delivery of culturally competent and sensitive medical treatment and HPDP services is that of evaluation, that is, the need to conduct regular evaluations of management, staff, target group, and the physical plant to ensure that the highest levels of culturally competent and sensitive care are being provided and that ongoing efforts are being made through in-service and continuing education to keep all agency personnel adequately trained in this arena. The authors recognize that this is a tall order, necessitating resources including staff and money, but feel that the benefits of such activity will far outweigh the costs in the long term, including litigation to settle disputes that may arise as a result of ignoring cultural differences.

USING THE CULTURAL ASSESSMENT FRAMEWORK

The CAF has been successfully used in a variety of community and health care settings. These included a rural mountain community that one of the author's was involved with that focused on helping youth and adults to better understand and appreciate the cultural diversity of the community and to reduce some of the racial tension that existed there. The CAF has also been used as the basis for conducting cultural assessments in a hospital, long-term care facility, a public health violence prevention project, a police department, and other community agencies in the Southern California area. As with all assessment efforts, the health promotion planner must start with clearly defined objectives for what it is they want to learn from the assessment process. Without clear objectives to guide development of the instrument, the potential for moving off track with questions that are not really relevant is highly likely.

Designing assessment instruments is a time-consuming process, and when you add a cultural overlay, the level of design difficulty can be greatly increased. Thus, doing some preliminary study, and reading about the target groups living in a community of interest, or who are using the services of an agency is essential. For example, developing a mammography project targeted to recent immigrant women would need to ask questions related to their cosmology and demographics; their perceptions and understanding of breast cancer; how and where they get their information about health issues; traditional concepts of health and disease including their explanatory models of disease causation; personal space and touching; decision making around health issues in the home; and even whether they have a concept about promotion of health and prevention of disease? Without addressing these and other culturally related questions, such a project might never get off the ground.

The CAF should be looked at as a menu of question options the health promotion planner can consider. Depending on what the focus of the assessment is, questions can be developed around any of the five major areas of the CAF. For instance, in the rural mountain community project noted above, the author worked with a group of teens to design a series of assessments that focused on cultural heritage, demographics such as language spoken in the home, education, length of time residing in the community, gender and gender roles in the home, decision making around health and other issues, traditional health beliefs and practices, perceptions of others living in the community and other associated concerns. Since this community had pockets of diversity, the CAF proved a useful

framework for considering the kinds of information that would be helpful in understanding what people in this community saw and felt about each other and where cultural sensitivity interventions could be structured to increase understanding and appreciation of differences.

CHAPTER SUMMARY

The need to adequately assess culture-specific variables when planning HPDP programming cannot be stressed enough. As has been repeatedly described throughout this book, there are many approaches that can be taken to assess, plan, implement, and evaluate HPDP programs for multicultural population groups. All these share common elements, including the need to accurately determine what the target population is, what group member's specific health needs and concerns are, what makes group members unique as a cultural or ethnic group, and what special planning efforts will be needed to deliver culturally competent and sensitive services to them.

This chapter has sought to provide a CAF that includes questions the health promoter should consider asking when designing programming for a multicultural population target group. The framework presents five major levels of assessment, including culture-specific demographic variables, culture-specific epidemiological and environmental influences, general and specific cultural characteristics, general and specific health beliefs and practices, and Western health care organization and service delivery variables. Each of these levels of assessment can help bring the health practitioner to a higher level of understanding about the cultural or ethnic group with which he or she is working and can help ensure that culturally appropriate, competent, and sensitive HPDP programs and services are planned for group members.

Chapter 7 is the culminating chapter of the foundation section of the book. All the preceding chapters have laid important stepping stones with regard to the important elements that HPDP planners must consider before embarking on the development of programs and interventions for a specific target group in a specific community. The following chapter echoes the messages of the previous chapters: Regardless of the target group, the health problem, or the setting, the selection of the intervention and educational activities must be based on a sound rationale that considers the relationship between the cultural characteristics of the target group and the health behaviors or changes sought. The chapter will reiterate that planning in multicultural HPDP settings must be a collaborative effort involving the planner and participants. The formidable task of developing and implementing a health promotion program will require the planner and participants to work together to accomplish a complex range of activities including (a) assessing the needs, problems, and resources of the target population; (b) developing appropriate goals and objectives; (c) devising strategies and interventions that consider the peculiarities of the settings; (d) implementing and monitoring the interventions; (e) evaluating the results; and (f) refining approaches toward greater program effectiveness and efficiency. All must be heard and represented in the decision-making processes.

Chapter 7 stresses to the health promotion student and practitioner that owing to the scope and complexity of the planning process, they will need to operate from some rational planning framework or model rather than solely on the basis of pragmatic, empirical, or expediency considerations. Program-planning models provide organizing frameworks that encourage a more systematic approach to the development of health promotion programs for specific target groups. The planner must be able to adapt these models to fit the needs of the planning situation and the cultural characteristics of the target group, setting, and health

problem. In addition, the planner must be extremely conscious of and sensitive to the need for building a comprehensive cultural assessment component into the planning process.

DISCUSSION QUESTIONS AND ACTIVITIES

1. Design a brief (one to two pages) cultural assessment instrument that each student could administer to his or her family members in an effort to better understand their cultural heritage, origins of their health beliefs and practices, etc. Consider the following:

   - What specific objectives will you use to guide development of your instrument?
   - What questions will you ask?
   - How will you use the information you gather to inform your own thinking about your cultural heritage?

2. *An alternate activity:* Working in small groups, design a cultural assessment instrument that would be administered to another class and that would be used to help in the design of an educational intervention related to college student alcohol use and abuse.

3. In either (1) or (2) above, share your activities and findings with the class when the activity is concluded, including your process and challenges related to design of the instrument.

REFERENCES

Andrews, M. M., & Boyle, J. S. (1995). *Transcultural concepts in nursing care* (2nd ed.). Philadelphia: J. B. Lippincott.

Bell, P., & Evans, J. (1981). *Counseling the black client.* Center City, MN: Hazelden Education Materials.

Borkan, J., & Neher, J. (1991). A developmental model of ethnosensitivity in family practice training. *Family Medicine, 23*(3), 212–217.

Brislin, R. W., & Yoshida, T. (Eds.). (1994). *Improving intercultural interactions: Modules for cross-cultural training programs.* Thousand Oaks, CA: Sage.

Brownlee, A. T. (1978). *Community, culture, and care: A cross-cultural guide for health workers.* St. Louis, MO: C. V. Mosby.

Campinha-Bacote, J. (1994). Cultural competence in psychiatric mental health nursing: A conceptual model. *Nursing Clinics of North America, 29*(1), 1–8.

Castro, F., Cota, M., Vega, S., & Valdez, E. (1997). Health promotion in Latino populations: A sociocultural model for program planning, development, and evaluation. In R. Huff & M. Kline (Eds.), *Promoting health in multicultural populations: A handbook for practitioners* (pp. 137–168). Thousand Oaks, CA: Sage.

Clark, A. L. (1978). *Culture, childbearing, health professionals.* Philadelphia: F. A. Davis.

Comings, J. P., & Kirsch, I. S. (2005). Literacy skills of US adults. In J. G. Schwartzberg, J. B. VanGeest, & C. C. Wang (Eds.), *Understanding health literacy: Implications for medicine and public health* (pp. 43–54). Chicago: American Medical Association Press.

Doak, C. C., Doak, L. G., & Root, J. H. (1996). *Teaching patients with low literacy skills* (2nd ed.). Philadelphia: J. B. Lippincott.

Farrales, S. (1996). Vietnamese. In J. G. Lipson, S. L. Dibble, & P. A. Minarik (Eds.), *Culture and nursing care: A pocket guide.* San Francisco: UCSF Nursing Press.

Fredericks, L., & Hodge, F. (1999). Traditional approaches to health care among American Indians and Alaska Natives: A case study. In R. Huff & M. Kline (Eds.), *Promoting health in multicultural populations: A handbook for practitioners* (pp. 313–326). Thousand Oaks, CA: Sage.

Friedman, M. M., Bowden, V. R., & Jones, E. G. (2003). *Family nursing: Research, theory, and practice* (5th ed.). Upper Saddle River, NJ: Prentice Hall.

Galanti, G. A. (1991). *Caring for patients from different cultures: Case studies from American hospitals.* Philadelphia: University of Pennsylvania Press.

Green, L., & Kreuter, M. W. (2005). *Health promotion planning: An educational and ecological approach* (4th ed.). Boston: McGraw-Hill.

Helman, C. (2000). *Culture, health and illness* (4th ed.). Oxford, UK: Butterworth-Heinemann.

Ishida, D. N., Toomata-Mayer, T. F., & Mayer, J. F. (1996). Samoans. In J. G. Lipson, S. L. Dibble, & P. A. Minarik (Eds.), *Culture and nursing care: A pocket guide.* San Francisco: UCSF Nursing Press.

Leddy, S. K. (2003). *Integrative health promotion: Conceptual bases for nursing practice.* Thorofare, NJ: Slack.

Leininger, M. (1995). *Transcultural nursing: Concepts, theories, research and practices* (2nd ed.). New York: McGraw-Hill.

Lipson, J. G. (1996). Culturally competent nursing care. In J. G. Lipson, S. L. Dibble, & P. A. Minarik (Eds.), *Culture and nursing care: A pocket guide* (pp. 3–6). San Francisco: UCSF Nursing Press.

Lipson, J. G., & Steiger, N. J. (1996). *Self-care nursing in a multicultural context.* Thousand Oaks, CA: Sage.

Lynch, E., & Hanson, M. (1992). Steps in the right direction: Implications for interventionists. In E. Lynch & M. Hanson (Eds.), *Developing cross-cultural competence: A guide for working with young children and their families.* Baltimore: Paul H. Brookes.

Marin, G., & Gamba, R. (1996). A new measurement of acculturation for Hispanics: The Bidirectional Acculturation Scale for Hispanics (BAS). *Hispanic Journal of Behavioral Sciences, 18*(3), 297–316.

Mo, B. (1992). Cross-cultural medicine a decade later: Modesty, sexuality, and breast health in Chinese-American Women. *Western Journal of Medicine, 9*(157), 260–264.

Office of Minority Health. (2001). *National standards for culturally and linguistically appropriate services in health care.* Washington, DC: U.S. Department of Health and Human Services.

Orque, M. S., Bloch, B., & Ahumada Monrroy, L. S. (1983). *Ethnic nursing care: A multicultural approach.* St. Louis, MO: C. V. Mosby.

Pasick, R. J., D'Onofrio, C. N., & Otero-Sabogal, R. (1996). Similarities and differences across cultures: Questions to inform a third generation for health promotion research. *Health Education Quarterly, 23*(Suppl. 12), S142–S161.

Purnell, L. D., & Paulanka, B. J. (2003). *Transcultural health care: A culturally competent approach* (2nd ed.). Philadelphia: F. A. Davis.

Ramirez, A. G., Cousins, J. H., Santos, Y., & Supic, J. D. (1986). A media-based acculturation scale for Mexican-Americans: Application to public health programs. *Family and Community Health, 9*(3), 63–71.

Roter, D. L. (2005). Health literacy and the patient-provider. In J. G. Schwartzberg, J. B. VanGeest, & C. C. Wang (Eds.), *Understanding health literacy: Implications for medicine and public health*. Chicago: American Medical Association Press.

Rudd, R. E., Renzulli, D., Pereira, A., & Daltroy, L. (2005). Literacy demands in health care settings: The patient perspective. In J. G. Schwartzberg, J. B. VanGeest, & C. C. Wang (Eds.), *Understanding health literacy: Implications for medicine and public* (pp. 69–84). Chicago: American Medical Association Press.

Seidel, H. M., Ball, J. W., Dains, J. E., & Benedict, G. W. (1995). *Mosby's guide to physical examination* (3rd ed.). St. Louis, MO: Mosby-Yearbook.

Spector, R. E. (2004). *Cultural diversity in health and illness* (6th ed.). Upper Saddle River, NJ: Pearson Prentice Hall.

Tripp-Reimer, T., Brink, P. J., & Saunders, J. M. (1984). Cultural assessment: Content and process. *Nursing Outlook, 32*(2), 78–82.

7

Planning Health Promotion and Disease Prevention Programs in Multicultural Populations

MICHAEL V. KLINE

Chapter Objectives

On completion of this chapter, the health promotion student and practitioner will be able to

- Identify and define levels of change sought by programs at the health promotion and health education levels

- Identify traditional and current health promotion and education program planning models to use as guides to practice and their limitations in multicultural health promotion and education program planning

- Formulate a conceptual framework for planning health promotion and education programs in multicultural populations

- Identify and differentiate between the levels of program objectives and levels of evaluation (i.e., impact, outcome, process, and formative) used for assessing those program objectives

- Identify and differentiate between the phases of program implementation (i.e., pre-implementation preparation, program implementation, and administration and monitoring) and discuss their application and limitations

The purpose of this chapter is to provide health practitioners with basic foundations for planning health promotion and education programs in multicultural populations. It cannot be all embracing, but the chapter can serve as a general primer for health promotion program planning. Topics related to current health promotion planning models, specific elements and issues of the planning process, and selected multicultural planning issues and concerns will be covered. Information will be drawn from other chapters in the volume for further illustration of the application of planning principles in several different target populations.

Consider this scenario. Deaths from breast cancer have been increasing for the past several years among Latinas living in a large metropolitan community. The local health jurisdiction, private providers, voluntary agencies, and community members are very concerned and want to reduce the number of deaths drastically. There are, however, severe financial limitations on initiating any new programs. Although increased screening, referral, and treatment programs are critically needed, monies will be made available for only providing health education programs to selected target groups of women. The following kinds of questions and the associated issues constitute the focus of this chapter:

- Who will the target groups be, and which should have priority?
- What are the specific health promotion and education needs, and how will they be identified?
- What types of education, screening, and treatment resources are currently available and accessible, and are they being used?
- Is one large multilevel community program or a series of educational programs needed?
- What should be the objectives of the programs?
- What cultural considerations does the planner need to be aware of when selecting and designing the programs' interventions?

- When programs are implemented, how will the administrator know whether the programs are having any effect on the problem?

This above planning scenario unfolds in a large community setting involving the need for health promotion and education activities targeted at Latinas at risk for breast cancer. The scenario could have considered any population of women located within any community, worksite, school, or health care program setting. The special needs posed by the target population and the particular setting and health problem are the types of challenges confronting the health promotion program planner in urban and rural communities, in inner cities, and on reservations.

DEFINING THE LEVEL OF PROGRAM CHANGE

Planning health promotion and education prevention programs in multicultural populations is a challenging endeavor that requires a systematic planning process, collection of accurate information, and selection of particular courses of action. The planning process requires the planner and participants to define the level of change sought as a result of their program—at the health education and/or health promotion level. For example, the focus of *health education level* interventions for a breast cancer education and screening program for Latinas could be to make specific kinds of educational and screening resources more available and accessible for enabling them to develop knowledge, attitudes, and skills for carrying out defined voluntary behaviors related to reducing the risk of a life-threatening disease.

On the other hand, the planning of strategies and interventions at the *health promotion program level* might seek to establish social ecological or environmental changes (supportive structures) in the form of policy changes, new or revised regulations, organizational arrangements encouraging access and availability to services, and health measures for encouraging, enabling, and reinforcing the practice of certain health-related risk-reduction behaviors among the target population (Green & Kreuter, 2005). The complexity of the community-level health promotion program risk reduction effort requires a greater scope of coordination, agency and citizen participation, commitment, and expense than does the breast cancer education and screening program that is aimed at a single target group.

HEALTH PROMOTION AND EDUCATION PROGRAM PLANNING MODELS AS GUIDES TO PRACTICE

Owing to the scope and complexity of planning activities, practitioners need to operate from some rational planning framework or model rather than solely on the basis of pragmatic, empirical, or expediency considerations. Using a well-tested organizing framework will encourage a more systematic approach to the development of health promotion programs for specific target groups. But, it remains that *there is no perfect health education or health promotion planning model because none offers consistently predictable relationships between means used and ends achieved in the planning process.* In spite of this limitation, several health promotion and education planning models have been widely used over time and serve as well-established frameworks for planning. If a particular model is used in multicultural health promotion planning situations, then the planner and participants must be extremely conscious of and sensitive to the need for building a rigorous cultural assessment component into the planning process. Last, a variety of necessary human capital and financial resources need to be available for carrying out these activities.

TRADITIONAL PLANNING MODELS

These models follow a traditional planning approach and generally divide planning

activities into three major parts: planning the program, implementing the program, and evaluating the program. Some of the health education or health promotion planning models (and their source references) that have served as the old "standbys" include the following:

- The Model for Health Education Planning (Ross & Mico, 1980)
- The Comprehensive Health Education Model (Sullivan, 1977)
- The Health Education/Promotion Planning Model (Dignan & Carr, 1992)
- The PATCH (Planned Approach to Community Health) framework (Kreuter, 1992; U.S. Department of Health and Human Services, 1996)
- The Multilevel Approach to Community Health (Simons-Morton, Greene, & Gottlieb, 1995; Simons-Morton, Simons-Morton, Parcel, & Bunker, 1988)

CURRENT PLANNING MODELS AND APPROACHES

The following five frameworks vary in depth, perspective, and terminology and are, as the old "standbys" listed above, intended to help move the planner and participants systematically through the planning process.

THE PRECEDE-PROCEED MODEL

The PRECEDE-PROCEED model is the single most frequently used planning framework for developing individual- and community-level interventions. The model uses a social ecological approach and its theoretical robustness derives from the hundreds of published applications of the model demonstrating its utility for planning, implementation, and evaluation of health promotion and health education programs (Green & Kreuter, 2005, p. xxi). PRECEDE is an acronym for *Predisposing, Reinforcing, and Enabling Constructs in Educational/ Ecological Diagnosis and Evaluation.* The second component of the model, PROCEED, is an acronym for *Policy, Regulatory, and Organizational*

Constructs in *Educational* and *Environmental Development* (Green & Kreuter, 2005). The model is based on the premise that health behaviors are very complex, multidimensional, and influenced by a variety of factors. The model is well described by Frankish, Lovato, and Poureslami (Chapter 4, this volume), and elements derived from the PRECEDE model will be referred to throughout this chapter. Users should recognize that the model heavily depends on data and may require additional funding and human resources to implement.

THE INTERVENTION MAPPING MODEL

The Intervention Mapping Model (IMM; Bartholomew, Parcel, Kok, & Gottlieb, 2001, 2006) provides a coherent step-by-step approach to the overall planning and development of health promotion and education interventions. And the model uses a social ecological approach. It can serve as another excellent tool for helping the planner design health education and promotion programs. Tortolero et al. (2005) provide support for the model's particular usefulness in adapting an existing intervention (for reducing adolescent pregnancy and sexually transmitted diseases) to a new population of high-risk minority youth. Fernandez, Gonzalez, Tortolero-Luna, Partida, and Bartholomew (2005) developed the Cultivando La Salud program, an intervention to increase breast and cervical cancer screening for Hispanic farmworker women.

SOCIAL ECOLOGICAL AND ENVIRONMENTAL MODELS

Health promotion professionals working in multicultural populations are also deeply involved in the development of social ecological and environmental models and components. PRECEDE (Green & Kreuter, 2005) and the IMM (Bartholomew et al., 2006) are good examples since they heavily incorporate consideration of the role of ecological and

environmental factors into the assessment process. Knowledge of these factors increase understanding about the roles that intrapersonal, social and cultural, and physical environment variables have in affecting risks and behavior; the interaction among these variables; the levels on which they operate; and their relationship to changing behaviors within the environmental context in which these people live and work toward preventing disease and improving health (Bronfenbrenner, 1979; Green & Kreuter, 2005; Green, Richard, & Potvin, 1996; Hovell, Walgren, & Gehrman, 2002; McLeroy, Bibeau, Steckler, & Glanz, 1988; Richard, Potvin, Kishchuk, Prlic, & Green, 1996; Sallis & Owen, 1997, 2002; Smedley & Syme, 2000; Stokols, 2000a, 2000b; Syme, 1986). This will be discussed further in Chapter 29.

The Person, Extended Family, Neighborhood Model (PEN-3)

Another planning model with a different focus, the PEN-3 model, grew out of the need to develop a more culturally appropriate planning framework for health promotion programs in Africa and for African Americans (Airhihenbuwa, 1995; Doyle & Ward, 2001). Abernethy et al. (2005) recently used the culturally based model in their efforts to recruit African American men for cancer prevention studies. Planning issues involving cultural appropriateness and cultural sensitivity are made explicit in PEN-3. Airhihenbuwa (1995), the model's developer, urges that culture should have a central role in the process of educational diagnosis and should be incorporated as a formal component when planning health promotion programs for any target group. PEN-3 is discussed further by Frankish et al. (Chapter 4, this volume).

The Social Marketing Model

Social marketing programs are increasingly being used to address such issues as HIV/AIDS, breast cancer, hypertension, nutrition, unintended/ unwanted pregnancies, alcohol and drug abuse, smoking, child abuse, depression, and many others. Social marketers use "commercial marketing techniques to promote the adoption of a behavior that will improve the health or well-being of the target audience or of society as a whole" (Weinreich, 1999, p. 3). Social marketing programs consist of at least four stages: "planning and strategy development; development of pretesting concepts, messages, and materials; implementation; assessment of in-market effectiveness; and feedback to the first stage" (Glanz & Rimer, 2005, p. 38). Audience (formative) research and environmental analysis drive the planning process (Maibach, Rothschild, & Novelli, 2002, p. 448). A major strength and tool of social marketing assessment is that target groups, through *market segmentation*, are broken down into smaller, more homogeneous and manageable subgroups (*target audiences*) classified by distinct characteristics and needs such as disease risk, gender, age, ethnicity, cultural considerations, residence location, habits,

readiness for change, and even common patterns of seeking and using the same sources of media where they live. The target audience is intimately involved via focus group methodology in the assessment and is also involved in the tailoring of the health message and identification of media sources to be used. *Hands-On Social Marketing* by Weinreich (1999) is an excellent step-by-step guide for planners. Other sources for learning more about this very powerful planning and intervention development tool include Andreasen (1995, 2005), Glanz and Rimer (2005), Maibach et al. (2002), and Novelli (1990).

A CONCEPTUAL FRAMEWORK FOR PLANNING HEALTH PROMOTION AND EDUCATION PROGRAMS IN MULTICULTURAL POPULATIONS

The framework conceptualized in Figure 7.1 by the author systematically portrays the sequence of detailed planning activities required in most planning efforts. This more traditional framework can help students and practitioners

---

Task 1: Planning the Program

    Subtask A: Involving those affected by the problem
    Subtask B: Assessing the needs of the community
    Subtask C: Diagnosing health-related concerns (problems and needs) in the community
    Subtask D: Prioritizing and selecting the target populations, problems, and settings
    Subtask E: Assessing the specific needs of the target group (targeted assessment)
    Subtask F: Developing appropriate target group goals and objectives
    Subtask G: Identifying health promotion program intervention activities that appropriately consider the needs of the target group, health problem, and setting

Task 2: Evaluating the Program

    Subtask A: Assessment of the long-term health and social outcomes of the target group (outcome evaluation)
    Subtask B: Assessment of the immediate impact of the program (impact evaluation)
    Subtask C: Assessment of the quality of program inputs during the development and implementation phases (process/formative evaluation)

Task 3: Implementing the Program

    Subtask A: Pre-implementation preparation
    Subtask B: Program implementation
    Subtask C: Implementation of administration and monitoring

---

Figure 7.1   Planning Framework

more systematically visualize the health education or health promotion planning process. It is also a framework that can be used by the author, at specific points of chapter discussion, to relate, integrate, and suggest various approaches and methods used in other planning models discussed above.

The planning framework in Figure 7.1 identifies three major tasks (planning, evaluation, and implementation), each with related subtasks. Each will be discussed in some depth, and the sequence of the tasks and subtasks may vary somewhat from other models depending on the problem, target population/group, setting, and circumstances. There is also an explicit assumption within this framework that review, discussion, and feedback should occur at every point, back and forth and from task to task by all players.

Task 1: Planning the Program

Subtask A: Involving Those Affected by the Problem

Subtask A identifies the need to involve those affected or concerned by the problem as the first formal step of the program planning process. This underlying principle of participation might well be the most important ingredient of successful program development (Bartholomew et al., 2006; Gielen & McDonald, 2002; Green & Kreuter, 2005; Minkler, 1990; Minkler & Wallerstein, 2002; Ross & Mico, 1980; Smedley & Syme, 2000; Sullivan, 1977; Chapter 4, this volume). Participation should occur from the time a problem or issue is first felt but not well defined to when it is well-documented and ultimately serves as a basis for writing program objectives, developing strategies, and implementing and evaluating the program. Planners need to recognize the needs, interests, and the social, cultural, and economic settings in which participants live and that there are many ways and reasons for how and why

people become involved. The planner and participants must identify the many possible points of collaboration and seek to formalize the relationship. The planner and participants need to be "culturally competent" (Huff & Kline, 1999a) as they interact and work together in the overall health promotion and disease prevention (HPDP) planning process. In this chapter, it is stressed that such competence needs to be a two-way obligation between the planner and participants.

Subtask B: Assessing the Needs of the Community or Target Population

Target Populations and Target Groups. The need for a health promotion program for a specific target population or target group in a community or setting should be based on the study of factual information and not on the hunches or biases of politicians, the planner, or participants. For the purpose of this chapter, "community" refers to a group of people (a target population) who may or may not share a common ethnic background, identity, values, norms, communication channels but who occupy an area, geographical or otherwise, within which their common and specific health-related problems and needs can be defined and dealt with, with them as collaborators in the planning process. The term *target group(s)* used in this chapter indicates a specific aggregate of individuals or aggregates of specific groups drawn from the target population after the assessment process identifies the relationships among their needs, problems, and resources (or resource gaps) and after priorities are defined and understood. Target groups within a community ultimately constitute the focus of assessment and planning efforts and will be discussed further in Subtask E.

SCOPE OF THE ASSESSMENT

The scope of the assessment activity will depend on the complexity of the problems and the needs of a target population. In some instances, understanding of the problem will be very limited, and assessment must begin with an intensive multilevel study process of the community. In other instances, the assessment's scope will be more focused and will precisely identify the setting, target group, health issue, and program intervention. At some level, then, an assessment is necessary to identify the problems and needs of a target population and to measure gaps between what is and what ought to be (McKenzie, Neiger, & Smeltzer, 2004; McKenzie & Smeltzer, 2001; Timmreck, 2002; Windsor, Clark, Boyd, & Goodman, 2004).

COMMUNITY NEEDS ASSESSMENT

Dignan and Carr (1992) view the *needs assessment* process as consisting of two related parts. The first segment, "community analysis," involves the collection of *extensive information* for investigating social and health-related problems, needs, and program resources of the community. "Community diagnosis" is the second segment and uses the information gathered in the first segment to identify specific health problems and resources that exist within specific target populations and HPDP programs to meet those needs. "Targeted assessment," a further intensive process involving a more focused target-group assessment and diagnosis, is conducted later and is discussed in Subtask E. Table 7.1 is used to list obvious and available categories of information and examples of types of information. Several good texts are available for helping practitioners develop needs assessment formats, including discussion of methods and techniques for collecting information (Bartholomew et al., 2006; Dignan & Carr, 1992; Gilmore & Campbell, 2004; Green & Kreuter, 1991, 1999, 2005; Green, Kreuter, Deeds, & Partridge, 1980; McKenzie et al., 2004). Concepts of disease mapping (i.e., identifying the geographical distribution of disease within a population) are useful, and

geographical information systems (GIS) methodology can be valuable tools in the assessment process (Gatrell & Loytonen, 1998; Goldman & Schmalz, 2000; Lawson & Williams, 2001).

The several categories of community assessment data presented in Table 7.1 provide the planner and participants with information to be synthesized and analyzed during the *diagnosis stage* (Subtask C).

THE NEED TO BUILD IN CULTURAL ASSESSMENT

Chapter 6 of this volume provides an in-depth assessment framework for helping the planner and participants better understand the similarities and differences between mainstream culture and the specific cultural/ethnic group targeted for intervention. These guidelines can be applied to the individual, small group, community, and organizational levels of assessment. And they can provide practitioners with a framework for identifying important demographics, epidemiological factors, cosmology, general and specific cultural characteristics, acculturation and generational factors, general and specific health beliefs and practices, environmental and biocultural factors, and organizational variables (Huff & Kline, 1999b; Chapter 6, this volume).

DIFFICULTIES IN DEFINING TARGET POPULATIONS

Interventions may fail miserably if the planner is not attentive to the need for differentiating among the many racial/ethnic subgroups, including their generational differences. McLeroy et al. (1995) observe that the difficulty of defining target populations such as older adults and diverse cultural groups may derive from the substantial heterogeneity within groups in terms of culture, racial/ethnic background, social norms, and generational and acculturation differences. The work

Table 7.1   Examples of Needs Assessment Information

Category of Information	Types of Information
1. "Eyeball" information for getting to know the physical-spatial character of the community (urban/inner city, rural, reservation)	Neighborhood pride, transportation, physical terrain, geographical isolation, parks, population density, physical condition of neighborhoods, traffic, congestion, pollution (air), allergens
2. General information about who lives in the community	Demographic data: age, sex, sex ratios, marital status, income, employment status, types of jobs, condition of housing, level of education, religion, nationality, generational information, poverty, in/out migration, family and household characteristics; vital events: births, deaths, marriages, divorces, mobility, dependency ratios, immigration status
3. General information about the community	Governmental structure (city, county, reservation, Federal); political and power structure; policy setting, trash and garbage pickup, quality of life: stress indicators (homicides, suicides, drunk driving, robberies, assaults, education and recreation facilities and resources); access to drugs, alcohol beverage outlets; gang problems, school drop-out, school absenteeism, self-esteem, spousal and child abuse, alienation, discrimination, feelings of hope, despair, anger; civic pride; gatekeepers community leadership, communication channels, opinion leaders, local economy, industry, perceived quality of life
4. Information about the state of health of the people who live in the community	Morbidity (illness) and mortality (death): total number/percentages by age, race/ethnicity, sex, cause; geographical area of occurrence; incidence and prevalence rates of chronic diseases and communicable diseases: distribution, intensity, duration; risk factors; disability by cause, days of work lost, occupational risks and diseases; mental illness, alcohol and drug problems, immunization levels, perceived quality of life; geographical information systems
5. Information about health care and social security	Health facilities numbers, types, location, and adequacy of service systems in the community (hospitals, emergency facilities, out-patient-urgent walk-in care, mental health alcohol-drug treatment programs, nursing homes; accessibility and availability of services; adequacy of numbers of trained public health and private health personnel; number covered by health insurance (Medicare, Medicaid, private insurance, supplemental security income); adequacy of local welfare programs in covering basic needs; scope and adequacy of local health department services; scope and adequacy of local voluntary health; operational health promotion programs (worksite, schools, community, health providers), satisfaction with health services
6. Preliminary baseline health-education-related information gathered from community target population	Level of health knowledge, health attitudes, and health behaviors/skills; identification of health risks and risk-taking behaviors; knowledge about location and availability of promotion/education programs and resources; patterns of using health promotion/health education resources
7. General culture-related information	See Chapter 6, this volume

of Chen and Hawks (1995) emphasizes that the model healthy Asian American/Pacific Islander (AA/PI) stereotype is a myth (see also Kagawa-Singer, Chapter 21, this volume). This is partly attributed to the practice of data collection systems clumping these ethnically heterogeneous populations into one or two broad categories (Asian American or Pacific Islander) that, in effect, masks their true health status. The planner and participants, in these instances, should collect ethnically specific data and avoid aggregation of AA/PI data (Chen, Diamant, Kagawa-Singer, Pourat, & Wold, 2004; Chen & Hawks, 1995; Ro, 2002). Amaro and de la Torre (2002) caution that several important Latina health disparities are not accurately reflected in global and aggregate measures of health status, for example, by specific cause of mortality. Williams and Flora (1995) demonstrate the value of disaggregating ethnic groups in assessing differences between Hispanic subgroups (e.g., education, income, health practices, communication channels). They found that there were different audience segments warranting different messages in a communication campaign. Padilla (1980; see also Padilla & Perez, 2003) strongly encourages the need to consider *acculturation* as an important cultural variable by which to segment intraethnic groups. Balcazar, Castro, and Krull (1995) provide the planner with a methodology for assessing key factors such as acculturation and educational status in various subgroups of Hispanics. Abraido-Lanza, Armbrister, Florez, and Aguirre (2006) offer several insights into the value of assessing acculturation and particular health outcomes in Latino populations in the United States. Such culture-related assessments can identify critical information, which, for example, could ultimately help in planning more culturally appropriate cancer reduction programs. The planner, then, needs to include an intensive cultural assessment component at this stage of planning

process and/or during the targeted assessment process (to be discussed further in Subtask E).

Subtask C: Diagnosing Health-Related Concerns (Problems and Needs) in the Community

Sometimes, the problem definition is easy, and collected information (as noted in Subtask B) may disclose obvious issues that require no protracted period of study. In these instances, of course, one should still verify the accuracy of the finding (McKenzie et al., 2004). More often, the plethora of information constitutes a giant puzzle in need of time-consuming study, synthesis, interpretation, and verification to make sense out of all the pieces.

The Diagnosis Process. The *diagnosis process* should provide the planner with at least the following information:

- Objective description of the health- and non-health-related problems and where they are concentrated as well as their nature, extent, and trends and how they contribute to the problem
- Identification of specific target groups within target populations that are affected
- Understanding why the target population or group is affected (e.g., as a result of taking or not taking specific personal health actions if those actions would prevent or ameliorate the problem)
- Identification of necessary health behaviors needed to be taken by the target population to prevent, ameliorate, or eliminate the health-related problem
- Identification of specific environmental interventions needed to prevent, ameliorate, or eliminate the health-related problem within the target population
- Identification and understanding of the degree of control the target population or agencies or institutions in the community actually have to prevent, ameliorate, or eliminate the health-related problem

- Understanding whether and how the problem was dealt with in the past
- Identification of the scope and adequacy, availability, and accessibility of resources necessary to deliver health and health promotion services to the target population related to preventing, ameliorating, or eliminating the health-related problem.

The PRECEDE model requires the planner to approach this diagnostic segment of the planning process in a systematic fashion and provides an excellent methodological format to follow (Green et al., 1980; Green & Kreuter, 2005). The planner is encouraged to seriously consider the role of *nonbehavioral factors* such as gender, age, family history of a specific disease as well as how these may contribute to the health problem even though these factors cannot be changed through a health promotion program (Gielen & McDonald, 2002; Green & Kreuter, 2005). The epidemiological assessment of PRECEDE also attempts to identify the role of environmental factors external to the individual and within the social, biological, and physical environments as they contribute to the problem. Some of these factors are often found to be beyond the control of the individual, but some can be identified and modified to support the behavior or influence the health outcome (Green & Kreuter, 2005).

Subtask D: Prioritizing and Selecting the Target Population or Group Health Problem and Setting

Communities do not possess the capacity to deal with all the health problems and target-group issues identified in the needs assessment and diagnosis phases. *The planner and participants must establish priorities concerning the problems, target groups, and program needs in a rational manner.* Techniques and approaches for prioritizing need range from simple discussion and consensus using nominal group process techniques to qualitative ranking procedures (Blum, 1974; Gilmore & Campbell, 2004; McKenzie et al., 2004; Timmreck, 2002).

It is also useful for the planner and participants to employ several preliminary questions for helping set priorities that were posed in the epidemiological, behavioral, and environmental assessment) of the PRECEDE model:

- Which problem(s) have the greatest impact in terms of death, disease, days lost from work, costs to the community?
- Which subpopulation is at specific risk?
- Which problem would be most amenable to program intervention?
- Which problem, when appropriately addressed, has the greatest potential for resulting in improved health status, economic savings, and the like? (Green & Kreuter, 2005)

Once these types of problems are identified and prioritized, informed decisions can be made as to which problems the planners will deal with. Also, health and health care disparities, including lack of access to HPDP programs and services among target groups (discussed in Chapter 5), would be considered in this process. It is from the answers to questions like these that the target groups and health problems are selected. *The process of diagnosis and setting of priorities provides the important foundations for later deriving program goals and objectives, and the ultimate selection of the strategies and methods to be used to accomplish the objectives!*

Subtask E: Assessing the Specific Health Promotion and Education Needs of the Target Group(s)

TARGETED ASSESSMENT

Now, planning efforts must move to an even more intensively focused level of assessment that investigates the status of the specific target group selected, their health-related knowledge, attitudes, and behaviors, and their relationship with the identified problems. This segment of the program planning process is referred to as the "*targeted assessment*" phase (Dignan & Carr, 1992). The primary challenge to the planner at this point is to identify how to deal with those problem behaviors/ lifestyles, genetic factors, and environmental factors that put the target group at risk of disease (identified in Tasks B, C, and D). The next challenge is to specifically identify how to change or modify behaviors and/or modify environmental targets to reduce the health risk of the target group and which of these are amenable to change through health education and promotion programs.

Predisposing, Enabling, and Reinforcing Factors: Their Value in Helping Identify the Target Group and Possible Program Intervention Activities

The PRECEDE model includes a detailed approach for conducting an ecological and educational assessment of the target group (Green & Kreuter, 1991, 2005). This assessment can help the planner to identify specific factors "that have the potential to influence a given health behavioral or environmental factor, or interaction of genes with behavior and environment" (Green & Kreuter, 2005, p. 14). These causal factors can be placed into three categories: *predisposing factors, reinforcing factors, and enabling factors* (Green & Kreuter, 2005).

The following example uses our earlier described target group of Latinas to illustrate how these three types of factors are involved and how the grouping of these factors according to the specific features of the situation can suggest the types of alternative program approaches to be explored. Assume that the assessment of the Latina target group disclosed that they do not possess *appropriate knowledge about the risk factors of breast cancer or about*

the availability of mammography screening in the community (predisposing factors). Perhaps its members also do not *know or believe that they need to obtain routine mammograms or that the practice of such behavior can help in the early detection of breast cancer* (predisposing factors). So they do not obtain routine mammograms (the problem behavior). Furthermore, the women's family and their neighborhood folk healer, owing to strongly held concepts of health and disease within their cultural milieu, *might view breast cancer fatalistically (fatalismo) or as a source of embarrassment, shame* (Fortenberry et al., 2002), *or "self-stigmatization"* (Corrigan & Penn, 1999) *that she has brought to her family or specifically her spouse* (negative reinforcing factors). This view might discourage the women from obtaining routine mammograms or even any other preventive action. Even if the health education program helps them to recognize the need to obtain screening, there still will be a *need for the behavior to be positively rewarded and supported by their peers, families, family physicians, and neighborhood folk healers* (positive reinforcing factors) who constitute yet other important target group in this scenario. The reader is encouraged to review the study conducted by Nguyen, McPhee, Nguyen, Lam, and Mock (2002) relevant to gaining the involvement and positive support by the men in the Vietnamese women's life. This element of positive reinforcement raises the likelihood that their wives would participate in cervical cancer screening programs and lower their risk of premature death (see also Lam et al., 2003). Also, the situation is worsened if there are *no health education programs in the community to serve as a resource where the women can gain accurate knowledge or the skills required to obtain screening* (enabling factor and a source of environmental need). Thus, there are also program *needs for making program resources available and accessible* (enabling factor).

The information derived above from the three types of factors can help the planner and participants to systematically identify alternative intervention program strategies for enabling the target group to carry out the needed risk-reduction actions. For example, the more obvious types of interventions needed become apparent and might include (a) health education sessions; and community media campaigns to strengthen the *predisposing factors* related to assisting the target group in acquiring appropriate knowledge and positive attitudes concerning the need to obtain routine mammogram screening and to recognize that the practice of such behavior can help them in the early detection of breast cancer; (b) indirectly working with physicians, peers, clergy, neighborhood healers, family and others to strengthen the *positive reinforcing factors*; and (c) target-group skill training related to strengthening the various *enabling factors* such as is needed for making and keeping clinic appointments for mammograms, political intervention within the community health service system/community organizations/ voluntary agencies, and cultural competence training for physicians and other health professionals, including the development of environmental support resources (Green & Kreuter, 1991, 2005). Intervention development will be the focus of Subtask G.

Subtask F: Developing Appropriate Health Promotion and Education

Goals and Objectives. The planner and participants are ready to formulate health promotion and education program goals and objectives when they understand more clearly the relationships between (a) the health problems, environment, and antecedent target-group behavior and (b) the role of predisposing factors, enabling factors, and reinforcing factors as they influence those target-group behaviors.

Program goals and objectives exist in a hierarchical relationship. Those at the top represent the major overall outcome a program strives to achieve. Figure 7.3 shows that objectives at the lowest level of the hierarchy must be achieved first to achieve the objectives at

the next highest level. Achievement then ascends up the hierarchy until the overall program objective is achieved. Goals and objectives, therefore, must be written coherently and must specify the various levels of program (and target group) activity and change sought.

PROGRAM GOALS AND EDUCATIONAL GOALS

Goals are formulated to identify what should happen as a result of the program. They are usually *not measurable,* but they are attainable, identify a desired future state or condition, are stated as occurring in the longer term rather than the shorter term, and lack a specific deadline for accomplishment (Bartholomew et al., 2006; Dignan & Carr, 1992; McKenzie et al., 2004; Timmreck, 2002). It is useful for the planner to formulate at least two types of goals: those for the overall program and those for services to be delivered as part of the overall program. This is helpful in clearly establishing the role of education in the program needed to achieve the program goals (Dignan & Carr, 1992). Figure 7.2 provides examples of a *program goal* and a related *educational goal.*

Program Objectives

Objectives, unlike goals, are written in measurable, time-bound, and realistic terms; are derived from the earlier detailed assessment of the target group; and stipulate the tasks needed for program and educational goal accomplishment. They also specify the magnitude and direction of the change sought (in terms of increasing knowledge, attitudes, or behavior or decreasing the occurrence of certain behavior or activity) within a certain time period. In this way, objectives serve as roadmaps for systematically reaching the goals. Behavioral outcomes of target-group performance are the most concrete and sought-after targets of the health promotion program's educational interventions (discussed in the Subtask G subsection). Well-written health promotion and education

Program Goal

Latinas in the target population of 55 years and above will increase their participation in mammography screening programs made available by the local health jurisdiction.

Educational Goal

Latinas in the target population of 55 years and above will

1. Learn the importance of early detection and breast cancer survival.
2. Learn the importance of family history and breast cancer.
3. Actively participate in community mammography screening clinics.

Figure 7.2   Example of a Program Goal and Educational Goals for a Breast Cancer Education and Detection Program

program plans should include a formal hierarchy of objectives. This hierarchy should include (a) the overall health promotion program outcome objective(s), (b) the overall health education target-group program objectives, (c) the health education (knowledge, attitude, and behavior) target-group objectives, and (d) the health education instructional learning objectives (see Figure 7.3). The overall health education program objectives are generally stated in behavioral terms. The instructional learning objectives are concerned with addressing the needs posed by the predisposing, enabling, and reinforcing factors identified earlier and which are necessary for effecting target-group-behavior change (Green & Kreuter, 2005). Figure 7.3 shows examples of each type and level of objective in the hierarchy.

The quality of the ultimate evaluation of the program will depend on how careful the program's goals and objectives are formulated.

Subtask G: Identifying Health Promotion Program Intervention Activities That Appropriately Consider the Needs of the Target Group, Health Problem, and Setting

DEFINING INTERVENTION

Bartholomew et al. (2001, 2006) define a health education or promotion *intervention* as

"a planned combination of theoretical methods delivered through a series of strategies organized into a program. An intervention can be designed to change environmental or behavioral factors related to health, but the most immediate impact of an intervention is on a set of well-defined antecedents or determinants of behavior and environmental conditions" (p. 1). Green et al. (1980) consider a health education *strategy,* as including one or more of a combination of *interventions* made up of methods and activities "that may be used to affect the *predisposing, reinforcing, and enabling factors* [italics added] which directly or indirectly influence behaviors" (p. 86). Green and Kreuter's (2005) most recent definition of an *intervention* is, "The part of a strategy, incorporating method and technique, that actually reaches a person or population" (p. G-5). However, they note, "the term 'intervention' will usually refer to a specific component of a more comprehensive 'program'" (p. 192). *Thus, a comprehensive community health promotion and education program could actually consist of several different intervention levels, including prevention and education; a social marketing component; mass media activities; skill practice and training; community organization; policy and legislative initiative development; and so on.* The PATCH approach, for example, encourages the use of multiple strategies in intervention

Overall Health Promotion and Education Program Outcome Objective

- The target population of Latinas aged 55 years or above obtaining mammography screening at local clinics will show an increase of __% at 1, 3, and 5 years of program implementation
- The number of mammography screening programs for Latinas in the target population will increase by __% within 2 years of program implementation
- Survival experience at 1, 5, and 10 years for those in the target group of high-risk Latinas attending the program who were diagnosed with early breast cancer

Overall Health Education Program Objectives

Educational: To increase the number of Latinas by __% in the target group attending breast cancer education programs who obtain screening at a community mammography clinic by the end of fiscal year 200_

Resource: To increase the number of breast cancer education programs for Latinas by __% in the target group by the end of fiscal year 200_

Health Education Target Group Objectives

- To increase the number of Latinas by __% in the target group who carry out *appropriate behaviors* related to obtaining a mammogram at a community clinic by *X* date
- To increase the number of Latinas by __% in the target group who possess *favorable attitudes* related to obtaining a mammogram at a community clinic by *X* date
- To increase the number of Latinas by __% in the target group who possess *appropriate knowledge* related to the need to obtain a mammogram at a community clinic by *X* date

Health Education Instructional Learning Objectives

Knowledge: By the end of the program, 80% of the Latinas in the target group

1. Will identify at least four risk factors associated with breast cancer
2. Can state that familial history of breast cancer is a risk factor associated with breast cancer
3. Will identify mammograms as necessary for detecting breast cancer
4. Can state that free mammograms are available at the clinic

Attitudes: By the end of the program, 70% of the Latinas in the target group

1. Will express the feeling that the consequences of breast cancer can be very serious
2. Will express the feeling that if one's mother or other close relative had breast cancer, there is a risk of having breast cancer
3. Will express the feeling that they can take action leading to the early detection and treatment of breast cancer

Skills: By the end of the program, 70% of the Latinas in the target group

1. Will be able to call the mammography screening clinic and make appointments
2. Will be able to arrange transportation to the mammography screening clinic to keep their appointments

Reinforcing: By the end of the program, 90% of the Latinas in the target group

1. Will have verbally encouraged women in their target group to make appointments for mammography screening at the clinic
2. Will have verbally encouraged women in their target group to keep their appointments for mammography screening at the clinic

Figure 7.3   Examples of a Hierarchy of Program Objectives for a Latina Breast Cancer Health Promotion and Education Program

activities at three levels of action: governmental, organizational, and individual (U.S. Department of Health and Human Services, 1996).

THE COMPLEX TASK OF INTERVENTION DEVELOPMENT

There is no foolproof way in which to select the right intervention or combination of interventions that will ensure the most effective results. An intensive effort has been made in the chapter thus far to help the planner clearly define the target group and to understand the roles and relationships of predisposing factors, reinforcing factors, and enabling factors, including environmental support needs and how these affect target-group behavior. Recognition and understanding of this information will give the planner and participant greater capacity to design appropriate health promotion and health education interventions for achieving the change specified in the target-group goals and objectives.

Development of a single or multiple-level intervention approach for any multicultural target group requires answers to several questions:

- At what level is change sought?
- Will the intervention be based on an appropriate theory? What theory(ies)? Why?
- What individual-level or community-level theories are important to consider (i.e., health education level, health promotion level, or both levels)?
- Has the intervention been used successfully elsewhere?
- Is the intervention design proposed appropriate for the target group's demographics (age, gender, and socioeconomic status), knowledge, skills, and behavior?
- Are the intervention activities tailored to fit the raison d'être of the program?

Studying other interventions that have been successful in particular settings and target groups can strengthen the rationale for the selection of an intervention approach. The notion of "best practices" implies that ideally the intervention selected for use in a program has been subjected to rigorous research and evaluation review that substantiates its repeated effectiveness in a particular target population or group (e.g., achieving the behavioral outcomes sought). Furthermore, it has been used in other populations and circumstances with similar outcomes (Green & Kreuter, 2005). There is much to draw from in terms of evidence-based practice with regard to past and existing program interventions and experiences (see also Zaza, Briss, & Harris, 2006).

IMPORTANT ELEMENTS TO CONSIDER IN THE DEVELOPMENT OF INTERVENTIONS

Steckler et al. (1995) noted that despite the range of methodological limitations in many studies of individual-level health education interventions, some of the well-designed and available studies could provide planners with valuable information about the efficacy of different approaches. For example, they cite four common elements in successful individual-level interventions. These elements that follow are particularly important for the planner and participants:

First, the intervention is grounded in a "*clearly operationalized underlying theoretical perspective . . . generally derived from the behavioral and social sciences and educational theory* [italics added]" (Steckler et al., 1995, p. 310). The reader is strongly urged to read Chapter 4 of this volume, where Frankish et al. examine and discuss specific health promotion and education theoretical foundations and their application to culturally related intervention development activities (see also DiClemente, Crosby, & Kegler, 2002; Glanz,

Lewis, & Rimer, 1990, 1997; Glanz, Rimer, & Lewis, 2002).

Second, the intervention uses *"a wide range of educational behavioral strategies suggested by the theoretical perspectives* [italics added]" (Steckler et al., 1995, p. 310), such as cognitive behavioral strategies, including shaping and guided practice, reinforcement control, behavioral contracting, commitment strategies, goal setting, and self-control strategies.

Third, the intervention incorporates the element of social support (Steckler et al., 1995, p. 310).

It is very important to understand the value of using social relationships, particularly in the provision of social support, as vehicles for encouraging and reinforcing positive health behaviors. Where possible, these kinds of supports should be built into the program. House (1981) identified and categorized four broad types of supportive behaviors or acts that others can provide to a person: emotional support (e.g., empathy, caring, trust); instrumental support (e.g., services that assist a person in need); informational support (e.g., advice, information, and suggestions that a person can use to deal with a problem); and appraisal support (e.g., positive feedback to strengthen the appropriate behavior) (see also Gallant, 2003; Heaney & Israel, 2002; Israel, 1982, 1985).

Fourth, the intervention combines diverse strategies, including multiple-component interventions (Steckler et al., 1995, p. 310).

The earlier study by Morisky, DeMuth, Field-Fass, Green, and Levine (1987) of health education for hypertensive patients using a combination of three strategies (consisting of interviewing following the visit to increase understanding of and compliance with the medical regimen, a home visit to encourage a family member to reinforce and support the patient, and small group sessions with the patient to help better self-manage his or her problems) increased compliance to the medical regimen (see also Gallant, 2003). Sallis and Owen (2002), from the perspective of the ecological models of health behavior, recognize that there is growing evidence that the multilevel approaches will have increased power to bring about at-risk population improvements in health. They note that "educational interventions designed to change beliefs and behavioral skills would be expected to work better when policies and environments support the targeted behavior changes" (p. 469).

TARGETING AND TAILORING

Pasick, D'Onofrio, and Otero-Sabogal (1996) cite the need to differentiate between the terms *tailoring* and *targeting*. Targeting implies the need to clearly identify the specific population subgroup that will be exposed to the intended intervention. The planner must be acutely aware of the group's and subgroup's diversity in history, cultural practices, including health beliefs and practices, language, socioeconomic status, and generational differences. Each subgroup, for example, may represent varying degrees of acculturation and assimilation in its current country of residence. Kreuter and Skinner (2000) defined targeting as the use of "a single intervention approach for a defined population subgroup that takes into account characteristics shared by the subgroups members" (p. 2). Kreuter, Lukwago, Bucholtz, Clark, and Sanders-Thompson (2003) cautiously add that since targeting implicitly assumes that there is sufficient target population homogeneity, one common approach could be used to reach all its members (p. 137). Social marketers, through segmentation of target markets (specific target groups) do not try to develop a "one size fits all" approach but rather "create programs targeted to the specific needs of each market" (Maibach et al., 2002, p. 449). Once the planner has targeted, he or she also needs to be able to tailor.

Tailoring, as espoused by Pasick et al. (1996), implies the need for the planner to be able to adapt the intervention and/or total design to "fit the needs and characteristics of a target audience" (p. S145). Interventions also need to incorporate the use of target-group-specific educational methods and techniques. In their use of the term *cultural tailoring,* then, the planner is encouraged to develop interventions, strategies, methods, messages, and materials that could be adapted to the specific cultural characteristics of the target group (Pasick et al., 1996; see also Resnicow, Braithwaite, Ahluwalia, & Baranowski, 1999; Resnicow, Braithwaite, Dilorio, & Glanz, 2002). The point being made is that tailoring must ensure that all specific cultural beliefs, health-related or otherwise, are held at a similar level. And in reality, individuals within cultural groups can have varying levels of certain cultural beliefs. This certainly implies that before any cultural-tailored health programs or messages can be undertaken, the planner and participants need to understand "how individuals perceive their own culture, the extent to which they identify with it, and the specific cultural values that are important to them" (Kreuter et al., 2003, p. 137).

Marin et al. (1995) believe that health education programs need to target and consider the unique conditions experienced by underserved groups. If the program is targeted only to the needs of the general population, then it might not reach the underserved groups or might not be effective in achieving the desired behavioral changes within these groups. The planner cannot expect that the same health education program found to be effective in one underserved population will be equally effective in another (Marin et al., 1995). Furthermore, the background factors that characterize a particular target group may affect its capability to participate in a program (e.g., knowledge, attitudes, beliefs, values, generational differences, language, socialization and family

roles, acculturation and assimilation, societal inequities, environment) and must be considered when planning any health education intervention (Marin et al., 1995; Resnicow et al., 2002).

Regardless of the level or direction in which program intervention focuses, it will have to be reached through a very intensive process of target-group-specific needs assessment and diagnosis and community familiarity. And, with regard to achieving specific behavior change or health-promotive environments, there is the need to view the cultural uniqueness of the target group because it relates to the way in which group members define health problems, how they identify proposed solutions to those problems, how they select types of activities to be initiated, and how favorable behavioral change, once achieved, can be sustained in that population. No easy task!

Task 2: Evaluating the Program

Did the program make a difference? The planner, participants, program administrators, and program staff want to know what their programs accomplish without being influenced by subjective judgments or political motives. Evaluation cannot be treated as an afterthought because planners need to learn what was achieved and what could have been improved. Evaluation is of critical importance to the continuation of program support and to account for how program funds were spent.

Israel et al. (1995) provide some useful observations concerning health education program-related evaluation issues. They note the complexities of evaluation issues associated with the conceptual design of the approaches and their limitations, and they stress the need to be aware of the different foci of health promotion and education programs and the implications for evaluation. There are some good texts that can assist the reader in gaining more in-depth information about the following important evaluation-related issues: selection of the evaluation study design use and its limitations, issues of instrument design and development, issues and conduct of evaluation-related data collection activities, and issues of measurement precision involving reliability and validity (Dignan, 1989; Dignan & Carr, 1992; Green & Kreuter, 2005; Green & Lewis, 1986; McKenzie et al., 2004; Mohr, 1992; Sarvela & McDermott, 2001; Suchman, 1967; Windsor et al., 2004).

LEVELS OF EVALUATION

Practitioners should be able to apply at least three dimensions of evaluation in their programs, but only if they understand the concept, limitations, and relationship of each—*impact evaluation, outcome evaluation,* and *process evaluation.* Each dimension is used to answer different questions about the program. Impact and outcome evaluation include direct measures associated with achieving the program's stated goals and objectives established earlier in Subtask F. Process evaluation constitutes a more indirect way to assess a program and examines the quality by which specific program inputs are produced as they are thought to be associated with achieving certain target-group outcomes. Process evaluation is conducted before and during the developmental and implementation stages of the program and seeks ways to improve the overall program and its health promotion and education component. Any one of the assessment dimensions may be used exclusively under certain conditions, but it will yield only limited information. When all three are used together, they form a fairly comprehensive approach to evaluation. Each level, it should be noted, is based on specific assumptions that need to be understood before making any judgments about program effectiveness. These three levels are briefly described next and, where appropriate, specific caveats are offered.

Subtask A: Assessment of the Long-Term Target-Group Health and Social Outcomes (Outcome Evaluation)

Outcome evaluation is concerned with examining health or social benefits over time. *The overall health promotion and education program outcome objectives formulated earlier in Figure 7.3 serve as the basis for this level of measurement.* The following kinds of questions can be answered:

- Does the target group of Latinas (at high risk owing to familial history of breast cancer) routinely obtain mammograms at 6 months, 1 year, and 5 years after completing the program?
- How many over a 3-year period or more of time died (in the target group who attended our program)?
- Of those in the target group attending the program that were diagnosed and treated early, how many survived for 1, 5, or 10 years?
- Are there increased numbers of new programs in place, which are available and accessible for breast cancer education and routine mammography screening?

The outcome level, unlike the assessment of impact (discussed next), usually reports program accomplishment at the end of a longer time period. It is more difficult to evaluate health and social benefits because trends or events are not discernible for long periods of time and most populations do not remain stable or geographically in place over long periods (Green et al., 1980). Thus, to evaluate the long-term effect of our community program in terms of a legitimate increase or decrease in cancer mortality, a greater level of funding and resources, a larger target group of program participants, and the capability of spending more time in follow-up would be required. *When using this level of evaluation, one must also be careful not to assume that the positive long-term behavioral, structural, or mortality changes related to the target group that occur are directly attributable to the effects of the program.* As in impact evaluation, all the possible conditions and variables to which the changes may be attributed cannot ever be completely controlled.

Subtask B: Assessment of the Immediate Impact of the Program (Impact Evaluation)

Impact evaluation examines the immediate or short-term impact of the program (or the interventions used) on changes in target-group knowledge, attitudes, and behavior as well as predisposing, enabling, and reinforcing factors (Green et al., 1980; Green & Kreuter, 2005). This is the level of evaluation used by most health program planners because it is amenable to measurement and can be used for reporting concrete results about the designated target group at different periods of time. *The overall health education objectives, health education target-group objectives, and the corresponding instructional objectives (knowledge, attitude, skill, and reinforcing objectives) formulated earlier in Figure 7.3 provide some useful examples to serve as the basis for this level of measurement.*

- By the end of the breast cancer education and screening program, how many in the target group of high-risk Latino women made appointments or obtained scheduled mammograms?
- By the end of the breast cancer education and screening program, how many new breast cancer education programs for Latinas were in place in the target area?
- By X date was there an increase in the number (by __%) of Latinas in the target group who carried out *appropriate behaviors* related to obtaining a mammogram at a community clinic?
- By X date was there an increase in the number (by __%) of Latinas in the target group

who possessed *favorable attitudes* related to obtaining a mammogram at a community clinic?
- By X date was there an increase in the number (by __%) of Latinas in the target group who possessed *appropriate knowledge* related to obtaining a mammogram at a community clinic?
- And so on for the knowledge, attitude, behavior, and reinforcing instructional objectives (see the earlier section Program Objectives)

The standards or criteria for accomplishment and for purposes of measurement are clear. When using this level of evaluation, one must be very careful not to assume that the knowledge, attitude, or behavior changes that occur, positive or negative, are necessarily and directly attributable to the effect of the program. It is simply too difficult to control all the possible conditions and variables to which the changes might be attributed. If care was observed in aspects of instrument design, data collection protocol, and efforts to build in reliability and validity, then one can make inferences more safely about program effect. If the program did not accomplish the objectives, then it is useful to go back and review aspects of the program at the process level to be discussed next.

Subtask C: Assessment of the Quality of Program Inputs During the Development and Implementation Phases (Process Evaluation)

Process evaluation is a more indirect way in which to assess the quality of the program elements that have been put in place. It is strongly desirable to base the process measures on predetermined and accepted practices related to what are thought to be the most appropriate inputs for achieving certain program outcomes. This requires evaluators to specify, as far as possible, the relevant dimensions, values, and standards to be used in the assessment of the development and implementation of the educational program. *Process evaluation, as viewed in the context of the questions posed below, is based on the assumption that if certain elements are present in the program and in the appropriate fashion (usually as defined by the planning participants), the program will have greater capability to achieve the desired outcome.*

How well is the breast cancer education and screening program being developed and implemented?

- Are the educational activities provided to the target group of Latinas *designed* in an appropriate manner and sequence to assist them in acquiring the knowledge, attitude, and skills related to obtaining a mammogram at the clinic?
- Are the educational activities provided to the target-group *implemented* in an appropriate manner and sequence to assist them in acquiring the knowledge, attitude, and skills related to obtaining mammograms at the clinic?
- Are the educational activities appropriately related to achieving the program's objectives?
- During the educational sessions, does the program staff achieve the *desired quality of interaction* with the target group for appropriately discussing and conveying required techniques related to obtaining a mammogram at the clinic?
- Are the educational activities designed and implemented in the appropriate sequence for enabling the "significant others" to acquire the knowledge and attitudes necessary to perform supportive roles for encouraging and reinforcing the target-group behavior (obtaining mammograms at the clinic)?

Owing to the assumption that this level of evaluation is based on, it is important to be able to identify as clearly as possible what represents the value or "standard" of measurement. Where possible, the planner should try to use a "Best Practice" and "Best Experience" approach in the design of program interventions (discussed in Task 1, Subtask G). Unfortunately, many times the "standard" may end up being a rule of thumb judgment arrived at through negotiation with planners, participants, staff, and implementers. Process evaluation, with its limitations, could be used to identify and examine the qualitative and quantitative aspects of the educational segment. Evaluators could look at, for example, the degree to which the rationale relating to the design and implementation of the educational segment is based on appropriate theoretical and programmatic foundations. Evaluators could also examine process variables related to the qualitative aspects of how and by whom the educational program is implemented, the appropriateness of the strategies and interventions selected in terms of their expected effect, staff and target-group interaction and performance during the sessions, and the levels of necessary and expected target-group participation. Saunders, Evans, and Joshi (2005) and Steckler and Linnan (2002) provide very useful and systematic approaches for developing process evaluation plans in different settings.

FORMATIVE EVALUATION

Information from process evaluation activities can also identify areas in which program changes, adjustments, or refinements may be needed to help the planner anticipate or prevent problems before the program starts and during program implementation. *Formative evaluation,* a type of process evaluation, is conducted early in the program's developmental stages and throughout implementation to provide immediate feedback about program performance and program dynamics (Gittelsohn et al., 2006; Herman, Morris, & Fitz-Gibbon, 1987; Sarvela & McDermott, 2001). Formative evaluation information can be obtained through focus group interviews, observations, surveys, and audits and could be used to answer the following types of questions:

- Is the breast cancer education and screening program for the target group located at accessible sites?
- Is the number of programs scheduled adequate in terms of the expected numbers of participants? Is program staff appropriately trained to teach the educational classes?
- Are there adequate numbers of (Spanish speaking and culturally competent) trained staff for conducting the sessions?
- Does the program have sufficient and appropriate equipment and culturally specific educational materials for conducting the planned activities?
- Have the educational materials been tested for appropriate content and readability?
- Are participants attending the educational sessions (making appointments to obtain mammograms) at the times they have been scheduled?
- How satisfied are the program participants with the program staff, the curriculum, and the educational materials?
- Are the educational sessions and screening clinics held at appropriate times for the target group? Does the program furnish transportation to those in the target group who need these services to reach and participate in the educational and screening programs?
- Do the program recipients truly represent the target group as it was identified in the targeted assessment phase of the needs assessment?

Task 3: Implementing the Program

Implementation begins before a health promotion and education program has been designed and initiated and also during and after its initiation. The paramount need here is for administrators and staff to carry out a necessary range of activities for mobilizing the program, keeping the program operational, and keeping it focused on accomplishment of its objectives. *The subject of implementation is approached much differently than the activities of planning and evaluation and has been left until this final section of the chapter.*

Effective implementation depends on the precision and completeness of the *formal program plan*, which should set forth a clear statement of the problem, needs, and priorities; a clear identification of the target group and the particular problem in need of change; an explicit statement of goals and objectives at all levels of the program; an explicit delineation of the strategies, interventions, and an accompanying description of planned activities and methods to be employed to achieve the objectives; and the evaluation plan related to assessing those objectives.

Implementation, then, is concerned with initiating the program; providing assistance to it and its planners, staff, and participants; and problem-solving issues that may arise, including reporting (or documenting) progress made (Ross & Mico, 1980). It is also described as the process of bringing programs into reality and includes "staff selection and training; the procurement of facilities, materials, and teaching aids; and the recruitment of learners (students, clients) into the program" (Greene & Simons-Morton, 1990, p. 33). Other planners have observed that implementation begins when the monies are allocated, authorization is given, administrative sanctions are established, and the management system required for project execution is in place (Timmreck, 2002).

THE COMPLEXITY OF IMPLEMENTATION

Implementation tasks can better be envisioned if they are divided into at least three subtask areas related to the different foci in the development and operation of the program: *pre-implementation preparation, program implementation, and administration and monitoring.* Some of the activities occur early in the program's developmental stages prior to initiation, some during the operational phases of the program, and some throughout the life of the program. A selected listing of major activities that should take place within each area is presented in Figures 7.4, 7.5, and 7.6. Readers are also encouraged to seek greater coverage on specific aspects of the topic from the texts cited here (Dignan & Carr, 1992; Green & Kreuter, 2005; Green & Simons-Morton, 1990; McKenzie et al., 2004; Ross & Mico, 1980).

Subtask A: Pre-Implementation Preparation

A program must have formal administrative (and community) support in the form of necessary capital and operating budgets. This support is needed early because many of the activities within this subtask area begin well before the initiation of the program, including selecting and training staff (e.g., needs and target-group assessment; cultural competency training; marketing and publicity activities for recruiting participants; identifying, purchasing, or acquiring cultural-specific educational and other materials; identifying space needs and acquiring program facilities; and acquiring

equipment. The planner needs to think about all the factors critical for effective program initiation. Timmreck (2002) advises administrators and staff to mentally walk through all the steps and activities needed to implement the program project, including the order of the activities and staffing needs and responsibilities. A selected listing of the scope of activities to be undertaken or completed within this phase is found in Figure 7.4.

Subtask B: Program Implementation

True implementation occurs after the program has been planned, publicized, marketed, and its initially required resources identified and allocated. Health education and promotion programs can be implemented by using a pilot or demonstration approach, phasing in the program over a specific period, or implementing the total program immediately. *Pilot approaches* are used to determine the feasibility of implementing on a larger scale and can be combined with either of the other two approaches. There is also a period of "working the bugs out" of the program through formative evaluation activities (discussed in

---

- Identification, contact, development, and maintenance of support (including financial fees, grants, gifts) and sponsorship for the program by community power bases
- Identification, contact, development, and maintenance of support (including financial fees, grants, gifts) and organizational sponsorship for the program by the professional, political, and administrative power bases
- Identification of staffing needs and specific program tasks to be performed (e.g., planning, identifying resources, advertising, marketing, conducting the program, evaluating the program, making arrangements for space and program materials, handling clerical work, keeping records for sign-up/collection of fees/attendance/budgeting)
- Identification of space needs and procurement of program facilities
- Identification and acquisition of program supplies and equipment
- Program curricula ready for instructional use; preparation of other related cultural-specific instructional/educational support materials acquired
- Development and initiation of media and marketing activities for getting the word out and for recruitment of participants
- Preparation and preliminary field-testing of evaluation instruments
- Provision of troubleshooting, consultation and/or technical assistance to planners and staff on as-needed basis to keep pre-implementation activities on track

---

Figure 7.4   Listing of Pre-Implementation Preparation Activities

Formative Evaluation). A selected listing of the scope of activities to be undertaken or completed within this phase is found in Figure 7.5.

Subtask C: Administration and Monitoring

Administration and monitoring activities related to implementing the program begin prior to initiation and continue through completion or continuation. These activities keep the program operational and promote the program to stakeholders and community through the routine preparation and dissemination of progress and performance reports. This subtask area also involves program management functions. A myriad of activities are conducted, including staff and volunteer supervision and maintenance of program records, program fee collection, monitoring of attendance, preparation of budgets, and providing emotional and intellectual support to the program. Green and Kreuter (1991, 2005) observe the critical need, prior to and during implementation, for the program to operate compatibly with the policies, regulations, and organization under which it is expected to function. Figure 7.6 presents a selected listing of additional activities to be maintained within this phase.

CHAPTER SUMMARY

Planning in multicultural HPDP settings must be a collaborative effort involving the planner and participants. The formidable task of developing and implementing a health promotion program requires the planner and participants to work together to accomplish a complex range of activities, including (a) assessing the needs, problems, and resources of the target population; (b) developing appropriate goals and objectives; (c) devising strategies and interventions that consider the peculiarities of the settings; (d) implementing and monitoring the interventions; (e) evaluating the results; and (f) refining approaches toward greater program effectiveness and efficiency. All must be heard and represented in the decision-making processes. All who are expected to function effectively in multicultural planning must be aware and accepting of cultural differences and should be culturally knowledgeable about the target group.

Owing to the scope and complexity of the planning process, practitioners need to operate from some rational planning framework or model rather than solely on the basis of pragmatic, empirical, or expediency considerations. Program planning models provide organizing frameworks that encourage a more systematic approach to the development of

---

- Continuing contact, development, and maintenance of support (including financial fees, grants, gifts) and sponsorship for the program by community power bases and/or administrative power bases
- Continuing review and needed modifications concerning all program activities, staff, and program participants
- As-needed maintenance of publicity, advertising, and marketing activities to encourage continuing involvement of participants
- Conducting the program; evaluating the program; continuing review of appropriateness of instructional curricula and preparation (as needed) of other needed cultural-specific instructional/educational support materials
- Continuing refinement of evaluation instruments
- Provision of continuing and as-needed troubleshooting, consultation and/or technical assistance activities to keep implementation activities on track

Figure 7.5   Listing of Program Implementation Activities

- Initiation and maintenance of the program's evaluation activities
- Development of overall implementation plan (including the specific timelines by event, anticipation of problems and barriers to implementing according to schedule)
- Timely and continuing review such as facilitation of needed modifications of the overall implementation plan (including the specific timelines by event, anticipation of and dealing with problems and barriers to implementing according to schedule)
- Development of a system for program management
- Recruitment, selection, hiring, and training of full-time and part-time program staff and volunteers
- Continuing review of needs related to recruitment, selection, hiring, and training of full-time and part-time program staff and volunteers
- Supervision of full-time and part-time program staff and volunteers
- Continuing coordination activities related to reducing duplication and achieving maximum efficiency in use of staff and materials
- Continuing review of space needs and procurement of program facilities as needed
- Continuing review of needs related to acquisition of program materials, supplies, and equipment
- Training for all staff and volunteers related to understanding legal concerns inherent in the program (e.g., informed consent and negligence)
- Provision of continuing and as-needed consultation and/or technical assistance activities to keep implementation activities on track
- Preparation of written and oral reports related to documenting and promoting the program; dissemination of reports to stakeholders and policy makers

Figure 7.6   Listing of Administration and Monitoring Activities

health promotion programs for specific target groups. The planner must be able to adapt these models to fit the needs of the planning situation and the cultural characteristics of the target group, setting, and health problem. In addition, the planner must be extremely conscious of and sensitive to the need for building a comprehensive cultural assessment component into the planning process. Regardless of the target group, the health problem, or the setting, the selection of the intervention and educational activities must be based on a sound rationale that considers the relationship between the cultural characteristics of the target group and the health behaviors or changes sought.

DISCUSSION QUESTIONS AND ACTIVITIES

Consider this scenario: (The scenario could have considered any population located within

any community, work site, school, or health care program setting.)

Mortality and morbidity from health-related causes have been increasing for the past several years among several population groups living in a large multicultural metropolitan community.

The local health jurisdiction, private providers, voluntary agencies and community members are very concerned and want to reduce the number of deaths and illnesses drastically. Local government officials recognize that increased screening, referral, and treatment programs are critically needed for identifying problems. Limited monies are available for providing *health promotion and education programs* to selected multicultural target groups. Select a specific target group in a specific geographical area in your county as a frame of reference to work from. Then, break into small (10–12 people) planning teams and consider the following questions relevant to the planning of a health promotion and education program:

1. How would you involve those affected by the problem?

2. How would you assess the needs of the community or target populations?

3. How would you diagnose and prioritize health-related concerns (problems and needs) in the community?

4. How would you assess the specific health promotion and education needs of the target group (i.e., targeted assessment)?

5. How would you use and apply your knowledge about the predisposing, enabling, and reinforcing factors as they can help your planning team identify the target group and select possible program intervention activities?

6. What levels of change would be sought in your program?

7. What specific health promotion and education program goals and objectives would be included in your hierarchy?

8. What factors would you consider relevant to identifying health promotion program intervention activities that would consider the special needs of the target group, the health problem, and setting?

9. What levels of evaluation (i.e., impact, outcome, process, and formative) would you use for assessing your previously stated program objectives?

10. What issues and elements should you be aware of when you use each phase of program implementation (i.e., pre-implementation preparation, program implementation, and administration and monitoring)?

REFERENCES

Abernethy, A. D., Magat, M. M., Houston, T. R., Arnold, H. L., Bjorck, J. P., & Gorsuch, R. L. (2005). Recruiting African American men for cancer screening studies: Applying a culturally based model. *Health Education & Behavior, 32*(8), 441–451.

Abraido-Lanza, A. F., Armbrister, A. N., Florez, K. R., & Aguirre, A. N. (2006). Toward a theory-driven model of acculturation in public health research. *American Journal of Public Health, 96*(8), 1342–1346.

Airhihenbuwa, C. O. (1995). *Health and culture: Beyond the Western paradigm.* Thousand Oaks, CA: Sage.

Amaro, H., & de la Torre, A. (2002). Public health needs and scientific opportunities in research on Latinas. *American Journal of Public Health, 92*(4), 525–529.

Andreasen, A. R. (1995). *Marketing social change: Changing behavior to promote health, social development, and the environment.* San Francisco: Jossey-Bass.

Andreasen, A. R. (2005). *Social marketing in the 21st century.* Thousand Oaks, CA: Sage.

Balcazar, H., Castro, F. G., & Krull, J. L. (1995). Cancer risk reduction in Mexican American women: The role of acculturation, education, and health risk factors. *Health Education Quarterly, 22*(1), 61–84.

Bartholomew, L. K., Parcel, G. S., Kok, G., & Gottlieb, N. (2001). *Intervention mapping: Designing theory and evidence-based health promotion programs.* Mountain View, CA: Mayfield.

Bartholomew, L. K., Parcel, G. S., Kok, G., & Gottlieb, N. (2006). *Planning health promotion programs: An intervention mapping approach.* San Francisco: Jossey-Bass.

Blum, H. (1974). *Planning for health: Development and application of social change theory.* New York: Human Sciences Press.

Bronfenbrenner, U. (1979). *The ecology of human development.* Cambridge, MA: Harvard University Press.

Chen, J. Y., Diamant, A. L., Kagawa-Singer, M., Pourat, N., & Wold, C. (2004). Disaggregating data on Asian and Pacific Islander women to assess cancer screening. *American Journal of Preventive Medicine, 27*(2), 139–145.

Chen, M. S., & Hawks, B. L. (1995). A debunking of the myth of healthy Asian Americans and Pacific Islanders. *American Journal of Health Promotion, 9*(4), 261–268.

Corrigan, P. W., & Penn, D. L. (1999). Lessons from social psychology on discrediting psychiatric stigma. *American Psychologist, 54*(9), 765–776.

DiClemente, R. J., Crosby, R. A., & Kegler, M. C. (Eds.). (2002). *Emerging theories in health promotion practice and research: Strategies for improving public health.* San Francisco: Jossey-Bass.

Dignan, M. B. (Ed.). (1989). *Measurement and evaluation of health education* (2nd ed.). Springfield, IL: Charles C Thomas.

Dignan, M. B., & Carr, P. A. (1992). *Program planning for health education and promotion.* Philadelphia: Lea & Febiger.

Doyle, E., & Ward, S. (2001). *The process of community health education and promotion.* Mountain View, CA: Mayfield.

Fernandez, M. E., Gonzalez, A., Tortolero-Luna, G., Partida, S., & Bartholomew, L. K. (2005). Using intervention mapping to develop a breast and cervical cancer screening program for Hispanic farmworkers: Cultivando la salud. *Health Promotion Practice, 6*(4), 394–404.

Fortenberry, J. D., McFarlane, M., Bleakley, A., Buli, S., Fishbein, M., Grimley, D. M., et al. (2002). Relationships of stigma and shame to gonorrhea and HIV screening. *American Journal of Public Health, 92*(3), 378–381.

Gallant, M. P. (2003). The influence of social support on chronic illness on self-management: A review and directions for research. *Health Education & Behavior, 30*(4), 170–195.

Gatrell, A., & Loytonen, M. (Eds.). (1998). *GIS and health. GISDATA VI.* London: Taylor & Francis.

Gielen, A. C., & McDonald, E. M. (2002). The PRECEDE-PROCEED planning model. In K. Glanz, B. K. Rimer, & F. M. Lewis (Eds.), *Health behavior and health education: Theory, research, and practice* (3rd ed., pp. 359–383). San Francisco: Jossey-Bass.

Gilmore, G. D., & Campbell, M. D. (2004). *Needs and capacity assessment strategies for health promotion and health education* (3rd ed.). Sudbury, MA: Jones & Bartlett.

Gittelsohn, J., Steckler, A., Johnson, C. C., Pratt, C., Grieser, M., & Pickrel, J. (2006). Formative research in school and community-based health programs and studies: "State of the art" and the TAAG approach. *Health Education & Behavior, 33*(2), 25–39.

Glanz, K., Lewis, F. M., & Rimer, B. K. (Eds.). (1990). *Health behavior and health education: Theory, research and practice.* San Francisco: Jossey-Bass.

Glanz, K., Lewis, F. M., & Rimer, B. K. (Eds.). (1997). *Health behavior and health education: Theory, research and practice* (2nd ed.). San Francisco: Jossey-Bass.

Glanz, K., & Rimer, B. K. (2005). *Theory at a glance: A guide for health promotion practice* (2nd ed., NIH Publication No. 05-3896). Washington, DC: National Cancer Institute, National Institutes of Health, U.S. Department of Health and Human Services.

Glanz, K., Rimer, B. K., & Lewis, F. M. (Eds.). (2002). *Health behavior and health education: Theory, research and practice* (3rd ed.). San Francisco: Jossey-Bass.

Goldman, K. D., & Schmalz, K. J. (2000). The gist of GIS (geographic information systems). *Health Promotion Practice, 1*(1), 11–14.

Green, L. W., & Kreuter, M. W. (1991). *Health promotion planning: An educational and environmental approach.* Mountain View, CA: Mayfield.

Green, L. W., & Kreuter, M. W. (1999). *Health promotion planning: An educational and ecological approach* (3rd ed.). Mountain View, CA: Mayfield.

Green, L. W., & Kreuter, M. W. (2005). *Health program planning: An educational and ecological approach* (4th ed.). New York: McGraw-Hill.

Green, L. W., Kreuter, M. W., Deeds, S. G., & Partridge, K. D. (1980). *Health education planning: A diagnostic approach.* Palo Alto, CA: Mayfield.

Green, L. W., & Lewis, F. M. (1986). *Measurement and evaluation in health education and health promotion.* Palo Alto, CA: Mayfield.

Green, L. W., Richard, L., & Potvin, L. (1996). Ecological foundations of health promotion. *American Journal of Health Promotion, 10*(4), 270–281.

Greene, W. H., & Simons-Morton, B. G. (1990). *Introduction to health education.* Prospect Heights, IL: Waveland Press.

Heaney, C. A., & Israel, B. A. (2002). Social networks and social support. In K. Glanz, B. K. Rimer, & F. M. Lewis (Eds.), *Health behavior and health education: Theory, research, and practice* (3rd ed., pp. 210–239). San Francisco: Jossey-Bass.

Herman, J. L., Morris, L. L., & Fitz-Gibbon, C. T. (1987). *Evaluator's handbook*. Newbury Park, CA: Sage.

House, J. S. (1981). *Work stress and social support*. Reading, MA: Addison-Wesley.

Hovell, M. F., Walgren, D. R., & Gehrman, C. A. (2002). The Behavioral Ecological Model: Integrating public health and behavioral science. In R. J. DiClemente, R. J. Crosby, & M. C. Kegler (Eds.), *Emerging theories in health promotion practice and research: Strategies for improving public health* (pp. 347–385). San Francisco: Jossey-Bass.

Huff, R. M., & Kline, M. V. (Eds.). (1999a). *Promoting health in multicultural populations*. Thousand Oaks, CA: Sage.

Huff, R. M., & Kline, M. V. (1999b). The Cultural Assessment Framework. In R. M. Huff & M. V. Kline (Eds.), *Promoting health in multicultural populations* (pp. 481–499). Thousand Oaks, CA: Sage.

Israel, B. A. (1982). Social networks and health status: Linking theory, research, and practice. *Patient Counseling and Health Education, 4*(1), 65–79.

Israel, B. A. (1985). Social networks and social support: Implications for natural helper and community level interventions. *Health Education Quarterly, 12*(1), 65–80.

Israel, B. A., Cummings, K. M., Dignan, M. B., Heaney, C. A., Perales, D. P., Simons-Morton, B. G., et al. (1995). Evaluation of health education programs: Current assessment and future directions. *Health Education Quarterly, 22*(3), 364–389.

Kreuter, M. (1992). PATCH: Its origin, basic concepts, and links to contemporary public health policy. *Journal of Health Education, 23*(3), 135–139.

Kreuter, M., & Skinner, C. (2000). What's in a name? *Health Education Research, 15*(1), 1–4.

Kreuter, M. W., Lukwago, S. N., Bucholtz, D. C., Clark, E. M., & Sanders-Thompson, V. (2003). Achieving cultural appropriateness in health promotion programs: Targeted and tailored approaches. *Health Education & Behavior, 30*(4), 133–146.

Lam, T. K., McPhee, S. J., Mock, J., Wong, C., Doan, H. T., Nguyen, T., et al. (2003). Encouraging Vietnamese-American women to obtain Pap tests through lay health worker outreach and media education. *Journal of General Internal Medicine, 18*(7), 516–524.

Lawson, A. B., & Williams, F. L. R. (2001). *An introductory guide to disease mapping*. Chichester, UK: Wiley.

Maibach, E. W., Rothschild, M. L., & Novelli, W. D. (2002). Social marketing. In K. Glanz, B. K. Rimer, & F. M. Lewis (Eds.), *Health behavior and health education: Theory, research, and practice* (3rd ed., pp. 437–461). San Francisco: Jossey-Bass.

Marin, G., Burhansstipanov, L., Connell, C. M., Gielen, A. C., Helitzer-Allen, D., Lorig, K., et al. (1995). A research agenda for health education among underserved populations. *Health Education Quarterly, 22*(3), 346–363.

McKenzie, J. F., Neiger, B. L., & Smeltzer, J. L. (2004). *Planning, implementing, and evaluating health promotion programs: A primer* (4th ed.). San Francisco: Benjamin Cummings.

McKenzie, J. F., & Smeltzer, J. L. (2001). *Planning, implementing, and evaluating health promotion programs: A primer* (3rd ed.). New York: Macmillan.

McLeroy, K. R., Bibeau, D., Steckler, A., & Glanz, K. (1988). An ecological perspective on health promotion programs. *Health Education Quarterly, 15*(4), 351–378.

McLeroy, K. R., Clark, N., Simons-Morton, B., Forster, J., Connell, C. M., Altman, D., et al. (1995). Creating capacity: Establishing a health education research agenda for special populations. *Health Education Quarterly, 22*(3), 390–405.

Minkler, M. (1990). Improving health through community organization. In K. Glanz, F. M. Lewis, & B. K. Rimer (Eds.), *Health behavior and health education: Theory, research, and practice* (pp. 257–287). San Francisco: Jossey-Bass.

Minkler, M., & Wallerstein, N. B. (2002). Improving health through community organization and community building. In K. Glanz, B. K. Rimer, & F. M. Lewis (Eds.), *Health behavior and health education: Theory, research, and practice* (pp. 279–311). San Francisco: Jossey-Bass.

Mohr, L. B. (1992). *Impact analysis for program evaluation*. Newbury Park, CA: Sage.

Morisky, D. E., DeMuth, N. M., Field-Fass, M., Green, L. W., & Levine, D. M. (1987). Evaluation of family health education to build social support for long-term control of high blood pressure. *Health Education Quarterly, 12*(1), 35–50.

Nguyen, T. T., McPhee, S. J., Nguyen, T., Lam, T., & Mock, J. (2002). Predictors of cervical Pap smear screening awareness, intention, and receipt among Vietnamese-American women. *American Journal of Preventive Medicine, 23*(3), 207–214.

Novelli, W. D. (1990). Applying social marketing to health promotion and disease prevention. In K. Glanz, F. M. Lewis, & B. K. Rimer (Eds.), *Health behavior and health education: Theory, research and practice* (pp. 342–369). San Francisco: Jossey-Bass.

Padilla, A. M. (1980). *Acculturation: Theory, models and some new findings*. Boulder, CO: Westview.

Padilla, A. M., & Perez, W. (2003). Acculturation, social identity, and social cognition. *Hispanic Journal of Behavioral Sciences, 25*(1), 35–55.

Pasick, R. J., D'Onofrio, C. N., & Otero-Sabogal, R. (1996). Similarities and differences across cultures: Questions to inform a third generation for health promotion research. *Health Education Quarterly, 23*(Suppl.), S142–S161.

Resnicow, K., Braithwaite, R., Ahluwalia, J., & Baranowski, T. (1999). Cultural sensitivity in public health: Defined and demystified. *Ethnicity & Disease, 9*(1), 10–21.

Resnicow, K., Braithwaite, R. L, Dilorio, C., & Glanz, K. (2002). Applying theory to culturally diverse and unique populations. In K. Glanz, B. K. Rimer, & F. M. Lewis (Eds.), *Health behavior and health education: Theory, research and practice* (3rd ed., pp. 485–509). San Francisco: Jossey-Bass.

Richard, L., Potvin, L., Kishchuk, N., Prlic, H., & Green, L. W. (1996). Assessment of the ecological approach in health promotion programs. *American Journal of Health Promotion, 10*(4), 318–328.

Ro, M. (2002). Moving forward: Addressing the health of Asian American and Pacific Islander women. *American Journal of Public Health, 92*(4), 516–519.

Ross, H. S., & Mico, P. R. (1980). *Theory and practice in health education*. Palo Alto, CA: Mayfield.

Sallis, J. F., & Owen, N. (1997). Ecological models. In K. Glanz, F. M. Lewis, & B. K. Rimer (Eds.), *Health behavior and health education: Theory, research, and practice* (2nd ed., pp. 403–424). San Francisco: Jossey-Bass.

Sallis, J. F., & Owen, N. (2002). Ecological models of health behavior. In K. Glanz, B. K. Rimer, & F. M. Lewis (Eds.), *Health behavior and health education: Theory, research, and practice* (3rd ed., pp.462–484). San Francisco: Jossey-Bass.

Sarvela, P. D., & McDermott, R. J. (2001). *Health education evaluation and measurement with powerweb: Health and human performance* (2nd ed.). New York: McGraw-Hill.

Saunders, R. P., Evans, M. H., & Joshi, P. (2005). Developing a process-evaluation plan for assessing health promotion program implementation: A how-to guide. *Health Promotion Practice, 6*(2), 134–147.

Simons-Morton, B. G., Greene, W. H., & Gottlieb, N. H. (1995). *Introduction to health education and health promotion* (2nd ed.). Prospect Heights, IL: Waveland Press.

Simons-Morton, D. G., Simons-Morton, B. G., Parcel, G. S., & Bunker, J. F. (1988). Influencing personal and environmental conditions for community health: A multilevel intervention model. *Family & Community Health, 11*(1), 25–35.

Smedley, B. D., & Syme, S. L. (Eds.). (2000). *Promoting health: Intervention strategies from social and behavioral research*. Washington, DC: National Academy Press.

Steckler, A., Allegrante, J. P., Altman, D., Brown, R., Burdine, J. N., Goodman, R. M., et al. (1995). Health education intervention strategies: Recommendations for future research. *Health Education Quarterly, 22*(3), 307–328.

Steckler, A., & Linnan, L. (Eds.). (2002). *Process evaluation for public health interventions and research*. San Francisco: Jossey-Bass.

Stokols, D. (2000a). Creating health promotive environments: Implications for theory and research. In M. S. Jamner & D. Stokols (Eds.), *Promoting human wellness: New frontiers for research, practice, and policy* (pp. 135–162). Berkeley: University of California Press.

Stokols, D. (2000b). The social ecological paradigm of wellness promotion. In M. S. Jamner & D. Stokols (Eds.), *Promoting human wellness: New frontiers for research, practice, and policy,* (pp. 21–37). Berkeley: University of California Press.

Suchman, E. A. (1967). *Evaluative research: Principles and practice in public service and social action programs*. New York: Russell Sage Foundation.

Sullivan, D. (1977). *Educating the public about health: A planning guide* (HEW Publication No. HRA 78–14004). Washington, DC: Public Health Service.

Syme, S. L. (1986). Strategies for health promotion. *Preventive Medicine, 15*(5), 492–507.

Timmreck, T. (2002). *Planning and program development, and evaluation: A handbook for health promotion, aging, and health services* (2nd ed.). Boston: Jones & Bartlett.

Tortolero, S. R., Markham, C. M., Parcel, G. S., Peters, R. J., Jr., Escobar-Chaves, S. L., Basen-Engquist, K., et al. (2005). Using intervention mapping to adapt an effective HIV, sexually transmitted disease, and pregnancy prevention program for high-risk minority youth. *Health Promotion Practice, 6*(3), 286–298.

U.S. Department of Health and Human Services. (1996). *Planned approach to community health: guide for the local coordinator.* Atlanta, GA: U.S. Department of Health and Human Services, Centers for Disease Control and Prevention, National Center for Chronic Disease Prevention and Health Promotion (updated 2003).

Weinreich, N. K. (1999). *Hands-on social marketing: A step-by-step guide*. Thousand Oaks, CA: Sage.

Williams, J. E., & Flora, J. A. (1995). Health behavior segmentation and campaign planning to reduce cardiovascular disease risk among Hispanics. *Health Education Quarterly, 22*(1), 36–48.

Windsor, R., Clark, N., Boyd, N. R., & Goodman, R. M. (Eds.). (2004). *Evaluation of health promotion, health education, and disease prevention programs* (3rd ed.). New York: McGraw-Hill.

Zaza, S., Briss, P.A., & Harris, K.W. (Eds.) (2006). *The guide to community preventive services: What works to promote health? Task Force on Community Preventive Services*. New York: Oxford University Press.

8

Tips for Students and Practitioners

Foundations of Multicultural Health Promotion

MICHAEL V. KLINE

ROBERT M. HUFF

The intent of the first seven chapters was to provide students and health promotion practitioners with general foundations, definitions, key terms, concepts, and theories that underlie the several sections which follow. They were concerned with assisting practitioners to better understand the processes, issues, dynamics, and challenges to be faced in the development of health promotion and disease prevention (HPDP) activities targeted at particular ethnic/cultural target populations. The chapters that follow use these foundations and provide information for practitioners working in the areas of multicultural HPDP. This "tips" chapter summarizes some of the more important ideas and concepts from these earlier chapters. These tips should not be viewed as mutually exclusive of one another; rather, they should be used as connected building blocks and skill anchor points for developing multicultural HPDP activities.

HEALTH PROMOTION IN THE CONTEXT OF CULTURE

The health practitioner needs to be aware that cultural forces, among other social forces, are powerful determinants of health-related behaviors in any group or subpopulation. Beliefs, ideologies, knowledge, institutions, religion, governance, and nearly all activities (including efforts to achieve health-related behavior change) are affected by the forces of the culture that dominates one's group or subgroup. The practitioner will need to identify the cultural factors that can be modified to facilitate the desired health-related behavior change. Thus, awareness and sensitivity to cultural diversity must be reflected in the planning, design, and implementation of health promotion programs. With these above suggestions, the HPDP practitioner should keep the following in mind:

- Be aware of the many ways of perceiving, understanding, and approaching health and

175

disease processes across cultural and ethnic groups and that cultural differences can and do present major barriers to effective health care intervention.

- Be careful in the assessment, intervention, and evaluation planning processes, and do not overlook, misinterpret, stereotype, or otherwise mishandle encounters with those who might be viewed as different from yourself.

- Be aware of the perceptions target groups might hold about your agency or planning group because these may impede the health promotion process.

- Be aware that the cultural diversity of the groups targeted for intervention may present problems that can disrupt the provision of services because of competing cultural values, beliefs, norms, and health practices in conflict with the traditional Western medical model (Brislin & Yoshida, 1994).

- Learn and understand the concepts of culture, ethnicity, acculturation, and ethnocentrism in terms of how these may affect your ability to assess, plan, implement, and evaluate HPDP programs for a variety of multicultural population groups.

- Be aware that ethnicity is used to stereotype diversity in human populations and frequently can lead to misunderstanding and/or distrust in all sorts of human interactions. Once a stereotype has been identified, one party or both parties might cease to look beyond the stereotype to find out who the other party really is.

- Reframe the term *race* to *multicultural*, *ethnic*, or *culturally diverse* to promote a greater sensitivity to the challenges, potentialities, and rewards of working with diverse cultural groups in HPDP activities.

- Assess the degree of acculturation in the target group when working in a multicultural setting, because there is a natural tendency on the part of many culturally diverse individuals to resist acculturation.

- Be aware of the possible barriers that might be encountered when the program is targeted to a community primarily composed of first-, second-, or even third-generation people. Acculturative processes affect the world view of these groups in different ways.

- Recognize that there are a variety of acculturation scales that can be used for assessment, depending on the ethnic group being targeted. These can assist in tailoring interventions that integrate health-promoting strategies into the learning that is occurring in both the culture of origin and the new culture (Abraido-Lanza, Armbrister, Florez, & Aguirre, 2006; Castro, Cota, & Vega, 1999; Marin & Gambia, 1996; Ramirez, Cousins, Santos, & Supic, 1986; Chapter 10, this volume).

- Be careful not to become caught in your own ethnocentrism, because culturally diverse target groups may view you as foreign, ignorant of illness or disease causality, or uneducated about proper social customs, forms of address, and nonverbal behaviors deemed appropriate by the groups for dealing directly or indirectly with their health problems or concerns.

- Seek to become more culturally competent and sensitive. The process is ongoing, and you should always be striving to increase and improve your abilities to work in a variety of cross-cultural settings.

- Be willing to step out of your current frames of reference and take the risk of discovering your own biases and stereotypes and opening yourself up to new and perhaps quite divergent points of view about the world in which you live.

- Become aware of the interpersonal and communication style from which the target group is operating when dealing with persons from other cultures, including factors such as overt hostility, covert prejudice, cultural ignorance, color blindness, and cultural liberation (Bell & Evans, 1981).

Cross-Cultural Communication

- Be acutely aware that, in an interaction between two or more individuals representing divergent cultural orientations, the rules governing the communication process may be different and the opportunity for miscommunication is significant.

- Remember that the typical Western medical model for communication in the health care encounter seeks to quickly establish the facts of the case and often relies on the use of negative and double-negative questions. This approach to the communication process may be seen as cold, too direct, or otherwise in conflict with a target group's more traditional beliefs, values, and ways of communicating and of seeking and receiving health care (Brislin & Yoshida, 1994).

- Remember that those involved in the process of communication should share a common set of rules prescribing how the communication will take place and through what channels, when it will occur, and even how feedback may or may not be provided between the message communicator and the message receiver (Northouse & Northouse, 1992).
- Seek to develop improved communication skills, and be aware that patience and persistence are the keys to unlocking these skills.
- Recognize that health care system variables (e.g., access to health care services, insurance, or financial resources, other demographics) can present potential barriers that you will need to consider when working in multicultural settings.
- Consider the views held by target groups that, culturally speaking, may be in conflict with the general health care system—for example, the concept of preventive health, fear of Western medical procedures, a strong distrust of Western medicine, and services involving referral to Western choices that may be considered irrelevant or inappropriate by many whose cultural or ethnic preferences conflict with the recommendations they may be given (Mull, 1993).
- Consider using strategies that have been demonstrated to be effective in overcoming barriers to HPDP efforts, such as (a) taking more time to explain Western concepts of health and disease prevention and treatment in terms that are culturally understandable and relevant to the target group and (b) designing and employing educational materials that are relevant and culturally appropriate to the target group, using well-trained bilingual/bicultural staff, employing indigenous health workers when working in and with diverse multicultural communities, and

seeking ways in which to improve access to services for multicultural populations.

CROSS-CULTURAL CONCEPTS OF HEALTH AND DISEASE

When viewed across a variety of multicultural groups, explanations for health and disease that characterize many traditional beliefs about disease causation, treatment, and general health practices can be seen as highly complex, dynamic, and interactive. These explanations often involve family, community, and/or supernatural agents in cause and effect, placation, and treatment rituals to prevent, control, or cure illness. A failure to understand and appreciate these "differences" can have serious implications for the success of any HPDP effort. Thus, the practitioner should consider the following:

- Be aware that the health concepts held by many cultural groups may result in people choosing not to seek Western medical treatment procedures because they do not view the illness or disease as coming from within themselves.
- Be aware that in many Eastern cultures and other cultures in the developing world, the locus of control for disease causality often is centered outside the individual, whereas in Western cultures, the locus of control tends to be more internally oriented (Dimou, 1995).
- Remember that if the more traditional person does seek Western medical treatment, then that person might not be able to provide or describe his or her symptoms in precise terms that the Western medical practitioner can readily treat (Landrine & Klonoff, 1992).
- Recognize that individuals from other cultures might not follow through with the health-promoting or other health-promoting encounter and may regard it as a negative or perhaps even hostile experience.
- Acknowledge that many individual patients and health care practitioners have specific notions about health and disease causality and treatment called *explanatory models*. These models are generally a conglomeration

of the respective cultural and social training, beliefs, and values; the personal beliefs, values, and behaviors; and the understanding of biomedical concepts that each group holds (Kleinman, 1980, 1988).

- Recognize that the more disparate the differences are between the biomedical model and the lay/popular explanatory models, the greater is the potential for you to encounter resistance to Western HPDP programs.

- Be aware of the need to be flexible in the design of programs, policies, and services to meet the needs and concerns of the culturally diverse population groups that are likely to be encountered.

Traditional Concepts of Illness Causality

- Be aware that folk illnesses are generally learned syndromes that individuals from particular cultural groups claim to have and from which their culture defines the etiology, diagnostic procedures, prevention methods, and traditional healing or curing practices.

- Remember that most cases of lay illness have multiple causalities and may require several different approaches to diagnosis, treatment, and cure, including folk and Western medical interventions.

- Recognize that folk illnesses, which are perceived to arise from a variety of causes, often require the services of a folk healer who may be a local *curandero,* shaman, native healer, spiritualist, root doctor, or other specialized healer.

- Recognize that the use of traditional or alternate models of health care delivery is widely varied and may come into conflict with Western models of health care practice. Understanding these differences may help you to be more sensitive to the special beliefs and practices of multicultural target groups when planning a program.

THE ETHICS OF HEALTH PROMOTION IN CULTURALLY DIVERSE POPULATIONS

The health promotion practitioner has the awesome responsibility of helping individuals, families, and communities make health decisions directed toward improving the quality of their lives. It is his or her obligation to pursue this outcome with moral and ethical conduct and at the highest level of professional competence, honesty, respect, confidentiality, and keeping one's word. One must be careful to do no harm to others and should not take any intentional risk that could result in doing harm to others. Student and practitioner must recognize that every person should be treated fairly and similarly; norms and rules must be applied to every member of a group consistently and continuously. With these above suggestions, the HPDP practitioner should keep the following in mind:

- Be aware that the potential for encountering health promotion issues that contain an ethical component is quite likely because of the vast differences in the cultural beliefs, values, and traditions of the many different multicultural population groups.

- Recognize that within or outside multicultural settings, the most important ethical principles for health promotion practitioners include (a) autonomy that allows an individual to make his or her own decisions toward self-determination; (b) beneficence—that is, the duty to do good in the client's or community's best interest; (c) confidentiality in respecting privacy of information; (d) nonmalificence—that is, to cause no harm to the client or target group; (e) respect for people and their rights; and (f) justice—that is, equity or fair treatment for all.

- Be attentive to the influences of a client's or the target group's culture when working within ethnically diverse communities because how we examine, interpret, judge, and subsequently act on another's actions is grounded within our own personal cultural identity and cultural framework concerning what is believed to be right and wrong.

- Be aware that in an ethical sense, cultural competence for the health promotion practitioner also refers to possessing the knowledge required for appreciating and respecting cultural differences and similarities within and between cultural groups and working in an unbiased manner to meet the client's or target group's needs.

- Recognize that it is virtually impossible to be a "cultural expert" of all cultures since there is a multitude of within-cultural differences such as levels of acculturation and assimilation, generational differences, and the degree to which each may adhere to his or her cultural beliefs and practices.
- Recognize that sometimes, to resolve an ethical dispute, cultural collaboration may sometimes necessitate working in partnership with traditional forms of medicine and healing (such as inviting traditional healers to the hospital to practice traditional healing techniques in conjunction with conventional medical health care practices).

MODELS, THEORIES, AND PRINCIPLES OF HEALTH PROMOTION WITH MULTICULTURAL POPULATIONS

All HPDP activities stem from a need to prevent, change, or modify risk within the context of individual, group, or community health-related behaviors. Frankish, Lovato, and Poureslami (Chapter 4, this volume) noted,

> Most health behavior theories can be applied to diverse cultural and ethnic groups, but health practitioners must understand the characteristics of target populations (e.g., ethnicity, socioeconomic status, gender, age, and geographical location) to use these theories correctly. (p. 65)

The focus of health promotion has been expanding to include social and cultural influences. To address health problems effectively, cultural factors and beliefs about health must be examined within a context that is relevant to the population of interest. Practitioners who are culturally sensitive in health promotion programs must be able to plan interventions that are relevant and acceptable within the cultural framework of

the population to be reached (Frankish, Lovato, & Shannon, 1999; Chapter 4, this volume). Therefore, HPDP practitioners should observe the following:

- Remember that there are a variety of frameworks, models, theories, and principles that can be used in planning health promotion and education programs. There is a critical need to take the time to study and determine which of these will have the best fit with respect to the cultural group, the health issue or risk behavior, the program setting, and the specific interventions needed.
- Use a theoretical framework in designing programs because this can provide researchers and program developers with a perspective from which to organize knowledge and interpret factors and events. In choosing an appropriate theory, you must first clarify the purpose of the proposed program or intervention.
- Be aware that health promotion or health behavior theories cannot tell you specifically how to plan a program or what interventions to use. They can guide your thinking as to the most promising approaches to planning intervention strategies (Hochbaum, Sorenson, & Lorig, 1992).
- Be aware that theories can be divided into groups according to the scope of their focus (e.g., intrapersonal, interpersonal, group, or community levels of interaction). Theories can also be organized according to their style of focus (e.g., cognitive-behavioral, social, reference group, ecological/environmental).
- Be aware that group- and community-level theories can include organizational change, diffusion of innovation, community organization, communication and media advocacy, social marketing, and many others.
- Recognize that theories can help us understand the nature of health behaviors and explain their dynamics, the processes for changing behavior, and the effects of external influences on the behavior. Theories can also help us identify the most suitable targets for programs, the methods for accomplishing change, and the outcomes for evaluation.

- Be aware that many theories of behavior change and health share a number of common elements, which can be distilled into several valuable principles that can usefully inform the design and evaluation of multicultural health promotion programs (Frankish et al., 1999, pp. 59–63; Green & Ottoson, 1994).

HEALTH DISPARITIES IN MULTICULTURAL POPULATIONS

In general, most individuals in multicultural populations are seeking and receiving appropriate health care. Most are working and relatively well educated, and most are striving to improve the quality of life for themselves and their families. However, many individuals and families in multicultural settings and target groups continue to be at higher risk of poor physical, psychological, and/or social health. The term *disparities* today is most often used to imply differences across racial/ethnic groups. The term is also used to describe differences in health across income, education, cultures, and gender groups (Shi & Stevens, 2005). And frequently, the term *health disparities* is used interchangeably with the term *health inequalities* and refers to patterns of differences in health care access, quality, utilization of health services, satisfaction, or outcomes. The causes of health disparities are not always obvious and are frequently rooted in the social context surrounding modern life. Be aware that personal social position and social class, racism and discrimination, social networks, and other relational community factors have a major impact on the health of populations. Perhaps most relevant to health promotion professionals is that while advances in health promotion strategies have contributed to improvements in population health, these gains in health have not necessarily benefited population groups equally. With the above information, the HPDP practitioner should keep in mind the following:

- Be cognizant, as a practitioner, that there is still a prevalent belief in this country among a majority of the population that health disparities do not exist. In light of improved and available data and research that now communicates the severity and breadth of health disparities, this belief needs to be corrected by increasing the public's awareness of the issue.
- Be aware that health education and promotion professionals are confronted with being able to focus increased attention on reducing health and health care disparities, to understand the major risk factors for the disparities, and to redesign health education and health care interventions to more comprehensively and simultaneously address these risk factors.
- Become increasingly familiar with the research and literature that demonstrate the relationships between health disparities and higher rates of mortality, shorter life expectancy, greater prevalence of chronic illness (such as diabetes and asthma), more frequent risk behaviors (such as smoking, not seeking early prenatal care, and not engaging in regular exercise), and generally poorer health status.
- Be aware that not all minority groups experience the same health deficits and that, depending on the condition, some groups have better health than whites.
- Be aware that there may be even greater variations in health found between specific subgroups of a racial/ethnic category than among the simplistic classifications (i.e., aggregated data) of Asian American, African American, Latino, and white.
- Be aware that there are major disparities across racial/ethnic groups seeking access to health care, including (a) not having or not being able to obtain health insurance coverage and (b) having a regular source of care that he or she can go to for the majority of their preventive and continuing health care needs.
- Recognize that in addition to health care disparities being related to reduced access, there are also very likely to be racial/ethnic disparities in the receipt of preventive health counseling

and referrals, health promotion and education programs, activities and materials.

- Recognize that culture may affect the ability of a patient to communicate comfortably and openly with health providers. Culture may also affect the patient's acceptance of and adherence to prescribed therapies and treatments. Also, in many instances, trained medical interpreters are not available to assist many patients who need them.

- Be aware that without informational materials and education commonly available in multiple languages, certain racial/ethnic minorities may be less likely to receive such materials and services.

- Be aware that rules and regulations have been implemented that require health plans and providers to offer information and materials in the language common within a geographic area or provider service network.

- Be aware that not all health education materials and health-related counseling services are tailored to reflect the diversity in cultures. This situation can make some health education resources unacceptable and even inappropriate to some groups while effective for others.

- Recognize that interventions and programs should build on existing knowledge of the risk factors for health disparities, address in a more comprehensive way the range of risk factors that contribute to health disparities, and unite and coordinate efforts across programs to strengthen the effectiveness of any interventions that are developed (Chapter 5, this volume).

CULTURAL ASSESSMENT FRAMEWORK

Assessment is the foundation for any program planning process as it provides formative evaluation data on which important decisions will be made that govern everything from setting measurable objectives to intervention design, implementation, and evaluation. In general, assessment data seek to gather a variety of information. Often, however, information

related to the effects of culture on the health issue or problem being addressed by the program plan is sketchy or nonexistent. The Cultural Assessment Framework (CAF) provides an opportunity to ask questions in one's assessment that can help the health promoter better target and tailor his or her program to account for cultural variables that could if overlooked result in a program that fails to achieve specified objectives. Given these concerns, the health promotion student and practitioner should do the following:

- Seek to identify culture-specific demographic characteristics of the target group to ensure that variables such as age and gender, social class and social status, education and literacy, language, religious preferences, occupation and income, patterns of residence and living conditions, and acculturation and assimilation are not overlooked.

- Identify culture-specific epidemiological and environmental influences that are playing a contributory role in the development of the health issue of concern to the health promoter.

- Consider the general and specific cultural characteristics of the target group, such as how the target group identifies itself and derives its cosmology and time orientation, perceptions of self versus community, social norms, values and customs, and communication patterns that can help the health promoter better understand how to structure interventions for his or her target group.

- Seek to identify how the target group makes sense of health and disease, including disease causality, responses to illness, use of Western medicine, and health behavior patterns.

- Consider whether the health promoter's agency is or is not prepared to support and/or deliver culturally competent health care services to its service area. This may help identify what agency and staff training may be needed, as well as what changes are needed within the physical setting to help their patients receive the best possible health care.

PLANNING HEALTH PROMOTION AND DISEASE PREVENTION PROGRAMS IN MULTICULTURAL POPULATIONS

Planning HPDP programs in multicultural populations is a dynamic and challenging process that requires systematic identification and selection of a particular course of action. Developing and implementing a health promotion program requires that planners and participants work together to accomplish a complex range of activities, including (a) assessing needs, problems, and resources of the target population; (b) developing appropriate goals and objectives; (c) devising strategies and interventions that consider the peculiarities of the settings; (d) implementing and monitoring the interventions; (e) evaluating the results; and (f) refining approaches toward greater program effectiveness and efficiency. Given these guidelines, the practitioner should note the following:

- Be able to define the level of change sought as a result of your program (i.e., the health education level or the health promotion level).
- Be aware that HPDP programs generally need to use different levels of interventions that respond to a broad level of community concern related to stimulating, establishing, and sustaining an appropriate combination of educational, organizational, political, and environmental strategies and supports needed to facilitate actions aimed at achieving the desired individual and community health.
- Remember that implementing a health promotion program at the community level requires that the planner identify specific health-related factors that affect health, the action strategy to be used (e.g., strengthen community action, build healthy public policy, create supportive environments that require or reinforce risk reduction behaviors, develop personal skills, reorient health services), and the level of action to be taken (e.g., society, a specific sector/system, community,

family, individual) (Chapters 4 & 7, this volume).
- Recognize that planners and participants need to be culturally competent and each must be sensitive to his or her own beliefs, values, patterns, and styles of interaction with other cultures, particularly as these styles could reflect biases or prejudices that could seriously disrupt the planning process.

Health Promotion Program Planning Models as Guides to Practice

- Be aware that planners must operate from some rational planning framework or model that can provide a systematic approach to the development of health promotion programs for specific target groups.
- Recognize that there are no perfect health education and health promotion planning models. You must adapt them to fit the needs of the planning situation and the cultural characteristics of the target group, setting, and health problem.
- Be aware that planning models, such as the traditional models and others including PRECEDE-PROCEED, PATCH, intervention mapping, and the PEN-3 models, can provide you with an overall framework for helping identify and apply intervention strategies for achieving change at the individual, group, community, or organizational level.

Planning Health Promotion Programs

- Be aware that planning in multicultural settings must be a collaborative effort involving planners, participants, governmental officials, and staff/workers involved in carrying out the program. All must be heard and represented in the decision-making process.
- Remember that planners working in multicultural settings always must build in a cultural assessment component.
- Be aware that after target group priorities in health and program needs have been identified, health promotion planners must initiate a more focused behavioral, educational, and cultural analysis and diagnosis.

- Be aware of the need to identify those target group behaviors, cultural factors, and environmental factors that are contributing to the health problem and are amenable to change through health promotion and health education programs.
- Recognize that the substantial heterogeneity (with regard to culture; ethnic background; social norms; and generational, acculturation, and assimilation differences) within diverse cultural groups may increase the difficulty of defining target groups and tailoring interventions.
- Recognize that clumping ethnically heterogeneous populations into one or two broad categories might mask their true health status.
- Recognize that planners and participants can be ready to establish health promotion and health education program goals and objectives only when they clearly understand the relationships among (a) the health problems, the environment, and antecedent target group behaviors and (b) the role of predisposing factors, enabling factors, and reinforcing factors as these influence target group behaviors.
- Be aware that there is no foolproof way to select the right combination of interventions that will ensure the most effective results.
- Remember that regardless of the target group, the health problem, or the setting, the selection of the intervention and educational activities should be based on a sound rationale that considers the relationship between the cultural characteristics of the target group and the health behaviors or changes sought.
- Be aware that program evaluation methods should reflect an understanding of cultural or ethnic preferences, interests, and experiences to ensure adequate and appropriate data collection efforts.
- Be aware that the quality of the ultimate overall evaluation of the program will depend on how carefully the practitioner and participants formulate the program's goals and objectives.
- Practitioners should be able to apply at least three dimensions of evaluation in their programs, including (1) *impact evaluation*, (2) *outcome evaluation*, and (3) *process evaluation*. Each level can be used to answer different questions about the program. When all three dimensions are used together, they form a fairly comprehensive approach to evaluation.

CHAPTER SUMMARY

There are a great many issues and factors to consider in planning, evaluating, and implementing programs for multicultural target groups. Although it is not possible to identify all the variables that can affect these processes, this chapter has sought to identify some of the key points that the practitioner should have in mind as he or she prepares to design programs for diverse cultural and/or ethnic groups. Chief among these are the variables related to cultural competence and sensitivity, including cross-cultural communication patterns, the explanatory models employed by all parties to a multicultural health promotion encounter, and the traditional health practices of the culturally diverse populations targeted for HPDP activities and services. In addition, the practitioner was reminded that the use of theories and models is critical to the planning of programs that will be relevant and acceptable to the target group being served. Finally, it was observed that planning HPDP programs for multicultural groups is a dynamic process requiring a systematic approach to the planning, implementation, and evaluation process and must include a comprehensive cultural assessment component. This can help ensure that the planner has an adequate understanding of the health issues, needs, interests, and potential barriers to successful implementation of the program or services to be offered to the target group.

The next five sections of the book, beginning with Chapter 9, consider five specific multicultural population groups: Hispanic/Latino, African American, American Indian and Alaska Native, Asian American, and

Pacific Islander. Each section includes three chapters followed by a customized "tips" chapter. The first chapter in each section presents an overview devoted to understanding this special population from a variety of perspectives and includes terms used to define the subgroups within the broader population, historical and demographic characteristics, immigration patterns, health and disease issues and concerns, and health beliefs and practices. The second chapter of each section is concerned with how to assess, plan, implement, and evaluate programs for each of the specific groups, including tips, models, and suggestions for more effective program design. The third chapter in each section presents a case study to emphasize points made in the overview and planning chapters. Chapter 9 provides an overview of the Latino/Hispanic population groups.

REFERENCES

Abraido-Lanza, A. F., Armbrister, A. N., Florez, K. R., & Aguirre, A. N. (2006). Toward a theory-driven model of acculturation in public health research. *American Journal of Public Health, 96*(8), 1342–1346.

Bell, P., & Evans, J. (1981). *Counseling the black client.* Center City, MN: Hazelden Education Materials.

Brislin, R. W., & Yoshida, T. (Eds.). (1994). *Improving intercultural interactions: Modules for cross-cultural training programs.* Thousand Oaks: Sage.

Castro, F. G., Cota, M. K., & Vega, S. C. (1999). Health promotion in Latino populations: A sociocultural model for program planning, development, and evaluation. In R. M. Huff & M. V. Kline (Eds.), *Promoting health in multicultural populations* (pp. 137–168). Thousand Oaks, CA: Sage.

Dimou, N. (1995). Illness and culture: Learning differences. *Patient Education and Counseling, 26,* 153–157.

Frankish, C. J., Lovato, C. Y., & Shannon, W. (1999). Models, theories, and principles of health promotion with multicultural populations. In R. M. Huff & M. V. Kline (Eds.), *Promoting health in multicultural populations* (pp. 41–72). Thousand Oaks, CA: Sage.

Green, L. W., & Ottoson, J. M. (1994). *Community health* (7th ed.). St. Louis, MO: Mosby-Yearbook.

Hochbaum, G. M., Sorenson, J. R., & Lorig, L. (1992). Theory in health education practice. *Health Education Quarterly, 19*(3), 295–313.

Kleinman, A. (1980). *Patients and healers in the context of culture.* Berkeley: University of California Press.

Kleinman, A. (1988). *The illness narratives: Suffering, healing and the human condition.* New York: Basic Books.

Landrine, H., & Klonoff, E. A. (1992). Culture and health-related schemas: A review and proposal for interdisciplinary integration. *Health Psychology, 11*(4), 267–276.

Marin, G., & Gambia, R. (1996). A new measurement of acculturation for Hispanics: The bidirectional acculturation scale for Hispanics (BAS). *Hispanic Journal of Behavioral Sciences, 18*(3), 297–316.

Mull, J. (1993). Cross-cultural communication in the physician's office. *Western Journal of Medicine, 159*(6), 609–613.

Northouse, P. G., & Northouse, L. L. (1992). *Health communications: Strategies for health professionals* (2nd ed.). Norwalk, CT: Appleton & Lange.

Ramirez, A. G., Cousins, J. H., Santos, Y., & Supic, J. D. (1986). A media-based acculturation scale for Mexican-Americans: Application to public health programs. *Family and Community Health, 9*(3), 63–71.

Shi, L., & Stevens, G. D. (2005). *Vulnerable populations in the United States.* San Francisco: Jossey-Bass.

PART II

Hispanic/Latino Populations

9

Hispanic/Latino Health and Disease

An Overview

LUIS F. VÉLEZ

PATRICIA CHALELA

AMELIE G. RAMIREZ

Chapter Objectives

On completion of this chapter, the health promotion student and practitioner will be able to

- Explain how the diversity among Hispanic/Latino population groups in America affects health outcomes

- Provide general background and historical information to help other students and practitioners become more familiar with the many ethnic subgroups of Hispanic/Latino Americans

- Describe how culture can affect both the focus and design of health promotion and health education efforts in the Hispanic/Latino populations

- Identify and illustrate why combining the heterogeneous Hispanic/Latino groups into one aggregated population is misleading for both practice and the scientific study of this population

(Continued)

AUTHORS' NOTE: The authors wish to thank Dani Presswood and Karen Stamm for their dedication in editing this chapter and Edgar Muñoz for his assistance with the graphs.

(Continued)

- Identify and give specific examples of traditional health beliefs and practices related to the cultural backgrounds of the many different subgroups of Hispanic/ Latino Americans

- Compare the patterns of the major diseases of Hispanic/Latino groups in their rates and health effects between the other racial or ethnic groups living in the United States

Latinos are persons of Cuban, Mexican, Puerto Rican, South or Central American, or other Spanish culture or origin, regardless of race. The federal government considers race and Latino/Hispanic origin to be two separate and distinct concepts; Latino/Hispanic Americans may be of any race. Latinos are the largest and fastest-growing minority group in the United States. In 2005, about 42.7 million Latinos lived in the United States (not including the 3.9 million residents of Puerto Rico), constituting 14% of the nation's total population. The overall health of Latinos is apparently better than that of non-Latinos, but Latinos suffer from health disparities more than other ethnic groups. This chapter describes the demographics and origins of Latinos in the United States, as well as the diseases that affect them the most and their health-related behaviors.

DEMOGRAPHICS

Population Size. It is estimated that by 2050 Latinos will number 102.6 million, constituting 24% of the total U.S. population (U.S. Census Bureau, 2006). In 1950, the Census reported the number of Latinos in the United States at 2.3 million. By 1970, the number more than tripled to 9.1 million. By 2000, the Latino population nearly quadrupled to 32.5 million, and by the year 2030, it is expected to be more than 73 million (U.S. Census Bureau, Public Information Office, 2007). Figure 9.1 shows the projected 100-year growth of the Latino population in the United States from 1950 to 2050.

Countries of Origin. More than 40% of Latinos are foreign-born, and only 28% of them are naturalized U.S. citizens (U.S. Census Bureau, 2005a). About two thirds (64%) of U.S. Latinos are of Mexican origin. An additional 10% are of Puerto Rican background, with about 3% each of Cuban, Salvadoran, and Dominican origins. The remaining 17% represent people from Central or South America, or other Hispanic or Latino origins (U.S. Census Bureau, 2006).

Age and Ethnicity. Latinos are also much younger than the population as a whole, with a median age of 27.2 years compared with 36.2 years. The youngest group is Mexican Americans, followed by Puerto Ricans, Central Americans, and Dominicans. South Americans and Spaniards have median ages closer to the general U.S. population, while the median age of Cubans is higher than the general population. About a third of Latinos are below 18 years, compared with one fourth of the total population (U.S. Census Bureau, 2006).

Population Centers. Almost half (49%) of U.S. Latinos live in California and Texas. Thirteen states have at least a half million Latino residents: Arizona, California, Colorado, Florida, Georgia, Illinois, Nevada, New Jersey, New Mexico, New York, North Carolina, Texas, and Washington (U.S. Census Bureau, 2006). Along the U.S.–Mexico border and in parts of California and South Florida, it is common for Latinos to be in the majority of a given local

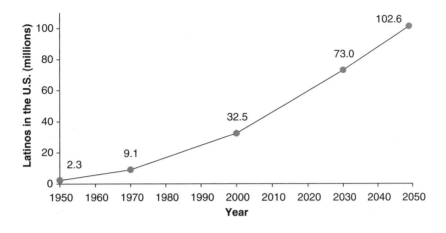

Figure 9.1 Estimated Growth of the Latino Population in the United States (1950–2050)

SOURCE: U.S. Census Bureau, Public Information Office (2007).

area (Natural Resource Defense Council [NRDC], 2004). Although the Latino population has spread throughout the country in recent years, four counties accounted for 21.9% of the total Latino population in 2000. There were 4.2 million Latinos in Los Angeles County, California; 1.3 million in Miami-Dade County, Florida; 1.1 million in Harris County, Texas; and 1.1 million in Cook County, Illinois. The largest Mexican American populations were found in Los Angeles, Chicago, Houston, San Antonio, and Phoenix. The largest Puerto Rican populations were in New York, Chicago, and Philadelphia. The largest Cuban populations were in Hialeah, Miami, New York, Tampa, and Los Angeles. The largest Central American populations were in Los Angeles, New York, Houston, Miami, and San Francisco. And the largest South American populations were in New York, Los Angeles, Chicago, and Miami.

Education. There are clear disparities in education attainment by race and ethnicity. In 2005, 87% of non-Latino whites had a high school diploma or higher, followed by Asians (86%), African Americans (80%), and Latinos (60%) (U.S. Census Bureau, 2007; U.S. Department of Education, 2006). Compared with non-Latino whites, three and a half times

as many Latinos of ages 16 to 24 are not enrolled in school and have not completed high school (7% vs. 24%) (Child Trends Data Bank, 2004). High school dropouts are more likely to be unemployed and earn less when they are employed than high school completers. Among adults aged 25 or older, dropouts reported worse health than high school completers, regardless of income (Wirt et al., 2004). Only 12% of Latinos have a bachelor's degree, compared with 49% of Asians, 29% of non-Latino whites, and 17% of African Americans (U.S. Census Bureau, 2005a, 2005b, 2005c, 2005d).

Employment. Most Latinos above 16 years of age (62%) are employed—the same rate as for non-Latino whites. According to the Census Bureau, Latinos are twice as likely as non-Latino whites to be employed in service jobs and twice as likely to be employed as laborers (U.S. Census Bureau, 2005a, 2005b). They are also the majority of the agricultural workforce. According to the Bureau of Labor Statistics, Latinos comprise 13% of the overall labor force but represent 83% of U.S. farm workers (U.S. Department of Labor, 2005).

Income. In 2005, the median Latino family income was $37,387, only 60% of the average white family income of $62,300 (U.S. Census Bureau, 2005a). About 22% of all Latinos were living in poverty, a slight increase from 2000. Of those, 29% were below 18 years. By ethnicity, the poverty rates vary greatly: 14% for Cuban Americans, 31% for Puerto Ricans, and 27% for Mexican Americans, compared with 13.5% of all Americans (U.S. Census Bureau, 2005a).

THE ORIGINS OF THE LATINO POPULATION IN THE UNITED STATES

Latinos are a culturally and genetically diverse group. Today's Latino population represents a blend of the common gene pool from Central Asia, numerous and varied adaptations, and further mixes with a large number of migrants from other continents.

There is significant debate about the different routes of the initial population into and through the American continent. However, genetic studies using mitochondrial DNA suggest that Native Americans are descendants of a group of individuals who lived in Mongolia some 20,000 to 30,000 years ago (Bonato & Salzano, 1997; Bortolini et al., 2003; Neel, Biggar, & Sukernik, 1994). Waves of migration along the American continent possibly took several routes at different times, some thousands of miles and years apart. This created diverse cultural patterns and biological adaptations among the various groups of early settlers. Many groups inhabited the Pacific coastal lands, while others settled in the mountains, the Amazon basin, and along the Atlantic coast and the Caribbean. The cultural and biological adaptations of these groups show more commonalities among those settling in similar environments (e.g., coasts vs. mountains), even if hundreds of miles apart, than among closer geographical neighbors (Kemp et al., 2007).

Europeans brought to the Americas their own varied genetic pool and diverse cultural patterns that evolved from Europe's active movement of groups of different ethnic characteristics, wars, and the creation and transformation of geopolitical units. On the Hispanic Peninsula (Portugal and Spain) in particular, this genetic and cultural exchange was strongly influenced by six centuries of Arab occupation (Payne, 1973). This Arab-Hispanic exchange is particularly important to the later mix that determined common characteristics among many Latinos in the Americas. The nomadic lifestyles of the Northern African peoples, accustomed to living in relative isolation from other groups and to long journeys through the desert, brought to southwest Europe unique biologic adaptations and their characteristic absence of private property and pluralistic means. After the fall of Arab rulers, most of the Arabian population that had already settled and mixed for several centuries remained in the peninsula. The territory then broke into small kingdoms that fought one another for almost three centuries. When the Spaniards reached the Americas, Queen Isabella and King Fernando had recently unified the territory under the Catholic religion (Payne, 1973). The Spaniards and Portuguese conquered the Americas in a way that resembled their own Arab occupation. Under their reign, disregard for the property and culture of the Amerindians was combined with a recently inaugurated strong, centralized, and religiously orthodox monarchy. For 300 years, they imposed on the colonies their medieval cultural and political structure from previous centuries, destroying the social structures of the Amerindians and isolating them from the transformations brought by the European Renaissance and the Industrial Revolution. Spain and Portugal themselves remained isolated from much of the social and technological gains of the Industrial Revolution and vested their economic stability in the exploitation of natural resources in the Americas and taxation of the natives and colonial settlers.

On realizing the weakness of the Amerindians, most likely due to their lack of immunity to European germs, the conquerors established a massive human trade, kidnapping more than 11 million people in Africa and taking them as slaves to the Americas (Thomas, 1997). The strongest of the African slaves were usually sold to North American plantation owners, while the weakest and shortest were sent to Central and South America and the Caribbean. Many slaves escaped to isolated communities known as *palenques* in Spanish America and *quilombos* in Brazil. In northeastern Brazil, several large communities of free slaves were established. For nearly 50 years in the second half of the 17th century, the largest *quilombo*, known as *Palmares* or *Angola Janga* (little Angola), was reassembled into a nation of more than 30,000 runaway slaves under the leader Ganga Zumba (Kent, 1965). *Palmares* was eventually defeated by the Portuguese and their people brought back into slavery.

Most of the European monarchies remained closely attached to the Roman Catholic Church. The Popes assumed the role of certifiers of the monarchs' authority and mediators of conflicts between different kingdoms. The Church and the monarchs considered it a duty to expand the Catholic faith to their colonies. Hundreds of priests arrived in the Americas to convert the Amerindians and the African slaves. The Church established European-style schools, but for centuries, education was available only to European colonists and their descendants, even though the new rulers had abolished the aboriginal educational systems. Nevertheless, some of the religious orders (e.g., the Jesuit missions in the upper Parana River) supported indigenous development projects and strongly voiced their disagreement with the cruel treatment given to the natives and the slaves (e.g., Fray Bartolome de las Casas, San Martin de Porres, and Santa Rosa de Lima). The ruling church also imported the Sacred Inquisition, an institution used to torture and kill thousands, which served as the main tool to force natives and slaves into submission to the Church and to the Spanish and Portuguese crowns.

The social class brought by the Hispanic conquerors was just as turbulent as the mix of biological characteristics, threats, and adaptations. Millions of natives died of the diseases that accompanied the Europeans (e.g., influenza, smallpox, measles, bubonic plague, typhoid fever, malaria, and diphtheria) (Watts, 1998). In addition, a large number of Amerindians (also probably in the millions) were violently exterminated by war, slavery, and the massive slaughtering of entire populations (e.g., natives in the islands of Espanola and Cuba [De las Casas, 2007]). The Spanish and Portuguese colonists were already a very diverse group, representing the genetic diversity of centuries of domination under the Romans, Goths, and Arabs. More recent waves of immigration to Latin America have included groups of Asians, Europeans, and Arabs. This genetic diversity was immensely multiplied with the subsequent mix with the Africans and the Amerindians. However, the genetic mixture was not generalized, and large groups of Amerindian and African populations remained isolated. The current population of Latin American origin features a wide variety of racial and genetic characteristics, ranging from purely Mongoloids, Negroids, and Caucasoids to mixes with different racial dominance. Today, most Latinos cannot claim racial purity or even the predominance of any particular racial background.

Many of the Amerindians and Africans lost not only their lives and goods, but those who survived the holocaust also lost their social structure and the fundamentals of their cultures. Additionally, most of the great scientific and technological advances of the Amerindians (e.g., highly advanced astronomical calculations, sophisticated agricultural techniques, and advanced crafting skills) as well as their system of preserving and passing on their knowledge were destroyed. The Amerindians' sustainable ways of exploiting natural resources were also replaced by voracious exploitation of gold, silver, and timber to finance the lavish lifestyles of the Spanish and Portuguese aristocracy and the Church's nobility. Under these circumstances, the resulting population was genetically diverse but politically submissive, uneducated, generally poor, disenfranchised, and technologically restrained. After gaining independence from Spain and Portugal, despite important gains in political participation, most Latin American nations reproduced the colonist model under the strong and often forceful dominance of the ruling elites that inherited power from the colonial rulers. The resulting cultures in what is today known as Latin America were decidedly at odds with the traditionally austere, planned, dominating, and empowered society inherited from the puritan settlers in North America. These diverse peoples of the American continent have now experienced several centuries of incredibly rich biological, social, and cultural interaction.

Since long before their territories became part of the Union, Latinos inhabited almost a third of the United States. Several Spanish explorers ventured into what is now the United States to places far north. Many Latin Americans and Spaniards settled here since the early 18th century, long before the American Revolution. With President James Monroe, the United States began a policy of expansion, purchasing Florida from Spain in 1819 and later annexing vast territories inhabited by Mexicans in today's Texas, New Mexico, Arizona, Colorado, Nevada, Utah, California, and part of Wyoming as part of the treaty of Guadalupe-Hidalgo in 1848 and the admission of Texas into the Union in 1845. In addition, as a result of the Spanish-American War at the turn of the 19th century, the United States gained control of the island of Puerto

Rico. Puerto Ricans received U.S. citizenship in 1920, but it was only after World War II that large numbers of Puerto Ricans migrated to the mainland, mostly to the New York City area. In essence, millions of Latinos in the United States never left their homeland; they simply found themselves within the redrawn boundaries of the country.

The frequent mobility of Latinos between their new country and the rest of Latin America never stopped either. In addition, since the Monroe Doctrine, the close—and often contemptuous—relationship between the United States and Latin American nations has created economic and social ties that have drawn millions more Latinos into this country in the last two centuries. For example, as a consequence of the Spanish-American War, Cubans gained their independence from Spain in 1898 and remained under strong U.S. dominance until the Cuban revolution in 1959. The United States was the main destination for the upper and middle classes that fled the island during the 1960s, as well as for smaller waves of immigrants that arrived later. Extreme poverty and lack of basic security in Latin America, an ever-expanding U.S. economy, and geographic proximity have created a strong magnet that brings both professionals and unskilled laborers to the country. The Latino immigrants have assimilated and reinforced a Latino culture that predated the American Revolution. Despite important differences among subgroups of Latinos and their acculturation into the dominating Anglo-European society, the Latino population shares strong commonalities, such as partial or full use of the Spanish language, close family structure, strong community and extended family ties, and highly emotive cultural expressions, among others.

In summary, Latinos are not a newly arrived group in the United States, although many have indeed migrated in recent decades. They are descendants of the first waves of migrants into the American continent and have mixed with groups from Africa and Europe, making it one of the most racially and genetically diverse populations in the world. U.S. Latinos have varied cultural expressions and have largely maintained strong interpersonal ties that provide support and protection for the entire community and serve as a significant health protective factor.

ACCULTURATION OF LATINOS INTO THE ANGLO-EUROPEAN DOMINANT CULTURE

Acculturation has been the subject of considerable debate in terms of its meaning and measurement. In the case of Latinos in the United States, it could be broadly defined as the assimilation into the system of memories, sentiments, and attitudes of the primarily dominant middle-class culture of predominantly white Protestants of Anglo-Saxon origins (Teske & Nelson, 1974). The concept of acculturation is easier to apply to other immigrant groups than to Latinos, given that for many Latinos in this country, theirs was the original dominant culture (e.g., Puerto Rico and the Southwest). For example, for millions of people along the U.S.–Mexico border, the Latino culture has added major elements of the dominant U.S. culture without losing their original roots. Studies of acculturation and health are affected by the difficulty inherent in measuring a change process that has not been uniform and that has undergone various degrees of adoption and preservation of values. Other factors affect the measurement of assimilation of U.S. Latinos. For example, the culture in Latin America is by no means uniform, and many of the immigrants come from highly mixed cultures with aboriginal, European, and African influences. In addition, the mix of English and Spanish, which may well be considered a third language in the future, seems to be the linguistic expression of a mixed rather

than an assimilated culture. Finally, the degree of assimilation is greatly confounded by poverty and lower education attainment; poor peoples share more in common among themselves than with those who are more affluent in their same ethnic group. So it's no surprise that the relationship between health and acculturation of U.S. Latinos is not yet well defined.

Most of the measures of Latino acculturation rely heavily on the cultural traditions maintained (food, family links, groups of friends, norms, etc.) and language preference (Marin, 1992). Overall, there are some trends in either positive or negative directions, but not always in the same direction and often with mixed effects. In general, acculturation measured as assimilation into the mainstream U.S. society at the expense of their Latino cultural values seems to have a negative effect on health behaviors. For example, more-assimilated Latinos show poorer substance abuse, diet, and birth outcomes (Lara, Gamboa, Kahramanian, Morales, & Bautista, 2005). On the other hand, acculturation may have a positive impact on the use of preventive services (e.g., cancer screening) and self-perception of health. With some other health issues, the evidence is not conclusive (e.g., immunization rates) (Lara et al., 2005). Although further research will help clarify the relationship between acculturation and health, the evidence from Latin America and other regions of the world suggests that health behaviors and health outcomes are more closely related to disparities in income, education, and access to health care than to cultural differences.

HEALTH CHALLENGES OF LATINOS IN THE UNITED STATES

Latinos face numerous difficult challenges, including lower educational attainment, lower income, poor living conditions, exposure to environmental pollution, limited access to health care services, and high prevalence of particular health problems. Although this chapter represents a comprehensive overview of the health problems affecting U.S. Latinos, a detailed description of each issue is beyond the scope of this chapter. Despite the many commonalities among all Latino subgroups, important differences exist in their morbidity and mortality profiles. For example, Puerto Ricans suffer disproportionately from asthma, HIV/AIDS, and infant mortality, while Mexican Americans suffer disproportionately from diabetes (National Centers for Health Statistics [NCHS], 2002). However, morbidity and mortality data for Latinos are underestimated by about 2% as a result of misreporting of race and Latino origin in the numerator of the rates (Rosenberg et al., 1999). It has also been hypothesized that morbidity and mortality for Latinos may be underestimated because of the so-called salmon bias: Individuals with life-threatening or expensive illnesses often seek treatment or die in their country of origin (Abraido-Lanza, Dohrenwend, Nq-Mak, & Turner, 1999).

Exposure to environmental hazards is an added problem with regard to the health of U.S. Latinos. According to the NRDC, a large percentage of Latinos live and work in urban and agricultural areas where they are exposed to the dangers of air pollution, unsafe drinking water, pesticides, and lead and mercury contamination. Most Latinos live in areas with air pollution above Environmental Protection Agency (EPA) standards, and one and a half million live in *colonias* along the U.S.–Mexico border, where a lack of potable water and sewage treatment contributes to waterborne diseases such as giardiasis, hepatitis, and cholera. In addition, the majority of farm workers in this country are Latinos and they (and their families) face regular exposure to pesticides, which can lead to increased risk of lymphoma, prostate cancer, and childhood cancers. Poor living conditions also contribute to environmental insecurity. For example, twice as many Latino children as non-Latino white children are likely to have lead in their

blood at levels higher than the action level established by the Centers for Disease Control and Prevention (CDC) (NRDC, 2004; U.S. EPA, 2006). Unfortunately, despite the serious risk that environmental pollution poses for the Latino population, government officials, scientists, industries, farm operators, and landlords often overlook the problem, leaving many Latinos without the information needed to evaluate and prevent those risks (NRDC, 2004).

Compounding the many health issues, Latinos often lack access to health care. In 2005, as in previous years, Latinos had the highest uninsured rate of all working-age adults. Nearly two thirds (62%) of Latino adults (about 15 million people) were uninsured at some point during 2005. This is due in part to relatively low rates of employer-sponsored and public insurance. Although employment rates among Latinos are similar to those of whites, Latino workers are much more likely to have employers who do not offer health benefits (Doty & Holmgren, 2006).

HEALTH DISPARITIES

Several reports indicate that Latinos have poorer quality of health care and worse access to care than non-Latino whites. According to the 2006 National Healthcare Disparities Report from the Agency for Healthcare Research and Quality (AHRQ, 2006), more disparities in quality of care are becoming larger for Latinos, as opposed to other ethnic minorities for whom more disparities became smaller. The report also noted that only Latinos and the poor faced disparities in access to care that were getting worse. Latinos of every income and education level are less likely than their non-Latino white counterparts to have health insurance, a usual primary care provider, a specific source of ongoing care, and to receive timely care for illness or injury and use most health care services, including routine care, emergency department visits, avoidable admissions, and mental health care. Latinos are also less likely to be immunized, to be recommended hospital care for pneumonia, and to be advised about smoking, drinking, and excess weight by their health providers (AHRQ, 2006).

One of the main problems for Latinos is limited cultural proficiency among health care providers. More Latino than non-Latino adults report that health providers seldom or never listened carefully, explained things clearly, respected what they had to say, and spent enough time with them. Only 5% of the U.S. physician population describes themselves as of Latino origin (AHRQ, 2006).

DISEASES THAT AFFECT LATINOS IN THE UNITED STATES

Chronic Diseases

Diabetes

Between 5 million and 7.5 million Latinos in the United States may have type 2 diabetes; apparently, less than half of them have been diagnosed (Burke, Williams, Haffner, Villalpando, & Stern, 2001). The estimated incidence of type 2 diabetes among Latinos is between 200,000 and 400,000 cases per year (Stern & Mitchell, 1995).

According to the CDC, overall, the age-adjusted diabetes prevalence among Latinos is approximately twice that among non-Latino whites (9.8% vs. 5.0%) (CDC, 2004d). There seems to be no gender difference in the prevalence of type 2 diabetes among Latinos (9.7% in men vs. 9.9% in women), compared with non-Latino whites (5.5% vs. 4.5%), but the age- and sex-adjusted prevalence decreases with education level and physical activity and increases with body mass index (BMI) (CDC, 2004d).

The prevalence of diabetes differs among Latino subgroups. Latinos in Puerto Rico, Texas, Illinois, and California have age-adjusted prevalence of about 10%, significantly lower than those in the New York–New Jersey area (8.0%)

and Florida (7.2%) (CDC, 2004d). These differences are most likely related to regional differences in ancestry and other factors.

Diet, physical activity, environmental factors, and genetic predisposition are involved in the development of type 2 diabetes. Overweight and obesity contribute to racial and ethnic disparities in the prevalence of the disease (Mokdad et al., 2001, 2003), but at each BMI level, Latinos have a higher prevalence of diabetes than non-Latino whites. Unfortunately, even though the onset of diabetes can be prevented or delayed (e.g., with 7% weight loss and moderate-intensity physical activity) (Knowler et al., 2002), the majority of Latinos exhibit low levels of exercise and diets high in saturated fats and simple carbohydrates (A. G. Ramirez et al., 1998; A. G. Ramirez & Suarez, 2001; Suarez & Ramirez, 1999).

Regarding genetic factors, the majority of Latinos have mixed racial origins involving Mongoloids (from Native Americans), Negroids (from Africans), and Caucasoids (from Europeans) (Hanis, Hewett-Emmett, Bertin, & Schull, 1991). Centuries of long migration journeys produced genetic adaptations that guaranteed survival under conditions of drought and scarce food. The adapted genes helped the body maximize water and caloric storage and minimize energy expenditure. These adaptations were extremely functional for Amerindians, whether enduring long trips along the deserts in Southwest North America, the hardship of living in the tall Andes, or the strong climatic changes in the Caribbean islands. In addition, many of the settlers who followed Columbus brought similar ancestry (e.g., nomadic or seminomadic tribes and subsistence farmers).

These genetic adaptations must have taken many centuries, and most likely several millennia. However, in the last half century, the lifestyle of Latinos in the United States, and to some extent in Latin America, has changed dramatically. Since people now have plenty of water and food and move around in motorized transportation, there is no longer the need for the body to store water and sugar and decrease energy expenditure. The modern diet of Latinos in this country tends to be high in refined carbohydrates and saturated fat, and meal portions tend to be large. Recent studies suggest that this diet adversely affects adolescents as well as adults: 16% of adolescent Latinas have a BMI greater than 30 kg/m^2 (Ogden, Flegal, Carroll, & Johnson, 2002).

The previously functional "thrifty" genes now promote obesity and contribute to insulin resistance. In turn, insulin resistance leads to a combination of hyperglycemia, hypertension, hyperlipidemia, renal dysfunction, and coronary artery disease, known as metabolic syndrome (Mazze, Strock, Simonson, & Berganstal, 2004; Meigs et al., 1997; Modan et al., 1985; Reaven, Lithell, & Landsberg, 1996). As body mass increases, insulin resistance increases, and the body produces more insulin to manage this resistance, until it is no longer possible to keep the glucose balance. A disproportionate number of Latinos (as many as 80% of those with type 2 diabetes and 50% of those at risk for diabetes) have metabolic syndrome (Gray et al., 1998; Haffner et al., 1996). It is estimated that half of adult Latinos and 1 out of 5 Latino adolescents with type 2 diabetes have metabolic syndrome (Ford, 2005).

The proportion of people with insulin resistance who develop type 2 diabetes every year is about 5% in the general U.S. population and 15% in Latinos. In addition, insulin resistance develops between the ages of 20 and 30 in Latinos, while it typically appears between 40 and 60 in the general population (Mazze et al., 2004). There is also an apparent increase in the number of Latino children and adolescents with obesity and prediabetes (Neufeld, Raffel, Landon, Chen, & Vadheim, 1998). The development of obesity and prediabetes among young Latinos could be related to the frequently undetected and untreated glucose intolerance among pregnant Latinas, leading to

newborns large for their gestational age (Dabelea et al., 2000). These children have a disproportionately high risk of childhood or adolescent obesity and insulin resistance, accompanied by increased arterial pressure and elevated levels of triglycerides and very low-density lipoprotein cholesterol (Meigs, 2003).

Early detection of Latinos at risk and rapid diagnosis of diabetes and associated metabolic disorders is a significant challenge (Knowler et al., 2002). The earlier age of onset, the high rates of noninsurance or underinsurance, and the high costs of diagnostic tests make timely diagnosis less likely among Latinos. The traditional parameters used to detect diabetes in a predominantly Anglo-European (e.g., blood glucose levels) do not necessarily fit the needs of Latino populations. Earlier and more frequent screening is needed. Since diabetes and prediabetes remain undiagnosed in more than half of Latinos at risk, family history is not a useful predictor. All persons of Latino origin should be screened, independent of age. In addition, since the rate of conversion from prediabetes to diabetes is high in Latinos, the traditional biochemical parameters are not appropriate. Latinos of any age or weight with a postprandial plasma glucose value greater than 160 mg/dl should be tested annually, and even lean Latinos with no signs of insulin resistance should have annual screenings beginning at 30 years of age (Knowler et al., 2002). Treatment of Latinos with type 2 diabetes is also different. Normally, selection of treatment is based on whether the patient's underlying impairment is insulin resistance or relative insulin deficiency, or both (Ferrannini, 1998). Because diabetes develops much earlier in Latinos and many of them are obese, insulin resistance is most likely their initial and significant underlying deficiency.

Diabetes represents the most important challenge to the health of Latinos in the United States. More precise diagnostic parameters, more affordable early detection tests, and better tailored treatment are needed to effectively address this challenge. In addition, genetic studies may provide a better understanding of this problem in Latinos and may eventually lead to more appropriate and permanent solutions. Unfortunately, despite the remarkably higher risk, evidence suggests that Latinos do not receive the care they need. For example, obese Latinos are less likely to be told by their provider that they are overweight than non-Latino whites; the proportion of adults with diagnosed diabetes who had three recommended services for diabetes was lower among Latinos than among non-Latino whites; and the proportion of adults who had their blood cholesterol checked was lower among Latinos compared with non-Latino whites (AHRQ, 2006).

Cardiovascular Disease

Data from the NHIS 2004 study of the NCHS showed that among Latinos age 18 and older, 9.2% have heart disease, 6% have coronary heart disease, 19.6% have hypertension, and 2.8% have had a stroke. Three percent of men and 2% of women of Mexican origin age 20 and older have had a myocardial infarction (MI), and 2.3% of men and 3.3% of women have had angina. Age-adjusted rates of MI have increased among Mexican American men but decreased among non-Latino white men and women (Ford & Giles, 2003). The death rate from coronary heart disease in Latinos is 1,130/100,000. In addition, 3.1% of men and 1.9% of women of Mexican origin age 20 and older have had a stroke. The death rate from stroke in Latinos is 43/100,000 in males and 38/100,000 in females.

Obesity, lack of physical activity, hypertension, and smoking are the four main risk factors for cardiovascular disease. Physical activity and smoking in Latinos are described in the section Behaviors Most Related to the Health of Latinos in the United States. As mentioned earlier, obesity is a major problem among Latinos. Almost 20% of preschool

children, 23% of elementary school students, and 16% of middle and high school students of Mexican origin are overweight. In addition, another 17% of Latino children and teens ages 2 to 19 are considered at risk of becoming overweight (Ogden et al., 2006). The elevated rates of childhood obesity are reflected in Latino adults, who exhibit among the highest rates of overweight (61.6%) and obesity (22.6%). Among Latino subgroups, adults of Mexican origin are particularly affected, with 40.1% being overweight and 32.6% obese. Gender and age differences exist, with the highest rates among females aged 40 to 59, with 33.2% overweight and 47.7% obese (Hedley et al., 2004; Schoenborn, Adams, & Barnes, 2002).

Hypertension. Hypertension is a major public health problem in the United States (CDC, 2002) and a key risk factor for heart disease and stroke. Hypertension also predicts premature death and disability from cardiovascular complications (Chobanian et al., 2003). In general, age-adjusted prevalence of hypertension is lesser among Latinos than among blacks or non-Latino whites (CDC, 2005a; R. R. Ramirez & de la Cruz, 2002). However, because early diagnosis and adherence to treatment are the two main determinants of future prognosis in hypertension, the low levels of hypertension awareness, treatment, and control are of great concern. Mexican Americans are less likely than non-Latino whites to be treated for hypertension (35% and 49%, respectively) (CDC, 2005a). Although Latinos seem to have lower blood pressure as a population, their risk of hypertension-related complications is higher, since they are treated for their hypertension only 50% of the time (Hyman & Pavlik, 2001).

In 2002, the age-standardized mortality rate related to hypertension was 127.2 per 100,000 population for all Latinos (similar to non-Latino whites: 135.9), with important gender differences (118.3 for women and

135.9 for men). Puerto Rican Americans show the highest hypertension-related mortality rates of all Latinos (154.0), 13% higher than non-Latino whites. Cuban Americans had the lowest (82.5), 39% lower than non-Latino whites (CDC, 2006a).

Respiratory Diseases

Air Pollution

Latinos have higher prevalence and death rates for the most common respiratory illnesses than non-Latino whites and experience greater exposure to substandard outdoor and indoor air quality. The majority of Latinos (80%) live in areas that have failed to meet at least one U.S. EPA air quality standard, compared with 65% of African Americans and 57% of whites. More than two thirds of the Latino population (71%) live in counties with high ozone concentrations, compared with 53% of non-Latino whites. More Latinos live in areas with excessive levels of carbon monoxide, sulfur dioxide, nitrogen dioxide, lead, and particulate matter (Perlin, Sexton, & Wong, 1999). In addition, because of low-quality housing, overcrowding, and lack of air conditioning, Latino children spend more time outdoors on smoggy summer days. Also, Latinos are more frequently exposed to other toxic chemicals, because they live, work, or attend schools near landfills, waste sites, bus depots, rail yards, industrial plants, or similar facilities, making the health risks from air pollution even more serious.

Asthma

In 2002, more than 2.9 million U.S. Latinos had been diagnosed with asthma. Studies suggest that Puerto Ricans may have higher asthma prevalence rates than any other Latino subgroup, while Mexican Americans may have the lowest rates of all racial/ethnic groups (Arif, Delclos, Lee, Tortolero, & Whitehead,

2003; Perez-Perdomo, Perez-Cardona, Disdier-Flores, & Cintron, 2003). In addition to high asthma prevalence rates, Puerto Ricans may also have higher asthma death rates (41 per million) compared with other Latino groups (16 per million among Cubans, 9 per million among Mexican Americans) and non-Latino whites (15 per million).

The age-adjusted asthma death rate in Latinos is 14% higher than in non-Latino whites. Unfortunately, Latinos are less likely to receive adequate health care and preventive medicine. A study found that Latino children received fewer medications than non-Latino white children, after adjusting for patient race, age, gender, insurance status, symptom severity, and the number of primary care visits for asthma (Ortega et al., 2002). The researchers reported that, overall, 94% of Latino children had not used preventive medications in the past year, compared with 73% of white children.

Chronic Obstructive Pulmonary Disease (COPD)

COPD is the fourth-leading cause of death in the United States. The disease is characterized by a blockage of air flow that prevents normal breathing and includes emphysema and chronic bronchitis, in addition to several other less-prevalent lung diseases. Cigarette smoking is the main cause of COPD, but other risk factors, including genetic predisposition, air pollution, occupational exposures, and secondhand smoke, can worsen the condition. The mortality rate of COPD for Latinos is around 19 per 100,000, and the prevalence is 28 per 1,000, lower than in other ethnic groups. This is most likely related to lower smoking rates in previous decades, but COPD prevalence is likely to rise because tobacco marketing has successfully increased smoking among Latino youth to levels not significantly different from non-Latino white youth and much higher than African American youth. Latinos have an additional occupational risk factor for COPD. Latinos who work in office building services, agriculture, construction, and personal services (hairdressers and cosmetologists) are two to four times more likely to develop COPD than those not working in those industries (Hnizdo, Sullivan, Bang, & Wagner, 2002).

Liver Cirrhosis

The development of liver cirrhosis is influenced by several factors, including alcohol consumption, exposure to various drugs and toxic chemicals, viral hepatitis, and other viral and infectious diseases (Dufour, Stinson, & Caces, 1993). It has been well established that alcohol consumption is a major contributor in deaths from cirrhosis and the related condition of alcoholic hepatitis (Mann, Smart, & Govoni, 2003). Latinos have increased mortality rates from alcohol-related cirrhosis compared with non-Latinos in general. Despite a 30% decrease in mortality rates since 1991, Latinos still have a twofold increased death rate over non-Latinos. Increased risk for liver cirrhosis death among Latino males may be explained by different drinking patterns among population subgroups or other factors. Some groups, especially those of Mexican and Central American heritage, have a drinking style marked by the periodic consumption of large amounts of alcohol. Other candidate factors include socioeconomic status and its component dimensions of income, occupation, and poverty status, all of which directly affect the use of medical care services (Stinson, Grant, & Dufour, 2001). Death rates from non-alcohol-related cirrhosis do not differ between Latinos and non-Latinos, but although Latinos have lower incidence of hepatitis B and C (as described below), they have poorer outcomes, developing cirrhosis and complications most likely associated with an already impaired liver function caused by diabetes and metabolic syndrome (Verma et al., 2006). Significant disparities in access to high-quality treatment

for cirrhosis among Latinos have also been documented (Nguyen, Segev, & Thuluvath, 2007).

Cancer

Almost 40,000 Latinos and 42,000 Latinas were expected to be diagnosed with cancer in 2006, and more than 12,000 men and 11,000 women were projected to die from the disease (American Cancer Society [ACS], 2006). Cancer is the second-leading cause of death among U.S. Latinos, accounting for 20% of all deaths. The median age at diagnosis is 62 years, and it is estimated that about 1 in 2 Latino men and 1 in 3 Latina women will be diagnosed with cancer in their lifetime. The most common cancer sites in Latinos are prostate in men and breast in women. Colon, rectum, and lung are the following more frequent cancer sites. Table 9.1 shows the age-specific proportional incidence ratio for selected cancers among Latino subgroups.

The main causes of cancer death in Latino men are lung (21%), colon (11%), and prostate cancer (9%). In Latina women, the main causes of cancer deaths are breast (16%), lung (14%), and colorectal cancer (9%). Table 9.2 shows the unadjusted mortality rates for the most common cancers for Latinos and non-Latino whites. Among all Latinos, lung cancer is the leading cause of cancer death in men and second in women. The number one cause of cancer death in Latinas is breast cancer (Howe et al., 2006). For the most frequent cancers, mortality rates in Latinos are lower than for non-Latino whites, but as mentioned earlier, many Latinos with terminal diseases migrate back to their country of origin, inducing an unknown bias to the mortality data. Nevertheless, Latinos have higher mortality rates from cancers of the stomach, liver and bile duct, and cervix, and of acute lymphocytic leukemia. It is important to note that stomach, liver, and cervical cancer are closely related to infections with *Helicobacter pylori*, hepatitis B and C, and

Table 9.1   Proportional Incidence Ratio (PIR) for Selected Cancers Among Latino Subgroups Using the Age-Specific Proportions Among the Non-Latino White Population as the Reference, 1999 to 2003

Site	Mexican		Puerto Rican		Cuban		South and Central American	
	Male	Female	Male	Female	Male	Female	Male	Female
Breast (female)	—	0.89	—	0.80	—	0.93	—	0.87
Lung and bronchus	0.86	0.62	0.80	0.74	0.93	0.58	0.63	0.49
Prostate	0.90	—	0.97	—	1.10	—	1.13	—
Colon and rectum	0.92	0.84	1.11	1.18	1.02	1.27	0.93	0.94
Stomach	3.03	3.53	2.22	3.65	1.11	1.26	4.31	5.07
Liver and intrahepatic bile duct	3.81	4.23	4.05	3.31	1.58	2.46	2.14	3.09
Gallbladder	3.26	4.62	2.14	2.95	1.99	1.36	3.95	6.30
Cervix	—	2.76	—	2.35	—	2.01	—	3.02

SOURCE: Ries et al. (2007).

Table 9.2   Death Rates by Selected Primary Cancer Site for Latinos and Non-Latino Whites, 2000 to 2004

Site	Latinos		Non-Latino Whites	
	Male	Female	Male	Female
Breast (female)	—	16.1	—	25.5
Lung and bronchus	36.0	14.6	75.4	44.3
Prostate	21.2	—	25.6	—
Colon and rectum	17.0	11.1	23.3	16.2
Stomach	9.1	5.1	4.9	2.4
Liver and intrahepatic bile duct	10.8	5.0	6.1	2.7
Cervix	—	3.3	—	2.2

SOURCE: Ries et al. (2007).

human papillomavirus (HPV), respectively (Howe et al., 2006).

Although Latinos have lower incidence rates for the most common cancers, they are more likely to be diagnosed with advanced-stage disease and experience lower overall survival rates than non-Latino whites. For all cancer sites, the survival-stage age-adjusted mortality relative risk for Latinos is about 18% higher than for non-Latino whites. For example, the risk of dying for Latino men is higher than for non-Latino whites for prostate (12%), lung and bronchus (8%), and stomach cancers (26%). For Latinas, the risk of dying is also higher than for her non-Latina counterparts for cancers of the breast (22%) and stomach (12%) (ACS, 2006).

Breast Cancer

Although breast cancer is the most frequently diagnosed cancer and the main cause of cancer death in Latinas, the incidence of breast cancer in Latinas is 40% lower than in non-Latina whites. This reduced incidence may be related to earlier age at first child, larger number of children, and less frequent use of hormone replacement therapy (ACS, 2006). However, breast cancer is more likely to be diagnosed at advanced stages in Latinas. Almost two thirds (63%) of non-Latina whites are diagnosed with localized tumors compared with more than half of Latinas (54%), and Latinas are diagnosed with larger tumors (ACS, 2006). This is probably due to low utilization of mammography services and delayed follow-up of abnormal screening results. Nevertheless, Latinas with breast cancer are 20% more likely to die of the disease than non-Latina whites of the same age and with the same tumor size (ACS, 2006). The disparities between Latinas and non-Latina whites in the lethality of breast cancer are influenced by poorer access to health care services and important comorbidities, such as metabolic syndrome and diabetes, but other potential biological factors adding to poorer outcomes in Latinas have not yet been thoroughly researched.

Lung Cancer

Lung cancer is the leading cause of cancer-related deaths in the world, and more than 4,000 Latinos die of this disease every year. Cigarette smoking is responsible for 87% of the deaths, which means that most cases of lung cancer—and deaths from the disease—could be avoided. Lung cancer is infrequently diagnosed at localized stages (14% in Latinos and 18% in non-Latino whites). Unfortunately, the 5-year survival rate for localized stages is less than 50%, 16% for tumor with regional extension, and 2% for tumors that have spread beyond. The Latino subgroup most affected is Cuban Americans, as a consequence of their higher rates of tobacco use (ACS, 2006).

Prostate Cancer

Approximately 12,000 Latinos are diagnosed with prostate cancer every year, and about 1,100 die from it, making this the most commonly diagnosed cancer in U.S. Latinos and the third-leading cause of cancer deaths (ACS, 2006). Incidence of prostate cancer is lower among Mexican Americans than among non-Latino whites but higher in Cubans and South Americans (Howe et al., 2006). Mortality rates from prostate cancer have been declining since the early 1990s for both Latino and non-Latino men (ACS, 2006), most likely due to the significantly easier and more precise diagnostic methods as well as more effective treatments.

Colorectal Cancer

Colorectal cancer is the second-leading cause of cancer death in Latino men and third in Latina women. Nearly 4,500 Latino men and 3,800 Latina women are diagnosed every year, and more than 1,300 Latino men and 1,000 Latina women die from the disease. Colorectal cancer is one of the diseases with significantly different rates in U.S. Latinos and Latin Americans. Although the incidence rate in U.S. Latinos is 20% lower for men and 30% lower for women than the general U.S. population, these rates are still much higher than in Latin America. The shared genetic background between these two groups suggests that diet and lifestyles adopted by Latinos in this country (higher intake of fat and refined carbohydrates, lower intake of fiber, and less physical activity) increase their risk of developing colorectal cancer. The incidence of colorectal cancer in U.S. Latinos has not changed in the last decade; however, the mortality rates have decreased for males but not for females (ACS, 2006). This is most likely due to improved early detection in men, although incidence and mortality were already lower among women. The 5-year survival rate for colorectal cancer is 90% if detected at a localized stage, but it drops to 68% with regional extension and to 10% with distant extension (ACS, 2006). As is similar to other types of cancer, significantly lower survival rates are seen for Latinos than for non-Latino whites when adjusted by age and stage. Less frequent use of screening services and limited access to timely and high-quality treatment are the probable causes of this disparity.

Stomach Cancer

Incidence of stomach cancer is up to seven times higher in several Latin American countries than in the United States, most likely due largely to dietary practices (eating roasted beans, smoking and salting meat and fish, etc.) and the high incidence and low rate of treatment of *Helicobacter pylori* infection. In the United States, Latinos have incidence rates up to 70% higher than non-Latino whites. About 2,500 new cases of stomach cancer are diagnosed

in Latinos every year, and nearly 1,200 Latinos die from it (ACS, 2006).

Liver and Bile Duct Cancer

Cancers of the liver and bile duct affect Latinos more than any other ethnic groups in this country. Latinos exhibit incidence and mortality rates from liver cancer twice as high as non-Latino whites. Each year about 2,300 Latinos are diagnosed with and just over 1,500 die from this disease. Mortality from liver cancer has increased 1.5% in Latino men and 2% in Latina women over the past 10 years (Howe et al., 2006). Liver cancer is associated with hepatitis B and C, as well as with the consumption of alcohol and grains contaminated with aflatoxins. Additionally, Latinos in the United States and Latin America have the highest incidence and mortality rates from gallbladder and extrahepatic bile duct cancer in the world. Women are affected more often than men. Risk factors affecting Latinos include obesity, hormonal factors, diet, and a possible genetic predisposition influencing the secretion of cholesterol into the bile and the consequent development of chronic gallstones. Liver cancer and cancer of the intra- and extrahepatic bile duct are often diagnosed at very late stages. Patients most frequently seek care for sudden jaundice and nonspecific symptoms, usually as a result of the obstruction of the bile duct caused by tumor growth. Liver and bile duct cancers also tend to have rapid regional and distant spread, further lowering survival rates. At present, the causes of liver and bile duct cancer incidence and mortality disparities have not been thoroughly investigated.

Cancer of the Uterine Cervix

Cervical cancer is closely associated with one or more of several strains of HPV. Women in Latin America have cervical cancer incidence and mortality rates three times higher than those of women in the United States, and Latinas in this country show rates of incidence twice as high and mortality 50% higher than non-Latina whites (Howe et al., 2006). Every year, about 2,000 Latinas are diagnosed with and 350 die of cervical cancer (ACS, 2006). The higher incidence of HPV among Latinas is often associated with marital promiscuity, high mobility of Latino men with low education, and cultural factors that make Latinas not only less likely to use condoms with their regular partners but also less likely to even discuss with them the risks of promiscuity. Early initiation of sexual activity is an added risk factor among Latinas of low socioeconomic status. In addition, the higher mortality rate in Latinas is associated with less frequent use of screening services and inadequate follow-up of abnormal results, as well as the aforementioned lack of access to quality cancer care (A. G. Ramirez, Suarez, Laufman, Barroso, & Chalela, 2000; A. G. Ramirez, Suarez, McAlister, et al., 2000). Thus, the elevated rates of HPV infection and cervical cancer in Latinas are primarily linked to low education, poverty, and social insecurity.

Cancer in Children and Adolescents

With the exception of leukemia, osteosarcoma (bone cancer), and germ cell tumors, Latino children and adolescents experience lower incidence of cancer than non-Latino whites. At approximately 350 deaths per year, cancer is the second-leading cause of death for Latino children and the fourth for adolescents. Although incidence of cancer in Latino children has not changed in the past decade, survival has increased enormously for Latinos and non-Latinos alike, primarily due to advances in treatment. Despite this improvement, however, Latino children still have lower 5-year survival rates than non-Latino whites.

Mental Health

The prevalence of mental disorders among Latinos in the United States is similar to that of non-Latino whites. One out of 10 Latinos 18

years or older reports a major depressive episode in their lifetime, and 7% in the last 12 months, compared with 15% and 8%, respectively, in the general population. Eleven percent of adult Latinos report symptoms that can be classified as serious mental illness, compared with 10% in the general population (Substance Abuse and Mental Health Services Administration [SAMHSA], 2006a, 2006b). Recent immigrants have lower reported rates of mental disorders than U.S.-born Latinos, and adult Puerto Ricans living on the island also tend to have reduced reported rates of depression than Puerto Ricans living on the mainland. Latinos tend not to seek direct attention for their mental health problems from mental health services. Among Latinos with mental health disorders, 1 in 11 U.S.-born and 1 in 20 foreign-born contact a mental health professional. Instead, mental ailments such as depression are often related to physical health and are more commonly reported to primary caregivers and even to religious ministers. Symptoms are usually not described as feeling depressed but as feeling nervous or tired, or as changes in sleeping or eating patterns, restlessness or irritability, and difficulty concentrating or remembering.

Barriers to using mental health care services among Latinos include low awareness of mental diseases, lack of insurance or of coverage for mental disorder treatment, need for transportation, language issues, and the stigma attached to mental health disease (AHRQ, 2006). It is extremely difficult for Spanish-speaking patients to find Spanish-speaking mental health practitioners, and lack of cultural competence in mental health services exacerbates the problem. The sensitive character of mental disorders makes translation services a less-than-ideal alternative. Bilingual patients are evaluated differently when interviewed in English as opposed to Spanish, and the lack of culturally appropriate and well-validated diagnostic instruments often results in misdiagnosis of mental health disease among Latinos (Añez, Paris, Bedregal, Davidson, & Grilo, 2005). In addition, Latinos may not respond to individual and group therapies in the same way as non-Latinos.

Injuries

Intentional and unintentional injuries are the third-leading cause of death among Latinos of all ages, with about 14,000 deaths in 2003. Unintentional injuries are the number one cause of death among those aged 1 to 34, while homicides are the second-leading cause of death among Latinos ages 10 to 24 (NCHS, 2005). Alcohol seems to be involved in automotive accidents more often among Latinos than among other ethnic groups. Suicide is the third-leading cause of death among 15- to 24-year-old Latinos, and men are nearly six times more likely to commit suicide than women (Mallonee, 2003). Seniors (65 years and older) show the highest suicide death rate, followed by persons 25 to 34 years. Nevertheless, suicide and homicide rates among Latinos have been declining since 1990.

Occupational Injuries

Latinos comprise a significant proportion of the unskilled labor force in the United States, and occupational injuries are a major problem. Non-agricultural Latino workers are reported to have a higher risk of occupational injuries than other workers (Pransky et al., 2002), and most of those who suffer disabling injuries lack health or disability insurance, becoming an enormous burden for their families. The number of Latino workers tripled between 1992 and 2003. During this period, three occupational groups accounted for nearly 77% of all fatal occupational injuries among Latino workers: operators, fabricators, and laborers (41.4%, or 3,128 cases); precision production, craft, and repair occupations (19.9%, or 1,504 cases); and farming, forestry, and fishing (16.2%, or 1,225 cases) (National Institute for Occupational Safety and Health, 2004). The proportion of Latino laborers in the construction workforce increased from 9% in 1992 to 21% in 2003.

During this time, the number of work-related deaths among Latino construction workers more than doubled, from 108 to 263 (Dong, Men, & Haile, 2005; Dong & Platner, 2004).

Maternal Health

In general, Latinas have shown better maternal outcomes and more protective behaviors than non-Latinas (Morales, Lara, Kington, Valdez, & Escarce, 2002; Phares et al., 2004). For example, pregnant Latinas have lower rates of tobacco and alcohol use and higher rates of breastfeeding (Franzini, Ribble, & Keddie, 2001; Rassin et al., 1994). Latinas have similar rates of preterm and very preterm delivery as well as of low birth weight and very low birth weight as non-Latina whites, and both groups exhibit much better outcomes than African Americans and Native Americans (CDC, 2004b; Martin et al., 2005). However, other practices put Latina mothers and infants at higher risk. For example, the percentage of pregnant Latinas who do not start prenatal care in the first trimester is twice as high as non-Latina whites (23% vs. 11%). In addition, pregnancy-related deaths occur more frequently in Latina women than in non-Latina whites. The pregnancy-related mortality ratio for Latinas is almost twice as high as the ratio for non-Latina whites (Hopkins et al., 1999). Latinas are also less likely to put their infants to sleep in the recommended back position (CDC, 2004b; Martin et al., 2005). A particular problem that has received little attention from the scientific community is the excess risk that Latina mothers and infants experience from delivering overweight babies, which is associated with elevated rate of gestational diabetes (e.g., complicated deliveries, postnatal hypoglycemia, and increased risk of the child developing diabetes during childhood or later).

Birth Defects

Latina women are at higher risk of delivering a child with life-threatening or disabling birth defects than non-Latina whites. For example, Latinas' risk of neural tube defects (spina bifida, hydrocephalus, and anencephaly) is 1.5 to 3 times higher than that of non-Latina whites. Most unborn children affected by neural tube defects do not survive to birth, and those who do are usually severely disabled. Neural tube defects are closely related to lower levels of folate in blood. Latinas are less likely to have heard about folic acid, to know it can prevent birth defects, and to take vitamins containing folic acid and consume fortified food (Phares et al., 2004). In addition, a significant proportion of Latinas may still consume unprocessed corn in their diets (tortillas and other maize products that contain whole ground corn). Unprocessed corn has been known to contain fumonisin, a toxin produced by fungi, which interferes with the cellular uptake of folic acid (Marasas et al., 2004). Possibly associated with the consumption of unprocessed maize, in the early 1990s Latina women in the Rio Grande Valley of Texas gave birth to babies with neural tube defects at a rate of 33 per 10,000 live births, approximately 6 times the U.S. national average for non-Latinas.

Place of maternal birth may have some influence on birth defects and perinatal mortality associated with birth defects. Foreign-born Latinas could have up to a 30% lower general risk of congenital malformations, 15% lower risk of cardiovascular defects, 25% lower risk of central nervous system defects, and 20% lower risk of multiple defects (Zhu, Druschel, & Lin, 2006). However, in general, this risk for Latinas is still higher than for non-Latina whites, and the disparity in perinatal mortality associated with birth defects between infants of Latina mothers and infants of non-Latina white mothers increased significantly from 1989 to 2002 (Yang, Greenland, & Flanders, 2006).

Infectious Diseases

Tuberculosis

Tuberculosis is a mycobacterial infection that typically affects the lungs, although other organs are sometimes involved. The disease is spread from person to person through the air. Infection usually requires close contact with someone with active tuberculosis over a long period of time. While most people who are infected with the disease will never become sick or have symptoms, some will develop the active disease. An estimated 10 million to 15 million people in the United States are infected with tuberculosis, and 10% of them will develop the active disease at some time in their lives (CDC, 2005b). Despite the decline in tuberculosis in this country, the rate in Latinos (9.5 per 100,000) is nearly eight times greater than in non-Latino whites (1.3 per 100,000). Although they represent only 13% of the total U.S. population, Latinos account for almost a third of all new cases of newly diagnosed tuberculosis and 45% of cases in foreign-born persons. In the past decade, many Latin American countries have installed private-based health care reforms that have impaired the appropriate functioning of disease prevention and control programs that depended heavily on community mobilization. Tuberculosis has been one of the most affected programs, with dispersion of efforts and lack of unified treatment protocols, leading to multidrug resistance. In fact, most cases (80%) of multidrug-resistant tuberculosis appear in recent immigrants. Most cases in Latinos concentrate along the U.S.–Mexico border in Arizona, Colorado, New Mexico, and Texas, and in Florida (CDC, 2005b). Nevertheless, the overall rate of tuberculosis in U.S. Latinos has decreased about 50% since 1992.

Influenza

Among all races/ethnicities, Latinos have the lowest age-adjusted mortality rates due to influenza and pneumonia. However, influenza/pneumonia is a leading cause of death, particularly among Latinos above 65 years (more than 80% of all pneumonia deaths among Latinos). Unfortunately, only about half (49%) of Latinos above 65 years receive influenza or pneumonia vaccinations, compared with over two thirds of non-Latino whites (69%) (CDC, 2004a). Lower rates of vaccination in Latino older adults are related to low access to health care, low socioeconomic status, low education level, large family size, language barriers, inadequate knowledge about vaccines and disease prevention, preconceived ideas about vaccines as being ineffective, and low motivation of primary care providers to recommend immunization to older Latinos (CDC, 2004a).

Acquired Immune Deficiency Syndrome (AIDS)

HIV/AIDS continues to disproportionately affect Latinos, who represent 15% of all AIDS cases in the United States. Sixteen percent of all women reported with AIDS are Latinos (CDC, 2004c). Men who have sex with men and, increasingly, heterosexual transmission are major factors in the spread of HIV in Latinos. In 2002, 3,321 (17%) of the 26,464 HIV-positive diagnoses occurred among Latinos. The AIDS incidence for Latinos was 19.2/100,000, more than three times the rate for non-Latino whites (5.9/100,000) (CDC, 2004c). In addition, Latinos with HIV infection are more likely than whites and African Americans to have their condition turn into AIDS within 12 months of diagnosis (AHRQ, 2006). Latino men are more than three times more likely to have AIDS than Latina women. In 2002, 3,056 Latinos died from AIDS, and there were 76,052 Latinos living with AIDS, which represents 20% of all AIDS cases.

Hepatitis

Hepatitis A. Hepatitis A is an acute and transitory inflammation of the liver caused by infection with hepatitis A virus (HAV). Infection with HAV most often occurs as a result of contact with an infected person or eating contaminated food or water. Hepatitis

A rates are higher among Latinos than among non-Latinos. Since the introduction of hepatitis A vaccine in the late 1990s, the number of hepatitis A cases in the United States has reached historic lows, but the vaccine is not universally given to all children in poor countries, and frequent international travel puts Latinos at higher risk (Weinberg et al., 2004). In addition, Latino children who live in urban areas of the U.S–Mexico border have one of the highest incidence rates of hepatitis A in the United States, which is associated with cross-border travel to Mexico and food-borne exposures during travel (CDC, 2007).

Hepatitis B. Infection with hepatitis B virus can cause long-term damage to the liver, including cirrhosis, liver cancer, and liver failure. The virus is spread by direct contact with the blood or body fluids of an infected person by having sex or sharing needles with an infected person or by mother-to-baby transmission during childbirth. Latinos have rates of hepatitis B infection approximately 30% lower than non-Latino whites in people aged 18 to 39 but 25% higher in people above 40 years (CDC, 2007). The incidence of hepatitis B in the United States has greatly decreased since the introduction of an effective vaccine; unfortunately, Latinos at high risk are less likely to receive the vaccine (AHRQ, 2006).

Hepatitis C. Hepatitis C results from infection with hepatitis C virus (HCV) and causes between 40% and 60% of the cases of chronic liver disease in the United States. The prevalence of hepatitis C among Latinos is estimated at 2.1%, significantly higher than the estimated 1.8% in the general population and 1.5% for non-Latino whites (CDC, 2007). The main risk factors for hepatitis C are high-risk sexual behavior and injection drug use, and tattooing has also been implicated among Latinos. Some reports suggest that Latinos have added factors that may worsen the condition and accelerate its progression, such as late diagnosis, obesity, and associated liver disease. Other problems include access to care and low awareness of hepatitis C among Latinos. Information about hepatitis C in the Latino community is surprisingly scarce, given the higher incidence, and clearly more studies with Latinos are needed.

BEHAVIORS MOST RELATED TO THE HEALTH OF LATINOS IN THE UNITED STATES

Diet

Latinos in the United States have adopted a combination of traditional dietary patterns and practices of their local communities. Despite several commonalities, there are many differences in the diet and food preparation practices among the Latino subgroups. Among the common features are the high consumption of grains and beans and the central role of the family in the preparation and consumption of meals (Romero-Gwynn et al., 1992, 1993). Latinos tend to eat more rice but less pasta and ready-to-eat cereals than non-Latino whites. Latinos are also less likely to consume vegetables, except tomatoes, and to eat fruits at a slightly higher rate. Latinos are more than twice as likely to drink whole milk and much less likely to drink low-fat or skim milk. They also tend to eat more beef, eggs, and legumes, and less processed meats, fats, oils, sugars, and candy. The Latino diet (especially that of Mexican Americans) provides lower total fat and higher dietary fiber intake. However, intake of vitamin E, calcium, and zinc are lower than the Recommended Daily Allowances (U.S. Department of Agriculture, 2007).

Acculturation and Diet

Acculturation is strongly linked to eating and physical activity patterns among Latinos. Latinos who use Spanish as their primary language tend to have less sedentary lifestyles and

consume less fat, saturated fat, and cholesterol (Aldrich & Variyam, 2000). The traditional Latino diets attached to cultural practices, rather than education or awareness of the food-disease relationship, seem to be the reason for some healthy eating practices among Latinos with low acculturation. For example, despite their lower socioeconomic status, first-generation Mexican American women tend to exhibit higher intake of protein, vitamins A and C, folic acid, and calcium than second-generation Mexican American or non-Latino white women. On the other hand, second-generation Mexican American women have diets closer to their non-Latino counterparts of similar socioeconomic status (Guendelman & Abrams, 1995). This is closely related to the risks of metabolic syndrome and diabetes described above, with the changing diet and the more sedentary lifestyles adding enormous risk to the genetic predisposition in Latinos. In addition, the diets of poor pregnant Latinas in the United States tend to be deficient in dietary iron, vitamin A, and calcium. These changes are common in all Latino subgroups but are more pronounced in some (e.g., Mexican Americans in large urban areas) and are associated with income, education, stress, and depression.

The Diets of Latinos of Mexican and Central American Origin

The majority of Latinos in this country are of Mexican and Central American descent, and their foods are more widely consumed by other Latinos. The diets of Latinos of Mexican and Central American origin (Guatemala, Nicaragua, Honduras, El Salvador, Belize, and Costa Rica) are closer to each other than to the diets of other Latino groups, although there are important differences in the methods of preparation. The basis of their traditional diet is corn and beans, adding animal products and some vegetables. Rice is also commonly consumed, as well as wheat, dairy products, and noodles. The consumption of meat and animal products is determined by their cost, not by their nutritional value. Beef, pork, chicken, fish, and eggs are all included, as well as milk and cheese in abundance. Sour cream is a common addition to many dishes, and pastries and other sweet wheat products are also frequently consumed. They also tend to eat fruits frequently, as well as chili peppers, tomatoes, and avocado and other vegetables, although their use of green leafy and cruciferous vegetables is very low (American Dietetic Association, 1998; Sanjur, 1995).

Generally, the diet of Mexican and Central Americans is nutritionally complete, thanks to the combination of corn/rice and beans, which provides an excellent supply of complex protein. When tortillas are made of limed corn, liming makes the calcium and niacin in the tortilla more bioavailable. In addition, traditionally prepared corn tortillas have added iron and zinc. Beans provide vitamins of the B complex, magnesium, folate, and fiber. The tomato and chili-based salsas, along with frequently used garlic and limes/lemons are important sources of vitamin C (Sanjur, 1995). Unfortunately, several unhealthy components have been added to the traditional diet of Mexican and Central Americans in the United States. They have a tendency to choose high-fat products such as sausage and fried pork rinds (*chicharron*), lard, processed foods, and large amounts of sugar, refined flour, and other hydrogenated fats (Romero-Gwynn et al., 1993). Comparing the diets of Mexican residents with newly arrived Mexican American immigrants and second-generation Mexican Americans, acculturated Mexican Americans consume less lard and somewhat more fruits, vegetables, and milk than either newly arrived immigrants or Mexican residents (Guendelman & Abrams, 1995). However, they also consume less corn tortillas, beans, soups, stews, gruels, and fruit-based drinks, and more meat, sweetened ready-to-eat breakfast cereals, soft drinks, candy, cakes, ice cream, snack chips, and salad dressings.

The Diets of Latinos of South American and Caribbean Origin

The eating habits of Latinos of South American and Caribbean origin vary from country to country (Kittler & Sucher, 2001). Some regions feature a largely maize-based diet, while other regions have a rice-based diet. Grilled meats are popular. Brazilian foods have heavy Portuguese, African, and native influences. The Portuguese contributed dried salt cod, *linguiça* (sausage), spicy meat stews, and desserts such as corn and rice pudding. African slaves brought okra, *dendê* oil (palm oil), and peppercorns. The most traditional Brazilian food is *feijoada completa*, which consists of black beans cooked with smoked meats and sausages served with rice, sliced oranges, boiled greens, and hot sauce. It is topped with toasted cassava meal (Hamre, 2007). Venezuelan and Colombian foods show a strong Spanish influence. Many foods are cooked or served with olive oil, cheese, parsley, cilantro, garlic, and onions. Chicken and beef stew with plantains, potatoes, yucca, and other starchy vegetables are popular among Colombians and Venezuelans (Hamre, 2007). As with Central Americans, they prepare a cornmeal bread (*arepa*) that accompanies many dishes and is served in different ways. Rice and various beans are also very frequently included in their diet, as well as plantain. Although Latinos from the southern cone also consume corn products, wheat bread is an important part of their diet. In addition, they eat significant quantities of beef and pasta. The diets of Peruvians and Ecuadorians include large amounts of potatoes and corn, and they tend to consume more seafood than other Latinos. Latinos from the Spanish-speaking Caribbean (Dominican Republic, Puerto Rico, and Cuba) also consume rice, beans, seafood, meat products, and plantain (Hamre, 2007). Coffee is a major beverage among all Latinos of South American and Caribbean origin, especially Colombians,

Ecuadorians, Brazilians, Cubans, and Argentinians. Yerba maté is a caffeinated, tealike beverage favored by Latinos from the Southern cone. Argentinians, Chileans, and Brazilians are also frequent consumers of wine.

Physical Activity

Latino adults have among the highest rates of overweight (54%) and obesity (24.6%), and of sedentary (46%) lifestyle. It has been argued that obesity stems from socioeconomic variables and not race and ethnicity, but even when these confounding variables are controlled for, Latinos sill show significantly higher BMIs (Winkleby, Gardner, & Taylor, 1996). While 49.9% of white women surveyed in the Behavioral Risk Factor Surveillance System (BRFSS) were meeting the recommendations for physical activity, only 36% of Latinas were compliant (Wilbur, Chandler, Dancy, & Lee, 2003). According to the CDC, the age-adjusted percentage of Latino adults 18 years and above engaging in regular physical activity decreased from 23% to 20% from 2000 to 2006, while those reporting no activity increased from 53% to 56% in the same period (NCHS, 2006). Unfortunately, obese Latino adults report being counseled about exercise less often than non-Latino whites (AHRQ, 2006).

Cancer Screening

Factors that influence participation of Latina women in the utilization of screening services include age, income, education, health insurance coverage, language proficiency, physician referrals, and system barriers. Other factors are cultural beliefs regarding modesty and sexual behavior, fatalism, acculturation factors unrelated to language use, family-centered values, and existing social support networks. The degree to which Latino population groups in each locale hold onto beliefs about

cancer may play an important role in levels of participation (CDC, 2004a; A. G. Ramirez, Suarez, Laufman, et al., 2000; A. G. Ramirez, Suarez, McAlister, et al., 2000; A. G. Ramirez, Talavera, et al., 2000).

Breast Cancer Screening

Since 1987, the use of breast cancer screening has been increasing among all racial and ethnic groups, and the gap in the prevalence of recent mammography use between Latinas and non-Latino white women has narrowed to about 5% (ACS, 2006). Two out of three Latinas aged 40 and older (66%) have had a mammogram within the past 2 years, compared with 71% of non-Latina whites. Among Latino subgroups, women of Central, South American, and Cuban origin show a higher prevalence of breast cancer screening (75%) than women of Mexican descent (64%). As noted earlier, despite great improvement in breast cancer screening rates, Latinas are often diagnosed with advanced-stage disease, largely due to lower frequency of and longer intervals between mammograms and lack of timely follow-up of suspicious mammograms (ACS, 2006).

Research shows that Latina women are less likely than non-Latina whites to believe that they are at risk for breast cancer and to incorrectly believe that mammograms are a method of preventing and treating breast cancer rather than detecting breast cancer. Breast cancer is perceived as a private matter among women in the Latino culture, and for this reason, many women do not seek out breast health services or receive the support they need when facing a possible breast cancer diagnosis. The lower rates of breast cancer screening among Latinas can also be attributed to low income, low educational attainment, lack of health insurance, language barriers, and lack of physician referrals. Distrust of doctors can also play a part in the decision of some women to forego basic breast health care (A. G. Ramirez, Suarez, Laufman, et al., 2000; A. G. Ramirez, Talavera, et al., 2000).

Colorectal Cancer Screening

Latinos aged 50 and older are less likely to have had a recent screening test for colorectal cancer than non-Latino whites—30% and 44%, respectively. There are differences in the recent use of colorectal cancer tests by country of origin among Latinos. Individuals of Mexican origin, for instance, are less likely than other Latinos to have had recent colorectal cancer screening. Machismo and other cultural barriers play a significant role in the lower rates of colorectal cancer screening, but lower income, lower education, and lack of health insurance are also important factors (ACS, 2006; Talavera et al., 2002).

Cervical Cancer Screening

While Latina women historically have been less likely to participate in cervical cancer screening compared with non-Latina whites, participation rates have improved in recent decades (ACS, 2006). The prevalence of recent Pap testing among Latinas 18 years and older increased from 64% in 1987 to 75% in 2003 (ACS, 2006). Although participation in cervical cancer screening is relatively similar across Latino subgroups, women of Mexican origin are the least likely to have had a Pap test. Additionally, uninsured women are less likely to have received a recent Pap test compared with women who have health care coverage (A. G. Ramirez, Suarez, Laufman, et al., 2000; A. G. Ramirez, Suarez, McAlister, et al., 2000).

Prostate Cancer Screening

In 2003, 53% of Latino men 50 years and older had a prostate-specific antigen (PSA) test within the past year, compared with 58% of non-Latino whites. Men of Mexican origin and those who lack health insurance had the lowest prevalence of PSA testing (American Cancer Society, 2006; Wilkinson et al., 2002).

Sexual Behaviors

Although the proportion of Latino teenagers who are sexually active has slightly decreased in the past 15 years, Latino adolescents are still more likely than non-Latino whites to have initiated sexual intercourse before age 13 (8% vs. 5%), and Latino boys are almost three times as likely as girls to have experienced sex (11% vs. 4%). Similarly, more Latino high school students report having sex than their non-Latino white counterparts (48% vs. 43%), and males are also more likely to have initiated sexual activity than females (53% vs. 44%) (CDC, 2006b).

Risky Sexual Behavior of Latino Teenagers

Risky sexual behavior is a significant problem in the Latino community, as reflected in the increased number of Latinos, particularly females, becoming infected with HIV and other sexually transmitted diseases (STDs). Latino male teens (21%) are significantly more likely to have had four or more sexual partners than their female counterparts (10%) (CDC, 2006b). About 1 of 4 Latino high school students (24%) has used alcohol or drugs at last sexual intercourse. Condom use among all youth increased during the 1990s, and while in 1991 Latinos were the least likely to have used a condom the last time they had sex, they now show rates similar to non-Latino whites, with 59% males and 48% females reporting using a condom during their last sexual intercourse.

Pregnancy and Abortion in Latina Teens

More than half of Latina teens (51%) become pregnant at least once before age 20, nearly twice the national average. Since 1995, Latina teens have recorded the highest birth rate of any major ethnic/racial minority in the country (Martin et al., 2005). African American girls have a higher pregnancy rate than Latinas, but the higher birth rate in Latina teens is related to lower rates of abortion. The proportion of Latina adolescents who choose abortion is about 24%, lower than non-Latina girls.

Sexual Behavior in Latinos Aged 15 to 44

More than 90% of Latinos are sexually active. The majority of Latinos aged 15 to 44 report having monogamous sexual relationships in the past 12 months, but 14% of Latinos and 6% of Latinas had three or more sexual partners in the previous year (Mosher, Chandra, & Jones, 2005). About 6% of Latino males and females report having sex with a partner of the same sex in the previous year.

Substance Abuse

Substance abuse seems to be strongly linked to social and family relations in Latinos. Family factors (including family bonds) predict the use of tobacco, alcohol, and other drugs in young Latinos, and they see great risk of upsetting their parents or losing the respect of family and friends (Ellickson, Collins, & Bell, 1999). Knowledge of friends' alcohol and tobacco use is highly predictive of personal use. Alcohol and tobacco marketing is an added environmental factor; Latino youth in the United States are overexposed to alcohol advertising as compared with non-Latino youth. For example, alcohol advertisement to young people in the San Antonio television market increased over 2.5 times from 2001 to 2005. Alcohol ads seen by youth and adults on San Antonio TV stations are shown on the top four ranked local stations among Latinos, including the Univision and Telemundo Spanish-language affiliates (The Center on Alcohol Marketing and Youth, 2007).

Alcohol and Illicit Drugs

In general, U.S. Latinos seem to have lower rates of alcohol and illicit drug use than non-Latino whites. However, age- and gender-adjusted rates show that Latinas have much lower rates of alcohol and drug use, while Latino men have higher rates than their non-Latino white counterparts. Despite lower overall substance use rates during adolescence compared with non-Latino whites, Latinos have higher rates of substance-related morbidity and mortality in adulthood (Gilliland Becker, Samet, & Key, 1995; Lee, Markides, & Ray, 1997). Alcohol consumption among young Latino adults has been associated with education, income, acculturation, family factors, and peer-oriented activities, among other factors (Turner & Gil, 2002; Vega & Gil, 1998). Acculturation is strongly related to alcohol use, but the relationship is rather complex. Substance abuse rates are twice as high for U.S.-born Latino men and seven times higher for Latinas than for their foreign-born counterparts. An increase in time since migration to the United States for foreign-born Latinos is associated with heavier alcohol use, as is having a more stable income. However, as U.S.-born Latinos reach higher educational levels, their use of alcohol decreases. For recent migrants, alcohol use is higher among the ones with lower education (Gil & Vega, 2001; Gil, Wagner, & Vega, 2000). Latino adults also seem more likely to drive under the influence of alcohol (Walker, Waiters, Grub, & Chen, 2005).

Latino Youth

Latinos aged 12 to 17 are less likely to report past-month alcohol and marijuana use than non-Latinos. About 1 in 6 (17%) Latino youth report alcohol use in the past month, and 1 in 10 (10%) report binge alcohol use, both slightly lower than non-Latinos. Among Latino youths, Cubans exhibit the highest rate of past-month alcohol use, while Puerto Ricans have the highest rate of past-month illicit drug use. Seven percent of Latino youth report marijuana use in the past month, compared with 8% of non-Latinos, and about 1%

report use of other drugs, similar to youth of other ethnic groups (SAMHSA, 2006a). Mexican Americans, Puerto Ricans, and Cubans report higher use of marijuana than Central and South Americans. Similar to adults, U.S.-born Latino youth are more likely to have used alcohol and illicit drugs in the past month than the foreign-born.

Latino Adults

Similar to other ethnic groups, young adults (18 to 25 years) show the highest rate of alcohol use, binge drinking, and illicit drug use among Latinos of all ages. Almost half (48%) report drinking alcohol at least once in the past month, 1 out of 3 (35%) report consuming five or more drinks on the same occasion in the last month, and 9% report heavy alcohol use (more than two drinks a day for men and one drink a day for women), compared with 63%, 43%, and 16%, respectively, among non-Latinos. Almost half (48%) report lifetime use of illicit drugs, 25% in the past year, and 14% in the past month, compared with 59%, 34%, and 19%, respectively, in the general population. Latinos older than 26 years report 43% use in the past month, 23% binge drinking, and 5% heavy alcohol use. One out of three (33%) admit lifetime use of illicit drugs, 8% in the past year, and 5% in the past month (SAMHSA, 2006a, 2006b).

Tobacco

A significant proportion of the Latino population in the United States is below 18 years of age, and tobacco companies have successfully increased their marketing strategies targeting Latino children. National data show evidence that the prevalence of current smoking among Latino middle school and high school males is not significantly different from non-Latino males, and despite lower rates than non-Latina females, smoking among Latina adolescents is increasing, contrary to the trends in other

groups. Three out of four Latino high school students try cigarettes at least once in their lifetime. They also showed a clearly increasing trend in smoking from 1993 to 1997. However, since 2000, cigarette use has slightly decreased among high school male students but has either increased or remained unchanged among Latina females. Latino adolescents seem to have earlier and faster initiation rates. The smoking rate in Latinos almost doubles from ages 12 to 13, peaks at 15 (Chalela, Vélez, & Ramirez, 2007), and seems to remain stable after age 15, suggesting that those who start smoking do so by the ninth grade and that it may be more difficult for them than for their non-Latino counterparts to age-out of the nicotine addiction. If the trend in smoking rates among Latinos has reached a plateau, stronger efforts are necessary to turn it into a descendent tendency, given the increased tobacco marketing to Latino children and their easier access to tobacco products. In addition, if Latino teenagers fail to age-out of smoking, there is an even more pressing need to find effective ways to target them with early messages to prevent initiation. Some studies on the effectiveness of antismoking campaigns show mixed results, and very little is known about the best way to reach Latino youth with smoking prevention messages.

Latinos are second to non-Latino whites in smoking rates among young adults (SAMHSA, 2006a, 2006b). Among Latinos, exposure to friends and siblings who smoke, parental approval of smoking, positive social outcome expectations, and low negative outcome expectations seem to be associated with transitioning into regular smokers from adolescence to young adulthood (Ellickson, Orlando, Tucker, & Klein, 2004; Ellickson, Perlman, & Klein, 2003; Tucker, Ellickson, & Klein, 2003). Major risk factors for Latinos include risk taking and depression, as well as parent, sibling, and peer tobacco use, while familism and Latino identity appear to be important protective factors (Brook, Pahl, Balka, & Fei, 2004).

ORAL HEALTH

The health disparities discussed throughout this chapter also include oral health. Latinos are more likely to lack access to dental care than non-Latino whites. Twice as many Latino children are likely to have untreated dental caries as non-Latino white children. Only 10% of Latino children age 8 receive sealants, compared with 29% of non-Latino white children. The percentage of untreated oral disease for adult Latinos (40%) is nearly double that for non-Latino whites (24%) (Dye et al., 2007).

Significance of the Health Situation of Latinos in the United States

Latinos are a genetically and culturally diverse group whose presence in the United States predates the American Revolution and whose migration to and from Latin American countries has been incredibly active since pre-Columbian times. Currently, Latinos constitute the largest ethnic minority group in the country. They are also the youngest and a group whose productive participation in society is of paramount importance for supporting the large proportion of people who are reaching retirement age in the coming decades. Unfortunately, despite important health problems that lower their productivity and lessen their quality of live, Latinos do not have access to the health care they need. In addition, as opposed to other ethnic groups, the disparity gap between Latinos and non-Latino whites is increasing. It is remarkable, though, that despite the higher exposure to environmental risks, the higher rates of serious illnesses, and the limited access to health care, the cohesiveness of the Latino community and the Latino family create a social support network that makes Latinos hard working, highly spirited, and strongly committed to the progress and well-being of American society.

Chapter 10, which follows, discusses several specific elements of the health promotion and disease prevention (HPDP) planning process unique to the Latino/Hispanic experience. These elements include planning frameworks, selected health issues, and cultural concerns. The authors also discuss, within a program-planning context, the importance of in-depth target group needs assessment, appropriate selection of program design, and particular aspects of program implementation and evaluation. They offer tips based on their extensive experiences, and make suggestions for more effective HPDP program design within the Latino/Hispanic populations.

DISCUSSION QUESTIONS AND ACTIVITIES

This chapter has highlighted a number of important issues related to Latino health and disease. Working in small groups, consider the following discussion items and activities and prepare your deliberations and activities for a full class discussion.

1. What are the predominant causes of morbidity and mortality among Latinos living in your community?

2. What is the ethnic distribution of Latinos living in your community and how are they similar and/or different in their cultural characteristics?

3. Select a health issue or problem and a particular ethnic Latino target group living in your community and discuss how you might intervene to reduce this problem within this particular target group. You may wish to review Chapters 10, 11, and 12 before starting this activity.

REFERENCES

Abraido-Lanza, A. F., Dohrenwend, B. P., Nq-Mak, D. S., & Turner, J. B. (1999). The Latino mortality paradox: A test of the "salmon bias" and healthy migrant hypotheses. *American Journal of Public Health, 89*(10), 1543–1548.

Agency for Healthcare Research and Quality. (2006). *National healthcare disparities report.* Rockville, MD: Author.

Aldrich, L., & Variyam, J. N. (2000, January/April). Acculturation erodes the diet quality of U.S. Hispanics. *Food Review, 23,* 51–55.

American Cancer Society. (2006). *Cancer Facts and figures for Hispanics/Latinos 2006–2008.* Atlanta, GA: Author.

American Dietetic Association, Diabetes Care and Education Dietetic Practice Group. (1998). *Mexican American food practices, customs, and holidays: Ethnic and regional food practices: A series* (2nd ed.). Chicago: Author.

Añez, L. M., Paris, M., Bedregal, L. E., Davidson, L., & Grilo, C. M. (2005). Application of cultural constructs in the care of first generation Latino clients in a community mental health setting. *Journal of Psychiatric Practice, 11,* 221–230.

Arif, A. A., Delclos, G. L., Lee, E. S., Tortolero, S. R., & Whitehead, L. W. (2003). Prevalence and risk factors of asthma and wheezing among U.S. adults: An analysis of the NHANES III data. *European Respiratory Journal, 21*(5), 827–833.

Bonato, S. L., & Salzano, F. M. (1997). A single and early migration for the people of the Americas supported by mitochondrial DNA sequence data. *Proceedings of the National Academy of Sciences USA, 94,* 1866–1871.

Bortolini, M., Salzano, F. M., Thomas, M. G., Stuart, S., Nasanen, S. P. K., Bau, C. H. D., et al. (2003). Y-chromosome evidence for differing ancient demographic histories in the Americas. *American Journal of Human Genetics, 73,* 524–539.

Brook, J. S., Pahl, T., Balka, E. B., & Fei, K. (2004). Smoking among New Yorican adolescents: Time 1 predictors of Time 2 tobacco use. *Journal of Genetic Psychology, 165*(3), 324–340.

Burke, J. P., Williams, K., Haffner, S. M., Villalpando, C. G., & Stern, M. P. (2001). Elevated incidence of Type 2 diabetes in San Antonio, Texas, compared with that of Mexico City, Mexico. *Diabetes Care, 24*(9), 1573–1578.

Center on Alcohol Marketing and Youth. (2007). *Alcohol advertising on television 2001–2005: Local market summary—San Antonio.* Retrieved January 27, 2007, from http://camy .org/tvt0012005/index.php?MarketID=641

Centers for Disease Control and Prevention. (2002). State-specific trends in self-reported blood pressure screening and high blood pressure—United States, 1991–1999. *Morbidity and Mortality Weekly Report, 51*(21), 456–460.

Centers for Disease Control and Prevention. (2004a). Access to health-care and preventive services among Hispanics and non-Hispanics— United States, 2001–2002. *Morbidity and Mortality Weekly Report, 53*(40), 937–941.

Centers for Disease Control and Prevention. (2004b). Health disparities experienced by Hispanics. *Morbidity and Mortality Weekly Report, 53*(40), 935–937.

Centers for Disease Control and Prevention. (2004c). *HIV/AIDS surveillance report* (Vol. 16). Retrieved January 20, 2007, from www.cdc.gov/hiv/stats/hasrlink.htm

Centers for Disease Control and Prevention. (2004d). Prevalence of diabetes among Hispanics: Selected areas, 1998–2002. *Morbidity and Mortality Weekly Report, 53*(40), 941–944.

Centers for Disease Control and Prevention. (2005a). Racial/ethnic disparities in prevalence, treatment, and control of hypertension: United States, 1999–2002. *Morbidity and Mortality Weekly Report, 54*(1), 7–9.

Centers for Disease Control and Prevention. (2005b). Trends in tuberculosis: United States, 2004. *Morbidity and Mortality Weekly Report, 54*(10), 245–249.

Centers for Disease Control and Prevention. (2006a). Hypertension-related mortality among Hispanic subpopulations: United States, 1995–2002. *Morbidity and Mortality Weekly Report, 55*(7), 177–180.

Centers for Disease Control and Prevention. (2006b). Youth risk behavior surveillance: United States 2005. Surveillance summaries. *Morbidity and Mortality Weekly Report, 55*(SS-5). Retrieved January 20, 2007, from www.cdc.gov/mmwr/PDF/SS/SS5505.pdf

Centers for Disease Control and Prevention. (2007). Surveillance for acute viral hepatitis: United States, 2005. *Morbidity and Mortality Weekly Report, 56*(SS03), 1–24.

Chalela, P., Vélez, L. F., & Ramirez, A. G. (2007). Social influences, and attitudes and beliefs associated with smoking among border Latino youth. *Journal of School Health, 77*(4), 187–195.

Child Trends Data Bank. (2004). *High school dropout rates.* Retrieved February 15, 2007, from www.childtrendsdatabank.org/ indicators/ 1HighSchoolDropout.cfm

Chobanian, A. V., Bakris, G. L., Black, H. R., Cushman, W. C., Green, L. A., Izzo, J. L., et al. (2003). The seventh report of the Joint National Committee on Prevention, Detection, Evaluation, and Treatment of High Blood Pressure: The JNC 7 report. *Journal of the American Medical Association, 289*(19), 2560–2572.

Dabelea, D., Hanson, R. L., Lindsay, R. S., Pettitt, D. J., Imperatore, G., Gabir, M. M., et al. (2000). Intrauterine exposure to diabetes conveys risks for Type 2 diabetes and obesity: A study of discordant sibships. *Diabetes, 49*(12), 2208–2211.

De las Casas, B. (2007). *A brief account of the destruction of the Indies.* Retrieved from www.gutenberg.org/files/20321/20321-8.txt

Dong, X., Men, Y., & Haile, E. (2005). *Work related fatal and nonfatal injuries among U.S. construction workers, 1992–2003.* Silver Spring, MD: The Center to Protect Worker's Rights. Retrieved March 3, 2007, from www.cpwr.com/publications/krtrendsfinal.pdf

Dong, X., & Platner, J. W. (2004). Occupational fatalities of Hispanic construction workers from 1992 to 2000. *American Journal of Industrial Medicine, 45*(1), 45–54.

Doty, M. M., & Holmgren, A. L. (2006). Health care disconnect: Gaps in coverage and care for minority adults. Findings from the Commonwealth Fund Biennial Health Insurance Survey (2005). *Issue Brief (The Commonwealth Fund), 21,* 1–12.

Dufour, M. C., Stinson, F. S., & Caces, M. F. (1993). Trends in cirrhosis morbidity and mortality: United States, 1979–1988. *Seminars in Liver Disease, 13*(2), 109–125.

Dye, B. A., Tan, S., Smith, V., Lewis, B. G., Barker, L. K., Thornton-Evans, G., et al. (2007). Trends in oral health status: United States, 1988–1994 and 1999–2004. National Center

for Health Statistics. *Vital Health Statistics, 11*(248). Retrieved March 15, 2007, from www.cdc.gov/nchs/data/series/sr_11/sr11_ 248.pdf

Ellickson, P. L., Collins, R. L., & Bell, R. M. (1999). Adolescent use of illicit drugs other than marijuana: How important is social bonding and for which ethnic groups? *Substance Use and Misuse, 34*(3), 317–346.

Ellickson, P. L., Orlando, M., Tucker, J. S., & Klein, D. J. (2004). From adolescence to young adulthood: Racial/ethnic disparities in smoking. *American Journal of Public Health, 94,* 293–299.

Ellickson, P. L., Perlman, M., & Klein, D. J. (2003). Explaining racial/ethnic differences in smoking during the transition to adulthood. *Addictive Behaviors, 28,* 915–931.

Ferrannini, E. (1998). Insulin resistance versus insulin deficiency in non-insulin-dependent diabetes mellitus: Problems and prospects. *Endocrine Reviews, 19*(4), 477–490.

Ford, E. S. (2005). Prevalence of the metabolic syndrome defined by the International Diabetes Federation among adults in the U.S. *Diabetes Care, 28*(11), 2745–2749.

Ford, E. S., & Giles, W. H. (2003). Changes in prevalence of nonfatal coronary heart disease in the United States from 1971–1994. *Ethnicity & Disease, 13*(1), 85–93.

Franzini, L., Ribble, J. C., & Keddie, A. M. (2001). Understanding the Hispanic paradox. *Ethnicity & Disease, 11,* 496–518.

Gil, A. G., & Vega, W. A. (2001). Latino drug use: Scope, risk factors and reduction strategies. In M. Aguirre-Molina, C. W. Molina, & R. E. Zambrana (Eds.), *Health issues in the Latino community* (pp. 435–458). San Francisco: Jossey-Bass.

Gil, A. G., Wagner, E. F., Vega, W. A. (2000). Acculturation, familism, and alcohol use among Latino adolescent males: Longitudinal relations. *Journal of Community Psychology, 28,* 443–458.

Gilliland, F. D., Becker, T. M., Samet, J. M., & Key, C. R. (1995). Trends in alcohol-related mortality among New Mexico's American Indians, Hispanics, and non-Hispanic whites. *Alcoholism, Clinical and Experimental Research, 19*(6), 1572–1577.

Gray, R. S., Fabsitz, R. R., Cowan, L. D., Lee, E. T., Howard, B. V., & Savage, P. J. (1998). Risk factor clustering in the insulin resistance syndrome: The Strong Heart Study. *American Journal of Epidemiology, 148*(9), 869–878.

Guendelman, S., & Abrams, B. (1995). Dietary intake among Mexican-American women: Generational differences and a comparison with white non-Hispanic women. *American Journal of Public Health, 85,* 20–25.

Haffner, S. M., D'Agostino, R., Saad, M. F., Rewers, M., Mykkanen, L., Selby, J., et al. (1996). Increased insulin resistance and insulin secretion in nondiabetic African-Americans and Hispanics compared with non-Hispanic whites: The Insulin Resistance Atherosclerosis Study. *Diabetes, 45*(6), 742–748.

Hamre, B. (2007). *Cuisine of South America.* Retrieved February 7, 2007, from http://gosouthamerica .about.com/od/cuisine/a/SouthAmerica.htm

Hanis, C. L., Hewett-Emmett, D., Bertin, T. K., & Schull, W. J. (1991). Origins of U.S. Hispanics: Implications for diabetes. *Diabetes Care, 14*(7), 618–627.

Hedley, A. A., Ogden, C. L., Johnson, C. L., Carroll, M. D., Curtin, L. R., & Flegal, K. M. (2004). Prevalence of overweight and obesity among US children, adolescents, and adults, 1999–2002. *Journal of the American Medical Association, 291*(23), 2847–2850.

Hnizdo, E., Sullivan, P. A., Bang, K. M., & Wagner, G. (2002). Association between chronic obstructive pulmonary disease and employment by industry and occupation in the U.S. population: A study of data from the Third National Health and Nutrition Examination Survey. *American Journal of Epidemiology, 156*(8), 738–746.

Hopkins, F. W., MacKay, A. P., Koonin, L. M., Berg, C. J., Irwin, M., & Atrash, H. K. (1999). Pregnancy-related mortality in Hispanic women in the United States. *Obstetrics and Gynecology, 94,* 747–752.

Howe, H. L., Wu, X., Ries, L. A. G., Cokkinides, V., Ahmed, F., Jemal, A., et al. (2006). Annual report to the nation on the status of cancer, 1975–2003, featuring cancer among U.S. Hispanic/Latino populations. *Cancer, 107*(8), 1711–1742.

Hyman, D. J., & Pavlik, V. N. (2001). Characteristics of patients with uncontrolled hypertension in the United States. *New England Journal of Medicine, 345*(7), 479–486.

Kemp, B. M., Malhi, R. S., McDonough, J., Bolnick, D. A., Eshleman, J. A., Rickards, O., et al. (2007). Genetic analysis of early Holocene skeletal remains from Alaska and its implications for the settlement of the Americas. *American Journal of Physical Anthropology, 132*(4), 605–621.

Kent, R. K. (1965). Palmares: An African state in Brazil. *Journal of African History, 6*(2), 161–175.

Kittler, P. G., & Sucher, K. P. (2001). *Food and culture* (3rd ed.). Stamford, CT: Wadsworth.

Knowler, W. C., Barrett-Connor, E., Fowler, S. E., Hamman, R. F., Lachin, J. M., Walker, E. A., et al. (2002). Reduction in the incidence of Type 2 diabetes with lifestyle intervention or metformin. *New England Journal of Medicine, 346*(6), 393–403.

Lara, M., Gamboa, C., Kahramanian, M. I., Morales, L. S., & Bautista, D. E. (2005). Acculturation and Latino health in the United States: A review of the literature and its sociopolitical context. *Annual Review of Public Health, 26,* 367–397.

Lee, D. J., Markides, K. S., & Ray, L. A. (1997). Epidemiology of self-reported past heavy drinking in Hispanic adults. *Ethnicity & Health, 2*(1/2), 77–88.

Mallonee, S. (2003). Injuries among Hispanics in the United States: Implications for research. *Journal of Transcultural Nursing, 14*(3), 217–226.

Mann, R. E., Smart, R. G., & Govoni, R. (2003). The epidemiology of alcoholic liver disease. *Alcohol Research & Health, 27*(3), 209–219.

Marasas, W. F. O., Riley, R. T., Hendricks, K. A., Stevens, V. L., Sadler, T. W., Gelineau-van Waes, J., et al. (2004). Fumonisins disrupt sphingolipid metabolism, folate transport, and neural tube development in embryo culture and in vivo: A potential risk factor for human neural tube defects among populations consuming fumonisin-contaminated maize. *Journal of Nutrition, 134,* 711–716.

Marin, G. (1992). Issues in the measurement of acculturation among Hispanics. In K. F. Geisinger

(Ed.), *Psychological testing of Hispanics* (pp. 23–51). Washington, DC: American Psychological Association.

Martin, J. A., Hamilton, B. E., Sutton, P. D., Ventura, S. J., Menacker, F., & Munson, M. L. (2005). *Births: Final data for 2003. National vital statistics reports* (Vol. 54, No. 2). Hyattsville, MD: National Center for Health Statistics. Retrieved January 23, 2007, from www.cdc.gov/NCHS/data/nvsr/nvsr54/nvsr54_02.pdf

Mazze, R., Strock, E. S., Simonson, G., & Berganstal, R. M. (2004). *Staged diabetes management: A systematic approach* (2nd ed.). London: Wiley.

Meigs, J. B. (2003). The metabolic syndrome. *British Medical Journal, 327*(7406), 61–62.

Meigs, J. B., D'Agostino, R. B., Sr., Wilson, P. W., Cupples, L. A., Nathan, D. M., & Singer, D. E. (1997). Risk variable clustering in the insulin resistance syndrome: The Framingham Offspring Study. *Diabetes, 46*(10), 1594–1600.

Modan, M., Halkin, H., Almog, S., Lusky, A., Eshkol, A., Shefi, M., et al. (1985). Hyperinsulinemia. A link between hypertension, obesity, and glucose intolerance. *Journal of Clinical Investigation, 75*(3), 809–817.

Mokdad, A. H., Bowman, B. A., Ford, E. S., Vinicor, F., Marks, J. S., & Koplan, J. P. (2001). The continuing epidemics of obesity and diabetes in the United States. *Journal of the American Medical Association, 286*(10), 1195–1200.

Mokdad, A. H., Ford, E. S., Bowman, B. A., Dietz, W. H., Vinicor, F., Bales, V. S., et al. (2003). Prevalence of obesity, diabetes, and obesity-related health risk factors, 2001. *Journal of the American Medical Association, 289*, 76–79.

Morales, L. S., Lara, M., Kington, R. S., Valdez, R. O., & Escarce, J. J. (2002). Socioeconomic, cultural, and behavioral factors affecting Hispanic health outcomes. *Journal of Health Care Poor Underserved, 13*(4), 477–503.

Mosher, W. D., Chandra, A., & Jones, J. (2005). *Sexual behavior and selected health measures: Men and women 15–44 years of age, United States, 2002.* Advance data from vital and health statistics; No. 362. Hyattsville, MD: National Center for Health Statistics. Retrieved from www.cdc.gov/nchs/data/ad/ad362.pdf

National Centers for Health Statistics. (2002). *A demographic and health snapshot of the U.S. Hispanic/Latino population: 2002 National Hispanic Health Leadership Summit.* Atlanta, GA: Author.

National Centers for Health Statistics. (2005). *Health, United States, 2005. With chartbook on trends in the health of Americans.* Hyattsville, MA: Author.

National Center for Health Statistics. (2006). *Physical activity among adults: United States, 2000 and 2005.* Retrieved February 2, 2007, from www.cdc.gov/nchs/products/pubs/pubd/hestats/physicalactivity/physicalactivity_tables.pdf

National Institute for Occupational Safety and Health. (2004). *Worker health chartbook 2004.* (DHHS [NIOSH] Publication No. 2004–146). Cincinnati, OH: Author. Retrieved February 2, 2007, from www.cdc.gov/niosh/docs/chartbook/pdfs/Chartbook_2004_NIOSH.pdf

Natural Resources Defense Council. (2004). *Hidden danger: Environmental health threats in the Latino community.* New York: Author.

Neel, J. V., Biggar, R. J., & Sukernik, R. I. (1994). Virologic and genetic studies relate Amerind origins to the indigenous people of the Mongolia/Manchuria/southeastern Siberia region. *Proceedings of the National Academy of Sciences, USA, 91*(22), 10737–10741.

Neufeld, N. D., Raffel, L. J., Landon, C., Chen, Y. D., & Vadheim, C. M. (1998). Early presentation of Type 2 diabetes in Mexican-American youth. *Diabetes Care, 21*(1), 80–86.

Nguyen, G. C., Segev, D. L., & Thuluvath, P. J. (2007). Racial disparities in the management of hospitalized patients with cirrhosis and complications of portal hypertension: A national study. *Hepatology, 45*(5), 1282–1289.

Ogden, C. L., Carroll, M. D., Curtin, L. R., McDowell, M. A., Tabak, C. J., & Flegal, K. M. (2006). Prevalence of overweight and obesity in the United States, 1999–2004. *Journal of the American Medical Association, 295*(13), 1549–1555.

Ogden, C. L., Flegal, K. M., Carroll, M. D., & Johnson, C. L. (2002). Prevalence and trends in overweight among US children and adolescents,

1999–2000. *Journal of the American Medical Association, 288*(14), 1728–1732.

Ortega, A. N., Gergen, P. J., Paltiel, A. D., Bauchner, H., Belanger, K. D., & Leaderer, B. P. (2002). Impact of site care, race and Hispanic ethnicity on medication use for childhood asthma. *Pediatrics, 109*(1), E1.

Payne, S. G. (1973). *A history of Spain and Portugal*. Madison: University of Wisconsin Press. Retrieved January 23, 2007, from http://libro.uca.edu/payne1/spainport1.htm

Perez-Perdomo, R., Perez-Cardona, C., Disdier-Flores, O., & Cintron, Y. (2003). Prevalence and correlates of asthma in the Puerto Rican population: Behavioral Risk Factor Surveillance System, 2000. *Journal of Asthma, 40*(5), 465–474.

Perlin, S. A., Sexton, K., & Wong, D. W. (1999). An examination of race and poverty for populations living near industrial sources of air pollution. *Journal of Exposure Analysis and Environmental Epidemiology, 9*(1), 29–48.

Phares, T. M., Morrow, B., Lansky, A., Barfield, W. D., Prince, C. B., Marchi, K. S., et al. (2004). Surveillance for disparities in maternal health-related behaviors: Selected states, pregnancy risk assessment monitoring system (PRAMS), 2000–2001. *Morbidity and Mortality Weekly Report, 53*(SS-4), 1–13.

Pransky, G., Moshenberg, D., Benjamin, K., Portillo, S., Thackrey, J. L., & Hill-Fotouhi, C. (2002). Occupational risks and injuries in non-agricultural immigrant Latino workers. American. *Journal of Industrial Medicine, 42*, 117–123.

Ramirez, A. G., McAlister, A., Villarreal, R., Suarez, L., Talavera, G. A., Perez-Stable, E. J., et al. (1998). Prevention and control in diverse Hispanic populations: A national initiative for research and action. *Cancer, 83*(Suppl.), 1825–1829.

Ramirez, A. G., & Suarez, L. (2001). The impact of cancer on Latino populations. In M. Aguirre-Molina, C. W. Molina, & R. E. Zambrana (Eds.), *Health issues in the Latino community* (pp. 211–244). San Francisco: Jossey-Bass.

Ramirez, A. G., Suarez, L., Laufman, L., Barroso, C., & Chalela, P. (2000). Hispanic women's breast and cervical cancer knowledge, attitudes, and screening behaviors. *American Journal of Health Promotion, 14*(5), 292–300.

Ramirez, A. G., Suarez, L., McAlister, A., Villarreal, R., Trapido, E., Talavera, G. A., Perez-Stable, E. J., & Marti, J. (2000). Cervical cancer screening in regional Hispanic populations. *American Journal of Health Behavior, 24*(3), 181–192.

Ramirez, A. G., Talavera, G. A., Villarreal, R., Suarez, L., McAlister, A., Trapido, E., et al. (2000). Breast cancer screening in regional Hispanic populations. *Health Education Research, 15*(5), 559–568.

Ramirez, R. R., & de la Cruz, G. P. (2002). *The Hispanic population in the United States: March 2002*. U.S. Census Bureau Publication No. P20–545. Washington, DC: U.S. Census Bureau.

Rassin, D. K., Markides, K. S., Baranowski, T., Richardson, C. J., Mikrut, W. D., & Bee, D. E. (1994). Acculturation and the initiation of breastfeeding. *Journal of Clinical Epidemiology, 47*, 739–746.

Reaven, G. M., Lithell, H., & Landsberg, L. (1996). Hypertension and associated metabolic abnormalities: The role of insulin resistance and the sympathoadrenal system. *New England Journal of Medicine, 334*(6), 374–381.

Ries, L. A. G., Melbert, D., Krapcho, M., Mariotto, A., Miller, B. A., Feuer, E. J., et al. (Eds.). (2006, November). *SEER cancer statistics review, 1975–2004*. Bethesda, MD: National Cancer Institute. Retrieved from http://seer.cancer.gov/csr/1975_2004/

Romero-Gwynn, E., Gwynn, D., Grivetti, L., McDonald, R., Stanford, G., Turner, B., West, E., & Williamson. E. (1993). Dietary acculturation among Latinos of Mexican descent. *Nutrition Today, 28*(4), 6–12.

Romero-Gwynn, E., Gwynn, D., Turner, B., Stanford, G., West, E., Willliamson, E., Grivetti, L., & McDonald, R. (1992). Dietary change among Latinos of Mexican descent in California. *California Agriculture, 46*(4), 10–12.

Rosenberg, J. M., Maurer, J. D., Sorlie, P. D., Johnson, N. J., MacDorman, M. F., Hoyert, D. L., et al. (1999). Quality of death rates by race and Hispanic origin: A summary of current research, 1999. *Vital and Health Statistics, Series 2, 128,* 1–13.

Sanjur, D. (1995). *Hispanic foodways, nutrition, and health.* Boston: Allyn & Bacon.

Schoenborn, C. A., Adams, P. F., & Barnes, P. M. (2002). *Body weight status of adults: United States, 1997–98.* Advance Data from Vital and Health Statistics. No. 330. Hyattsville, MD: National Center for Health Statistics.

Stern, M. P., & Mitchell, B. D. (1995). Diabetes in Hispanic Americans. In National Diabetes Data Group (Eds.), *Diabetes in America* (2nd ed., pp. 631–659, NIH Publication 95–1468). Bethesda, MD: National Diabetes Data Group.

Stinson, F. S., Grant, B. F., & Dufour, M. C. (2001). The critical dimension of ethnicity in liver cirrhosis mortality statistics. *Alcoholism: Clinical and Experimental Research, 25*(8), 1181–1187.

Suarez, L., & Ramirez, A. G. (1999). Hispanic/ Latino health and disease: An overview. In R. M. Huff & M. V. Kline (Eds.), *Promoting health in multicultural populations: A handbook for practitioners* (Vol. 17, pp. 115–136). Thousand Oaks, CA: Sage.

Substance Abuse and Mental Health Services Administration, Office of Applied Studies. (2006a). *2004 National survey on drug use and health: Detailed tables.* Retrieved February 7, 2007, from www.oas.samhsa.gov/nsduh/ 2k4nsduh/2k4tabs/2k4tabs.pdf

Substance Abuse and Mental Health Services Administration, Office of Applied Studies. (2006b). *Results from the 2005 national survey on drug use and health: National findings* (NSDUH Series H-30, DHHS Publication No. SMA 06–4194). Rockville, MD: Author.

Talavera, G. A., Ramirez, A. G., Suarez, L., Villarreal, R., Marti, J., et al. (2002). Predictors of digital rectal examination in U.S. Latinos. *American Journal of Preventive Medicine, 22*(1), 36–41.

Teske, R. H. C., Jr., & Nelson, B. H. (1974). Acculturation and assimilation: A clarification. *American Ethnologist, 1*(2), 351–367.

Thomas, H. (1997). *The slave trade. The story of the Atlantic slave trade: 1440–1870.* New York: Touchstone.

Tucker, J. S., Ellickson, P. L., & Klein, D. J. (2003). Predictors of the transition to regular smoking during adolescence and young adulthood. *Journal of Adolescent Health, 32*(4), 314–324.

Turner, R. J., & Gil, A. G. (2002). Psychiatric and substance use disorders in South Florida: Racial/ethnic and gender contrasts in a young adult cohort. *Archives of General Psychiatry, 59,* 43–50.

U.S. Census Bureau. (2005a). *S0201—Selected population profile in the United States: Hispanic or Latino. 2005 American Community Survey.* Retrieved February 10, 2007, from http:// factfinder.census.gov/servlet/IPTable?_bm=y& -geo_id=01000US&-qr_name=ACS_2005_ EST_G00_S0201&-qr_name=ACS_2005_ EST_G00_S0201PR&-qr_name= ACS_2005_EST_G00_S0201T&-qr_name= ACS_2005_EST_G00_S0201TPR&-ds_ name=ACS_2005_EST_G00_&-reg= ACS_2005_EST_G00_S0201:400;ACS_2005_ EST_G00_S0201PR:400;ACS_2005_EST_G0 0_S0201T:400;ACS_2005_EST_G00_S0201T PR:400&-_lang=en&-redoLog=false&- format=

U.S. Census Bureau. (2005b). *S0201—Selected population profile in the United States: white alone, not Hispanic or Latino. 2005 American Community Survey.* Retrieved Retrieved February 10, 2007, from http://factfinder.cen sus.gov/servlet/IPTable?_bm=y&geo_id=0100 0US&-qr_name=ACS_2005_EST_G00_ S0201&-qr_name=ACS_2005_ EST_G00_ S0201PR&-qr_name= ACS_2005_EST_G00_ S0201T&-qr_name=ACS_2005_EST_ G00_S0201TPR&-ds_name=ACS_ 2005_EST_G00_&-reg=ACS_2005_EST_ G00_S0201:451;ACS_2005_EST_G00_S0201 PR:451;ACS_2005_EST_G00_S0201T:451;A CS_2005_EST_G00_S0201TPR:451&- _lang=en&-redoLog=false&-format=

U.S. Census Bureau. (2005c). *S0201—Selected population profile in the United States: Black or African American alone. 2005 American Community Survey.* Retrieved February 9, 2007, from http://factfinder.census.gov/servlet/ IPTable?_bm=y&-geo_id=01000US&- qr_name=ACS_2005_EST_G00_S0201&- qr_name=ACS_2005_EST_G00_S0201PR&-q

r_name=ACS_2005_EST_G00_S0201T&-qr_name=ACS_2005_EST_G00_S0201TPR&-ds_name=ACS_2005_EST_G00_&-reg=ACS_2005_EST_G00_S0201:004;ACS_2005_EST_G00_S0201PR:004;ACS_2005_EST_G00_S0201T:004;ACS_2005_EST_G00_S0201TPR:004&-_lang=en&-redoLog=false&-format=

U.S. Census Bureau. (2005d). S0201—*Selected population profile in the United States: Asian alone. 2005 American Community Survey.* Retrieved February 11, 2007, from http://factfinder.census.gov/servlet/IPTable?_bm=y&-geo_id=01000US&-qr_name=ACS_2005_EST_G00_S0201&-qr_name=ACS_2005_EST_G00_S0201PR&-qr_name=ACS_2005_EST_G00_S0201T&-qr_name=ACS_2005_EST_G00_S0201TPR&-ds_name=ACS_2005_EST_G00_&-reg=ACS_2005_EST_G00_S0201:012;ACS_2005_EST_G00_S0201PR:012;ACS_2005_EST_G00_S0201T:012;ACS_2005_EST_G00_S0201TPR:012&-_lang=en&-redoLog=false&-format=

U.S. Census Bureau. (2006). *Facts for features: Hispanic heritage month.* Retrieved February 11, 2007, from www.census.gov/Press-Release/www/releases/archives/facts_for_features_special_editions/007173.html

U.S. Census Bureau. (2007). *Educational attainment in the United States: 2006. Detailed tables.* Retrieved February 15, 2007, from www.census.gov/population/www/socdemo/education/cps2006.html

U.S. Census Bureau, Public Information Office. (2007). *More diversity, slower growth.* Retrieved February 15, 2007, from www.census.gov/Press-Release/www/releases/archives/population/001720.html

U.S. Department of Agriculture, Agricultural Research Service. (2007). *What we eat in America, NHANES 2003–2004.* Retrieved February 5, 2007, from www.ars.usda.gov/Services/docs.htm?docid=13793

U.S. Department of Education, National Center for Education Statistics. (2006). *The Condition of Education 2006.* NCES 2006–071, Washington, DC: Government Printing Office. Retrieved February 15, 2007, from http://nces.ed.gov/pubs2006/2006071.pdf

U.S. Department of Labor. (2005). *Findings from the National Agricultural Workers Survey (NAWS) 2001–2002: A demographic and employment profile of the United States workers. Research Report No. 9.* Burlingame, CA: Author.

U.S. Environmental Protection Agency. (2006). *Environmental justice: Frequently asked questions.* Retrieved February 12, 2007, from www.epa.gov/compliance/resources/faqs/ej/index.html#faq4

Vega, W. A., & Gil, A. G. (1998). *Ethnicity and drug use in early adolescence.* New York: Plenum Press.

Verma, S., Bonacini, M., Govindarajan, S., Kanel, G., Lindsay, K. L., & Redeker, A. (2006). More advanced hepatic fibrosis in Hispanics with chronic hepatitis C infection: Role of patient demographics, hepatic necroinflammation, and steatosis. *American Journal of Gastroenterology, 101*(8), 1817–1823.

Walker, S., Waiters, E., Grube, J. W., & Chen, M. J. (2005). Young people driving after drinking and riding with drinking drivers: Drinking locations—what do they tell us? *Traffic Injury Prevention, 6*(3), 212–218.

Watts, S. J. (1998). *Epidemics and history: Disease, power and imperialism.* New Haven, CT: Yale University Press.

Weinberg, M., Hopkins, J., Farrington, L., Gresham, L., Ginsberg, M., & Bell, B. P. (2004). Hepatitis A in Hispanic children who live along the United States–Mexico border: the role of international travel and food-borne exposures. *Pediatrics, 114*(1), e68–e73.

Wilbur, J., Chandler, P. J., Dancy, B., & Lee, H. (2003). Correlates of physical activity in urban Midwestern Latinas. *American Journal of Preventive Medicine, 25*(3, Suppl. 1), 69–76.

Wilkinson, J. D., Wohler-Torres, B., Trapido, E., Fleming, L. E., MacKinnon, J., Voti, L., et al. (2002). Cancer trends among Hispanic men in South Florida, 1981–1998. *Cancer, 94,* 1183–1190.

Winkleby, M. A., Gardner, C. D., & Taylor, C. B. (1996). The influence of gender and socioeconomic factors on Hispanic/white differences in body mass index. *Preventive Medicine, 25*(2), 203–211.

Wirt, J., Choy, S., Rooney, P., Provasnik, S., Sen, A., & Tobin, R. (2004). *The condition of education, 2004* (NCES Publication No. 2004–077). Washington, DC: Government Printing Office. Retrieved February 15, 2007, from http://nces.ed.gov/programs/coe/2004/pdf/12_2004.pdf

Yang, Q., Greenland, S., & Flanders, W. D. (2006). Associations of maternal age- and parity-related factors with trends in low-birth weight rates: United States, 1980 through 2000. *American Journal of Public Health, 96*(5), 856–861.

Zhu, M., Druschel, C., & Lin, S. (2006). Maternal birthplace and major congenital malformations among New York Hispanics. *Birth Defects Research (Part A): Clinical and Molecular Teratology, 76*(6), 467–473.

10

Health Promotion in Latino Populations

Program Planning, Development, and Evaluation

FELIPE G. CASTRO

HECTOR BALCAZAR

MARYA COTA

Chapter Objectives

On completion of this chapter, the health promotion student and practitioner should be able to

- Identify and discuss the importance for program planners to understand the diversity that exists within Latino/Hispanic populations and communities and the major cultural beliefs, values, familial, and community characteristics that exist within these diverse communities relevant to motivating the involvement and participation of Latino/Hispanic consumers in community health promotion programs

- Identify health promotion and education program planning models to use as guides to practice and discuss their limitations in Latino/Hispanic tailored health promotion and education program planning

- Explain why "culturally relevant" Latino/Hispanic community health promotion and education programs should emphasize the Principle of Relevance (starting where the people are) and the Principle of Participation (eliciting the participation of community residents) to encourage their learning, support, and sense of ownership in the program

- Formulate a conceptual framework for planning health promotion and education programs within several different Latino/Hispanic subgroups (e.g., Mexican, Guatemalan, Puerto Rican, Cuban) that offer health information, motivates healthy behavior change, and promotes such change in a culturally relevant manner using interventions that build on the existing cultural strengths of each subgroup

- Identify and differentiate between program goals and program objectives and identify evaluation methods for assessing those program goals and objectives

- Explain the importance and usefulness of assessing "acculturative status" among Latinos/Hispanics in the initial assessment of health needs

- Differentiate between and describe at least the three following aspects of program implementation as it encourages an effective Latino/Hispanic-based health promotion program:

  1. Client preparation by advising them on guidelines for their active participation

  2. Enhancing the cultural competence of program staff

  3. Enhancing the cultural competence of the program's administrative staff and infrastructure

INTRODUCTION

A Latino Perspective on Health Promotion

This chapter presents a Hispanic/Latino[1] perspective on the design of effective and culturally relevant health promotion programs. Generally, the process of program design involves four basic steps: Step 1—Program Planning, Step 2—Program Development, Step 3—Program Implementation, and Step 4—Program Evaluation (McKenzie, Nieger, & Smeltzer, 2005). This stepwise approach is outlined further within a "User-Friendly Worksheet for Developing Health Promotion Programs"[2] (see Appendix A). The observations presented in this chapter include insights gained by the authors in their many years of research and program development within the field of health promotion. A major aim of this chapter is to provide scholarly and practical information for helping health professionals design and work with health promotion programs that serve Latino populations, in efforts to reduce or eliminate health disparities (Carter-Pokras & Baquet, 2002; National Alliance for Hispanic Health, 2001; U.S. Department of Health and Human Services [DHHS], 2000). This perspective recognizes that enacting healthy behavior change is not easy. It requires the acceptance of the need for change, motivation, and commitment to this change, as well as guided and sustained effort. These setting conditions for healthy behavior change are typically more difficult for many Latino and other racial/ethnic minority persons, especially when they reside within low-income neighborhoods or within unstable familial or other high stress living situations.

Cultural Enhancement of Program and Staff. In a quest to improve health promotion program effectiveness and staff capacity, culturally enhanced health promotion programs can be referred to as being *culturally relevant*

(designed for relevance) or *culturally respon-sive* (designed for responsiveness) to the cultural needs of members of a targeted or special population. In contrast, health educators, health providers, or other program staff can be described as being *culturally sensitive, culturally competent,* or even *culturally proficient,* in their *cultural capacity* to understand, appreciate and actively engage members of a targeted or special population. The hallmark of cultural capacity among program staff requires their abiding respect for diversity and for the well-being of members of a special population (Sue & Sue, 1999). Cultural capacity is then translated into culturally responsive services when program staff deliver culturally relevant services or program activities. In addition, enhancing the cultural capacity of program staff involves increasing their clinical skills for being more responsive to diverse participant or patient needs. Thus, respect for diversity and community collaborations are key elements of culturally responsive health services and programs. The ultimate goal is to increase patient treatment adherence, satisfaction, and positive health outcomes.

Devoid of programmatic attention to cultural issues, many mainstream health promotion programs have exhibited limited success in attracting, involving and retaining Latino consumers/clients[3] (Hirachi, Catalano, & Hawkins, 1997; Kumpfer, Alvarado, Smith, & Bellamy, 2002). Motivating Latino consumer involvement and participation in a health promotion program remains a major challenge. Nonetheless, this challenge can be met if program planners appreciate the cultural diversity that exists within a Latino community by understanding its prevailing cultural beliefs, values, and cultural norms, while also understanding the within-group variability on these characteristics that also exists among members of that community (Castro et al., 2006).

Characteristics of Health Promotion Programs. Initiating and sustaining health change efforts to reduce health disparities involves programmatic interventions that mobilize personal, interpersonal, and environmental resources in a unified and integrated manner. A well-designed and culturally responsive health promotion program helps sustain these efforts across time to produce genuine health-related changes and improvements in health. Health promotion programs typically focus on healthy change to reduce risks or the severity of one or more of the *lifestyle disorders:* cardiovascular disease (reducing elevated lipids, reducing high blood pressure), the cancers (screening for breast, cervical, colorectal, or other cancers), diabetes mellitus (promoting weight reduction, management of blood glucose levels), arthritis and other musculoskeletal diseases (Brownson, Remington, & Davis, 1998), as well as reducing the disease burden of addictive disorders (alcohol abuse, tobacco use, use of illegal drugs, excessive food consumption, other addictions). In general, one goal of health promotion programs is to reduce health disparities on one or more of the 10 leading health indicators: physical inactivity, overweight and obesity, tobacco use, substance use, responsible sexual behavior, mental health, injury and violence, environmental quality, immunization, and access to health care (U.S. DHHS, 2000).

Thus, a health promotion program consists of a multisession program of organized activities designed to promote healthy *lifestyle changes.* A well-designed health promotion program will typically include several components: (1) informational knowledge to provide health information and to change maladaptive beliefs about health, (2) motivational messages to prepare the participant for behavior change efforts, (3) skills development via techniques that build capacity for change, (4) social supports that elicit the aid of significant others, and (5) environmental changes to reduce barriers to change and to mobilize resources for making health-related changes.

Infusing Cultural Responsiveness Into Program Design

The Principles of Relevance and of Participation. Culturally relevant community-based programs should be designed according to two important systems principles: (1) the *principle of relevance,* "starting where the people are" and (2) the *principle of participation,* eliciting the participation of community residents, thus promoting their "sense of ownership" in the program, while also fostering "active learning" through participation (Minkler, 1990). The use of this approach operates as a *community-grounded needs assessment* to identify and respond actively to the most pressing health needs within a local community. Accordingly, from the perspective of the participatory social action research approach (Minkler & Wallerstein, 2003), community residents are invited to participate in the conceptualization and design of a health promotion program. Under the principle of participation, program developers elicit the views of community leaders, stakeholders, and residents regarding the nature and extent of important community health needs. This approach establishes a *health partnership,* while also challenging health professionals to apply their social, psychological, and medical knowledge toward addressing the community's expressed needs (Rawson, Martinelli-Casey, & Ling, 2002). In summary, this health partnership "grounds" the health promotion program within the contemporary health needs and desires of local community residents.

A Principle of Cultural Relevance. An emerging principle for health promotion may be identified as the principle of cultural relevance. A health promotion program that is designed to effectively reduce or eliminate health disparities within a specific minority population requires that the health planner be deeply knowledgeable of the culture of the targeted group, while also having respect for members of that group, and consulting with members of that group to more fully understand the group's cultural diversity and complexity in its values, major beliefs, customs, and traditions (Orlandi, Weston, & Epstein, 1992). In this regard, health promotion programs can contribute significantly toward reducing health disparities in Latino populations in several ways. These include the following: (1) facilitating consumer access to program activities in Spanish, as needed; (2) employing bilingual/bicultural staff and training them to become culturally competent; (3) integrating Latino cultural factors into core program components (family-oriented values, i.e., familism, *personalismo, respeto, simpatia*) (Castro & Hernandez-Alarcon, 2002; Marin & Marin, 1991); (4) adjusting program activities in accord with *levels of acculturation,* as these exist among program consumers; and (5) developing sensitivity to features of the local Latino community and its culture. A health promotion program can "work" when it offers health information, motivates and sustains healthy behavior change, and promotes this change in a culturally relevant manner using intervention activities that build on existing *cultural strengths.* The design of such interventions should also be guided by empirically based health promotion research that informs program developers and staff about empirically validated interventions "that work" in changing *mediators* of healthy behavior change (Kellam & Langevin, 2003; MacKinnon, Lockwood, Hoffman, West, & Sheets, 2002).

STEP 1: PROGRAM PLANNING

Contrasting Roles of Theory, Models, and Grassroots Approaches

Contrasting Approaches to Health Promotion Program Planning. In the field of prevention science, a dynamic tension exists regarding competing approaches toward prevention program planning. Generally, the "academic approach" emphasizes a theory- or model-driven "top-down" strategy that consists of an organized plan for program design. In contrast, the "grassroots community approach" builds a program from the "bottom-up," based on sensitivity and responsiveness to current community needs. The strength of the "academic approach" involves its focused organization and planning; its weakness lies in a possible lack of fit with contemporary community needs and preferences, while its emphasis on fidelity in program delivery may introduce inflexibility to changing community needs. In contrast, the strength of the grassroots community approach lies in its closeness and sensitivity to local community needs and a sensitivity to the community culture; its weakness lies in a utilization of activities or interventions that may not be empirically validated and may be ineffective in producing healthy behavior change on targeted behaviors or on other important health outcomes (Schinke, Brounstein, & Gardner, 2002).

Importance of Theory to Guide Program Design. In the applied setting, many social service and health interventions are delivered based on units of service to address a specific presenting problem. Unfortunately, such interventions are seldom governed by a well-specified theoretical, conceptual, or logic model; they often focus concretely on service delivery with limited efforts to address the underlying "causal" disease mechanisms that this intervention purports to change. In contrast, the contemporary academic approach to health promotion program planning is based on several health promotion theories and models. Among these models, the most popular are the Health Belief Model (Becker, 1974; Hochbaum, 1958; Rosenstock, 1990), the Theory of Reasoned Action (Ajzen & Fishbein, 1980; Fishbein, 1967), the Theory of Planned Behavior (Ajzen & Madden, 1986), Social Learning Theory (Bandura, 1986; Perry, Baranowski, & Parcel, 1990), Green's

PRECEDE model (Green, Kreuter, Deeds, & Partridge, 1980), and Diffusion of Innovation (Orlandi, Landers, Weston, & Haley, 1990; Rogers, 1983), the Stages of Change Model (the Transtheoretical Model) (Prochaska & DiClemente, 1992), Motivational Interviewing (Miller & Rollnick, 1991), and the Ecodevelopmental Model (Szapocznik & Coatsworth, 1999). Details of these theories and models as applied to health promotion have been described in detail by others (DiClemente, Crosby, & Kegler, 2002; Glanz, Rimer, & Lewis, 2002).

These classical theories and models of health and behavior offer important tools to guide health promotion program design, because they summarize the cumulative scientific knowledge gained from epidemiology, prevention science, health promotion, and other academic fields, as it describes and explains "what works" and "how it may work," by "mapping out" processes that govern healthy behavior change. Understanding the major factors that influence healthy behavior change, as described by these theories and models, is essential to the design of a health program curriculum that incorporates the strongest scientific and evidence-based knowledge to design more effective health promotion programs.

The Challenge of Programmatic Integration. A contemporary challenge in the field of health promotion involves integrating these "academic" and "grassroots" approaches by using theory and models to guide program planning and service delivery, while also grounding these academic models within the "real world" context of local community needs and preferences.

Furthermore, in the spirit of the *community-based participatory research* (CBPR) approach, and also to avoid a "one-size-fits-all" approach, it is desirable to obtain, "the best of both worlds," by integrating the academic and grassroots approaches. This is accomplished by drawing from a combination of theories that use traditional individual-focused behavior-change strategies, as well as by using social ecological and culturally relevant approaches (Glanz et al., 2002). In this regard, CBPR has served as a unifying translational framework, and under its basic social ecological model, it can be used as a framework for including cultural factors to restructure consumer environments, to eliminate barriers, and to facilitate healthy behavior change (Castro & Balcazar, 2000; Castro & Hernandez-Alarcon, 2002).

Anders, Balcazar, and Paez (2006) provide an example of designing a CBPR program that features a *Promotoras de Salud Model* as applied to cardiovascular disease risk reduction among Latinos/Hispanics. The *Promotoras de Salud Model,* a "natural helpers" model (Eng & Parker, 2002), builds from this ecological paradigm and incorporates cultural factors into a unified approach that addresses factors hypothesized to effect changes in health-related behaviors (Anders, et al., 2006).

Promotoras (lay health workers) are members of a local community who can be recruited and trained to administer a program or to offer health education or health promotion activities (Castro et al., 1995). They function as "cultural brokers" who serve the community and can translate bidirectionally from community to program and vice versa (Balcazar et al., 2006). Many programs have found *Promotoras* to be useful adjuncts to program recruitment and implementation because they offer personalized support (*personalismo*) that removes barriers to health care and promote self-care behaviors among women who are reached by these *Promotoras* (Reinschmidt et al., 2006). Often *Promotoras* enjoy greater trust from the local community (*mas confianza de la comunidad*). *Confianza* is a Latino cultural concept and refers to deep trust that is earned through established caring relationships. *Confianza* is often hard for new programs and program providers to attain, whereas *Promotoras* can facilitate the process of gaining *confianza* from the community and from individual program participants.

Concepts of moderators and mediators. A core question in the design of health promotion programs is "To effect changes in behavior that enhance health, where and how should we focus our intervention efforts?" The design of effective health promotion programs builds on epidemiological and other scientific evidence, on "what works." Such program design efforts are enhanced by understanding the effects of moderators and mediators as intermediate "causal" factors that operate within the "causal chain" of events that produce health-related outcomes. A basic goal in the science of prevention is to eliminate or reduce risk factors that lead to disease, and/or to increase or strengthen protective factors that safeguard against disease (Hawkins, Catalano, & Miller, 1992). To illustrate this, Figure 10.1 presents a model that describes the temporal sequence of events involving types of factors that occur in three stages: (1) antecedents, initial factors or starting conditions; (2) intermediate factors, that include moderators or mediators; and (3) outcomes, that constitute results of this causal process.

In this simple model (Panel A), the presence of various *setting conditions,* for example, *tobacco availability,* operate as initial factors that directly prompt subsequent tobacco use. This model is presented in a compact and simplified form, given that in actuality a larger combination of factors operate in the manner summarized by this simplified model. For example, factors such as socioeconomic status (SES) and an urban/rural community setting are presented here succinctly under the general category of "Setting Conditions." Thus, the physical and social environment in which a person lives presents specific "setting conditions" that can influence health-related behavior (D. A. Cohen, Mason, et al., 2003).

In the case of a *moderator variable* (an effect modifier), the influence of setting conditions on a health outcome can be moderated (can be modified) by levels of a moderator variable. Examples of moderator variables include the following: *gender*—male, female; *race/ethnicity*—Hispanic, African American, white nonminority; *levels of acculturation*—low, bicultural, high; and *traditionalism*—traditional or modernistic. For example, based on epidemiologic survey data, gender can operate as a moderator variable related to an outcome variable such as heavy alcohol use. For example, in response to setting events (being in high school or being in college), the rate of *binge drinking* (consuming five or more drinks in a row) when in high school (12th grade), and also when in college,

have been observed to differ consistently by gender. Epidemiological data confirm that for the period of the past 2 weeks, young males exhibit higher rates of binge drinking (33% in high school and 50% in college) relative to young females (23% in high school and 34% in college) (Johnson, O'Malley, Bachman, & Shulenberg, 2006). Thus, in this case, gender (male, female) operates as a moderator variable (an effect modifier) of the influence of the community setting (being in school) and the targeted outcome, binge drinking. As noted, this

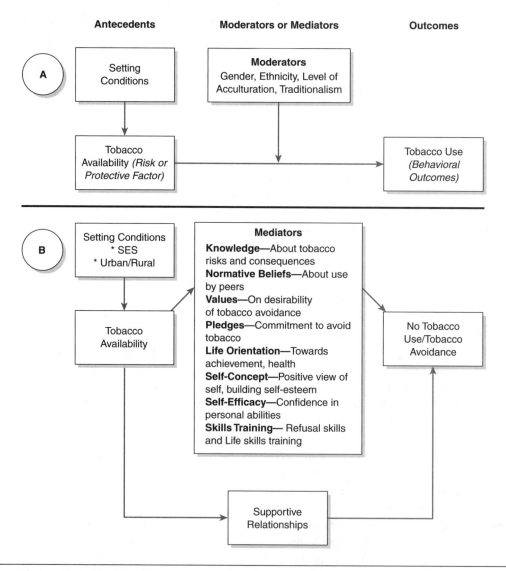

Figure 10.1   Basic Models of Moderators and Mediators of Tobacco Use

gender effect is observed both within a high school setting and within a college setting.

Furthermore, Panel B presents a set of psychosocial *mediators,* intermediary factors that can aid in preventing tobacco use among adolescents. Mediators are "intermediate" or "in-between" variables that occur in time between the setting condition and the outcome (MacKinnon, Krull, & Lockwood, 2000). Mediators are part of a stagewise sequence of events that can be targeted for modification to attenuate this disease-related "causal process." In a review of several intervention studies, Tobler (1986) noted that certain interventions can operate as mediators that aid in reducing alcohol, tobacco, and other drug (ATOD) use among adolescents. Along these lines, Hansen (1992) developed a comprehensive review of various types of interventions to prevent substance use among adolescents within school-based settings. These include (1) giving informational knowledge; (2) changing values, normative beliefs, and/or life orientations; (3) making a commitment via a public pledge to avoid ATODs; (4) enhancing self-concept, self-esteem, or self-efficacy; and/or (5) teaching refusal and life skills (see Figure 10.1). Within an effective prevention program, one or more of these specific mediating interventions are ideally combined into a coherent "prevention intervention program."

It must be noted that solely providing factual informational knowledge regarding the dangers of substance use has been shown to be a weak intervention and is usually not sufficient for motivating adolescents to avoid ATOD. In contrast, changing *normative beliefs* about the extent to which adolescent peers use tobacco may change current misconceptions regarding tobacco use, and this operates as a more potent intervention of avoidance of cigarette and other substance use. Similarly, increasing a youth's *self-esteem* or changing *self-concept* (self-image) of the self as a "nonsmoker" has a weak effect in discouraging tobacco use. A more potent intervention involves increasing *self-efficacy* and

refusal skills for avoiding tobacco use. The strategy of increasing skills to avoid tobacco use, in the form of *life skills training* (Botvin, Schinke, Epstein, Diaz, & Botvin, 1995) and *refusal skills training* (Kulis et al., 2005; Marsiglia, Kulis, Hecht, & Sills, 2004) have been shown to be the strongest mediators that help youth avoid the use of alcohol, tobacco, and illegal drugs.

In this regard, Anders et al. (2006) have used the CBPR approach with Latinos to change relevant health-related "mediators" to prevent chronic diseases such as cardiovascular disease or diabetes. This approach also includes attention to moderators that operate as contextual factors (level of acculturation, immigration status), social resources (social support, family cohesiveness, coping mechanisms), psychological responses (individual values or beliefs), and social supports (*Promotora* support and health education), as well as addressing multiple behavioral outcomes (diet, smoking, physical activity, alcohol consumption). The application of the *Promotora model* when integrated into a CBPR approach, and with a focus on changing "mediators," contributes scientific capacity and cultural content to the design of health promotion programs. This also involves a focus on changing *culturally specific mediators,* such as *family traditionalism, ethnic identity* enhancement, teaching *traditional cultural norms,* and *biculturalism,* with the aid of *Promotora*-led activities.

The Role of Staff Cultural Competence

The *cultural competence* of program staff also serves as an important factor for increasing the effectiveness of health promotion programs. *Cultural competence* refers to the capacity of health professionals or of health service delivery systems to understand *deep structure* (Resnicow, Soler, Braithwait, Ahluwalia, & Butler, 2000) and to respond with cultural sensitivity to the health needs of a specific cultural subgroup (National Alliance for Hispanic Health, 2001).

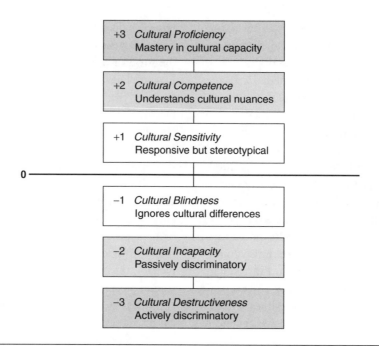

Figure 10.2   A Cultural Competence Continuum

Capacity for Cultural Competence. Figure 10.2 presents a series of cultural attitudes and capabilities ordered in sequence according to progressive levels of *cultural capacity.* From this perspective, the capacity for cultural competence varies along a graded continuum. A variation of this *cultural competence continuum* has been proposed previously by various scholars (Cross, Bazron, Dennis, & Isaacs, 1989; Kim, McLeod, & Shantzis, 1992; Orlandi et al., 1992), and has been modified and expanded elsewhere (Castro, 1998).

Along this cultural capacity continuum, the lowest capacity level is *cultural destructiveness* (−3), which involves overt discrimination and openly destructive attitudes that emphasize the "superiority" of the dominant culture and the "inferiority" of indigenous cultures. Next on this continuum, *cultural incapacity* refers to passive discrimination. This incapacity is superseded by *cultural blindness* (−1), an orientation which asserts that "all cultures and people are alike and equal." Although universal equality is an ideal, it is not a reality, and this perspective glosses over the presence of health disparities and other forms of sociocultural

inequity. Beyond these negative orientations, the first level of positive cultural capacity is *cultural sensitivity* (+1). Cultural sensitivity is characterized by having a *basic* understanding and appreciation for the importance of cultural factors in the delivery of health services.

Beyond cultural sensitivity, *cultural competence* (+2) involves the capacity to work effectively with members of a specific cultural group. Beyond cultural sensitivity, progressing to cultural competence requires greater depth in skills and experiences, thus moving beyond a superficial analysis of cultural features toward the capacity to understand and to work with *cultural nuances.* Cultural nuances are subtle but real cultural differences "that make a difference." Understanding cultural nuances facilitates an accurate interpretation of the communications and behaviors exhibited by an ethnic minority client. Thus, the health provider can accurately infer correct meaning from such thought and behavior, as interpreted within the client's unique *cultural context.* For example, among Latinos, a culturally competent health program planner would understand and appreciate the role of *personalismo,* the importance ascribed to trust and personalized communications in interpersonal relationships. Accordingly, a culturally competent program planner would incorporate aspects of *personalismo* into a health promotion program to make it more culturally relevant for initiating and maintaining program involvement among Latinos.

Finally, *cultural proficiency,* refers to the highest and idealized level of cultural capacity. It is characterized by the health professional's *deepest understanding* of cultural issues and their nuances for a specific cultural group. This would be reflected also in a health professional's capacity for leadership in the design of effective health promotion interventions for ethnic minority populations. As noted, *cultural proficiency* (+3) is the highest expression of cultural capacity, and it serves as an ideal level of capacity, a state of *high mastery* that health professionals should aspire to attain (Castro, 1998). Here, it has been noted that cultural capacity is a skills level that is specific for a particular racial/ethnic or cultural group. For example, a Latino health provider may have attained the level of cultural proficiency when working with Mexican American clients, although may only have developed the level of cultural sensitivity when working with Chinese American clients (Castro & Garfinkle, 2003).

Origins of Health Promotion Programs

Health promotion programs originate under a variety of different "starting conditions" that determine a program's purpose, identity, and developmental trajectory. Among the many possible starting conditions, the most typical ones are (1) local epidemiologic need, (2) a call for proposals, (3) tailoring of an existing program, and (4) community demand.

Local Epidemiologic Need. The direct approach to the establishment of a health promotion program emphasizes program development based on *local epidemiologic need.* In this approach, several observed cases of disease within a geographic area will signal the presence of a health-related problem. For example, low rates of vaccinations among Latino children within a local community might emerge as a potential public health problem based on clinical or epidemiologic evidence of higher rates of disease among children from a specific community.

A Call for Proposals. Response to a *call for proposals* is a second approach rooted in observed epidemiologic needs that can prompt the design of a health promotion program in response to such a call. In this approach, a sponsoring agency (the federal government, a state or county health agency, or a private foundation) identifies a particular health problem, identifies a targeted population or populations, and describes a relevant health promotion program that it seeks to fund. For example, a request for applications (RFA) or a request for proposals (RFP) from the federal government may announce the availability of federal funds to support health promotion research/service delivery projects to provide mammography screenings to low-income populations, such as among low-acculturated Latino women. The RFA announces available levels of funding and presents basic guidelines for program design and development. Under these basic starting conditions, a team of researchers/interventionists could develop a health promotion program proposal that includes a rationale for the program, a proposed curriculum, an implementation design, a timeline, and a budget. The sponsoring agency reviews the proposals submitted for scientific and programmatic merit, and the best proposals are funded based on sufficient merit as determined by a panel of expert reviewers.

Tailoring of an Existing Program. A third mechanism in the origin of a health promotion program involves tailoring of *an existing program* to create a modified program (Castro, Barrera, Martinez, 2004; Collins, Murphy, & Bierman, 2004) that better fits the needs of a specific group or community. For example, a community-based AIDS prevention program that has served Mexican Americans/Chicanos in five cities in the southwestern United States may be adapted to serve Puerto Rican populations in the New England area and in Puerto Rico, along with Cuban populations in the greater Miami area. In this case, the target population remains Hispanics, but an intervention originally designed for Mexican Americans in the Southwest should be modified to serve Puerto Ricans and Cubans in other regions of the country. Here, cultural competence in program design and adaptation involves modifying the prior AIDS prevention curriculum to address somewhat differing needs and environments experienced by the local groups of Latinos/Hispanics.

Community Demand. Finally, a fourth mechanism for developing a health promotion program is *community demand.* Based on community organization and political action by a local group of concerned citizens and community leaders, this group may demand resources to solve a local public health problem. For example, a group of residents from an inner-city housing project that has been ravaged by drug abuse and violence lobbies the city council for funds earmarked to address this problem. United as a local housing coalition, this group ultimately procures funding for a 2-year project aimed at consolidating the citizens' coalition and at educating all housing project residents on strategies for drug and violence prevention. In this case, the population targeted for this health promotion intervention is restricted geographically to those who are residents of the local housing project. Then, after this project is funded, community experts from the local university and from local community-based social service agencies may be hired as consultants to further design, monitor, and evaluate the program. In this case, a general program plan is funded and experts acceptable to the local community are subsequently hired to work out the details that aim to make the program successful.

These four types of "starting conditions" for health promotion programs, which have been observed in various Latino communities,

illustrate the diversity of conditions that influence the identity, character, and development of a given health promotion program. In each case, the deeper goal is to develop and implement a health promotion program that is effective in meeting complex and pervasive health problems that affect members of a particular Latino community.

Facilitating Problem Conceptualization and Assessment

A Verbal Logic Model. A major problem in health promotion program planning is the challenge of conceptualizing clearly the set of conditions that may lead to disease, and consequently in further conceptualizing and planning a proposed intervention or program that can arrest or counter that disease-inducing process. In other words, the problem involves developing a clear conceptualization or *logic model* during the program planning phase by "capturing the story" (modeling the causal process) that describes this process. Figure 10.3 presents a simple descriptive "causal model" framework to help health promotion program planners and health educators to think about (conceptualize) and plan a prevention intervention that can be tailored to the needs of a targeted group or population. This *verbal logic model* is used as part of the *User-Friendly Worksheet for Developing a Health Promotion Program* (see Appendix A). The *User-Friendly Worksheet* has been used as a framework to help university graduate and undergraduate students in planning and designing a viable health promotion program.

A Disease Risk Model. This "descriptive causal model" consists of two related parts: (A) a Descriptive Disease Risk Model and (B) a Descriptive Prevention Intervention Model. This verbal logic model uses conventional sentence structure to help guide program planners in conceptualizing a plausible chain of events, "a likely causal process." Part A, the *Descriptive Disease Risk Model*, describes a progressive disease process, whereas Part B, the *Descriptive Prevention Intervention Model*, presents a similar process while introducing a proposed prevention intervention. This model framework helps answer the question "What can be done programmatically in the design of a program for members of a targeted population to effectively counter the effects of a naturally occurring disease process?" The process that is "modeled" may or may not be entirely accurate, although the aim is to use theoretical and empirical health promotion knowledge and available local data as evidence regarding the events actually occurring within the local community. As shown in Figure 10.3, the sentence completion format prompts the identification of a specific "target group" by describing the group's ethnicity, age, gender, community of residence, and other defining factors, for example, Latino 10- to 12-year-old males from El Barrio. The *risk event(s)* prompts information regarding events or conditions to which members of the target group are exposed, for example, adult family members who smoke cigarettes. The subsequent *risk behavior(s)* reflect reactions to the risk event, for example, as these youths would experiment with cigarette smoking. Then, future *disease outcome(s)* can be that these youths will develop lung cancer and/or coronary heart disease in adulthood.

A Prevention Intervention Model. Following this Descriptive Disease Risk Model analysis, under the Descriptive Prevention Intervention Model analysis, the program planner is challenged to identify and describe a competing healthy "causal" process. Here, the *target population* remains the same, and thus this item is automatically carried over as the starting point within the Prevention Intervention Model. However, in this model, a specific prevention intervention is proposed. For these Latino 10- to 12-year-old males (in the fifth and sixth grades) from El Barrio, this prevention intervention could consist of [culturally relevant information and refusal skills training]. The aim is to promote certain health behavior(s), whereby these youths would [learn how to respond assertively and to refuse and avoid offers to smoke cigarettes]. And accordingly, desirable health outcome(s) would be that these youths can [actively avoid early addiction to tobacco, as well as lung cancer and coronary heart disease developing later in life as linked to cigarette smoking].

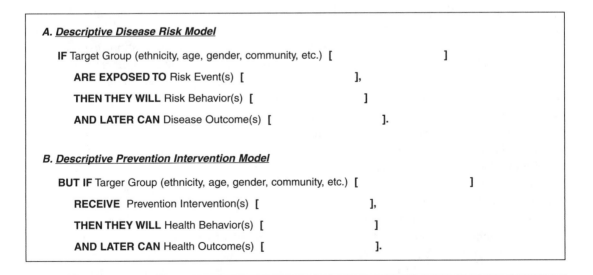

A. ***Descriptive Disease Risk Model***

   IF Target Group (ethnicity, age, gender, community, etc.) [   ]

      ARE EXPOSED TO Risk Event(s) [   ],

      THEN THEY WILL Risk Behavior(s) [   ]

      AND LATER CAN Disease Outcome(s) [   ].

B. ***Descriptive Prevention Intervention Model***

   BUT IF Targer Group (ethnicity, age, gender, community, etc.) [   ]

      RECEIVE Prevention Intervention(s) [   ],

      THEN THEY WILL Health Behavior(s) [   ]

      AND LATER CAN Health Outcome(s) [   ].

Figure 10.3   A Descriptive "Causal" Model Framework

As a second example, the Descriptive Disease Risk Model could state that: IF [adolescent Mexican American females (aged 13–18) (high school adolescents) from El Barrio] ARE EXPOSED TO [family cooking practices that feature high-fat foods], THEN THEY WILL [prepare high-fat meals for self and family] AND LATER CAN [develop obesity and non-insulin-dependent diabetes mellitus (NIDDM) by age 40]. In contrast, the Descriptive Prevention Intervention Model may state, BUT IF [adolescent Mexican American females (aged 13–18) from El Barrio] RECEIVE [training in heart healthy meal preparation], THEN THEY WILL [prepare low-fat, high-fiber meals for self and family and exercise regularly] AND LATER CAN [maintain normal weight and avoid the development of type 2 diabetes mellitus].

Key Factors in a Cultural Assessment of Health Needs

Acculturative Status. A major factor that describes the within-group variability existing among a Latino population is *level of acculturation*. For Latino/Hispanic clients, *acculturative status* refers to the client's cultural orientation and level of involvement within their Latino culture, for example, Mexican, Cuban, etc. Here, it is noteworthy that most "acculturation scales" do not measure the *process* of acculturation (cultural change), but instead measure a current level of *acculturative status*, as measured on a hypothetical dimension (continuum) that ranges from an identity that is "very Mexican" (or very Hispanic/Latino) to an identity which is "very Euro-American" (Cuellar, Harris, & Jasso, 1980).

Within the past two decades, several second-generation acculturation scales for Latinos have been developed that examine acculturation as conceptualized according to two distinct and perhaps independent (orthogonal) dimensions (Cuellar, Arnold, & Maldonado, 1995; Marin & Gamboa, 1996).

A related descriptive model of acculturation identities has also been presented based on this two-factor model (Balcazar, Castro, & Krull, 1995; Castro & Garfinkle, 2003; Castro, Nichols, & Kater, 2007). Recently, many scholars have criticized the original unidimensional measurement of acculturation among Hispanics/Latinos and other ethnic minority populations (Escobar & Vega, 2000; Hunt, Schneider, & Comer, 2004). However, despite the limitations of this elementary single-dimension conceptualization and measurement of acculturation, this simple approach still provides a useful indicator for assessing within-group variability in acculturative status among Latinos and other ethnic minority people. This approach adds useful information beyond the "ethnic gloss" (Trimble, 1995) involved in simply classifying persons as members of an ethnic minority group, such as being categorized simply as "Hispanic," "Latino," or "Mexican American," etc.

As summarized in Figure 10.4, for the acculturation continuum, recurring thematic content within these scales involves five factors: the linguistic capabilities of the participant in English and in Spanish, that is, (1) speaking capabilities, and (2) reading capabilities, (3) their level of exposure to the Euro-American (non-Hispanic white) and to the Mexican or native Latino cultures (Mexican, Puerto Rican, Cuban, etc.), (4) the ethnic identity of the person's current circle of friends (e.g., entirely Latino, from both, or entirely Euro-American or other), and (5) the level of pride that the person has toward his or her own cultural group.

As measured by a typical acculturation scale for Latinos, a prevailing concept in the literature about Latinos is that there exist three basic levels or types of acculturative status: low-acculturated, bilingual bicultural, and high acculturated (see Figure 10.4). In terms of the major sociocultural characteristics of members of these three subpopulations, low-acculturated clients are primarily Spanish speaking, have a cultural attachment with

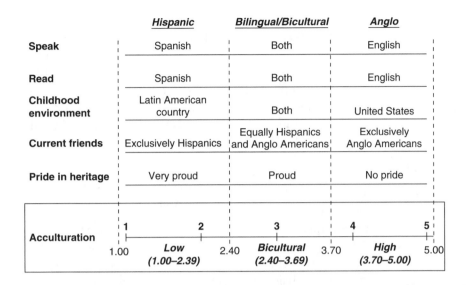

	Hispanic	**Bilingual/Bicultural**	**Anglo**
Speak	Spanish	Both	English
Read	Spanish	Both	English
Childhood environment	Latin American country	Both	United States
Current friends	Exclusively Hispanics	Equally Hispanics and Anglo Americans	Exclusively Anglo Americans
Pride in heritage	Very proud	Proud	No pride

Acculturation

1   2   3   4   5

1.00   *Low* (1.00–2.39)   2.40   *Bicultural* (2.40–3.69)   3.70   *High* (3.70–5.00)   5.00

Figure 10.4 The Acculturation Continuum: A Conceptual Framework to Accompany the General Acculturation Index

SOURCE: Felipe G. Castro, Hispanic Research Center, Arizona State University.

their native Latino culture, maintain mostly Latino friends, and tend to express pride in their native cultural background. In contrast, high-acculturated Latinos are those who primarily or exclusively speak English, feel a closer attachment toward the non-Hispanic white (Euro-American) culture, have primarily or exclusively Euro-American friends, and may express little pride in being from a Latino culture. Here also, some high-acculturated persons who are strongly oriented toward *assimilation* into the Euro-American culture may no longer identify with Latino cultural activities. Such clients may also self-identify as being "white" or "American." Furthermore, more complex ethnic identity patterns have emerged within contemporary American society with the increase in the numbers of mixed-ethnic heritage young adults, for example, youth having a Euro-American mother and a Mexican American father, based on ethnic intermarriages that increased in prevalence during the 1980s and thereafter.

Despite the limitations of a unidimensional measurement of this acculturation construct

(Rogler, Cortes, & Malgady, 1991), this variable offers useful detail in measuring levels of the within-group variability that exists among Hispanics/Latinos, as compared with only using a demographic-level categorical label, for example, "Hispanic." In summary, for Latinos(as), level of acculturation can be measured by using one of various scales that have been developed (Barona & Miller, 1994; Cuellar et al., 1980, 1995; Marin & Gamboa, 1996; Marin, Sabogal, Marin, Otero-Sabogal, & Perez-Stable, 1987).

The present authors have developed and used a short scale in telephone survey research, in community-based studies, and in the clinical setting (see Appendix B; Castro, 1988; Balcazar et al., 1995). This acculturation index (the General Acculturation Index) can be used in conjunction with the acculturation continuum (Figure 10.4) to describe a Latino client's level of acculturation. This index has exhibited sound psychometric properties (coefficient ranging from Cronbach's $\alpha \geq .70$ to .85) with various Latino populations, and it can be administered by self-report or by interview with Euro-Americans as well as with Latinos (Balcazar et al., 1995; Castro & Gutierres, 1997; see Appendix B).

Socioeconomic Status. SES is a frequently used composite indicator of socioeconomic position based on indicators of education and income. Within many Latino communities, low level of acculturation is often correlated with low SES. Indeed, with *upward social mobility,* as some Latinos acquire new skills for economic growth (education, language, social contacts) and advance upwardly in SES within the mainstream American society, their level of acculturation also tends to increase concurrently, although some develop and maintain a bilingual/bicultural identity.

Thus, as observed at a population level, the association (correlation) between level of acculturation (toward mainstream American society) and SES is often positive. For example, in one community study with a total sample of 571 Latino women, among the subgroup of immigrant Latino women (*Latinas*) ($n = 256$), level of acculturation was correlated ($r = +.22$, $p < .001$) with these women's highest level of education in Latin America (Balcazar et al., 1995). And, among a subgroup of U.S.-born Latinas ($n = 315$), level of acculturation was correlated ($r = +.21$, $p < .001$) with these women's highest level of education in the United States (Balcazar et al., 1995). Both results illustrate how among Latinas, higher levels of education are associated with higher levels of acculturation. Also, in this total sample of women, level of acculturation was correlated positively with monthly household income ($r = +50$, $p < .001$), underscoring the significant positive association often observed between higher levels of acculturation and greater incomes. However, it should also be noted that for most Latinas when observed at the individual level, this correlated process does not necessarily indicate the eventual occurrence of complete *assimilation* into mainstream American society, which refers to an ethnic person's total immersion into the mainstream culture, and that person's complete loss of

identification with his or her own native ethnic culture. In other words, at the population level, these correlations reflect the apparent movement of Latinos across the acculturation continuum as they rise in SES, although this does not necessarily indicate that an individual Latina or Latino is motivated entirely by a desire to fully assimilate.

Identifying and Segmenting the Population: A Basic Schema

Most descriptive accounts of the characteristics of Hispanics/Latinos(as) emphasize the fact that Hispanics are a heterogeneous population (Marin & Marin, 1991). In fact, the U.S. Hispanic/Latino population actually consists of clusters of related *subpopulations,* identifiable by *nationality*—that is, Mexican American, Puerto Ricans, Cubans, Dominicans, and so on (U.S. Department of Commerce, 1993; Marin & Marin, 1991)—and by other indicators—for example, urban-rural characteristics, and so on. While nationality identifies meaningful subgroups within the Hispanic population, nationality alone is too coarse a category to yield distinct and meaningful subgroups in relation to health needs and for health promotion program design. Instead, health needs covary more meaningfully in relation to SES and levels of acculturation when assessed jointly (Balcazar et al., 1995). The availability of a meaningful and easy to use method for *segmenting* the Hispanic/Latino population would be useful for program planners who work with various members of this general population.

As noted previously, specific consumer or client needs experienced by various Hispanics/Latinos may be conceptualized using this two-factor model that jointly examines levels of acculturation and levels of SES, in a 2 × 2 schema (Balcazar et al., 1995; see Figure 10.5). Level of acculturation when segmented (for simplicity) into low level ($X = 1.00$ to 2.39) and into higher levels ($X = 2.40$ to 5.00) identifies, respectively, the need for health education and services as delivered in Spanish (for

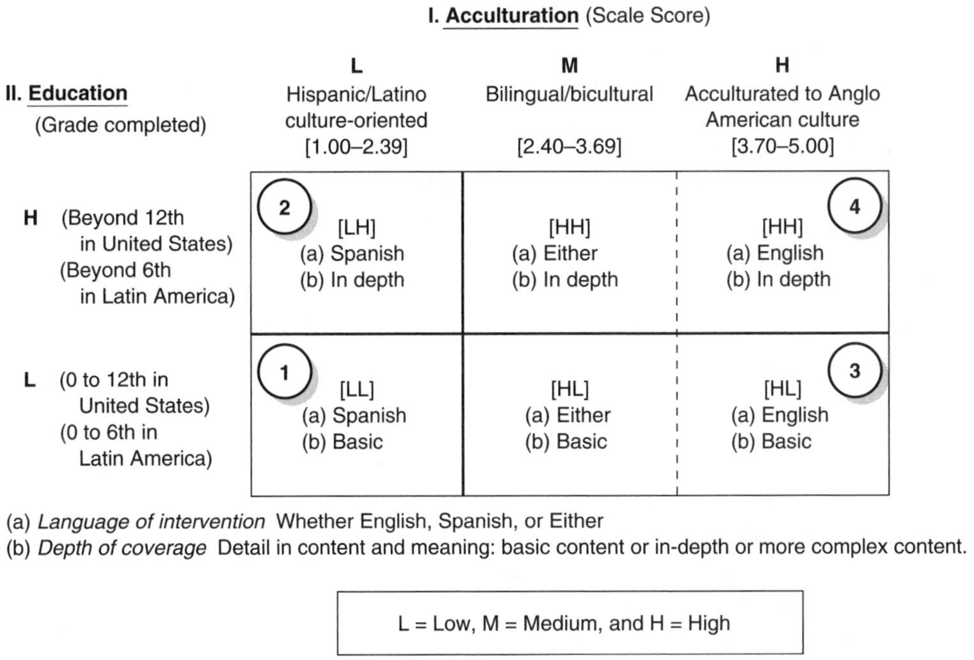

I. **Acculturation** (Scale Score)

	L Hispanic/Latino culture-oriented [1.00–2.39]	M Bilingual/bicultural [2.40–3.69]	H Acculturated to Anglo American culture [3.70–5.00]
II. **Education** (Grade completed)			
H (Beyond 12th in United States) (Beyond 6th in Latin America)	② [LH] (a) Spanish (b) In depth	[HH] (a) Either (b) In depth	[HH] (a) English (b) In depth ④
L (0 to 12th in United States) (0 to 6th in Latin America)	① [LL] (a) Spanish (b) Basic	[HL] (a) Either (b) Basic	[HL] (a) English (b) Basic ③

(a) *Language of intervention* Whether English, Spanish, or Either
(b) *Depth of coverage* Detail in content and meaning: basic content or in-depth or more complex content.

L = Low, M = Medium, and H = High

Figure 10.5   A Two-Factor Schema for Health Promotion With Latino Populations

low-acculturated clients) or as delivered in English (for higher-acculturated clients). A proxy but less accurate measure that approximates this segmentation is a client's self-report of whether he or she typically speaks in English or in Spanish. As also indicated by Figure 10.5, based on established group cut-points, a six-group segmentation can also be conducted.

These two levels of acculturation can then be cross-tabulated with a Latino client's lower or higher level of educational preparedness to comprehend programmatic information, by using the client's highest level of education. Here, *lower* educational level (6 years or less in Latin America or 12 years or less in the United States) is distinguished from a *higher* educational level. When cross-tabulated with level of acculturation, as defined previously, this can yield four distinct Latino sociocultural groups (in a 2 × 2 figure) that segments the general Latino population into four distinct and more homogeneous subpopulations that have differing health and health-educational needs (see Figure 10.5 and Balcazar et al., 1995, p. 65).

Within this schema, the low-acculturated, low-educated group (Group 1) is the "least advantaged" Latino subgroup, both socially and economically, and this subgroup typically requires more intense health promotion program planning to fully address their needs. In contrast, the higher-acculturation, higher-education group (Group 4) is the "most advantaged" group and will respond to a health promotion program that is much different in design and implementation (Lopez & Castro, 2006). Here, it might be noted that Group 4 Latino clients would be able, linguistically and by health needs, to participate in a health promotion program that is designed for middle-class Euro-American clients, while Group 1 Latinos would not.

After specific sectors or population subgroups have been identified based on this 2 × 2 factor schema, this classification can be used *to plan specific prevention interventions* that take into account the subgroup's distinct health information needs, such as language of intervention, as well as types and complexity of information that can be presented to them. In addressing the specific needs of each subgroup, it is clear that cultural competence in program planning and evaluation requires concurrent attention to both level of education and level of acculturation (Balcazar et al., 1995).

Another classification approach for Latinos examines peer group characteristics based on acculturation status and family variables such as *family cohesion*. For example, new studies have found that peer-group differences in family cohesion and acculturation are associated with different levels of cigarette smoking (Balcazar, Peterson, & Krull, 1997) and diabetes severity (Moayad, Balcazar, Pedregon, Velasco, & Bayona, 2006). It is currently postulated that high family cohesiveness that is often observed among low-acculturated peer groups may function as a protective factor against high-risk-taking behavior, a view described by some as being an *Hispanic paradox* (Castro & Coe, 2007; Palloni & Morenoff, 2001).

Taking Stock of Resources: Financial and Staffing

In assessing a program's capacity for intervention or service delivery, a proposed health promotion program must establish a balance between program scope relative to two programmatic resources: (1) the available budget for program delivery and (2) the staff who are available to deliver the intervention. Even for a specific health problem, for example, weight management among overweight Latino men and women, the health service needs of most indigent groups or populations and their lack of resources create conditions of overall need that can far outweigh the programmatic resources available to meet those needs. Thus, it is often necessary to narrow the *scope of the intervention* to define, "a feasible, manageable, affordable set of behaviors and outcomes to address and measure in a program" (Windsor, Baranowski, Clark, & Cutter, 1994, p. 83).

Limiting the amount of staff-client contact, in terms of number of program sessions offered is one strategy to reconcile program offerings with available staff resources. In addition, offering programmatic content in a group format aids in maximizing the numbers of clients reached given the available program resources. Here also, a balance must be established in program design between (1) maximum numbers of clients that the program aims to reach; (2) the duration and intensity of program activities offered, that is, the "program dose" (e.g., number of sessions); and (3) the quality of program content. The best designed health promotion programs seek to maximize coverage in all three areas while also balancing this with the limitations of staff size, staff expertise and experience, and the number of hours of face-to-face contact that the staff can offer these clients/consumers.

STEP 2: PROGRAM DEVELOPMENT

Focusing the Program's Curriculum

Regarding the conceptual steps involved in planning a health promotion program for various Latino populations, it is important to define the target group explicitly and to use public health and health psychology knowledge to design a culturally relevant curriculum that is appropriate in terms of level of acculturation, age or developmental stage, gender, health needs and preferences, etc. For these clients, the program curriculum for a disease-specific intervention, for example, diabetes prevention, may set a goal of reducing the prevalence of obesity within a targeted group of disadvantaged (low-acculturated, low-educated; Group 1) Latinas, aged 25 to 40. In addition, the proposed program's curriculum of program content must also consider the complex of health risk factors and environmental barriers that co-occur with obesity among these disadvantaged Latinos and Latinas (Marks, Garica, & Solis, 1990). Such co-occurring factors may include limited access to health care, an exposure to impoverished living conditions that impose high levels of stress, limited access to healthier foods, comorbidity with other health problems, for example, tuberculosis, and so on (Carter-Pokras, 1994; Giachello, 1994).

For example, in planning a program for diabetes risk reduction among disadvantaged Latinos (Group 1), the apparent "individual" problem of being overweight must be conceptualized and defined within the broader context of a family system, both core and extended, in which family members may regularly consume high fat foods when attending various cultural family activities and traditional celebrations, such as baptisms, *quinceneras,* weddings, birthday parties, etc.

Defining Program Goals and Objectives

Defining and setting goals and objectives of a health promotion program are an important task in translating health promotion theory and intervention strategies into a specific curriculum of program activities. Program *goals* are broad aims that give direction to the health promotion program, whereas program *objectives* consist of specific details that specify how each program goal will be reached. In other words, program goals are *general*—for example, "to increase rates of exercise among Latinas in the local community." In contrast, program objectives are *specific*: "during the forthcoming month, participating Latinas, ages 25 to 40, will increase walking exercise from zero to three days a week, by walking for 15 minutes or more at each session." Program objectives are stated to include four specific components: (1) the targeted population, (2) the timeframe or conditions, (3) a specific outcome, and (4) a criterion for achieving that outcome (McKenzie et al., 2005). Typically, each goal will have one or more objectives (see Appendix A, the User-Friendly Worksheet for Developing Health Promotion Programs).

Proposing Ideal Versus Achievable Program Goals

In the development of a culturally relevant health promotion curriculum to address health disparities among racial/ethnic minority populations, dedicated program developers tend to propose ambitious programmatic goals and objectives. This may be prompted by their desires to improve the health status of disadvantaged (Group 1) Latino populations (those least acculturated, least educated, and poorest Latinos), in light of their existing health disparities. In contrast, setting modest but attainable goals while also addressing barriers to full program participation constitute a prudent approach for designing a viable health promotion program that is more likely to succeed. As one practical issue, a participant's acquisition of program knowledge and skills does not always progress in a cumulative and linear manner. For example, in a 10-session cancer prevention program that covers issues of prevention through screening self-examinations, healthy diet, and healthy lifestyles, a typical Latino program participant from the disadvantaged Latino group (Group 1) might miss attendance at 3 to 6 out of the 10 sessions due to transportation problems, unexpected family emergencies, personal illness, competing family priorities, or waning interest. Thus, a 10-session program may only succeed in imparting half its program content and skills, that is, a 50% exposure to the full "program dose," with even less than that in the form of actual learning of program content. Having fewer sessions does tend to increase attendance per session (Kumpfer et al., 2002), whereas in contrast, a limit exists in the amount of information, skills development and overall learning can be incorporated into each of these individual sessions.

This situation prompts the need for program planners to incorporate *repetition and review* into the design of the health promotion program curriculum, as well as to set modest program goals. A general rule of thumb is to anticipate that clients from the most disadvantaged group may only exhibit a 50% acquisition (learning) rate of program content, relative to an ideal learning and/or skills development rate of 100%, if learning had occurred efficiently and in a cumulative fashion.

Accordingly, such experiences should prompt the program planner to set *achievable goals* and *realistic learning objectives,* relative to this ideal or complete mastery of program content.

In contrast, in working with the more advantaged Latinos, Latinos with higher education, high SES, and high acculturation (Group 4), and perhaps for those of high education and lower acculturation (Group 2; see Figure 10.5), goals and learning objectives may be set at 80% of the ideal. For example, among these *more advantaged* Latinos, an 80% attendance rate (8 of 10 sessions), and 80% correct learning on a knowledge test, skills acquisition at 80% of maximum, or course passage by 80% of the group of participants, constitute realistic goals, whereas setting these goals at 50% may be more realistic for Latinos from the disadvantaged group (Group 1).

Strategies for Strengthening the Intervention

A major but elusive goal in the design of effective health promotion programs is to design an effective intervention, one that yields empirical evidence-based data that it truly "works" in effecting a significant change on the targeted behavior or health outcome that the program purports to change, for example, weight loss in an obesity treatment program. This effectiveness is measured in terms of the magnitude of change from baseline to postintervention observations, on targeted health-related beliefs, attitudes, and/or behaviors. In other words, the intervention exhibits a significant *effect size* (Tobler, Lessard, Marshall, Ochshorn, & Roona, 1999), a measure of the strength of effect of the intervention on a specified health outcome (J. Cohen, 1988; J. Cohen, Cohen, West, & Aiken, 2003). In other words, "How much change did the program produce as compared with an inert program or placebo group?" For example, for a weight reduction program, how much weight loss was achieved per individual client, and across all participating clients? Many school-based prevention intervention programs exhibit *small to*

moderate effect sizes on targeted outcomes (Tobler et al., 1999). In contrast, as community-based prevention interventions typically lack the controlled conditions of school-based interventions that foster consistent consumer participation, community-based programs are typically expected to exhibit intervention effects in the range of *small effect sizes.* In the extreme case, if an intervention program for weight loss produces no weight loss among program participants, then the effect size will be zero, leading to the conclusion that the program "did not work." Changing specific health-related behaviors among residents of a small community poses a major health promotion challenge, and this challenge is even greater when working with disadvantaged populations.

A few strategies have been proposed that may strengthen a health promotion intervention. One strategy, (1) *maintaining intervention fidelity*, focuses on delivering a planned (often a manualized) intervention consistently and in the exact manner in which it was designed (Hansen & Collins, 1994). This quality control activity seeks to ensure that all clients receive the same and a complete "dose" of the tested and effective health intervention protocol. Clearly, a complementary strategy to ensure that a client receives the maximum intervention "dose" is to promote (2) *full client participation and adherence* with the intervention's activities. However, as noted previously, among many Latinos, the effectiveness of these two strategies for promoting healthy behavior change is contingent on the availability of an accessible, well-designed, and culturally relevant intervention protocol that engages their interest and participation.

In this regard, a strategy for enhancing the magnitude of program effect is to (3) *develop a culturally effective intervention,* one that appeals and greatly motivates participation and learning among members of the targeted audience. A related strategy for enhancing program effect that is based on cultural relevance is to (4) *target appropriate mediators* of relevant behavior change (Hansen & Collins,

1994). Here, also, this strategy includes identifying culturally relevant mediators, which is possible when a program planner is culturally competent and fully understands the culture of the targeted group.

Another strategy to enhance intervention effect is to (5) *establish environmental contingencies that prompt or reward healthy behavior change* (Kazdin, 1994). For a given cultural group, this also requires in-depth knowledge of the cultural and environmental conditions that govern the occurrence of a targeted behavior and the use of these natural reinforcing consequences that produce change in a targeted health-related behavior or behaviors. Finally, another key strategy is to (6) *develop a system of social supports,* a system that will prompt and maintain healthy behavior change within a given community setting. Given the central role of *la familia* (the family) within Latino cultures, a culturally effective health promotion program curriculum for Latinos(as) should explicitly include family-related issues. Accordingly, the program curriculum would do well to include a module that devotes a complete session to Latino family issues and dynamics and that mobilizes family support.

STEP 3: PROGRAM IMPLEMENTATION

Flexibility in Program Development

Once a program operates effectively by developing "programmatic momentum," a program tends to evolve and even develop "a program identity" as it establishes recognition within the local community. Although programmatic guidelines may give a program its direction, in time a program can serendipitously develop in a few unique and unexpected ways. This may be a positive or a negative occurrence as related to program effectiveness. Proactive program managers will detect such serendipitous and perhaps unexpected developments as related to initial program goals and objectives. Some of these unique developments can then be considered in relation to principles of prevention science and health promotion, and within the context of the original program goals and objectives, when considering possible program modifications for use in a new program cycle. In this regard, a major program challenge involves making indicated adjustments in program curriculum and activities, procedures and forms of delivery (program adaptation), provided that such changes do not detract from attaining established program goals and objectives and intended program outcomes (Castro et al., 2004; Collins et al., 2004).

Staff Development and Administrative Leadership

Role of Administrative Leadership. One factor that is seldom discussed in health promotion program design and implementation, yet which is critical to program effectiveness, is administrative leadership. The best administrators or program directors of health promotion programs with Latino populations appear to be those who (1) have a knowledge of the local community and an organized vision of the program's purpose and direction; (2) can communicate this vision to program staff on a regular basis; (3) can build commitment and morale among program staff; (4) give staff members an appropriate voice regarding program policies and procedures; (5) plan meetings as needed to speak personally with community leaders and other community stakeholders; (6) maintain a balance between scientific agendas and cultural agendas in the ongoing evolution of the program; (7) are *proactive* in anticipating problems, and in searching for solutions that optimize program effectiveness given the available resources; (8) inspire confidence and trust among staff and community members as a dedicated leader whose agenda is driven by the goal of enhancing the health and welfare of the local community; and (9) exhibit strength and integrity in responding forcefully on behalf of the program, as needed.

A program director's attention to these issues, in consultation with staff and/or with the program's advisory board, will prompt effective decision making on behalf of the project. Effective administrative leadership and oversight also involves making programmatic decisions that enhance the project by (1) garnering support for the program from the local community and from the funding agency; (2) strengthening staff morale and commitment to project goals; (3) maintaining fidelity in program implementation to the extent possible; (4) identifying serendipitous developments that may improve program effectiveness by making informed program adaptations when needed; (5) ensuring an effective program evaluation that documents program development as well as its effectiveness; and (6) meeting regularly with staff to assess program activities, engaging in problem solving, and planning for future activities and program growth. Effective program administration and management is often a "hidden factor" not examined closely in the past, a factor that may contribute significantly to a health promotion program's overall effectiveness.

Eliminating Barriers to Participation

Specifically targeting *treatment barriers* in advance (*de ante mano*) will avoid major design errors and serve to inform program planners/ providers of critical barriers to program adherence. There are a number of barriers that have been identified when working with Latinos(as)/ Hispanics. These barriers can be grouped into categories such as (1) personal, (2) systemic, and (3) community-based. Personal barriers include, but are not limited to, a client's or patient's mental health status, cultural and linguistic background, education level, and family structure. For example, cognitive or educational capacity to follow through with program or treatment recommendations is critical. Among Latino populations, limited English-speaking abilities constitute an obvious barrier to understanding programmatic activities or treatment guidelines, unless program content is available in Spanish. Also, cultural beliefs that are in conflict with program information or treatment

might not be so easily identifiable (e.g., use of herbal remedies). Furthermore, family structure may appear one way in a clinical or community program setting but may be completely different in the participant's home. For example, the mother may bring the children for appointments or program sessions, but it may be the father who determines what is done at home. A "treatment boss" conceivably could be a family member, spiritual leader, or other influential individual. In that case it would be a good idea to know who that person is what she or he exactly will support in terms of program planning.

Regarding systemic barriers, access to the program site or clinic, bus lines, clinic or program hours, and physical appearance of a program location can all operate as barriers to participation in a program or treatment. White Memorial Hospital in Los Angeles serves as an example of a complete systemic makeover that led that hospital out of bankruptcy and into a successful inpatient and outpatient medical practice. The strategies used included community outreach, community needs assessment, and a public relations makeover. The hospital reinvented itself from a private, elitist hospital to a community-oriented hospital. It originally had been a private hospital, although the surrounding neighborhood changed to a mainly Hispanic, Asian, and African American population. The facilities are now attractive and culturally inviting and include ethnic art and signs in multiple languages that reflect the cultures of the local community. The hospital also has remarkable staff diversity.

Community barriers may be political in nature or simply a matter of tradition. Courting community leaders and collaborating with community needs may constitute the difference between program success and failure. *Centro de Amistad,* a community-based health services center located in the township of Guadalupe, Arizona, has united Yaqui Indian, Mexican Immigrant, and Mexican American populations to create a number of successful community-based health campaigns, such as a *Promotora-*led diabetes screening and management program. Their success stems from collaborations with community leaders and representatives who participate in their program planning and implementation.

STEP 4: PROGRAM EVALUATION

Considerations in Program Evaluation

The Single-Group Repeated Measures Design. A program's evaluation plan should be developed during the program planning stage and should serve as a core component of the total health promotion program. In formal program evaluation research, an experimentally sound evaluation design typically features an *intervention group* and *a control group* and the randomization of clients or schools to each of these groups depending on the unit of analysis (McKenzie et al., 2005). However, for many community-based health promotion programs, such design elegance is seldom possible. Typical in such programs is the absence of a *control group* and of *randomization*; in contrast, the opportunity to obtain multiple measures across specific time points to examine client progress is often possible. These conditions naturally yield a *one-group repeated measures design*. While this design has evaluation weaknesses, it does offer a viable program evaluation design that is applicable within many community settings (Windsor et al., 1994).

This one-group repeated measures design only allows program evaluators to draw limited but, nonetheless, useful conclusions regarding program effects. Given that internal validity is *not* an all-or-nothing condition, but rather a matter of degree, a well-developed and well-implemented single-group repeated measures design can yield a useful and reasonably valid outcome data regarding effects that are likely attributable to the program intervention. For many community service programs, such evidence of program effect, whether or not attributable exclusively to the intervention itself, serves as viable evidence that points to program effectiveness.

In addition, under this one-group design, much valuable *process-related data* can be gathered regarding the manner in which the program was delivered and the possible mechanisms of program effect. Such data can, "tell the story" of the program's development and possible sources of program effectiveness. The well-planned and regular collection of specific measured variables along with qualitative *narrative data* (e.g., on a weekly basis), as obtained from key program participants (clients, health educators, administrators, etc.), can generate a stream of programmatic data that can describe the temporal growth of the program and its possible effects (Ulin, Robinson, & Tolley, 2005). Thematic extraction methods, such as those described from grounded theory (open coding, axial coding, in vivo coding, selective coding, process analysis, case analysis, and model building), can be used to build a rich and informative account of program process (Castro & Coe, 2007; Miles & Huberman, 1994; Strauss & Corbin, 1990). The popular program for the coding and analysis of qualitative text data, *Atlas.Ti* (Muhr, 2004), and other related programs can be used to conduct the analysis of such data (Castro & Coe, 2007).

Relating Evaluation Design to Programmatic Realities

Specific details on fundamental aspects and approaches for program evaluation of health promotion programs have been presented elsewhere (McKenzie et al., 2005). As noted previously, along with program design and implementation, cultural competence in the evaluation of community-based health promotion programs for Latino populations also requires an in-depth knowledge and appreciation of issues that affect program effectiveness with various Latino populations (Skaff, Chesla, de los Santos, Mycue, & Fisher, 2002). The evaluation program itself should include *culturally relevant measures*, for example, measures of acculturation that aptly evaluate population characteristics as well as program effects on relevant outcomes, as specifically relevant for members of a targeted group of Latinos(as). Accordingly, the assessment protocol must consist of survey or interview items or questions that are matched to the linguistic and educational aptitudes of members of the targeted population. In working with various Latino populations, developing conceptually parallel assessment forms in Spanish as well as in English is often necessary (Geisinger, 1994; Gonzalez, Stewart, Ritter, & Lorig, 1995) (e.g., see Appendix B). The availability of simple, easily administered, and clinically useful measures that are reliable and valid for use with various Latino populations (i.e., available in English and in Spanish) remains as an important area for research and development that can aid in the design and implementation of health promotion programs for Latinos (Marin & Marin, 1991).

Process and outcome information that aids in program evaluation includes the systemic collection of brief but specific information on consumer/client adherence, information on barriers to program participation, and information on program-related health outcomes. In turn, when used under a *formative evaluation* approach, initial results, when used as early stage evaluative feedback, can aid in improving or fine-tuning program content and activities. Moreover, four types of client *baseline information* (collected at intake) will aid in describing and understanding the characteristics of the participating clientele. These major types of data are (1) group cultural characteristics, (2) sociocultural resources, (3) subjective health culture, and (4) access to health services. In particular, simple descriptive data on the acculturative and sociocultural characteristics of Latino program participants, as compared with those who have declined participation or who have dropped out, can yield valuable programmatic information on which clients the program has reached effectively and which clients the program has failed to engage (Lopez & Castro, 2006).

A similar strategy in the use of baseline and ongoing monitoring data can be implemented, perhaps more easily within a clinical setting. As clients complete a treatment or a follow-up session, the administration of a brief treatment summary form can generate significant data for monitoring the client's progress and for evaluating program-related outcomes. The goal is to administer a simple form on a regular basis, so that it becomes a routine and standard aspect of a client's clinical visit. Unfortunately, many clinical settings typically do not plan nor implement even this simple evaluation activity.

In contrast, invoking the principle of participation, while involving program or clinic staff in the planning, design, and implementation of a program's evaluation plan can build their sense of ownership and participation. This is a particularly useful strategy during the present *era of accountability* in which program funding and a program's survival is often contingent on documenting program effectiveness. Thus, beyond the issue of funding, program staff who are committed to the delivery of effective services to their clients can be encouraged to participate in the design and implementation of a program evaluation protocol. They can be advised that their effectiveness as interventionists and their contributions toward enhancing the health of their clients and community can be documented and their efforts refined, based on their active participation in the overall evaluation effort.

CHAPTER SUMMARY

In guiding the design of culturally effective health promotion programs for Latinos(as), many dimensions of cultural relevance and scientific intervention should be considered. Designing culturally relevant programs for a specific community involves "starting where the people are." This means knowing well the culture of the targeted community and then building a framework from which to infuse "cultural relevance" into each of the four steps involved in program design, and as outlined within the *User-Friendly Worksheet for Developing a Health Promotion Program* (see Appendix A). A thorough community-grounded needs assessment involves that community leaders and residents lay the foundation for culturally relevant program design.

Designing a culturally relevant program can also involve *innovation,* which involves introducing new cultural components based on identified community needs but added to the program curriculum in relation to an empirically based theoretical or scientific rationale and with design rigor. Thus, when infusing a program with culturally relevant activities for Latino populations, it is helpful to incorporate certain cultural features into program design. These cultural features can include the following: (1) specific cultural factors (*personalismo, respeto,* familism, gender issues, etc.), integral components of the health promotion program; (2) specifying cultural characteristics beyond demographics (i.e., level of acculturation, family cohesiveness, ethnic identity); (3) targeting specific subgroups and tailoring to their needs, without compromising program effectiveness; (4) incorporating CBPR methods for relevance and innovation to program design; (5) incorporating and building new conceptual frameworks or logic models based on cultural relevance and innovation yet based also on a scientific foundation; (6) establishing a mix and balance of quantitative rigor with depth and richness of qualitative cultural assessment; and (7) aiming toward both innovation and efficacy into the program design. Reaching communities with culturally relevant programs requires the "art of designing" health promotion programs that are relevant, innovative, and efficacious. Enhancing program design with the appropriate *infusion of cultural factors* is an emerging prerequisite for successful program planning, development, implementation, and evaluation of health promotion programs that effectively reach and inspire Latino/Hispanic communities with a combination of cultural responsiveness and strong science.

The next chapter presents a case study where the author tries to emphasize points made in the overview and planning chapters. The study is concerned with the application of concepts and approaches for bridging the gap between theory and practice. They provide an opportunity for the student and practitioner to get a "bird's-eye" view of some of the specific methods and techniques of HPDP program planning, application, and problem solving.

NOTES

1. The *Hispanic/Latino* population of the United States numbered 41.32 million as of July 1, 2004, constituting 14.07% of the U.S. population, thus making Hispanics/Latinos the largest racial/ethnic population of the United States (U.S. Census Bureau, 2005). In this chapter, we will use the terms *Latinos* and *Hispanics* interchangeably, based on the dual usage that occurs within the contemporary literature. These terms refer to people living in the United States, primarily Mexican Americans, Chicanos or Chicanas who live in the southwestern United States, as well as Puerto Ricans (both from the Island of Puerto Rico and from the mainland United States), and Cubans, as well as other Hispanics/Latinos, which include Colombians, Guatemalans, Nicaraguans, and other immigrants and naturalized persons from Central America and South America.

2. This *user-friendly worksheet* has been used for several years in a graduate/undergraduate course titled Health Promotion in Minority Populations. This outline presents a series of questions that "walk through" the student across major steps and activities involved in health promotion program design.

3. The terms *participant, consumer, client,* and *patient* will be used interchangeably as participants or consumers who are the recipients of community-based health promotion programs, and clients or patients who are the recipients of agency-based health promotion programs. We are discussing program design as relevant to both settings and to persons who receive the health promotion program within these various settings.

REFERENCES

Ajzen, I., & Fishbein, M. (1980). *Understanding attitudes and predicting social behavior.* Englewood Cliffs, NJ: Prentice Hall.

Ajzen, I., & Madden, T. J. (1986). Prediction of goal-directed behavior: Attitudes, intentions, and perceived behavioral control. *Journal of Experimental Social Psychology, 22,* 453–474.

Anders, R., Balcazar, H., & Paez, L. (2006). Hispanic community-based participatory research using a Promotores de Salud model. *Hispanic Health Care International, 4,* 71–78.

Balcazar, H., Alvarado, M., Hollen, M. L., Gonzalez-Cruz, Y., Hughes, O., Vazquez, E., et al. (2006). *Salud Para Su Corazon*—NCLR: A comprehensive *Promotora* outreach program to promote Herat-healthy behaviors among Hispanics. *Health Promotion Practice, 7,* 68–77.

Balcazar, H., Castro, F. G., & Krull, J. L. (1995). Cancer risk reduction in Mexican American women: The role of acculturation, education, and health risk factors. *Health Education Quarterly, 22,* 61–84.

Balcazar, H., Peterson, G., & Krull, J. (1997). Acculturation and family cohesiveness in Mexican American pregnant women: Social and health implications. *Family & Community Health, 20,* 16–31.

Bandura, A. (1986). *Social foundations of thought and action: A Social Cognitive Theory.* Englewood Cliffs, NJ: Prentice Hall.

Barona, A., & Miller, J. A. (1994). Short acculturation scale for Hispanic youth (SASH-Y): A preliminary report. *Hispanic Journal of Behavioral Sciences, 16,* 155–162.

Becker, M. H. (1974). The Health Belief Model and personal health behavior. *Health Education Monographs, 2,* 324–473.

Botvin, G. J., Schinke, S. P., Epstein, J. A., Diaz, T., & Botvin, E. M. (1995). Effectiveness of culturally-focused and generic skills training approaches to alcohol and drug abuse prevention among minority adolescents. *Psychology of Addictive Behaviors, 9,* 183–194.

Brownson, R. C., Remington, P. L., & Davis, J. R. (1998). *Chronic disease epidemiology and control* (2nd ed.). Washington, DC: American Public Health Association.

Carter-Pokras, O. (1994). Health profile. In C. W. Molina & M. Aguirre-Molina (Eds.), *Latino health in the U.S.: A growing challenge* (pp. 45–79). Washington, DC: American Public Health Association.

Carter-Pokras, O., & Baquet, C. (2002). What is a "health disparity"? *Public Health Reports, 117,* 426–434.

Castro, F. G. (1988). *Southern California social survey.* Unpublished manuscript.

Castro, F. G. (1998). Cultural competence training in clinical psychology: Assessment, clinical intervention, and research. In A. S. Bellack & M. Hersen (Eds.), *Comprehensive clinical psychology: Sociocultural and individual differences* (Vol. 10, pp. 127–140). Oxford, UK: Pergamon.

Castro, F. G., & Balcazar, H. (2000, April). *Cultural considerations in prevention practice: Bringing prevention into practice.* Paper presented at the Northern California Conference on Prevention Technology, San Jose, California.

Castro, F. G., Barrera, M., & Martinez, C. (2004). The cultural adaptation of prevention interventions: Resolving the tensions between fidelity and fit. *Prevention Science, 5,* 41–45.

Castro, F. G., Barrera, M., Pantin, H., Martinez, C., Felix-Ortiz, M., Rios, R., et al. (2006). Substance abuse prevention intervention research with Hispanic populations. *Drug and Alcohol Dependence, 84S,* S29–S42.

Castro, F. G., & Coe, K. (2007). Traditions and alcohol use: A mixed-methods analysis. *Cultural Diversity & Ethnic Minority Psychology, 13,* 269–284.

Castro, F. G., Elder, J., Coe, K., Tafoya-Barraza, H. M., Moratto, S., Campbell, N., et al. (1995). Mobilizing churches for health promotion in Latino communities: *Compañeros en la Salud. Journal of the National Cancer Institute Monographs, 18,* 127–135.

Castro, F. G., & Garfinkle, J. (2003). Critical issues in the development of culturally relevant substance abuse treatments for specific minority groups. *Alcoholism: Clinical and Experimental Research, 27,* 1–8.

Castro, F. G., & Gutierres, S. (1997). Drug and alcohol use among rural Mexican Americans. In E. R. Robertson, Z. Sloboda, G. M. Boyd, L. Beatty, & N. J. Kozel (Eds.), *Rural substance abuse: State of knowledge and issues* (pp. 499–533). NIDA Research Monograph No. 168. Rockville, MD: National Institute on Drug Abuse.

Castro, F. G., & Hernandez-Alarcon, E. (2002). Integrating cultural variables into drug abuse prevention and treatment with racial/ethnic minorities. *Journal of Drug Issues, 32,* 783–810.

Castro, F. G., Nichols, E., & Kater, K. (2007). Relapse prevention with Hispanic and other racial/ethnic populations: Can cultural resilience promote relapse prevention? In K. Witkiewitz & G. A. Marlatt (Eds.), *A therapist's guide to evidence-based relapse prevention* (pp. 257–290). Burlington, MA: Elsevier.

Cohen, D. A., Mason, K., Bedimo, A., Scribner, R., Basolo, V., & Farley, T. A. (2003). Neighborhood physical conditions and health. *American Journal of Public Health, 93,* 467–471.

Cohen, J. (1988). *Statistical power analysis for the behavioral sciences* (2nd ed.). Hillsdale, NJ: Lawrence Erlbaum.

Cohen, J., Cohen, P., West, S. G., & Aiken, L. S. (2003). *Applied multiple regression/correlation analysis for the behavioral sciences* (3rd ed.). Mahwah, NJ: Lawrence Erlbaum.

Collins, L. M., Murphy, S. A., & Bierman, K. L. (2004). A conceptual framework for adaptive prevention interventions. *Prevention Science, 5,* 185–196.

Cross, T. L., Bazron, B. J., Dennis, K. W., & Isaacs, M. R. (1989). *Toward a culturally competent system of care.* Washington, DC: Georgetown University Child Development Center.

Cuellar, I., Arnold, B., & Maldonado, R. (1995). Acculturation rating scale for Mexican-Americans II: A revision of the original ARMSA scale. *Hispanic Journal of Behavioral Sciences, 17,* 275–304.

Cuellar, I., Harris, L. C., & Jasso, R. (1980). An acculturation rating scale for Mexican American normal and clinical populations. *Hispanic Journal of Behavioral Sciences, 2,* 199–217.

DiClemente, R. J., Crosby, R. A., & Kegler, M. C. (2002). *Emerging theories in health promotion practice and research.* San Francisco: Jossey-Bass.

Eng, E., & Parker, E. (2002). Natural helper models to enhance a community's health and competence. In R. J. DiClemente, R. A. Crosby, & M. C. Kegler (Eds.), *Emerging theories in health promotion practice and research* (pp. 126–156). San Francisco: Jossey-Bass.

Escobar, J. I., & Vega, W. A. (2000). Mental health immigration's AAA's: Where we are and where do we go from here? *Journal of Nervous and Mental Disease, 188,* 736–740.

Fishbein, M. (Ed.). (1967). Attitude and the prediction of behavior: Results of a survey sample. In *Readings in attitude theory and measurement* (pp. 477–491). New York: Wiley.

Geisinger, K. F. (1994). Cross-cultural normative assessment translation and adaptation issues influencing the normative interpretation of assessment instruments. *Psychological Assessment, 6,* 304–312.

Gonzalez, V. M., Stewart, A., Ritter, P. L., & Lorig, K. (1995). Translation and validation of arthritis outcome measures into Spanish. *Arthritis and Rheumatism, 38,* 1429–1446.

Giachello, A. L. (1994). Issues of access and use. In C. W. Molina & M. Aguirre-Molina (Eds.), *Latino health in the U.S.: A growing challenge* (pp. 83–111). Washington, DC: American Public Health Association.

Glanz, K., Rimer, B. K., & Lewis, F. M. (2002). *Health behavior and health education: Theory, research and practice* (3rd ed.). San Francisco: Jossey-Bass.

Green, L. W., Kreuter, M. W., Deeds, S. G., & Partridge, K. D. (1980). *Health education planning: A diagnostic approach.* Mountain View, CA: Mayfield.

Hansen, W. B. (1992). School-based substance abuse prevention: A review of the state of the art in curriculum, 1980–1990. *Health Education Research, 7,* 403–430.

Hansen, W. B., & Collins, L. M. (1994). Seven ways to increase power without increasing N. In L. M. Collins & L. A. Seitz (Eds.), *Advances in data analysis for prevention intervention research* (pp. 184–195). NIDA Research Monograph No. 142. Rockville, MD: National Institute on Drug Abuse.

Hawkins, J. D., Catalano, R. F., & Miller, J. Y. (1992). Risk and protective factors for alcohol and other drug problems in adolescence and early adulthood: Implications for substance abuse prevention. *Psychological Bulletin, 112,* 64–105.

Hirachi, T. W., Catalano, R. F., & Hawkins, J. D. (1997). Effective recruitment for parenting programs within ethnic minority communities. *Journal of Child and Adolescent Social Work, 14,* 23–39.

Hochbaum, G. M. (1958). *Public participation in medical screening programs: A sociopsychological study*. Public Health Service Publication No. 572. Washington, DC: U.S. Public Health Service.

Hunt, L. M., Schneider, S., & Comer, B. (2004). Should "acculturation" be a variable in health research? A critical review of research with U.S. Hispanics. *Social Science & Medicine, 59,* 973–986.

Johnson, L. D., O'Malley, P. M., Bachman, J. G., & Shulenberg, J. E. (2006). *Monitoring the future national survey results on drug use, 1975–2005: Vol. 1. Secondary school students* (NIH Publication No. 06–5883). Bethesda, MD: National Institute on Drug Abuse.

Kazdin, A. (1994). *Behavior modification in applied settings* (5th ed.). Pacific Grove, CA: Brooks/Cole.

Kellam, S. G., & Langevin, D. S. (2003). A framework for understanding "evidence" in prevention research programs. *Prevention Science, 4,* 137–153.

Kim, S., McLeod, J. H., & Shantzis, C. (1992). Cultural competence for evaluators working with Asian American communities: Some practical considerations. In M. A. Orlandi, R. Weston, & L. G. Epstein (Eds.), *Cultural competence for evaluators* (pp. 203–260). Rockville, MD: Office of Substance Abuse Prevention.

Kulis, S., Marsiglia, F. F., Elek, E., Dustman, P. A., Wagstaff, D. A., & Hecht, M. L. (2005). Mexican/Mexican American adolescents and keepin' it REAL: An evidence based substance abuse prevention program. *Child and School, 27,* 133–145.

Kumpfer, K. L., Alvarado, R., Smith, P., & Bellamy, N. (2002). Cultural sensitivity and adaptation in family-based prevention interventions. *Prevention Science, 3,* 241–246.

Lopez, V., & Castro, F. G. (2006). Participation and program outcomes in a church-based cancer prevention program for Hispanic women. *Journal of Community Health, 31,* 343–362.

MacKinnon, D. P., Krull, J. L., & Lockwood, C. M. (2000). Equivalence of mediation, confounding, and suppression effect. *Prevention Science, 1,* 173–181.

MacKinnon, D. P., Lockwood, C. M., Hoffman, J. M., West, S. G., & Sheets, V. (2002). A comparison of methods to test mediation and other intervening variable effects. *Psychological Methods, 7,* 83–104.

Marin, G., & Gamboa, R. J. (1996). A new measurement of acculturation for Hispanics: The Bidimensional Acculturation Scale for Hispanics (BAS). *Hispanic Journal of Behavioral Sciences, 18,* 297–316.

Marin, G., & Marin, B. V. (1991). *Research with Hispanic populations.* Newbury Park, CA: Sage.

Marin, G., Sabogal, F., Marin, B. V., Otero-Sabogal, R., & Perez-Stable, E. J. (1987). Development of a short acculturation scale for Hispanics. *Hispanic Journal of Behavioral Sciences, 9,* 183–205.

Marks, G., Garcia, M., & Solis, J. M. (1990). Health risk behaviors of Hispanics in the United States: Findings from HHANES, 1982–84. *American Journal of Public Health, 80*(Suppl.), 20–26.

Marsiglia, F. F., Kulis, S., Hecht, M. L., & Sillis, S. (2004). Ethnicity and ethnic identity as predictors of drug norms and drug use among preadolescents in the U.S. Southwest. *Substance Use & Misuse, 39,* 1061–1094.

McKenzie, J. F., Nieger, B. L., & Smeltzer, J. L. (2005). *Planning, implementing and evaluating health promotion programs* (4th ed.). San Francisco: Pearson.

Miles, M. B., & Huberman, A. M. (1994). *Qualitative data analysis: An expanded sourcebook* (2nd ed.). Thousand Oaks, CA: Sage.

Miller, W. R., & Rollnick, S. (1991). *Motivational interviewing: Preparing people to change addictive behaviors.* New York: Guilford Press.

Minkler, M. (1990). Improving health through community organization. In K. Glanz, F. M. Lewis, & B. K. Rimer (Eds.), *Health behavior and health education: Theory, research, and practice* (pp. 257–287). San Francisco: Jossey-Bass.

Minkler, M., & Wallerstein, N. (2003). *Community-based participatory research for health.* San Francisco: Jossey-Bass.

Moayad, N., Balcazar, H., Pedregon, V., Velasco, L., & Bayona, M. (2006). Do acculturation and family cohesiveness influence severity of diabetes among Mexican Americans? *Ethnicity & Disease 16,* 452–459.

Muhr, T. (2004). Atlas.ti (Version 5.0) (Computer software). Thousand Oaks, CA: Sage.

National Alliance for Hispanic Health. (2001). *Quality health services for Hispanics: The cultural competency component* (DHHS Publication No. 99–2L). Rockville, MD: Department of Health and Human Services.

Orlandi, M. A., Landers, C., Weston, R., & Haley, N. (1990). Diffusion of health promotion innovations. In K. Glanz, F. M. Lewis, & B. K. Rimer

(Eds.), *Health behavior and health education* (pp. 288–313). San Francisco: Jossey-Bass.

Orlandi, M. A., Weston, R., & Epstein, L. G. (1992). *Cultural competence for evaluators.* Rockville, MD: Office of Substance Abuse Prevention.

Palloni, A., & Morenoff, J. D. (2001). Interpreting the paradoxical in the Hispanic paradox: Demographic and epidemiological approaches. *Annals of the New York Academy of Sciences, 954,* 140–174.

Perry, C. L., Baranowski, T., & Parcel, G. (1990). How individuals, environments, and health behavior interact: Social Learning Theory. In K. Glanz, F. M. Lewis, & B. K. Rimer (Eds.), *Health behavior and health education* (pp. 161–186). San Francisco: Jossey-Bass.

Prochaska, J., & DiClemente, C. (1992). Stages of change in the modification of problem behaviors. *Progress in Behavior Modification, 28,* 183–218.

Rawson, R. A., Marinelli-Casey, P., & Ling, W. (2002). Dancing with strangers: Will U.S. substance abuse practice and research organizations build mutually productive relationships? *Addictive Behaviors, 27,* 941–949.

Reinschmidt, K. M., Hunter, J. B., Fernandez, M. L., Lacy-Martinez, C. R., de Zapien, J. G., & Meister, J. (2006). Understanding the success of Promotoras in increasing chronic disease screening. *Journal of Health Care for the Poor and Underserved, 17,* 256–264.

Resnicow, K., Soler, R., Braithwait, R. L., Ahluwalia, J. S., & Butler, J. (2000). Cultural sensitivity in substance abuse prevention. *Journal of Community Psychology, 28,* 271–290.

Rogers, E. M. (1983). *Diffusion of innovation* (3rd ed.). New York: Free Press.

Rogler, L. H., Cortes, D. E., & Malgady, R. G. (1991). Acculturation and mental health status among Hispanics. *American Psychologist, 46,* 585–597.

Rosenstock, I. M. (1990). The Health Belief Model: Explaining health behavior through expectancies. In K. Glanz, F. M. Lewis, & B. K. Rimer (Eds.), *Health behavior and health education* (pp. 39–62). San Francisco: Jossey-Bass.

Schinke, S., Brounstein, P., & Gardner, S. (2002). *Science-based prevention programs and principles, 2002* (DHHS Publication No. [SMA] 03–3764). Rockville, MD: Center for Substance Abuse Prevention, Substance Abuse and Mental Health Services Administration.

Skaff, M. M., Chesla, C. A., de los Santos, Mycue, V., & Fisher, L. (2002). Lessons in cultural competence: Adapting research methodology for Latino participants. *Journal of Community Psychology, 30,* 305–323.

Strauss, A., & Corbin, J. (1990). *Basics of qualitative research: Grounded theory procedures and techniques.* Newbury Park, CA: Sage.

Sue, D. W., & Sue, D. (1999). *Counseling the culturally different: Theory and practice.* New York: Wiley.

Szapocznik, J., & Coatsworth, J. D. (1999). An ecodevelopmental framework for organizing the influences on drug abuse: A developmental model of risk and protection. In M. Glanz & C. Hartel (Eds.), *Drug abuse: Origins and interventions* (pp. 331–366). Washington, DC: American Psychological Association.

Tobler, N. S. (1986). Meta-analysis of 143 adolescent drug prevention programs: Quantitative outcome results of program participants compared to a control or comparison group. *Journal of Drug Issues, 16,* 537–567.

Tobler, N. S., Lessard, T., Marshall, D., Ochshorn, P., & Roona, M. (1999). Effectiveness of school-based drug prevention programs for marijuana use. *School Psychology International, 20,* 105–137.

Trimble, J. E. (1995). Toward an understanding of ethnicity and ethnic identity, and their relationship to drug use research. In G. Botvin, S. Schinke, & M. Orlandi (Eds.), *Drug abuse prevention with multiethnic youth* (pp. 3–27). Thousand Oaks, CA: Sage.

Ulin, P. R., Robinson, E. T., & Tolley, E. E. (2005). *Qualitative methods in public health: A field guide for applied research.* San Francisco: Jossey-Bass.

U.S. Census Bureau. (2005). *Race and Hispanic or Latino origin of the population of the United States: 2003 and 2004.* Retrieved November 29, 2005, from www.census.gov/press-release/www/ releases/archives/natrecepop2004_tb1.pdf

U.S. Department of Commerce. (1993). *We the American Hispanics.* Washington, DC: Government Printing Office.

U.S. Department of Health and Human Services. (2000). *Healthy people 2010* (2nd ed., Vols. 1 and 2). Washington DC: Government Printing Office.

Windsor, R., Baranowski, T., Clark, N., & Cutter, G. (1994). *Evaluation of health promotion, health education, and disease prevention programs* (2nd ed.). Mountain View, CA: Mayfield.

Appendix A

USER-FRIENDLY WORKSHEET FOR
DEVELOPING A HEALTH PROMOTION PROGRAM

This user-friendly worksheet guides you through major steps involved in program planning, design, implementation, and evaluation by having you respond to questions in a brief "sentence completion" format. By answering each question, you will address a series of program design issues. In addition, the items not easily answered now will prompt you to think further about what you might do to complete the design of your proposed health promotion program.

This user-friendly guide has four major sections:

I. Program Planning

II. Program Design/Development

III. Program Implementation

IV. Program Evaluation

I. Program Planning
  A. Identifying the Health Problem
    1. What is the targeted health problem or disease entity, and why is it important to eliminate or reduce it?
    2. What are the known or likely risk and protective factors for this problem?
  B. Identifying the Population
  Describe your identified population in terms of
    1. Age group(s)
    2. Ethnic/racial identity
    3. Gender(s)
    4. Geographic area or residence within a local community
    5. Unique aspects of this problem for members of this identified group
  C. Needs and Resource Assessment
    1. Generally, the *needs and resource assessment* will be conducted
      a. In the form of
      b. To ask about
  D. Stakeholders
    1. The main constituencies or groups of *stakeholders* are
    2. The corresponding *key informants* from these constituencies are

  E. Archival and Community-Level Data
    1. Community-level indicators of the problem are
    2. The most important archival data to be obtained are
    3. The most important variables to be examined are

II. Program Development
  A. Guiding Model(s)
    1. Basically, the theoretical or logic model that can serve as the program's guiding framework is
    2. Provide the *logic model* as a set of statements that describe the factors that logically "cause" the disease and the interventions that can break this causal process
  B. Conceptual or Theoretical Framework
    1. The behaviors targeted for change are
    2. More specifically, the major theoretical framework(s) that can guide healthy behavior change in your program is/are
    3. Relevant concepts (constructs) or variables from this/these theory/theories are

4. Describe how each of these constructs may contribute to healthy behavior change
5. Culture-specific factors to be considered in your program are

C. Goals and Objectives
1. Program *goals* and *objectives* will be to
   a. Goal 1. To
   * Objective 1.1: To
   * Objective 1.2: To
   b. Goal 2. To
   * Objective 2.1: To
   * Objective 2.2: To
   (Goals 3, 4, . . ., N, as needed)
   n. Goal N: To
   * Objective *n*.1: To
   * Objective *n*.2: To

D. Design Format
1. The experimental (involving randomization), quasi-experimental, or other proposed program design is
2. The group or groups to be involved in this project are
3. Observation points (pretest, posttest, follow-up) for data collection will be
4. Major *outcome variables* will be

E. Intervention/Curriculum, Social Marketing, and Diffusion of Innovation
1. Proposed name for the program
2. This program will fit the needs of the targeted group by
3. What are the major proposed intervention strategies
4. Number of program sessions will be
5. The major theme for each session will be
   (1)
   (2)
   (3)
   (4)
   (5)
   (6)
   (*n*)
6. Program delivery site(s) will be
7. What social marketing approaches will be used?
8. How will this program be implemented and its use sustained?

F. Outcomes and Outcome Variables
1. The major outcomes will be to increase and to decrease
2. Thus, scales or measured indicators of these outcomes will be

III. Implementation
A. Program Implementation
1. What are some practical aspects for implementing this program?
B. Program Administration
1. This program will be directed or overseen by
C. Program Staffing
1. The major staff who will administer, for example, Project Director, who will deliver the program, for example, lay health educators, peer counselors, etc.
2. Staff training will involve
3. Other staff-related issues are

IV. Evaluation
A. Outcome Evaluation
1. The basic evaluation program approach will be
2. Expected short-term changes on specific outcomes will be
B. Process Evaluation
1. Indicators of *fidelity in implementation* and/or of quality in program implementation will be
2. Problems in program delivery or effectiveness will be identified by
3. Anticipated types of *cultural adaptations* that may be needed to make the program more culturally relevant are
4. Participant satisfaction and responses to the program will be evaluated by
5. Other issues
C. Data Analysis
1. What data analyses will be conducted to evaluate the extent of successful program effects?
D. Additional Comments
1. What other issues not yet covered need commentary?

Appendix B

GENERAL ACCULTURATION INDEX

Please circle the choice that is true for you. Then add the circled scores to obtain the SUM below. Then divide the SUM by 5 to obtain the General Acculturation Index (AI) value.

1. I speak
   1. Only Spanish
   2. Spanish better than English
   3. Both English and Spanish equally well
   4. English better than Spanish
   5. Only English

2. I read
   1. Only Spanish
   2. Spanish better than English
   3. Both English and Spanish equally well
   4. English better than Spanish
   5. Only English

3. My early life from childhood to 21 years of age was spent
   1. Only in Latin America (Mexico, Central America, South America) or the Caribbean (Cuba, Puerto Rico, etc.)
   2. Mostly in Latin America or the Caribbean
   3. Equally in Latin America/the Caribbean and in the United States
   4. Mainly in the United States and some time in Latin America/the Caribbean
   5. Only in the United States

4. Currently my circle of friends are
   1. Almost exclusively Hispanics/Latinos (Chicanos/Mexican Americans, Puerto Ricans, Cubans, Colombians, Dominicans, etc.)
   2. Mainly Hispanics/Latinos
   3. Equally Hispanics/Latinos and Americans from the United States (Anglo Americans, African Americans, Asians/Pacific Islanders, etc.)
   4. Mainly Americans from the United States
   5. Almost entirely Americans from the United States

5. In relation to having a Latino/Hispanic background, I feel
   1. Very proud
   2. Proud
   3. Somewhat proud
   4. Little pride
   5. No pride (or circle 5 if you are *not* of Latino/Hispanic background)

SUM =

Acculturation Index (AI) = SUM/5 = _____

INDICE GENERAL DE ACULTURACION

Por favor, circule el número de la selección que sea más correcta para usted. Luego calcule la SUMA. Divida la SUMA entre cinco para obtener su Índice General de Aculturación.

1. Yo hablo
   1. Solamente español (castellano)
   2. El español mejor que el inglés
   3. El inglés y el español por igual
   4. El inglés mejor que el español
   5. Solamente inglés

2. Yo leo
   1. Solamente español (castellano)
   2. El español mejor que el inglés
   3. El inglés y el español por igual
   4. El inglés mejor que el español
   5. Solamente inglés

3. Mi juventud desde la infancia hasta los 21 años de edad la viví
   1. En Latinoamérica (México, Centroamérica, Sudamérica) o en el Caribe (Cuba, Puerto Rico, etc.)
   2. Principalmente Latinoamérica o el Caribe
   3. En Latinoamérica/el Caribe y en los Estados Unidos por igual
   4. Principalmente en los Estados Unidos y un tiempo en Latinoamérica/el Caribe
   5. Solamente en los Estados Unidos

4. Actualmente mi círculo de amigos está formado de
   1. Casi exclusivamente hispanos/latinos (chicanos, méxico americanos, puertorriqueños, cubanos, colombianos, dominicanos, etc.)
   2. Principalmente hispanos/latinos
   3. Mexicanos/hispanos y angloamericanos (norteamericanos, áfrico americanos [negros], asiático americanos, etc.)
   4. Principalmente angloamericanos
   5. Casi exclusivamente angloamericanos

5. En relación con mis raíces latinas/hispanas me siento
   1. Muy orgulloso(a)
   2. Orgulloso(a)
   3. Algo orgulloso(a)
   4. Un poco orgulloso(a)
   5. Nada orgulloso(a), o no tengo raíces latinas/hispanas

SUMA =

Índice de Aculturación = SUMA/5 = _____

11

Case Study—Diffusion Acceleration

A Model for Behavior Change and Social Mobilization

AMELIE G. RAMIREZ

LUIS F. VÉLEZ

PATRICIA CHALELA

KIPLING GALLION

ALFRED L. MCALISTER

Chapter Objectives

On completion of this chapter, the health promotion student and practitioner will be able to

- Discuss Social Cognitive Theory as this applies to the Diffusion Acceleration Model

- Define the major features of the Diffusion of Innovation Model

- Define the similarities and differences between traditional models of communication and the Diffusion Acceleration Model

AUTHORS' NOTE: The authors wish to thank Dr. Kimberly Wildes for her careful editorial review of this chapter. We also thank Ms. Jessica Flores for her assistance with some of the background research in preparation for the manuscript.

Social communication is an essential component of public health programs, but it has limited effectiveness as a lone intervention (MacDonald, 1998; World Health Organization, 1986). Communication interventions are most effective when they are part of comprehensive programs that address policy changes, environmental modifications, and community mobilization. Many programs use social marketing and paid advertisement, and this strategy has shown to be effective, although developing these communications campaigns tends to be expensive (Hershey et al., 2005; McAlister, 1995a; Nettleton & Bunton, 1995; Seigel & Doner, 2004). Audience preferences are moving targets for commercial and social advertisers, and several studies suggest that many of these campaigns are only partially successful. Several comprehensive health promotion programs have chosen a communication strategy that uses mass and interpersonal channels, but differs significantly from the traditional social marketing approach. This strategy has been labeled "diffusion acceleration" and involves community mobilization, and often policy changes (McAlister, 1991, 1997). This chapter includes four case studies of programs that have used the Diffusion Acceleration Model as part of comprehensive health promotion interventions.

Our conceptualization of diffusion acceleration builds on the pioneering work in interpersonal and social communication and adoption of innovations by Lazarsfeld, Berelson, and Gaudet (1948), as well as on the earlier studies in group decision making and the role of opinion leaders as gate keepers by Kurt Lewin (1951). However, throughout this chapter, we primarily refer to the systematic way in which these concepts were presented and improved on in Social Cognitive Theory (SCT) and the Diffusion of Innovations Theory (Bandura, 1977, 1986, 1996; Rogers, 1962, 2003). The concept has been applied to several public health communication programs

in different parts of the world (McAlister, 1997; McAlister et al., 1992; Puska et al., 1985; Ramirez & McAlister, 1988; Vélez, 1998; Vélez, Giraldo, Unás, Prada, & Arango, 1998). The basic theoretical hypothesis is that the diffusion of health practices or situations that are not widely present in a population can be accelerated by presenting examples of relevant individuals who have already acquired the practice, synchronically using mass and interpersonal communications. Accelerating the diffusion of health practices requires more than simply combining communication channels; it is primarily about giving a voice to the audience themselves. It blends cognitive and social processes. Members of the community who have already undergone the proposed changes hold the best knowledge and experience about what it takes to achieve success, although they are rarely aware they have such knowledge. Using classical journalistic techniques and SCT parameters to obtain the stories from these innovators, the Diffusion Acceleration Model can be used to expand the number of people to whom the storyteller's experience is passed in a credible and empowering manner. The experience then simultaneously reaches "early adopters" and "early and late majorities" according to the characteristics of each one of these groups, as described by the Diffusion of Innovation Theory (these terms are further elaborated in the section titled Diffusion of Innovations Theory).

Although the Diffusion Acceleration Model is based on solid theoretical premises, just like those premises, the model mostly systematizes a process that has been present as the fundamental human learning method. The beauty of the concepts presented by the SCT and Diffusion of Innovations Theory is their simple, yet profound understanding of basic human behavior. Diffusion acceleration simply proposes applying modern communication logic to the traditional learning processes systematized by those theories.

In antiquity, the transmission of behavioral patterns happened by word of mouth and through religious and philosophical writings. Nowadays, this is very effectively done through the media; innovations are introduced and modeled, adopted, and then modeled directly through interpersonal connections. This is certainly the case in the adoption of new technologies and use of new services and has been masterly perfected in political campaigning, among other social interactions (Barberich, 2002; Lewin, 1951; Mutz, Sniderman, & Brody, 1996). However, the passing on of daily practices that influence health still largely happens through word of mouth or selected media available mostly to those with better education and income.

Despite all the health-related information available, current political and communication processes give priority to macrosocial means such as technology, power, and security above basic health, individual, and community needs (United Nations Development Program, 2005). The accelerated transmission of macrosocial patterns in part competes against the diffusion of daily behaviors that may help us live better and happier lives. As the adoption of new technologies and services speeds up, previously accepted behaviors become obsolete. Humans need to quickly adapt to the new biological and social challenges. The problem, though, is that naturally occurring genetic and biological adaptations may take hundreds of years, but social and behavioral changes can happen at a faster pace if the appropriate communication processes are used. The Diffusion Acceleration Model proposes a commonsense approach to disseminating these behavioral changes through what are current natural communication channels.

THEORETICAL BASIS OF THE DIFFUSION ACCELERATION MODEL

Social Cognitive Theory

Albert Bandura's (1977, 1986, 1996) SCT says that people's behaviors are not definitively determined by internal forces or external stimuli, but by a network of factors that operate as determinants of each other. Behavior, environmental events, and cognitive and other personal forces are crucial factors that can explain human functioning.

Bandura defines the nature of people in terms of their symbolizing, forethought, self-regulatory, and vicarious capabilities. Symbolizing capability is the ability to transform experiences, through symbols, into a framework for decisions to be made in the future. Actions are then based on these symbols and thoughts. This structure is not permanent, and therefore can be influenced and altered, which is evident in changing behavior. Forethought capability is the tendency to anticipate and model behavior according to the anticipated consequences. It is important to note that it is these expected outcomes, and not positive or negative incentives, that dictate actions. People do not act to please others, but act based on internal standards and self-evaluative reactions. This is known as self-regulatory capability. Vicarious capability is the ability to learn through observation. This allows people to make generalizations and rules based on other people's actions. Most behaviorists maintain that learning can only result from direct experience. However, observing behavior is safer, permitting the individual to learn from other people's dangerous mistakes, and it is more efficient, allowing the individual to save time that might be wasted on tedious trial and error. The more costly and hazardous the mistakes, the more reliance is placed on observational learning.

Modeling is the term used to characterize the psychological matching process. The process is much more intricate than describing it as "imitation" or "mimicry" might imply. Modeling, also known as observational learning, allows people to acquire cognitive skills and new patterns of behavior by observing the performance of others. A behavior is modeled and the individual, who possessed no previous knowledge, is able to imitate and reproduce it simply through observing. This allows the simultaneous transmission of knowledge to many individuals. An additional purpose of modeling is to strengthen or weaken previously learned behavior. Modeling provides the individual with very valuable information that affects her or his perception of the modeled behavior, including possible outcomes that the viewer may expect, as well as performance expectations. The actions of others can also serve as a cue to action, known as response facilitation effects. These effects are distinguished from observational learning in that they do not present a new behavior. Modeling can be inhibitory, where people reduce behavior after seeing negative consequences, or disinhibitory, where they increase behavior after seeing threatening or prohibited activities performed without punishment. The environment also sends signals to the individual. The observer pays attention to objects or settings that are favored by others and react to them. People also react to the emotions portrayed by a model in a specific scenario and subsequently associate the emotion and scenario.

Affecting performance expectations by enhancing the individual's trust in her or his capacity to act as the model is a key element in the diffusion acceleration concept. A role model who resembles the audience is more likely to empower them to imitate the behavior by conveying the idea that they are just as capable as the model is. Enhancing performance expectations through role modeling is a key element of Albert Bandura's Self-Efficacy Theory (1996).

Diffusion of Innovations Theory

The study of innovations diffusion began in the first part of the 20th century and became a widely used theoretical model after Everett Rogers published his *Diffusion of Innovations* book in 1962 (Lazarsfeld et al., 1948; Lewin, 1951; Rogers, 1962, 2003). Rogers stated that new ideas are not uniformly adopted, but rather follow a predictable pattern of adoption.

Some individuals are more likely to initially try certain innovations, while others take longer, and some may even never adopt it, or adopt it when a revised version of the innovation is already beginning a new adoption cycle. He called the first adopters of any new innovation or idea "innovators" and based on series of studies estimated that they composed about 2.5% of the total pool of potential adopters. After them come early adopters (13.5%), early majority (34%), late majority (34%), and laggards (16%). Each adopter's willingness and ability to adopt an innovation would depend on their awareness, interest, evaluation, trial, and adoption.

Diffusion of Innovations Theory states that each group of adopters has certain identifiable characteristics. Innovators tend to be very well educated and informed, venturesome, and capable of tolerating important levels of uncertainty and risk. Innovators may try something new without much assessment of the risks, because its possible benefits make it exciting. They may also overestimate their own capacities, and it is important to note that failure is not infrequent for innovators. On the other hand, early adopters also tend to be educated and well informed, but they are also leaders. They tend to be active information seekers and do not trust a single source. To maintain the respect of their social group they must make careful, well-informed decisions. To do so, early adopters assess the innovation and its implementation using information provided by innovators. If it has been effective for the innovators, then they will be encouraged to adopt it. They act also as innovation filters: If the risk/cost-benefit balance and utility of the innovation make it worth adopting, they are also likely to pass it on through their often extensive communication networks (Lewin, 1951). As opinion leaders, the majority of the community trusts the evaluation that they made. Adoption of the innovation becomes more important to the rest of the social group as it produces social and/or economical benefits to earlier adopters. In some cases, the innovation brings such vital or visible advantages that nonadopters risk losing viability or social status. In the next group, early majorities are usually those in the immediate or extended network of the early adopters. They tend to rely a lot on the judgment of opinion leaders and are highly exposed to mass communications and informal social contacts. The late majorities tend to rely less on the mass media and are more skeptical and traditional. They adopt innovations that are already frequently being used by others. Finally, the laggards are more isolated people that mostly rely on neighbors and friends as their main sources of information. They also tend to be more fearful of risks.

This theory also describes how the characteristics of innovations are judged in the adoption process. One of the most remarkable elements of diffusion theory is that, for most members of a social system, the adoption depends heavily on the decisions of other members of the system and their communication networks. The risk-benefit analysis made by some members of the group is decisive to overcome uncertainty among the rest. In addition, the connections between opinion leaders and the rest of the group determine the extent to which the leaders' judgments are known. This is a critical junction for diffusion of innovations and social cognitive theories. Many good innovations never get diffused and cost-effective health innovations such as preventive behaviors or the use of new services may take many years, and even decades, to be widely adopted. The diffusion of health innovations can be accelerated using role models as sources of information, activating community interpersonal communication networks, and adding social validation through the mass media.

Diffusion Acceleration: A Working Model Based on Social Cognitive and Diffusion of Innovation Theories

We can summarize the acquisition of new behaviors as a process in which influential people (opinion leaders) take new ideas from innovators and from the media and pass them on to followers through personal contact. Different theorists and experiments have sought to illustrate whether the media or personal contact are superior, but the consensus is that the media is not necessarily less persuasive than interpersonal contacts; the source's utility depends on how accessible it is and the likelihood that it will give the individual useful information (Chaffee & Mutz, 1988; Reardon & Rogers, 1988). Our Diffusion Acceleration Model facilitates contacts between opinion leaders and individuals who have already acquired a healthy behavior (role models as innovators). Since early adopters learn about the experience of innovators through interpersonal networks and the mass media, we can accelerate the diffusion of health innovations by strategically disseminating role model stories through these channels. In our health promotion projects, we synchronically present role model stories through the mass media and interpersonal channels at the same time (McAlister et al., 1992; Ramirez et al., 1999; Ramirez & McAlister, 1988; Vélez et al., 1998).

Although opinion leaders may eventually acquire enough information about a health innovation from the traditional health informational sources, we consider role models a more efficient source of such information (McAlister, 1995a). According to SCT, modeling serves as a major vehicle for information transmission as it instructs people about new ways of thinking and behaving by demonstration and description (Bandura, 1986). Role models motivate and inform. They display the possible outcomes that could result if the individual should choose to adopt the modeled practice, and in doing so, exemplify and legitimate the practice. Unfortunately, many people who have adopted healthy behaviors are not opinion leaders, and they may not pass on their experience to others, or at least not fast enough to produce significant social change. However, if we visualize these role models as successful innovators, we can help opinion leaders learn about their experience. Their testimony per se provides the risk/cost-benefit assessment that opinion leaders as early adopters seek, thus abbreviating an essential part of the diffusion process. Our Diffusion Acceleration Model helps opinion leaders learn about health innovations from role models, similar to the "two-step" model originally proposed by Lazarsfeld et al. (1948).

An additional major element of our model is bridging connections between opinion leaders and the early and late majorities, augmenting the "two-step" model into a multistep model. Since the early majority relies primarily on the judgment of opinion leaders, we propose to purposefully identify and activate the interpersonal networks naturally developed around leaders. This requires canvassing the communities to identify these networks and producing materials to facilitate their passing of health information to others. The intention is not to create new interpersonal networks, but to identify and enable opinion leaders to discuss relevant health information with their usual contacts. If these leaders are carefully identified, diffusing information does not create an additional burden for them. It simply provides new topics for the usual opinion leader-community interaction and new sources for the leaders to reaffirm their credibility in the community. However, as for any other innovation, the proposed practice has to be worthy of the opinion leaders' consideration, adoption, and dissemination; otherwise, they won't even participate in the program. As explained in detail later, we usually produce some simple printed materials containing role model stories to facilitate this process, but as the communication technologies evolve, these enabling materials may take other formats.

In summary, the Diffusion Acceleration Model essentially consists of finding successful role models, composing their stories and disseminating them through the mass media and community networks based on opinion leaders.

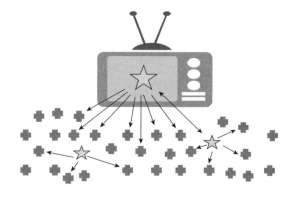

Figure 11.1   Diffusion Acceleration Model Dual Link

This process takes the commanding voice away from health planners and gives it to the community, letting the audience themselves be the message (McAlister, 1995a). Figure 11.1 illustrates these communication links.

Health Promotion Programs Using Diffusion Acceleration

Several programs have used the diffusion acceleration models. Some of these programs are briefly described in this chapter, and in this section we present basic program implementation principles that guided their development. These programs include the North Karelia Project in Finland (Karvonen, 1995; McAlister, 1995b; Puska, 1995a, 1995b; Puska et al., 1985), the *A Su Salud* (To Your Health) (Amezcua, McAlister, Ramirez, & Espinoza, 1990; McAlister et al., 1992, 1995; Ramirez et al., 1995; Ramirez & McAlister, 1988), and the AIDS Community Demonstration Projects (ACDPs) in the United States (Curran, 1997; Fishbein & Rhodes, 1997; McAlister, 1997; Pulley, McAlister, Kay, & O'Reilly, 1996), and *Mejor Hablemos* (Let's Talk!) in Colombia (McAlister & Vélez, 1999; Vélez, 1998; Vélez, McAlister, & Hu, 1997; Vélez et al., 1998), which are described in detail in this chapter, as well as many other programs such as *Salud En Acción* (Ramirez et al., 1998), Speak-up (Ramirez, Vélez, Chalela, Grussendorf,

& McAlister, 2006), *Sin Fumar* (smoke-free) (Chalela, Vélez, Ramirez, 2007), and some components of the Texas Tobacco Prevention Initiative (McAlister, Huang, & Ramirez, 2006; Meshack et al., 2004; Shegog et al., 2005), among others not included in this chapter.[1]

As described above, this model combines the most powerful elements of mass media and interpersonal communication to influence learning new information and to change health practices. It includes the use of various media (e.g., newspapers, television, radio, community newsletters) as channels. The model also includes engaging local opinion leaders to discuss media messages with their personal contacts and to provide positive reinforcement for any health change effort. The model, which requires very little training for these opinion leaders, is well suited to reaching specific audiences and a large number of people in the community.

Program Organization

Applying the model requires careful planning and a solid organizational structure as for any community-based health promotion program. However, although empirical evidence suggests that this is an efficient model to promote health, several aspects of diffusion acceleration can be applied separately to different programs, and planners may choose to use just what fits their current or future programmatic plans.

Key organizational elements include funding, logistics, relations with the community, and message planning, development and delivery. In the past, public health agencies have often served as the sources of financial, office space, equipment, and minimal personnel support. Depending on the goals set during the planning stages and the type of community, one or more individuals may be required to implement the program. For purely community-based programs with just

basic evaluation instead of a major research component, implementation may require at least one full-time person capable of conducting all the program tasks. A modest array of office equipment to enable record keeping and the creation of monthly newsletters is also needed. With cost savings by joining an existing organization, the total investment could be equivalent to a social worker position with a college education and at least 3 years of experience.

In the case of North Karelia (see example in Box A on p. 266), the ambitious goals, the geographically disperse community, the experimental character of the program, and the decisive government support and corresponding accountability required a complex organizational structure (Karvonen, 1995; McAlister, 1995b; Puska, 1995a, 1995b; Puska et al., 1985). However, once the main scientific and public accountability questions were answered and the basic processes were well established, the program was sustained with a relatively simple and straightforward organizational structure. In *A Su Salud* in South Texas (see example in Box C on p. 270), the field work required two community organizers, a media coordinator, a part time program coordinator, and basic clerical support to implement the program in two different locations covering around 50,000 people. *Mejor Hablemos* in Cali, Colombia (see example in Box D), required two community coordinators, two full-time journalists, and a program coordinator, besides the staff purely dedicated to research.

It is important to notice that the programs above were research based, and their purpose was to implement and document the implementation and impact of the intervention model. Later developments of the three programs have typically required, at the minimum, a part-time media coordinator and a part-time community coordinator. Under some conditions, one person can manage both jobs; however, these tasks are typically distributed between two people. Media production does not require exceptional journalistic skills, but strong command of language and ability to articulate the messages clearly are necessary. Community outreach normally requires an individual with strong interpersonal communication skills, an outgoing and amiable personality, and thorough familiarity with the community.

Role Models

As described in detail before, role modeling is at the center of our Diffusion Acceleration Model. The three examples mentioned and all the programs derived from them rely on learning through observation and imitation of others. Instead of having an expert mandate certain actions to the audience, these programs simply disseminate stories of people in the community who have adopted the recommended practice.

Different aspects are involved in modeling. The first one is defining who could be an effective role model. People are more likely to imitate others who they feel are doing a little better than them. In this regard, a role model should be similar to the audience and appealing enough to match some of their aspirations. Besides basic personal information to describe the normal daily activities and joys of the role model, it is important to include in their stories basic information, new attitudes, and new perceptions about the social desirability of the particular behavior promoted, as well as the essential skills necessary for performing it. Individuals from the community who already have made the changes sought by the program are identified and featured in the media materials, including discussions or demonstrations of how and why they took steps to protect their health. This strategy virtually guarantees that messages are understandable and relevant to the audience.

Messages from peers are credible and deal with the problems and barriers that are most relevant to the community. It is important to note that the emphasis is on individuals who have made changes toward the healthy behavior, rather than on individuals who have already suffered the consequences of the disease and wish they had done something differently in the past. Some researchers also suggest including some stories of role models that had negative consequences from not doing the recommended actions. However, there needs to be careful balance using just a few of these negative outcome stories to raise awareness accompanied by clear action clues to help the audience overcome possibly discouraging feelings of fear and many more stories with positive outcomes from the proposed healthy behavior.

In general, role models should "represent the community" by having the various social characteristics found in the audience, "have experienced the behavior" so that they can articulate a positive story about the particular change they have made or are making, and be able to "articulate their feelings," thus identifying the thoughts and emotions they had prior to and during the process of making the behavior change. Finding people with these characteristics is often challenging at the beginning. In our current and previous experiences, often the first role model stories come from contacts of members of the program staff in the community. Health professionals are also good sources of role models, and they may be willing to ask their patients to tell their stories. Role models may also come from the peer network, and other volunteer, religious, social, or civic organizations. Eventually, the program staff becomes very proficient at identifying good role models in many situations and motivating them to provide their stories.

McAlister (1995a) and others have coined the term *behavioral journalism* to define the journalistic approach to presenting real stories about behavior change that are explicitly designed to stimulate imitation. Behavioral journalism uses real-life stories in the hope that members of the audience will imitate them because they address the factors that are theoretically related to a particular behavior change. For example, a good role model to promote mammography screening might be a middle-aged woman who learned to overcome familiar barriers and thus obtained screening exams in a timely manner, because she knew that breast cancer is highly treatable if found early. This role model would also highlight the alternative that delayed screening increases the severity of the cancer, possibly leading to death, and ultimately to the loss of her children's mother. By explaining how she overcame those barriers familiar to the audience, she is modeling factors critical for behavior change in screening and early detection of breast cancer.

Interpersonal and Mass Communications

People don't always tune in to what is presented via the mass media, and even when they do, they may or may not respond. SCT sustains that a critical element in the effects of communication is whether the person receives social reinforcement, or encouragement and praise for intentions and actions to change behavior. These days behavior change most commonly involves learning about things from the media or other sources, mentioning them to people we know, and processing the feedback that we receive from them (social reinforcement). The direction and amount of the reinforcement and prompting help us decide whether to try or abandon the behavior. This is what Albert Bandura calls "dual link" communications (Bandura, 1986). The combination of mass media and personal contact makes it possible to influence almost any kind of behavior. And it can be done very efficiently on a large-scale basis.

Mass and Small Media

Social marketing campaigns require detailed audience segmentation and usually involve paid advertisement, both affecting its impact and reach. The Diffusion Acceleration Model, on the contrary, is a self-segmented strategy in which the model represents an array of characteristics and aspirations of the community. The real human character of the role model stories helps different segments of the audience identify and apply different aspects of the story to their own experiences and needs. Researchers and practitioners who have used the Diffusion Acceleration Model have found that different segments of the population assimilate the story in their own way, and when asked to reproduce it, they embellish it in ways that seem as if several unique stories carrying the same message have been presented.

Also, the Diffusion Acceleration Model is based on journalistic techniques, as opposed to advertisement, and relies on partnerships with the local media to present role model stories. The demonstrational studies that have used the model have proven that healthy behaviors are newsworthy when presented appropriately and that the journalistic media are eager to participate, as long as their collaboration includes doing what they usually do: reporting. The North Karelia, *A Su Salud, Mejor Hablemos,* and other similar programs have all collaborated with local news sources, including television and radio newscast, opinion programs, newspaper articles, and even a weekly photo-novella developed in collaboration with a local tabloid in Colombia. The program staff is involved in the production process according to the characteristics of each media outlet, but none of these programs have involved paid advertising.

Media outlets are initially invited to participate according to the size and demographics of their audience (media reach). Another basic consideration is the types of media and the particular media outlets preferred by the audience. Newspapers or radio and television stations that have the largest reach are good channels, but sometimes smaller outlets are better at reaching specific subpopulations.

Health-related role model stories usually fit better the news and human interest sections. News sections often carry health sections centered on the opinion of health experts, but newspapers, radio, and TV stations are very receptive to stories centered on role models, as long as these stories are of value to their audiences and fit their programming types and schedules. However, media partners may easily get tired of the same topic. Different topics and angles, varied role model characteristics, and personalized stories help sustain media interest. Although every role model story is different for the program's team, they can be seen as repetitious or "old news" to journalists. Rotating themes was not so difficult for multirisk projects such as the North Karelia and *A Su Salud,* but it has been more challenging for single-risk programs such as *Mejor Hablemos* (violence prevention) and those focused primarily on cancer screening (*Salud En Acción*).

Establishing partnerships with the media is an important challenge. Once the program establishes the desired media, their interest is not at all guaranteed, and their internal dynamics may not fit what the program proposes. Preparation, flexibility, and patience are necessary. Media managers like to see brief and well-prepared materials that inform them about the program. It is also important to bring to mind different alternatives when contacting them. Finally, getting the attention of media editors or managers may take several attempts. The staff of *Mejor Hablemos* in Colombia, for example, repeatedly tried to gain the attention of *El Caleño*, a local sensationalist tabloid that carries stories about criminal activity in the city, besides some stories of human interest. The paper does not place any advertisement, sells over 20,000 copies a day, is written at a low reading level, and has four readers for every buyer. It is also the paper that reaches the poorest neighborhoods in Cali. After many unsuccessful attempts to meet with the team, the chief editor was invited to lunch with them and was asked to provide advice to the program's team. This opened the door to a very successful partnership that took peaceful conviviality stories to the most violent neighborhoods in the city for several years.

Sometimes, the media outlet is willing to participate but wants assistance with something else from the team. In the case of *A Su Salud* in South Texas, the radio station with the best penetration among the audience was *La Rancherita del Norte,* a station with a powerful transmitter in the town across the border in Mexico. A long-lasting collaboration was established, but it implied crossing the border from the United States and assisting them with other health information that they wanted to provide their audience.

The optimal working relationship with media personnel is probably one of coproduction, but each medium follows different production protocols, and they want to keep absolute control of the essential parts. The best arrangement is when the program staff (media coordinator and community coordinator) and the media personnel work together to develop, produce, and distribute the messages. In San Antonio Texas, the *A Su Salud* program's collaboration with the main Spanish television station lasted for many years. As part of the agreement project staff were in charge of identifying the role models, contacting the health reporter, and arranging the interview, including preinterviewing the role model, and producing a brief informational sheet about the topic and the role model for the reporter. The cameraman and the reporter took care of videotaping, editing, and of course, broadcasting the interview. Although occasionally the contents of the stories can be slightly changed during the editing, thoroughly preparing the interview will prevent any significant distortion, and reporters quickly learn the foundations of the program.

Finally, any relationship established with the media must be cultivated in the friendliest terms possible, and they need to be acknowledged as a key program partner. In Cali, Colombia, a carefully managed collaboration with a television newscast team and a radio morning news section turned into a multistation program that involved, at one time, seven radio stations and two local newspapers.

Print Materials

All the programs that have used the Diffusion Acceleration Model included some type of small media or print materials, such as brochures, flyers, calendars, newsletters, and posters, as well as audio and video formats. The use of small media can provide a point of reference for personal contacts and face-to-face communications about adopting healthy behaviors. The newsletters produced in the North Karelia Project were simple but contained powerful role model stories and other necessary information to facilitate behavioral change. *A Su Salud* produced a monthly calendar featuring a role model story and highlighting the times at which the same role models appeared in the mass media. These calendars also included clinic information and other resources. *Mejor Hablemos* printed a monthly bulletin with a role model story in the form of a photo-novella.

The production of small media materials does not need to be sophisticated, and in many occasions, it is done and printed in-house using a simple word processor or basic media publisher software. Although these materials still need to be attractive, the most important consideration is not the high quality, but its function of serving as conversation openers for the peer networkers or opinion leaders. As new communication technologies emerge as enablers of interpersonal communications, these "small media" may take many different formats such as Internet-based discussion groups, cellular phone messaging, PDF-based content, Web sites, etc.

Interpersonal Communications

As mentioned before, involving opinion leaders is crucial to accelerate the diffusion of any innovation. Field programs using the Diffusion Acceleration Model begin this process canvassing the communities to identify natural interpersonal communication networks. The people at the center of these networks are undoubtedly opinion leaders, although many of them may not be recognized community leaders. For example, in the case of *Mejor Hablemos* in Colombia, hair dressers and community agents working for the National Institute of Family Welfare were some of the most active and trusted information gate keepers, but only a few of them were politically active as community leaders. In *A Su Salud* in Texas, church groups, school teachers, and clinic staff were identified as opinion leaders, as well as some hair dressers and other community members. In the North Karelia Project, store owners and clinic staff were among the most active opinion leaders.

The Diffusion Acceleration Model relies on volunteer local opinion leaders who serve as "peer networkers" by contacting friends, relatives, coworkers, and neighbors with whom they share program information. Other people may eventually join and gain capacity as trusted opinion leaders in their community, but building new peer networks may prove to be a difficult and a time- and resource-consuming effort. Our experience indicates that it is better to invest in identifying, motivating, and involving already existing networks from the beginning of the program.

Peer opinion leaders are people who are just like the men and women that the program wants to influence, from the same social group and community. They are organized to systematically distribute some of the behavioral journalism materials and provide social reinforcement for imitation of the role models. Community networking is a very simple action, and it's relatively easy to train large numbers of people to accomplish it. Although these programs are by no means the first ones to involve community leaders and volunteers, there is a fundamental difference with other approaches. The Diffusion Acceleration Model does not ask of them any action different than just talking to their own interpersonal networks about the proposed health innovation, as they commonly would talk about any other issue of importance to the community. The unsophisticated print materials mentioned above as "small media" facilitate the opening of these conversations.

Invariably, this process also empowers opinion leaders beyond the goals of the program, and they gain satisfaction and solidify their position of respect in the community. However, these programs have also involved symbolic incentives as simple as social events that recognize volunteer efforts and other gestures of appreciation. Long-term satisfaction and low attrition are achieved when incentives are thoughtfully created and judiciously distributed throughout the program's life.

Program Results

The results of these programs have varied according to the health issue promoted, the community, the resources available, and the goals that are set. In the case of cancer screening, for example, as soon as implementation is under way and reasonable goals have been set, clinic usage typically increases within 2 months of program initiation. In the North Karelia Project, some changes were clearly visible within a year, but others took much longer to realize. However, these changes tend to be enduring as long as implementation is consistently maintained.

The programs often also take force of their own. For example, in Brownsville, Texas, a network of more than 100 volunteer opinion leaders had been involved in cancer prevention for 3 years. In the second year, after learning about the risks of early childhood sun exposure, a few of the parents in the network decided to ask the local elementary school to make some changes. Eventually, most of the network expressed support of a friendly "lobbying" campaign aimed at the school board and administrators. As a result, sunshades were installed over some play areas and recess times were shifted to avoid the midday sun. When a network has been active for some time, it can influence more complex institutional policies that shape behavior.

Conclusions

Accelerating the diffusion of health innovations is a public health goal as important as developing new vaccines and improving basic hygiene. There are several planning models to develop health communication programs, each one with its merits and applications. We described here a theory-based approach that has shown to be cost-effective in changing behavior and mobilizing communities. This model is particularly suitable for efforts aimed at developing strong local action and giving a voice to the community (Smedley & Syme, 2000), and also moving the adoption of health practices to a point where their diffusion takes a force of its own. It is founded on the use of interpersonal and mass communications as the modern way of evaluating the value of health practices as new ideas and incorporating them into established cultural patterns. Further developments of the Diffusion Acceleration Model will test its implementation in different settings and with different problems, as well as test the inclusion of new mass and interpersonal communication means in light of the ever-changing technology and processes of social interaction.

BOX A   The North Karelia Project

Background: Communities in eastern Finland found that the mortality rates due to cardiovascular disease (CVD) were exceptionally high, especially those in the area of North Karelia. The North Karelia Project was developed after local people voiced their concern and submitted a petition to reduce CVD in January, 1971. Finnish experts, the World Health Organization, and representatives from North Karelia formed a council that planned the strategies for the new project. The council outlined two basic objectives: to reduce mortality from CVD in the local population in the first period (1972–1978) and to reduce major chronic disease mortality and promote health in the local population in a second phase. The intermediate objective was to promote secondary prevention of CVD. Smoking, elevated serum low-density lipoprotein cholesterol, elevated blood pressure, and an emphasis on general lifestyle changes were targeted as the main risk factors to be addressed in the study.

Program Implementation: The North Karelia Project incorporated many innovative services that have since been modeled by many public health projects. It was the first major public health program to use the Diffusion Acceleration Model in a systematic way. The program disseminated its messages through the mass media and interpersonal networks supported by print materials. In an 11-year period, about 50 hours of programming directed against smoking and advocating healthy lifestyles were aired on the television and radio. In the first 5-year span of the project, they printed over half a million media materials. The campaign distributed posters, leaflets, antismoking signs, newspaper articles, and aids for developing social contacts. A magazine that dealt with topics related to cholesterol was founded. The local press was kept informed of the latest activities and findings. Local journalists attended training seminars and wrote their own columns and reviews, giving the articles a more credible viewpoint to the communities. Collaboration with other groups on the production of many of the materials helped offset the cost and more widely distribute them.

The lay opinion leader component of the program focused its attention on the dual-link model of information flow. Opinion leaders participated influencing and reaching the grassroots communities. Project leaders interviewed local informants to identify the most respected and influential individuals in the community. These people were then found and recruited as project assistants; their association with the project furthered the publicity and positive image of the health innovations. The project assistants attended a weekend seminar and returned for follow-ups. Collaborative efforts between the project and institutions were very active and effective. These two aspects, the media and preventive services, have been relatively consistent with the other projects discussed, such as the AIDS Community Demonstration Project.

Environmental changes were necessary to support the behavior modifications. Because many of the project managers were active with local decision makers, municipal health care workers, and local organizations before assuming roles in the project, they were very effective in their encounters in the community. The North Karelia Project did a very exhaustive job in trying to create change through many resources. The project encouraged work sites, schools, and homes to be smoke-free. They emphasized smoke-free zones and not the negative "no smoking" zones. The group distributed many signs and stickers that were received with much support; the most popular was the one that said "no smoking here—we participate in the North Karelia Project." Later, it evolved into "smoke-free area—smoke-free Karelia." These signs replaced smoking signs and advertisements. The project had a significant effect on national policy. In 1977, Parliament passed a legislation to eliminate all tobacco advertisements and ban smoking in indoor public places. Children under 16 years of age could not purchase cigarettes. Labels on the cigarette boxes now required health warnings. A portion (0.5%) of the tobacco taxes were set aside to go toward antismoking programs and research.

To address the excessive fat consumption, there was an effort to collaborate with many of the food manufacturers and supermarkets. Dairies assisted by promoting low-fat dairy products; sausage factories promoted low-fat sausage. Manufacturers worked with project members to address issues like legislation, labeling, advertising, and information exchange. Campaigns with manufacturers led to new products such as the domestic rapeseed oil. Efforts with supermarkets resulted in "health days." Health care workers presented information at grocery stores so that shoppers could make healthy choices as they selected and purchased groceries. The goal was to decrease the purchasing of saturated fat and increase consumption of vegetables and berries. This was seen as an economic threat as most vegetables were imported. The farmers whose only source of income was dairy products opposed this, but special measures were taken to teach them to grow currants and strawberries. With new sales campaigns and advertisements, berry consumption went up. Many of the farmers switched to these crops and were able to maintain their independent farms.

Outcomes: Mortality rates in North Karelia were generally higher than the rest of the population at the start of the program. There was a significant decline in CVD and cancer mortality in males aged between 35 and 64 years of age when compared with the 3-year period before the program was initiated (preprogram period). The average numbers of annual deaths for men and women between the preprogram period and the end of the project declined by 82% in North Karelia and 89% in all of Finland due to improvements in cardiovascular health. In the overall project period, there were 50,000 fewer deaths in Finland and 3,800 less in North Karelia than there would have been had they continued at the original death rate. Overall, it was found that the total serum cholesterol and blood pressure dropped more in North Karelia than it did in Kuopio. The number of male smokers decreased over the project. Female smokers, however, increased. This could be due to the fact that the target population of most of the antismoking promotion was middle-aged men. There was also a switch in fat consumption—a significant replacement from full-fat to low-fat milk and a lower total energy intake from fats. The participation rates in the project also declined over time. The overall findings showed a major decline in risk factors.

The North Karelia Project set a foundation for public health initiatives in the future. Programs worldwide have since reproduced all or part of the model. As more concerns emerge in the public health arena, it is essential to continue to build on the existing framework to develop better models and continue to make progress.

| BOX B | Community HIV Prevention: The Long Beach AIDS Community Demonstration Project |

Background: Funded by the Centers for Disease Control and Prevention, the ACDPs were developed to produce change in risk behavior among "high-risk" and "hard-to-reach" populations. Multiple sites were initiated across the country. All sites operated with a common protocol based on recommendations from the Unicoi Conference, a forum made up of nationally recognized leaders in community intervention and social and behavioral sciences.

Program Implementation: Research of the target community *before* implementing any sort of program was essential, and solid behavior change theories were used as a framework for the intervention. A "diffusion acceleration" strategy was chosen using small media materials to illustrate role model stories of community individuals who were changing or had changed their risk behaviors. A network of community lay opinion leaders distributed these materials and reinforced change among the at-risk community members. A joint evaluation protocol was developed and implemented across the project sites as well. Using common methods was essential to the study, allowing the methods to be tested across diverse populations. It also resulted in firmer conclusions since the data were able to be pooled, increasing the population size, and thus increasing the strength of the statistical analyses. Eventually, these factors allowed them to provide framework for a successful HIV prevention program. The behavioral goals of the intervention were to maintain consistent condom use for intercourse, consistent condom use with main and "other" partners, and the consistent use of bleach for cleaning shared injection equipment among intravenous drug users. By the end of the project, the researchers had interviewed close to 10,000 individuals. The community members who had been exposed to the intervention made significant changes in the state of change continuum toward changing their risk behaviors.

The structure, content, and activities incorporated in the project reflect the assumptions of well-accepted social theories that describe the mechanisms for changing behavior and risk reduction beliefs in target populations. By employing formal theories as the framework, the project became more credible; these theories have already undergone scrutiny through evaluation and empirical testing in other arenas and maintain some degree of confidence in their validity and generalizability. This allowed the researchers to develop an objective strategy based on ideas that are more concrete than informal beliefs and opinions. One of the more important theories seen in the structure of the ACDP is the Stages of Change Model (Prochaska & DiClemente, 1992; Prochaska, DiClemente, & Norcross, 1992; Prochaska & Velicer, 1997). The model held that a person progresses through stages when adopting or changing a behavior; it is not an "all or nothing" process, but a sequence of steps to change. Behavior and the state of change are dependent on the individual's intention to change. Intentions are influenced by personal attitudes, perceived norms, perceived risks, and belief in the individual's ability to change (self-efficacy). This is why it is critical to understand the common perceptions, needs, and beliefs of the target population. Different approaches and interventions are necessary at each stage to be effective.

The intervention materials were created in an attempt to put forth messages that show different circumstances, behavioral intentions, and stages of change that exist in the target population. Role models from the target community shared their experiences with the changed risk behaviors or the process of changing risk behaviors. Brochures, pamphlets, flyers, and trading cards illustrating their stories were distributed by volunteers throughout the community. Based on the formative research, the design and format of the media were created to be the most appealing to the community. The information could be standardized to emphasize the same message to all of the population. If they chose to display numerous messages, they could easily address heterogeneous cultures and diverse behaviors. The materials could be modified as often as needed and distributed easily and cost-effectively. Portable media allowed readers to take the information with them so that they could review at a later time and possibly even share with others. By virtue of being media, the material gained acceptance as it appeared more mainstream. The small media was also appropriate for topics that might be considered unsuitable for the general public. Role models allow a way to present behavioral alternatives without directly advocating the illegal or inappropriate practice. The goal was to encourage intravenous drug users to clean their equipment, since it posed a threat to disease transmission, but not to promote intravenous drug use itself. Restraints in literacy posed a problem to using this type of media, but by designing comic book–like stories and pictures, the message is brought out in the open. Awareness is diffused where it otherwise would not be.

The interventional materials were delivered by recruited volunteers in the target community. They were to focus on the role model literature, praise attempts to change, and were encouraged to share personal changes. This was known as the peer network. Peer networks address modeling communication by distributing and promoting the model and providing social reinforcement. The peer network was a supplement to the role model stories and mainly served to reinforce the issues presented. Peer volunteers were recruited through contact with outreach workers, trained in basic education, and given advice on how to reach out to people. The volunteers were not required to adopt the behavior goal to participate. In addition to being distributors, they also served as role models. Modeling makes the behavior acceptable as it appears that "everyone is doing it." Because the volunteers were from the community, it lent some credibility to the ability to change in their environment. Self-efficacy and acceptance increased as the individuals saw other community members had the ability to change.

Outcomes: The goal in the ACDP was to move individuals closer to changing the risk behavior. The role model stories served as social models for observational learning. Empirical data were gathered in the early stages to determine the exact beliefs about the behavior—the perceived risks, outcomes, attitudes, and stereotypes. Each story targeted a single risk reduction behavior and was a sincere, earnest personal account of how and why the role model began a change. An important aspect in AIDS prevention is that the individual be able to identify with the model. By using a member from the community, the material was able to focus on perceived barriers, finding new social support, and beliefs and factors that correlated with the intent to change. Stories were written in

(Continued)

(Continued)

colloquial language and had a photo of a role model. The type of story released was based on where the community was on the continuum of behavior change. As the community slowly shifted toward adopting the behavior, different role model stories were released portraying the new situations. Printed materials also had instructions for condoms and bleach cleaning, basic AIDS information, notices of special events, and information on health and social services.

The peer network was important for distributing materials, but more important for serving as social reinforcement to the community. The mass media acted as supplementary material that allowed the volunteer opinion leaders to show concrete details of the "hows" and "whys" members can and do change. Through all these channels, the ACDPs accelerated the diffusion of the behavior changes, and individuals exposed to the intervention had significant behavioral changes. The diffusion accelerator was very effective and could be customized to other behavioral changes and health interventions in hard-to-reach communities in the future.

BOX C   *A Su Salud*

Background: A broad program of community health promotion was initially implemented in the low-income community of Eagle Pass, on the Mexican–American border. Eagle Pass is located in southwest Texas, and the estimated population at the time of the study was 23,100. More than 90% were of Mexican American origin, 7% Anglo-Europeans, and less than 1% African Americans. A similar border town (Del Rio) was chosen as no-intervention control. The purpose of the study was to demonstrate the effectiveness of a health promotion intervention powered by a Diffusion Acceleration Model. The main goals of *A Su Salud* included reducing cigarette smoking, modifying eating habits, reducing alcohol abuse, increasing use of preventive services, increasing physical activities, and increasing seat belt use. Among adult males in the community, 38% were smokers, and 38% reported heavy drinking. Among women more than 30 years old, 55% reported no Pap smear and 48% reported no self-breast examination within the last year. Among population 50 years and older, 79% reported no colorectal exam within last year. Finally, among the general population, 41% reported not having had their blood pressure taken within the last year, 57% reported no physical activity, 85% reported no fat avoidance in their regular diets, and 82% did not always use seat belts.

Program Implementation: The project followed the lay opinion leader concept illustrated in the North Karelia Project. Two community workers were hired to recruit volunteer opinion leaders and train them in simple skills they could use to encourage and reinforce positive health behaviors among people in their natural social network. The project also produced, printed, and televised materials containing explanations and modeled behavior changes.

Community lay opinion leaders referred to these materials in their interaction with their networks. These leaders needed no expertise other than enthusiasm and good nature to encourage others to look at the role models shown on the television programs and newspapers and the ability to tactfully suggest and reinforce imitations of models.

A one-page printed flyer titled *Seis Asesinos Importantes Andan Sueltos en el Condado de Maverick* (Six Important Assassins are Loose in Maverick County) was circulated. The flyer described the "six killers" as avoidable risk factors associated with premature death in the county. It was placed in the local newspaper and distributed to 5,000 homes. In addition, two sets of television programs were developed and produced. The first one consisted of 15 programs ranging in length from 5 to 10 minutes. In these programs, role models and some additional health information were presented in a news format. The second television series consisted of four 30-minute programs presented in a mini documentary format, with a health education specialist serving as narrator and role models as the central interest. These television presentations were followed by periodic role model stories presented on the local newspaper and a Spanish radio station broadcasting from the Mexican town across the border. In addition, at the beginning of each month, community bulletins were distributed throughout the community by the opinion leaders. These bulletins contained a brief story and a picture of a role model, a calendar of role model mass media stories listing the channel, time, and program title, and important information about clinic schedules, fees, phone numbers, etc.

The volunteer lay opinion leaders simultaneously represented the project goals, as well as the community reaction to those goals. They received brief training to pass around the bulletins, providing minimal social reinforcement and encouraging friends and acquaintances to pay attention to media events. Opinion leaders came from neighborhoods, business settings, government institutions, social clubs, health care providers, educational settings, and religious organizations.

Using the same diffusion acceleration strategy, *A Su Salud* program included policy advocacy promoting voter and consumer action. The process followed three different elements: consumer/voter awareness, mobilization, and consultation with policy and decision makers. Community members presented the city council with a proposal to limit smoking in public places, followed by letters of support from the volunteer opinion leaders and others in key positions in the community. Businesseswere also approached. After a year of effort, a smoking restriction ordinance was finally approved.

Outcomes: The project continued in Eagle Pass from 1984 to 1989. Results showed that, in the study community exposed to the mass media and opinion leader network, an 18% smoking cessation (1 year without smoking) rate was seen, as compared with 7.5% in a control community with no organized campaign. The program was later extended as *Salud En Acción* to San Antonio and Brownsville, two larger metropolitan areas in South Texas, focusing on nutrition and cancer screening behaviors. Control communities were designated in Laredo and Houston, Texas. Additional media materials were produced including a periodic flyer with original healthy recipes from the kitchens of role models. These recipes were eventually turned into a 180-page cookbook. Media use was expanded to an average of 1 hour of radio per month, weekly English language columns (role model stories) in two

(Continued)

(Continued)

major newspapers with a circulation of more than 200,000, a biweekly section in a Spanish language newspaper with a circulation of 50,000, regular evening television newscasts on the local Spanish station, as well as stories over a local cable free access network.

To evaluate results with women exposed to the media and interpersonal communications program, the women were surveyed at the beginning of the campaign and again 2 years later. These evaluations showed that the Pap test adherence rate (screening every 2 years according to then-current recommendations) increased from 54% to 61% among women who had recently received the screening for cervical cancer. In the control community of Laredo, the rate for the same period changed only from 46% to 47%. Among women who had not obtained a Pap test recently and didn't intend to get another one, the Brownsville study group showed a decrease from 23% to 13%. This meant the percentage of women in this category, who had avoided Pap screening for years, was cut nearly in half. Meanwhile, in the Laredo control group, the percentage of women in this category dropped only slightly.

This program was further extended to major cities of high concentration of Hispanic/Latino populations nationwide, including Puerto Ricans in New York City, New York; Cuban Americans in Miami, Florida; Central and South Americans in San Francisco, California; and Mexican Americans in San Diego, California; San Antonio, Texas; and Brownsville, Texas. The group of researchers involved in this extension of the program, eventually developed it into *Redes En Acción*, the most active national network of Hispanic/Latino cancer prevention research, training, and outreach.

BOX D   *Mejor Hablemos* (Let's talk!)

Background: Cali is the second largest city in Colombia with a population of more than 2 million people. The city attracts high numbers of migrants from the southwestern region of the country. The city has high unemployment rates and large areas of severe poverty. Cali experienced an increase in violence rates from 23 to 106/100,000 per year from 1983 to 1995. *Mejor Hablemos* was a communication intervention based on the Diffusion Acceleration Model, developed within the larger framework of DESEPAZ, a comprehensive violence prevention program established in the city of Cali, Colombia. The word DESEPAZ is a Spanish acronym for "development, security and peace." The program aimed to restore public safety through social development, prevention of violence, community political empowerment, respect for human rights, and enhancement of social cohesion. The guiding principles of DESEPAZ acknowledged that violence is a multi-causal problem that requires multiple and comprehensive interventions, these interventions must be based on permanent and solid scientific research, violence prevention must be a priority in efforts to restore public safety, and public safety is the responsibility of both government and citizens.

Program Implementation: The program included the following: a unit to study the epidemiology of violence (Vélez et al., 1998); an effort to improve the effectiveness of law enforcement agents and restore trust between them and the citizens; the improvement of the well-being and capacity of the police force; the creation of judiciary precincts specialized in family issues and conciliation centers that provided conflict resolution assistance; building "Houses of Peace" from all the public institutions involved in public safety (police, army, courts, family precincts, etc.); setting up computer networks between courts, police and other law enforcement agencies; and training of special murder investigation brigades. The mayor also took legal actions restricting the times of alcohol sales and instituted temporary bans on weapon-carrying permits. Other programs included employment and training of the work force, increasing elementary and secondary school coverage and extending the network of public libraries, self-built housing developments, and education for peace through social communications and other community-based interventions.

In 1996, as a further development of the social communication efforts to promote peaceful conviviality, the CISALVA Institute for the Research and Development of the Prevention of Violence and the Promotion of Social Conviviality at the Universidad del Valle in Cali developed a program titled *Mejor Hablemos*. Using the Diffusion Acceleration Model, *Mejor Hablemos* aimed to change attitudes, abilities, intentions, and behavior that influence peaceful conviviality. The program was based on sustained, rigorous ethnographic and epidemiological research. Tolerance, forgiveness, personal control, and dialogue were the main points addressed with the communities who participated as main partners in the conception and design of the project's strategies and processes.

With the auspices of the Colombian Ministry of Health, the Mayor's Office and the City Secretary of Health, *Mejor Hablemos* involved agreements with 10 radio stations belonging to large national radio conglomerates, as well as individually owned local stations, and several community owned radios. The most popular local television newscast broadcasts also presented weekly notes dealing with these stories, as did *El Caleño*, a daily tabloid paper with gruesome images of violence with the highest circulation in the city. *El Caleño* published the *Mejor Hablemos* story every week as its central page, right next to the topless pin-up girl of the week, which was exactly the highly visible place where the program leaders wanted to reach young adult males with the role model stories. Traditional regional papers such as *El País* also contributed to the strategy. All the stories were written at a low reading level. In the course of 3 years, the program reached over 300 hours of radio and television air time, and more than 200 newspaper articles featuring role model stories, all provided for free by the media partners. The program staff, which included two journalists, two sociologists, and two community workers, identified the role models, preproduced the stories for the newspapers and radio, and collaborated with the television crew in the production of the TV stories.

The program involved and briefly trained lay opinion leaders through alliances with over 200 owners of corner shops and popular hairdressers in beauty parlors, as well as hospitals, schools, and community day cares. Other spaces for message dissemination included

(Continued)

(Continued)

schools' sports areas and football/soccer matches—where the concept of the "blue card," "time out" for overly aggressive conduct was implemented. The community networks reinforced the contents of the mass media through dialogue triggered by using the monthly bulletin *Con-Vivencias* (sharing life experiences). The four-page bulletin, coproduced with the community, contained an introduction to the specific theme written by a community leader (e.g., bullying in school, youth gangs, sexual abuse inside families, marital violence, heavy drinking and arms use, conflict resolution in sports' situations), and all the relevant telephone numbers of institutions that dealt with violence in the city. The two center pages always portrayed a photo-novella, called real stories (*Historias Reales*), narrating in a simple way a real case story of a conflict and its peaceful resolution, sometimes with institutional help, but always with the main concept of dialogue and conversation as the way to prevent conflict. This bulletin also invited readers to tune in to the role model stories on the mass media. The distribution of 10,000 monthly bulletins was done via alliances with barrio associations and leaders, and dialogue and debate was pursued via audio and radio forums (workshops accompanied by tapes and discussion guides).

While the comprehensive DESEPAZ intervention was sustained throughout the city, there was a decrease of 20% in the rates of homicides, an increase of 10% in the detention of murder suspects, and a several-fold increase in the use of mediation services. Program evaluation of *Mejor Hablemos* also documented more favorable attitudes toward peaceful conflict resolution and a decrease in self-reported family violence. Unfortunately, later city administrations drastically reduced the funding for the program. *Mejor Hablemos* has served as a model for similar projects in other places, and the Colombia Ministry of Health sponsored the extension of the program to the cities of Bogotá and Medellín, covering in total one third of the total population of Colombia. Similarly, the model developed to study the epidemiology of violence has been adopted nationwide in Colombia and in several major cities in Latin America under the auspices of the Pan American Health Organization.

NOTE

1. Although these programs are repeatedly mentioned throughout the chapter, for the sake of reading fluency, the corresponding in-text bibliographic citations will not be referenced again.

DISCUSSION QUESTIONS AND ACTIVITIES

1. How does the Diffusion Acceleration Model differ from traditional communication models used by health promoters to change behaviors in multicultural communities?

2. In small groups, select a health problem and target group and discuss how you would apply the Diffusion Acceleration Model to that problem and target group. Be prepared to share your discussions with the rest of the class.

REFERENCES

Amezcua, C., McAlister, A. L., Ramirez, A., & Espinoza, R. (1990). *A Su Salud*: Health promotion in a Mexican-American border community. In N. F. Bracht (Ed.), *Health promotion at the community level* (pp. 257–277). Newbury Park, CA: Sage.

Bandura, A. (1977). *Social Learning Theory.* Englewood Cliffs, NJ: Prentice Hall.

Bandura, A. (1986). *Social foundations of thought and action: A Social Cognitive Theory.* Englewood Cliffs, NJ: Prentice Hall.

Bandura, A. (1996). *Self-efficacy: The exercise of control.* New York: W. H. Freeman.

Barberich, M. W. (2002). Fireside politics: Radio and political culture in the United States, 1920–1940. *Journal of Interdisciplinary History, 33,* 147–149.

Chaffee, S. H., & Mutz, D. C. (1988). Comparing mediated and interpersonal communication data. In R. P. Hawkins, J. M. Wiemann, & S. Pingree (Eds.), *Advancing communication science: Merging mass and interpersonal processes* (pp. 19–43). Newbury Park, CA: Sage.

Chalela, P., Vélez, L. F., & Ramirez, A. G. (2007). Social influences, attitudes and beliefs associated with smoking among border Latino youth. *Journal of School Health, 77,* 187–195.

Curran, J. W. (1997). The primary role of HIV interventions at the community level. In N. H. Corby & R. J. Wolitsky (Eds.), *Community HIV prevention: The Long Beach AIDS community demonstration project* (pp. 1–4). Long Beach: The University Press, California State University.

Fishbein, M., & Rhodes, F. (1997). Using behavioral theory in HIV prevention. In N. H. Corby & R. J. Wolitsky (Eds.), *Community HIV prevention: The Long Beach AIDS community demonstration project* (pp. 21–30). Long Beach: The University Press, California State University.

Hershey, J. C., Niederdeppe, J., Evans, W. D., Nonnemaker, J., Blahut, S., Holden, D., et al. (2005). The theory of "truth": How counterindustry campaigns affect smoking behavior among teens. *Health Psychology, 24*(1), 22–31.

Karvonen, M. (1995). Prehistory of the North Karelia Project. In P. Puska, J. Tuomilehto, A. Nissinen, & E. Vartiainen (Eds.), *The North Karelia project: 20 year results and experiences* (pp. 17–22). Helsinki, Finland: The National Public Health Institute, Helsinki University Printing House.

Lazarsfeld, P. F., Berelson, B., & Gaudet, H. (1948). *The peoples choice. How the voter makes up his mind in a presidential campaign.* New York: Columbia University Press.

Lewin, K. (1951). *Field theory in social science; selected theoretical papers* (D. Cartwright, Ed.). New York: Harper & Row.

MacDonald, T. H. (1998). *Rethinking health promotion: A global approach.* London: Routledge.

McAlister, A. L. (1991). Population behavior change: A theory-based approach. *Journal of Public Health Policy, 12*(3), 345–361.

McAlister, A. (1995a). Behavioral journalism: Beyond the marketing model for health communication. *American Journal of Health Promotion, 9*(6), 417–420.

McAlister, A. L. (1995b). The role of the North Karelia Project in modern public health. In P. Puska, J. Tuomilehto, A. Nissinen, & E. Vartiainen (Eds.), *The North Karelia Project: 20 year results and experiences* (pp. 319–326). Helsinki, Finland: The National Public Health Institute, Helsinki University Printing House.

McAlister, A. (1997). The diffusion accelerator: Combining media and interpersonal communication in community-level health promotion campaigns. In N. H. Corby & R. J. Wolitsky (Eds.), *Community HIV prevention: The Long Beach AIDS community demonstration project* (pp. 31–44). Long Beach, CA: The University Press, California State University.

McAlister, A. L., Fernandez-Esquer, M. E., Ramirez, A. G., Trevino, F., Gallion, K., Villarreal, R., et al. (1995). Community level cancer control in a Texas barrio: Part II—baseline and preliminary outcome findings. *Journal of the National Cancer Institute Monographs, 18,* 123–126.

McAlister, A. L., Huang, P., & Ramirez, A. G. (2006). Settlement-funded tobacco control in Texas: 2000–2004 pilot project effects on cigarette smoking. *Public Health Reports, 121*(3), 235–238.

McAlister, A. L., Ramirez, A. G., Amezcua, C., Pulley, L., Stern, M. P., & Mercado, S. (1992). Smoking cessation in Texas-Mexico border communities: A quasi-experimental panel study. *American Journal of Health Promotion, 6*(4), 274–279.

McAlister, A., & Vélez, L. F. (1999). Behavioral sciences concepts in research on the prevention of violence. *Pan American Journal of Public Health, 5*(4), 316–321.

Meshack, A. F., Hu, S., Pallonen, U. E., McAlister, A. L., Gottlieb, N., & Huang, P. (2004). Texas tobacco prevention pilot initiative: Processes and effects. *Health Education Research, 19*(6), 657–668.

Mutz, D. C., Sniderman, P. M., & Brody, R. (1996). Political persuasion: The birth of a field of study. In D. C. Mutz, P. M. Sniderman, & R. Brody (Eds.), *Political persuasion and attitude change* (pp. 1–16). Ann Arbor: University of Michigan Press.

Nettleton, S., & Bunton, R. (1995). Sociological critiques of health promotion. In R. Bunton, S. Nettleton, & R. Burrows (Eds.), *The sociology of health promotion: Critical analyses of consumption, lifestyle and risk* (pp. 41–58). London: Routledge.

Prochaska, J. O., & DiClemente, C. C. (1992). Stages of change in the modification of problem behavior. In M. Hersen, R. Eisler, & P. M. Miller (Eds.), *Progress in behavior modification* (pp. 184–214). Sycamore, IL: Sycamore.

Prochaska, J. O., DiClemente, C. C., & Norcross, J. C. (1992). In search of how people change: Applications to addictive behaviors. *American Psychologist, 47,* 1102–1113.

Prochaska, J. O., & Velicer, W. F. (1997). The transtheoretical model of health behavior change. *American Journal of Health Promotion, 12*(1), 38–48.

Pulley, L. V., McAlister, A. L., Kay, L. S., & O'Reilly, K. (1996). Prevention campaigns for hard-to-reach populations at risk for HIV infection: Theory and implementation. *Health Education Quarterly, 23*(4), 488–496.

Puska, P. (1995a). Experience with major subprogrammes and examples of innovative interventions. In P. Puska, J. Tuomilehto, A. Nissinen, & E. Vartiainen (Eds.), *The North Karelia Project: 20 year results and experiences* (pp. 273–288). Helsinki, Finland: The National Public Health Institute, Helsinki University Printing House.

Puska, P. (1995b). Main outline of the North Karelia Project. In P. Puska, J. Tuomilehto, A. Nissinen, & E. Vartiainen (Eds.), *The North Karelia Project: 20 year results and experiences* (pp. 24–30). Helsinki, Finland: The National Public Health Institute, Helsinki University Printing House.

Puska, P., Salonen, J. T., Koskela, K., McAlister, A., Kottke, T. E., Maccoby, W., & Farquhar, J. W. (1985). The community-based strategy to prevent coronary heart disease: Conclusions from ten years of the North Karelia Project. *Annual Review of Public Health, 6,* 147–193.

Ramirez, A. G., & McAlister, A. L. (1988). Mass media campaign: *A Su Salud. American Journal of Preventive Medicine, 17*(5), 608–621.

Ramirez, A. G., McAlister, A., Gallion, K. J., Ramirez, V., Garza, I. R., Stamm, K., et al. (1995). Community level cancer control in a Texas barrio: Part I—theoretical basis, implementation, and process evaluation. *Journal of the National Cancer Institute Monographs, 18,* 117–122.

Ramirez, A. G., McAlister, A., Villarreal, R., Suarez, L., Talavera, G. A., Perez-Stable, E. J., et al. (1998). Prevention and control in diverse Hispanic populations: A national initiative for research and action. *Cancer, 83*(8), 1825–1829.

Ramirez, A. G., Vélez, L. F., Chalela, P., Grussendorf, J., & McAlister, A. L. (2006). Tobacco control policy advocacy attitudes and self-efficacy among ethnically diverse high school students. *Health Education & Behavior, 33*(4), 502–514.

Ramirez, A. G., Villareal, R., McAlister, A., Gallion, K., Suarez, L., & Gomez, P. (1999). Advancing the role of participatory communication in the diffusion of cancer screening among Hispanics. *Journal of Health Communication, 4*(1), 31–36.

Reardon, K., & Rogers, E. (1988). Interpersonal versus mass media communication: A false dichotomy. *Human Communication Research, 15*(2), 284–303.

Rogers, E. (1962). *Diffusion of innovations.* New York: Free Press of Glencoe.

Rogers, E. (2003). *Diffusion of innovations* (5th ed.). New York: Free Press.

Seigel, M., & Doner, L. (2004). *Marketing public health: Strategies to promote social change.* Sudbury, MA: Jones & Bartlett.

Shegog, R., McAlister, A. L., Hu, S., Ford, K. C., Meshack, A. F., & Peters, R. J. (2005). Use of interactive health communication to affect smoking intentions in middle school students: A pilot test of the "Headbutt" risk assessment program. *American Journal of Health Promotion, 19*(5), 334–338.

Smedley, B. D., & Syme, S. L. (Eds.). (2000). *Promoting health: Intervention strategies from social and behavioral research.* Washington, DC: National Academy Press.

United Nations Development Programme. (2005). *Human development report 2005: International cooperation at a crossroads—Aid, trade and security in an unequal world.* New York: Author.

Vélez, L. F. (1998). Violencia y medios de comunicación. *Revista Latinoamericana de Comunicación: Chasqui, 64,* 73–77.

Vélez, L. F., Giraldo, J. C., Unás, V., Prada, M. A., & Arango, O. A. (1998). Crónica roja: Hacia un periodismo del abrazo. *Revista Latinoamericana de Comunicación: Chasqui, 62,* 58–61.

Vélez, L. F., McAlister, A., & Hu, S. (1997). Measuring attitudes toward violence in Colombia. *American Journal of Social Psychology, 137*(4), 533–534.

World Health Organization. (1986). *Ottawa charter for health promotion.* Geneva, Switzerland: Author.

12

Tips for Working With Hispanic/Latino Population Groups

ROBERT M. HUFF

MICHAEL V. KLINE

There are many terms used to describe persons who trace their ancestry back to Spain, the most common of which are *Hispanic* and *Latino*. Suarez and Ramirez (1998) commented that it is more appropriate to use terms that actually identify the country of origin of the individual or population group (e.g., Mexican American, Guatemalan American) because this recognizes that these diverse ethnic groups have customs and behaviors that are unique to them despite the fact that they might share a common ancestral language and other more general cultural characteristics (also see Chapter 9, this volume). Thus, the health promoter is urged to consider this suggested approach not only because it is a more accurate way in which to describe Hispanic population groups and individuals but also because it can serve as the first step in becoming more culturally competent and sensitive to the diversity of peoples who have been labeled as having Hispanic or Latino origins.

This brief "tips" chapter seeks to provide comments, suggestions, and recommendations

for working with these different ethnic groups in health promotion and disease prevention (HPDP) activities. These tips are taken from Chapters 1, 2, 9, 10, and 11 of this volume and are meant to be only general starting points when thinking about designing HPDP programs for Hispanic population groups.

CULTURAL COMPETENCE

As noted in Chapter 1, health promoters need to develop cultural competence skills for working across multicultural population groups. This is an especially important issue when working with Hispanic populations because there is a great diversity of ethnic differences that must be considered if one hopes to be successful in one's HPDP efforts. The following tips for the health promoter and the student can help facilitate that process:

- Seek to learn the history and immigration patterns of the specific ethnic group you will be targeting for HPDP interventions or services.

278

- Become familiar with the group's specific cultural values, beliefs, and ways of life, including forms of address and other verbal and nonverbal communication patterns, food preferences, attitudes toward health and disease, and related cultural characteristics that differentiate this group from other Hispanic populations.
- Seek to incorporate these cultural values, beliefs, and ways of life into the HPDP programs or services wherever appropriate and possible.
- Be aware that the degree to which Spanish is used as the primary language of the specific ethnic group will depend on a variety of factors including generational level, age, and gender. Assessment is the key to understanding.
- Be aware that acculturation is a critical factor in explaining risk behavior and health status. The more traditional the individual or group, the less likely the individual or group is to know about, understand, or practice Western approaches to HPDP.
- Understand that the measurement of acculturation is an important activity for understanding how traditional, acculturated, and assimilated a specific ethnic group may be. There are a variety of scales that can be used, and you are urged to read Chapters 1, 9, 10, and 11 for a more detailed discussion of this process.
- Understand that family and family support are extremely important core values among Hispanic population groups.
- Be aware that avoiding conflict and achieving harmony in interpersonal relationships is a strong cultural value.
- Be aware that respect is an extremely important factor in all relationships and especially in HPDP encounters.
- Examine your own perceptions, stereotypes, and prejudices toward the target group and be willing to suspend judgments (where they exist) in favor of learning who these people really are rather than who or what you might think they are. This is a critical first step in developing cultural competence and sensitivity.
- Take the time to make multiple visits to the community where the target group lives. Talk with community leaders and residents, visit important cultural sites within the community, eat at local restaurants, attend local events, and otherwise become familiar with the community's ways of life.
- Seek to establish early and continuing support from the community for any HPDP programs and services that are to be offered.

HEALTH BELIEFS AND PRACTICES

There are a variety of health beliefs and practices that characterize the many different Hispanic population groups residing in the United States. An understanding of these can help the health promotion students and practitioners develop an increased understanding of and sensitivity to the differences he or she is likely to encounter and also can provide for opportunities to incorporate these differences into his or her HPDP intervention and treatment programs and services.

- Recognize that belief in folk illnesses is still a strong cultural characteristic among many traditional Hispanic population groups. Developing an understanding of some of these illnesses and their traditional treatments can help you to be more effective in the design of specific HPDP intervention and treatment services.
- Recognize that *fatalism*, the belief that one has no control over one's health outcomes, is a common attitude among many traditional Hispanic population groups.
- Understand that there are a number of explanatory models used to make sense of health and disease and that these are generally associated with the social, psychological, or physical domains.
- Where differences exist between the explanatory models of the target group and yourself, you will need to make efforts to ameliorate or otherwise find ways to work within these different frames of reference.
- Consider becoming more familiar with traditional healing practices where these exist in the community because this may provide opportunities to bring beneficial practices into the biomedical framework while also

of cultural tailoring that may be useful to the health promoter because it encourages the recognition of the need to design interventions that are specific to the cultural characteristics of the target group. The health promoter may also wish to consider the following comments and suggestions as he or she begins the design phase of the program-planning process:

- Recognize that the development of culturally appropriate interventions requires consideration of available community resources and inclusion of important cultural themes of the target group. For example, *family* is one of the strongest core values of traditional Hispanic culture, so interventions that have a family focus might prove more effective than those that focus on the individual.
- Be aware that "one size fits all" is not a useful approach to intervention design. Programs and services need to be tailored to the target groups they will serve.
- Linguistic, literacy, gender relevance, and other cultural factors must be considered in the design of the intervention to be carried out in the community.
- Remember that using captive audiences and unconventional sites for the delivery of HPDP programs and services can be a highly effective approach to reaching and involving the community. This may involve home parties, parks and other recreation areas, social groups, block parties, and other locations where community members might gather.
- Be aware that interventions such as role modeling and use of community social networks can be useful approaches for demonstrating and reinforcing individual behavior change.
- Be aware that developing partnerships with the local media (e.g., radio, television, newspapers) for the dissemination of health education and health promotion information can be a valuable and effective approach for both marketing the program or service and reinforcing the successes of program participants, who may be recruited as role models for the community in which the program or service has been targeted.

- Recognize that the use of behavioral theory to guide development of intervention approaches is central to well-conceived and appropriately designed intervention strategies (see Chapter 4, this volume).
- Recognize that the recruitment and training of a group of community peer networkers who can distribute program materials and reinforce messages can be an extremely effective method for maintaining community involvement and support for the HPDP program or service.
- Seek to develop interventions that focus on positive health changes rather than on negative or fear-arousing consequences.
- Remember that the development of educational materials must reflect relevant cultural values, themes, and learning styles of the target group for which they are designed.
- All materials used in the HPDP program that are written in a language other than English must be *back translated* and pilot tested to ensure that they say what is meant and that the messages are clear and understandable to the target group.
- Always assess the cultural appropriateness of any pictures, slang, models, dolls, or other educational materials prior to their inclusion in the program because some materials may be in bad taste or may make the target group uncomfortable.
- Remember that employing and training community members to facilitate educational programs in the community is a valuable and effective approach for implementing an HPDP program or service.

EVALUATION CONSIDERATIONS

Evaluation is central to understanding how well a program or service is doing in meeting the needs of the clientele it is serving. For this reason, the health promoter is urged to consider the following recommendations:

- Seek to develop evaluation strategies, methods, and instruments that reflect an understanding of current theory and practice in the evaluation and research literature.

- Evaluation of HPDP programs and services should include culturally relevant measures for evaluating the impact of the program or service on the target group.
- Assessment and evaluation items must be tailored to the educational and linguistic capabilities of the target group for which they are intended. Here, again, back translation of items will be an important consideration in the development of the assessment and evaluation instruments.
- Recognize that evaluation and assessment are processes for which it frequently is difficult to gain support, even from the most sophisticated of groups. Efforts to explain the underlying assumptions governing these processes, as well as the methods and anticipated outcomes from these activities, can help make explicit what is often unclear to those inexperienced in evaluation and can motivate increased interest and support for evaluation and assessment methods and procedures.
- Recognize that providing evaluation and assessment training for community members who will be involved in the provision of the HPDP program or service can help promote increased input and support for evaluation efforts. This can also extend the number of staff and community supporters who can be involved in data collection activities related to assessment and evaluation activities.
- Evaluation efforts should consider the needs and interests of the stakeholders, both in the community and in the agency providing the HPDP program or service.
- Evaluation criteria should be elicited from the community in which the program or service is being offered because its members are the ones who know what is important to them.
- Evaluators should recognize that HPDP participants from the community might have limited test-taking skills or abilities. Thus, efforts to design evaluation methods should reflect these potentialities by seeking approaches that are within the relevant experiences and skills of the target group.
- Be sure to design evaluation and assessment reporting and feedback mechanisms to ensure that the target community is regularly informed about how well the program or service is functioning to improve the health issue or problem for which it was designed.

The next section of the book considers Black American population groups. This section includes three chapters followed by a customized "tips" chapter. The first chapter in this section presents an overview devoted to understanding this special population from a variety of perspectives and includes terms used to define the subgroups within the broader population, historical and demographic characteristics, immigration patterns, health and disease issues and concerns, and health beliefs and practices. The second chapter of the section is concerned with how to assess, plan, implement, and evaluate programs for Black American groups, including tips, models, and suggestions for more effective program design. The third chapter in this section presents a case study to emphasize the points made in the overview and planning chapters. This section begins with Chapter 13.

REFERENCES

Pasick, R. J., D'Onofrio, C. N., & Otero-Sabogal, R. (1996). Similarities and differences across cultures: Questions to inform a third generation for health promotion research. *Health Education Quarterly, 23*(Suppl.), S142–S161.

Suarez, L., & Ramirez, A. G. (1999). Latino health and disease: An overview. In R. M. Huff & M. V. Kline (Eds.), *Promoting health in multicultural populations: A handbook for practitioners* (pp. 115–136). Thousand Oaks, CA: Sage.

PART III

African American Populations

13

Promoting Health Among Black American Populations

An Overview

JOYCE W. HOPP

PATTI HERRING

Chapter Objectives

On completion of this chapter, the health promotion student and practitioner should be able to

- Identify, differentiate, and discuss the various subcultures represented by the term *Black Americans*
- Analyze and discuss health problems of Black Americans with regard to health services availability and accessibility in the United States
- Recognize what the effect of slavery had (and continues to have) on the health beliefs and practices of Black Americans in the 21st century
- Identify and describe the three main historical phases of Black American health care in the United States
- Identify and give specific examples of traditional health beliefs and practices related to cultural backgrounds of Black Americans
- Compare the patterns of the major diseases in their rates and health effects between Black and White Americans living in the United States
- Assess the positive ways in which Black churches assist their parishioners in health promotion and disease control

Black Americans, according to the 2000 census, constitute 12.9% of the U.S. population (Centers for Disease Control and Prevention [CDC], 2005a); by 2020, they will constitute 15% according to a prediction by the U.S. Bureau of the Census (1992). Blacks, however, suffer disproportionately from preventable diseases and premature deaths. This chapter explores the extent of this disparity and the historical and current factors that may contribute to it. It also alerts the health professional to the health beliefs, behaviors, and cultural content in which Black Americans function as a basis for understanding their health promotion and health care needs.

In the year 2020, nearly one out of five children of school age and one out of six adults of prime working age (25 to 54 years) will be Black. Thomas (1992) points out that although rising numbers of Blacks will be represented in both influential occupations and positions, they will also be among the poorest, the least educated, and the jobless. Throughout the 20th century, Blacks have lagged behind Whites in terms of life expectancy; whereas life expectancy has risen to 76 years for the overall population, it has fallen to 69 years for the Blacks (U.S. Bureau of the Census, 1992).

For Blacks in the United States, health disparities can mean earlier deaths, decreased quality of life, loss of economic opportunities, and perceptions of injustice (CDC, 2005a). Achieving a healthy nation is impossible without healthy minority populations and elimination of racial disparities (CDC, 2004). The extent of the disparity between Black and White populations was first documented in 1980. The *Report of the Secretary's Task Force on Black and Minority Health* (Heckler, 1985) documented that Blacks suffered nearly 60,000 excess deaths per year. Although the prevalence of cardiovascular disease and stroke are similar in both populations, the mortality rates are higher for Black American (Magnus, 1991). Black men, in particular, are twice as likely as White men to die from strokes or

heart attacks (Caplan, 1991). Hypertension is higher among Black Americans than among Whites. Black American men below 45 years of age have a 10 times greater chance of dying from high blood pressure than do White men (Magnus, 1991). Although the top 3 causes of the 10 leading causes of death are the same for non-Hispanic Whites, the risk factors, morbidity and mortality rates for these diseases, and injuries are often greater among Blacks than Whites. Three of the 10 leading causes of death for Blacks are not among the leading causes of death for Whites, namely, homicide, HIV/AIDS, and septicemia (CDC, 2005a).

Maternal mortality rates for Black women are three times higher than those for White women (Aday, 1993). Black babies born in the United States have an increased risk of low birth weight and perinatal mortality (Cabral, Fried, Levenson, Amaro, & Zuckerman, 1990).

More Black Americans than Whites smoke, although Black Americans smoke an average of 20% fewer cigarettes; however, they have a higher incidence of lung cancer (Magnus, 1991). More than 44% of Black women above 20 years of age are overweight, compared with 27% of women in general (U.S. Department of Health and Human Services [U.S. DHHS], 1990b).

Black Americans come from a wide variety of backgrounds and cultural experiences, which in turn influence their health behaviors. But they share traditional health beliefs and practices, which can affect many aspects of their interactions with the health care delivery system and public health.

BLACK SUBCULTURAL DIVERSITY

Although all Blacks in the United States are often labeled *African Americans*, foreign-born and immigrant Blacks who have not become acculturated into the American culture might not identify with American-born Blacks and therefore might not classify themselves as African Americans. Many Blacks, who immigrated to the United States from Africa, Great

Britain, and the islands of the Caribbean, even though their ancestors may have been enslaved prior to emigration, might not identify with the descendants of slaves in the United States. Some Blacks are Spanish speaking, emigrating from Central American countries. Thus, Blacks in the United States represent a wide range of backgrounds with a variety of beliefs and customs, so that a single label does not fit all Blacks. Following are definitions used in the literature:

African Americans: This term usually refers to American-born Blacks only, excluding foreign-born Blacks.

Afrocentricity: This is a way of interpreting the history, culture, and behavior of Blacks around the world. From this perspective, African history is seen as a diaspora and the history of Black Americans is understood as a part of the story of that dispersion (Coughlin, 1987).

Blacks: This term is used by the U.S. Bureau of the Census to denote the race of individuals. The labels for Black and White will be capitalized in this chapter because when they are not, we believe that they are used as adjectives, describing the color of people's skin. We use these terms to identify population classifications.

Non-Hispanic Whites: This is used interchangeably with Whites and Caucasians.

Race and Ethnicity: Race and ethnicity are classifications currently used for various purposes, such as tracking morbidity and mortality statistics, defining group characteristics, and exploring the health characteristics of individuals and groups. Most current data consider four racial groups in the United States: Black/African American, American Indian and Alaska Natives, Asian American and Pacific Islander, and White; additionally, there are two ethnic categories: Hispanic and non-Hispanic (CDC, 1998).

Minority: Vander Sanden (1972) describes this as a "sociological term that refers to a culturally or physically distinctive social group whose members experience various disadvantages at the hands of another social group" (quoted in Adams, 1995, p. 6).

HISTORICAL PERSPECTIVE: A BRIEF OVERVIEW OF BLACK AMERICAN HISTORY IN THE UNITED STATES

Slavery in the United States

No discussion of Black culture would be complete without mentioning the effect of slavery on this group of Americans. Black Americans' cultural personality and breeding are strongly shaped by the slavery experiences of their ancestors. Slavery has shaped Black culture more than has any other factor.

Slavery, according to Sowell (1994), "is one of the oldest and most widespread institutions on Earth" (p. 186). The practice affected the lives of countless people of various ethnic groups around the world for generations. Slavery existed in the Western Hemisphere before Columbus's ships appeared on the horizon, and it existed in Europe, Asia, Africa, and the Middle East for thousands of years.

What, then, distinguishes the Black American slavery experience? Blacks did not consensually come to America seeking a land of freedom, as did other migrants. During their more than two centuries of bondage, however, their many ancestral languages and cultures faded away and the genetic differences were combined to produce the American Black. Thus, American Blacks were a cultural and biological product of the New World rather than direct descendants of any given African nation or culture (Sowell, 1994).

American Blacks also have different histories according to the time of acquiring freedom. Although the Emancipation Proclamation of 1863 freed most American Blacks, about half a million were free before then. These "free persons of color" had a history, a culture, and a set of values that continue to distinguish their descendants from other Blacks well into the 20th century. A third small, but important, segment of the Black population consists of emigrants from the West Indies. They, too, have had an economic and social history very different from that of other Blacks (Sowell, 1981).

A variety of ceremonial or ritual behaviors accompanied the slaves from Africa. Most African religions were tribal; however, some tribes practiced Islam and voodoo. Voodoo is a blend of Christian, African, and other beliefs related to both religion and health practices. Researchers report that medical care for ill slaves was, at best, inconsistent (Guillory, 1987). Most slave owners insisted that slaves immediately inform them of any illness. Many Blacks, however, preferred self-treatment or treatment by Black herb/root doctors or influential conjurers. Slave owners always watched for malingerers; one way of dealing with the potential of faked illness was to make the medicine worse than the complaint (Guillory, 1987).

Because of slavery, the level of trust that Blacks had for White physicians was either very low or nonexistent. This mistrust survives, to a certain extent, even today. Individuals who survived the experience of slavery formed a society that had little resemblance to the proud and independent stance of their ancestors (Guillory, 1987).

Social and psychological means of control by slave owners, in addition to armed guards, were not sufficient to control the potential for rebellion or runaways. An additional means was the maintenance of ignorance among the slaves. This ignorance included not only the absence of formal education but also the lack of knowledge of the geographical area. Unfamiliarity with the area reduced the risk of successful escapes (Sowell, 1994).

Urban slaves, often domestic servants, were different from rural field hands. Urban slaves were much more likely to be able to read and write because of their wider access to resources. They were also more likely to have social contact with free Blacks in the cities. Frederick Douglas observed that urban slaves were almost free citizens. He knew this from personal experience as an urban slave before he escaped to the North to become a leader of his people (Sowell, 1994).

Following the abolition of slavery, many Blacks continued to live on farms. Families depended on extended family members for health care. Many older family members served as midwives and root doctors. Health care rarely was sought outside the community because of lack of trust, money, knowledge of available health care, and transportation. Reliance on ethnomedicine flourished.

Slavery as an institution is gone from the United States, but its effects continue to be felt in the 21st century.

Post-1950s Health Care Reform and Black America

Important events that led to more equal access to medical care and improved health status for Black Americans were (a) the Civil Rights Act of 1964, (b) Medicaid-Medicare legislation of 1965, and (c) Title VI of the Civil Rights Act, which prohibited racial discrimination in any institution receiving federal funds, giving hospitals a power incentive to alter their practices. In spite of increased access to medical care services, however, Black Americans continue to have disproportionately large numbers of premature and excess deaths compared with the White majority (Thomas, 1992).

McCord and Freeman's (1990) study of excess mortality in Harlem, New York, shows that, due largely to high levels of homicide, drug- and alcohol-related deaths, and cardiovascular disease, the men of this inner-city community were less likely to reach their 65th birthdays than were men in Bangladesh, a resource-poor nation. Blacks are more often the victims of crime; Page, Kitchin-Becker, Solovan, Golec, and Hebert (1992) found that Black city residents were four times as likely to die from homicide than were White city residents and that Blacks represented two thirds of all known murder suspects.

McBride (1993) postulates that the history of Black health care has occurred in three main phases: *engagement* (mid-1960s to mid-1970s), *submersion* (late 1970s to mid-1980s), and *crisis recognition* (late 1980s to present). During the engagement phase, a community health policy orientation prevailed as the national government targeted resources to health care programs for needy Black and other poor Americans. Neighborhood health centers were replaced by community health centers, which included a variety of ambulatory multidisciplinary services. In the submersion phase, health professionals and political leaders experienced a newfound inclusion in health policy, but the government reduced medical resources for the inner-city poor. By the time of the crisis recognition phase, leaders of the Black community were able to make the point that the specific disease problems and access needs of the Black poor were intertwined with the many general sources of stress in the Black community, namely, high unemployment, overburdened community services and public hospitals, drug abuse, fear and violence in the neighborhood, and the overburdening of single mothers.

URBANIZATION

Just as the urban and rural Blacks had different experiences during slavery, so too do the urban and rural Blacks of today. In the early part of the 20th century, many Blacks migrated to the northern cities from rural areas in the South. This migration increased after World War II. In 1910, 73% of all Black Americans lived in rural areas; by 1960, 73% lived in urban environments (Guillory, 1987). Similarly, in 2005 a natural disaster, the hurricane named "Katrina," resulted in a forced evacuation of thousands of Black residents of New Orleans, Louisiana, a city which had been two thirds Black. Many Black residents found themselves in places as far away as Alaska, struggling to fit into new communities.

Health care is more available to Blacks in the cities but still was inferior to that available to Whites. Cancer incidence is higher among Blacks living in urban areas as opposed to rural areas. Although the reasons for this difference are unclear, it appears that urban Blacks are exposed to more environmental hazards and other risk factors. Urban Blacks seek health care more frequently and practice more preventive measures, whereas rural Blacks, especially those who are poor, do not seek medical care until the problems are serious. Often, the Black client's response to the history of poor health care and inhumane treatment in the past is to stay away from health care facilities (Guillory, 1987).

TRADITIONAL HEALTH BELIEFS AND PRACTICES

Just as there is diversity among Blacks in terms of heritage, background, and culture, so too are there individual variations in beliefs. Congress and Lyons (1992) attribute these variations to the duration of stay in the United States, age, and economic status. New immigrants tend to share beliefs directly related to their cultural backgrounds, whereas those who have lived in America longer tend to possess a greater belief in the scientific medical model. Few studies differentiate among subgroups of Black Americans, although recent usage of the term *non-Hispanic Black* indicates that researchers are recognizing that difference.

Congress and Lyons (1992) also point out that socioeconomic status is a significant factor in diverse cultural beliefs on health and treatment. The economically deprived are more likely to retain the beliefs and values of their countries of origin than are their middle-class counterparts from the same culture. It is important that the practitioner understands the effect of socioeconomic factors on his or her clients' health beliefs and their ability to use health care services. Many health care

practitioners tend to treat the poor in a pater-
nalistic fashion.

American-born Blacks share many traditional beliefs with foreign-born Blacks, but the
reasons why they continue to use traditional
healing methods and self-treatment regimens
are somewhat different. Traditional health
was perhaps the only health system accessible
to everyone in Africa. Some 80% of Africans
used traditional healing methods, which have
been sustained over the years partly because
they are acceptable, available, and affordable
(Airhihenbuwa & Harrison, 1993). The use
of traditional remedies to prevent, treat, and
cure illness dates back to the dawn of time.
The reliance on informal folk healers by the
American Black population has roots in the
fact that their access to more formalized
American health care was denied, first by
slavery and then by segregation. Second- and
third-generation Blacks raised in northern
urban areas since civil rights legislation may be
less influenced by these southern Black beliefs
(Congress & Lyons, 1992).

Caribbean Blacks may be especially influenced by their native countries, particularly if
they are undocumented immigrants, because
of their recent arrival in the United States, with
limited access to the formal health care system.
The beliefs of some Haitians regarding the
causes, treatment, and prevention of illness
differ significantly from U.S. practices. Many
attribute diseases to supernatural causes.

Snow (1983), in her extensive research of
traditional health beliefs among Blacks, reports
that individuals who come into contact with
orthodox medicine contrary to their traditional
health beliefs often will react by ignoring the
prescribed treatment, misusing the treatment,
complaining about the quality of care they are
receiving, or seeking treatment from a folk
healer. Folk healers often become the only
health care providers for low-income Blacks.

Some folk healers are considered to be sorcerers with magical powers either to cause or

to cure illness. They acquire this special gift
when they are "born with the veil," the veil
being the amniotic sac that surrounds and pro-
tects the baby during pregnancy. It is believed
that a child born with the veil will have power
to see and hear ghosts and to foretell the future
(Rich, 1976).

Folk healers often offer themselves to the
Blacks in urban ghettos by advertising their
services (Snow, 1978). Although some provide
useful services, others use their acclaimed
power to manipulate and swindle money from
the gullible. Sometimes their treatment works;
when it fails, believers are convinced that it
failed because the victim was beyond hope.
Webb (1971) reports that folk medicine is
grounded on belief, not knowledge; thus, it
requires only occasional success for it to maintain its power and control over believers.

Good health is considered harmony with
nature; illness and bad health, on the other
hand, are viewed as disharmony with nature
that may be caused by a variety of factors
(Jacques, 1976). Therefore, Blacks tend to classify illness into two categories: natural and
unnatural (Congress & Lyons, 1992). This categorization affects the methods that traditional
health practitioners use to treat or cure an illness. The majority of practitioners and followers believe that illness can be cured if only
special care is taken to follow the prescribed
plan of the master (God). Thus, causes of illness generally fall into three domains: divine
punishment, environmental hazards, and
impaired social relationships (Snow, 1974).

Natural illnesses can result from stress;
cold; impurities in the water, air, or food;
improper eating habits or diet; weakness; or
lack of moderation in daily activities. They are
considered nature's calling card as punishment
for sin; natural illnesses can be visited on sin-
ners directly or on their children. Hence, disorders such as mental retardation, seizures, and
deformities demonstrate that innocent children
suffer the consequences of their parents'

misdeeds or sins. It is believed that illness is predictable and is according to God's plan (Gregg & Curry, 1994).

Rotter's (1966) external locus of control construct explains the traditional Black belief that evil influences may be blamed for illnesses or mishaps. This is matched by the belief that magical means are needed to bring about the desired behavior. Snow (1974) maintains that sympathetic magic is believed to link the body with forces in nature, whereas external forces are thrust on individuals who must learn to manipulate them for their own well-being. Natural illnesses can occur at any time; individuals are susceptible at various times, depending on factors such as drinking too much, staying out too late, eating the wrong types of foods, fighting with neighbors, failing to pay, failing to wear protective charms during certain periods of life, and lunar or planetary cycles (Flaskerud & Rush, 1989).

The cause of an illness is more important than its manifestation in the body. For example, stroke is variously believed to be caused by taking a bath during the menstrual period, eating red meat, or punishment by God. An illness such as this is considered to be a test of faith that might not be explained in the lifetime of those afflicted; they might only learn the reason when they reach heaven. Because the illness is regarded as God's punishment, it cannot be treated or cured by human medicine. Gregg and Curry (1994) quote the philosophy expressed thusly: "You got to die with something; one day you got to leave here . . . When it's time to go, it's time to go" (p. 522). The only prescription to follow to obtain a cure is to admit the sin, be sorry for having committed it, and vow to improve in the future.

Unnatural illnesses are caused by the evil influences of the devil, and many times they are induced by witchcraft or caused by demons or bad spirits (Jacques, 1976). Unnatural illness can be terrifying to individuals because they usually do not respond to self-treatment or remedies administered by friends, relatives, or practitioners (Snow, 1978). In such cases, the use of conjurers or voodoo doctors is needed to manipulate the spirits or demons (Guillory, 1987). As Snow (1978) explains, magic gives people the illusion that they have a measure of control over events.

Specific aids, such as soap, incense, lotions, aerosol sprays, candles, and oils have been sold in lower-class Black neighborhoods for the purposes of keeping away evil spirits, bringing luck at bingo games or the races, and keeping spouses at home. Webb (1971) reports that some of these seemingly primitive remedies are successful because of the psychotherapeutic quality of such medicine to heal or destroy, as in voodoo deaths.

Worry, according to traditional beliefs of many Blacks, is the main component in the course of unnatural illness. When worry is prolonged, the individual cannot sleep, eat, or perform everyday activities. According to folk healers, too much worry causes someone to "go crazy" (Snow, 1978).

The remedies for treating calamities caused by evil influences include food, medicine, antidotes, healing, and prayer proposed to God by a medium with unusual powers (Snow, 1974). Other cures and treatments include external aids such as magic and visible protection in the form of prayer, cards, charms, and asafetida bags (Snow, 1983). Guillory (1987) reports that other folk remedies include eating garlic for hypertension, drinking teas made from herbs for colds, applying tallow to the chest and covering it with a cloth for colds, pouring kerosene into cuts as a disinfectant, and wearing garlic around the neck to keep from catching disease. Use of vinegar, Epsom salts, Bengay, and copper wire or bracelets for arthritis; horehound tea or buttermilk for diabetes; and tea made of rabbit tobacco and pine top for asthma is common.

The health practitioner should acquaint himself or herself with the cultural beliefs and practices of the Black Americans the practitioner treats and should determine which may be beneficial or potentially hazardous. Replacing dangerous practices with alternatives is possible if done sensitively. For example, the use of marijuana teas for respiratory conditions can be discouraged by explaining the reason for concern and then recommending an alternate herb tea acceptable to the patient and family.

How does a health practitioner learn the specific cultural beliefs and practices of individuals? The best sources are patients themselves. Another source is office staff members who reside in the community or who are of the same ethnocultural background as the patients. Probing into nonbiomedical illness customs may initially be met with apprehension, but if the topic is approached in a sincere and nonjudgmental style, it is surprising how much information can be obtained from patients themselves.

Williams (1996) points out that Black American churches have been the most important social institutions in the Black community. Churches frequently offered the only respite from the continuous repression of slavery and afforded the only places where members could exercise leadership. Black churches today function as centers for health screening, promotion, and counseling. Clergies deal with marital and family problems, drug and alcohol problems, financial problems and HIV/AIDS, all of which directly affect the health of their parishioners.

Spirituality and religion are key sources of strength for Black Americans. Black women in recovery from substance abuse identified spirituality as a key component of the Black personality and culture; it had a significant correlation with positive mental health outcomes for these patients (Minority Nurse, 2004). The Black church is where many Blacks learn important aspects of socialization. It offers positive modeling by older members of the congregation, important lessons in managing life, and transmission of values. The high esteem with which

Blacks hold their churches suggests that religiosity may be an important coping resource for Black Americans (Minority Nurse, 2004).

The health practitioner needs to be sensitive to the religious beliefs of his or her patients and be alert for opportunities to learn of potential treatment of prevention. The health practitioner does not need to hold the same religious beliefs but needs to recognize their effect on patients' lives and prognoses. Open-ended questions such as "What does your belief in God mean to you now?" and "How does your belief in God's direction in your life make a difference?" may be used to elicit the patient's beliefs in relation to a health problem.

SOCIODEMOGRAPHIC CHARACTERISTICS OF BLACK AMERICAN POPULATIONS

Black Americans live in all regions of the country and are represented in every socioeconomic group. One third live in poverty, a rate three times that of the White population. More than half live in central cities, areas often typified by poverty, poor schools, crowded housing, and unemployment and exposed to a pervasive drug culture, periodic street violence, and high levels of stress (U.S. DHHS, 1990b).

Population Growth. The Black population in the United States increased an average of 1.4% per year between 1980 and 1992, compared with 0.6% for the White population and 0.9% for the total population. Fully 84% of the growth in the Black population was from natural increase or the excess of births over death. Immigration, which increased substantially since 1980 for the Black population, accounted for the remaining 16% (U.S. Bureau of the Census, 1992).

Sex and Age Distribution. Both Black and White populations have aged since 1980. The Black population had a median age of 28.2 years in

1992, compared with 24.8 years in 1980. The corresponding median ages for Whites were 34.3 and 30.8 years, respectively. Compared with the White population, a larger proportion of the Black population was below 18 years of age, and a smaller proportion was aged 65 years or more. Only 15% of the Black population was aged 55 or more, compared with 22% of the White population. Among both Blacks and Whites, there were more females in this older age group (U.S. Bureau of the Census, 1992).

Marital Status and Households. Since 1980, the number of Black households has risen at a faster pace (29%) than the number of White households (15%). This differential growth can be attributed in part to greater increases in Black householders than White householders who are separated, divorced, or never married as well as the higher growth rate of the adult Black population. Black families maintained by women with no spouses present rose from 40% to 46%, and those maintained by men with no spouses present from 4% to 7%; this increase in Black families maintained by women was slower than the sharp rise of the 1970s, during which the rate jumped from 28% to 40%. The proportion of children living with two parents has declined since 1980 for both Blacks and Whites; in 1992, 36% of Black children below 18 years of age lived with both parents, compared with 42% in 1980, a 16% decline. In the same time period, White families had a 6% decline, going from 83% in 1980 to 77% in 1992 (U.S. Bureau of the Census, 1992).

Economic Characteristics. In 1992, Blacks made up 11% of the total labor force in the United States and accounted for 21% of the unemployed. They comprised twice the proportion of the unemployed as they did of the employed, a condition unchanged from 1980 to 1992. The per capita income of the Black population in 1992 ($9,170) was about 60%

that of the White population ($15,510), with a similar ratio (0.59) in both 1979 and 1989. Black median family income in 1991 ($21,550) was 57% that for Whites ($37,780).

A person's earning power is positively correlated to educational attainment. A substantial difference is evident in comparing workers with high school diplomas to those with bachelor's degrees. Blacks with bachelor's degrees or more had earnings 66% higher than those possessing only high school diplomas. In 1992, Black males earned 80% of what White males earned. When education was taken into consideration, however, Black males with college educations attained earnings parity with comparably educated White males in several occupations but not in executive, administrative, or managerial positions (U.S. Bureau of the Census, 1992).

Educational Attainment. Black adults made notable progress in attaining high school diplomas during the 1980s. In 1980, 51% of Blacks aged 25 years or more had attained high school diplomas; by 1992, 68% had done so. The corresponding rates for Whites were 71% and 81%, respectively. In 1980, 8% of Black adults had bachelor's degrees or more; by 1992, this proportion had increased to 12% (U.S. Bureau of the Census, 1992).

Poverty Rates. The proportion of Black persons in poverty has fluctuated little since the mid-1960s. The 1991 poverty rate for Blacks (33%) was three times that for Whites (11%), compared with the corresponding 1979 rates of 31% and 9%, respectively. Approximately 4.5 million (46%) of all Black-related children below 18 years of age were in poor families, compared with 8.3 million (16%) of White-related children. Three times as many Black persons (29%) as White persons (9%) aged 55 years or more were poor in 1991. Approximately 34% of all poor Black persons lived in the South, whereas White persons aged 55 years or more who were below the poverty level were more likely to reside in the North or West region (62%) (U.S. Bureau of the Census, 1992).

The Homeless. Black Americans are disproportionately represented among the homeless.

In New York City, about 25% of the population is Black, but Black Americans comprise 73% of the city's homeless people (Institute of Medicine, 1988). Similarly, Blacks make up 7.5% of Ohio's population but 11% of the state's homeless (Braithwaite & Taylor, 1992).

HEALTH AND DISEASE PATTERNS AMONG BLACK AMERICANS

Differences in health status of Blacks and Whites have been documented in the United States as long as health data have been collected. These differences persist in spite of large increases in life expectancy and improvements in the health status of the general population (Thomas, 1992).

Diabetes. Diabetes was the sixth leading cause of death in the year 2000. More than 17 million American have diabetes, and more than 200,000 people die each year of related complications. Black Americans are twice as likely to have type 2 diabetes as Whites of similar age. Additionally, Blacks and American Indians have higher rates of diabetes-related complications such as kidney disease and amputations (Centers for Disease Control and Prevention, Office of Minority Health [CDC-OMH], 2005a).

The highest rates of type 2 diabetes are among Black women, especially those who are overweight. Black women with diabetes are nearly seven times more likely to die from ischemic heart disease than are Black women without diabetes (Will & Casper, 1996). Among Blacks 65 to 74 years of age, one in four has diabetes.

Physicians should take advantage of their patient's routine office visits to conduct food and kidney exams and recommend eye screening once a year. Health care professionals should teach patients to make proper diabetes management a part of their daily lives. Reducing high blood pressure among people with diabetes could prevent one third of diabetes-related eye, kidney, and nerve diseases. Approximately 60% of diabetes-related blindness could be avoided with good glucose control or by early detection and laser treatment. Half of all lower extremity amputations can be prevented by properly caring for the feet and reducing risk factors such as abnormally high blood sugar, cigarette smoking, and high blood pressure (CDC-OMH, 2005a).

Studies indicate that type 2 diabetes, usually thought of as adult-onset diabetes, is increasingly being diagnosed in children and adolescents, particularly Blacks, American Indians, and Hispanic/Latino Americans (CDC, 2005b).

Since the development of diabetes is associated with obesity, primary prevention should include lifestyle changes in diet (a plant-based, low-fat diet) and increasing regular physical activity (CDC-OMH, 2005a).

Gestational diabetes is a form of glucose intolerance diagnoses in some women during pregnancy. It occurs more frequently in Blacks, Hispanic/Latino Americans, and American Indians. It is also more common among obese women and women with a family history of diabetes.

Cardiovascular Disease and Stroke. Cardiovascular diseases are the leading cause of death for Black Americans, as they are for the entire U.S. population. Between 1972 and 1992, the coronary heart disease death rate declined about 49%, and stroke death rate declined about 58% (U.S. DHHS, 1996). Despite these gains, for Black Americans the death rates for coronary heart disease and stroke were 155 and 45 per 100,000, respectively, compared with 113 and 26 per 100,000 for the total population. End-stage renal disease actually increased from 13.9 to 14.4 per 100,000 for the total population and 34 to 43 per 100,000 for Blacks (U.S. DHHS, 1995).

Hypertension. Hypertension is defined as sustained blood pressure of 140/90 mmHg in individuals aged 18 years or more. Hypertension is a significant component of the relative risk for heart disease, stroke, and end-stage renal disease. The single most powerful determinant for hypertension is ethnicity. High blood pressure is much more common among Blacks of both genders than among the total population. Severe hypertension is present four times as often among Black men as among White men (U.S. DHHS, 1990b). Hypertension kills 15 times as many Black males as White males in the 15- to 40-year age group and 7 times as many Black females as White females in any age group.

Genetic and physiological differences alone are unlikely to explain race differences in blood pressure. There are cultural variations in the relationship between age and blood pressure levels (Williams, 1992). Cross-cultural studies indicate that blood pressure within racial groups varies by geographical or social context. Williams (1992) points out that blood pressure levels in West Africans are generally lower than those in U.S. and Caribbean Blacks. When Black populations in Africa move from their original communities to large urban centers, their blood pressure increases.

Livingstone and colleagues report that church affiliation was inversely related to blood pressure among Black residents sampled in Maryland (Livingstone, Levine, & Moore, 1991). A study of Blacks and Whites in North Carolina provides direct evidence that social support is related to blood pressure among Blacks (Williams, 1992). Health behaviors, such as excessive intake of alcohol, sodium, and dietary fat, as well as inadequate physical activity, are also determinants of high blood pressure (Williams, 1990b). Many of the preferred foods among Black Americans, including pork products, fried foods, and baked goods, are high in saturated fat, total fat, and sodium content (Magnus, 1991). Changing the types of foods, and the methods of food preparation, as well as an increased level of physical activity, could potentially control hypertension without medication.

Stroke. Stroke is the third leading cause of death for both Blacks and Whites; however, between 1992 and 2002, Black males and females aged 20 to 74 had higher age-adjusted rates of stroke per 100,000 individuals than their White counterparts (CDC, 2005c). Black men die from stroke at almost twice the rate of men in the total population, and Black men's risk of nonfatal stroke is also higher (U.S. DHHS, 1990b). The incidence of stroke among southern Blacks is nearly double that of southern Whites, especially among the rural poor. The so-called Stroke Belt, encompassing the southeastern United States, largely owes its higher stroke mortality to the Black population living there.

Stroke death rates increase dramatically with age, but the age distribution of stroke deaths differs among racial and ethnic groups. Among Whites, only 25% of the stroke deaths occur before age 75, while the percentage of deaths before age 75 ranges from 45% for Asians/Pacific Islanders to 37% for Blacks (CDC, 2005c). Blacks have the highest stroke death rates among U.S. racial and ethnic groups (2.1 times higher than for Hispanics and American Indians/Alaska Natives, 1.6 times higher than for Asians/Pacific Islanders, and 1.4 times higher than for Whites [CDC, 2005c]).

Sickle Cell Anemia. This genetic blood disease, in which abnormal hemoglobin molecules fail to release sufficient oxygen to the tissues, affects more than 80,000 Black Americans. The sickle cell trait, although more common in Blacks, appears to result not from race but rather from geographic origin (Williams, Lavizzo-Mourey, & Warren, 1994). Sickle cell anemia is an autosomal recessive genetic disorder; the presence of two defective genes (S) is needed for sickle cell anemia. If each parent carries one sickle hemoglobin gene (S) and one normal gene (A), each child has a 25% chance of inheriting two defective genes and having sickle cell anemia; a 25% chance of inheriting two normal genes and not having the disease; and a 50% chance of being an unaffected carrier (U.S. Department of Energy, Biological and Environmental Research, 2005).

Every year about 1 in 500 Black Americans are born with sickle cell anemia. It can result in severe pain, stroke, organ failure, and a life span shortened by 30 years. Children affected with sickle cell disease (SCD) are at increased risk for severe morbidity (e.g., severe hemolytic anemia, splenic dysfunction, pain crises, and bacterial infections) and mortality, especially during the first three years of life (CDC, 2000). Although there is no cure for sickle cell anemia, physicians can help patients through the painful crises with painkilling drugs and oral and intravenous fluids to reduce or prevent complications (CDC, 2000).

In 1972, Congress passed the National Sickle Cell Anemia Control Act, which included newborn screening programs for SCD to be done by the states; however, states did not widely adopt newborn screening for SCD until 1986. A randomized trial demonstrated that oral penicillin significantly reduced SCD-related morbidity and mortality in children; this study spurred states to adopt newborn screening (CDC, 2000). By the year 2000, most states were screening newborns for SCD.

Cancer. The incidence of cancer and the mortality rate for cancer have increased at an unprecedented rate in the Black community over the past 40 years. The overall cancer incidence rate for Blacks went up 27%, compared with an increase of 12% for Whites. The cancer mortality rate is 27% higher for Blacks than for other racial groups and has increased by nearly 50% over the past 40 years. This figure represents a 10% increase among Black

women and a 77% increase among Black men (American Cancer Society, 1989).

Cancer sites in which Blacks have significantly higher increases in incidence and mortality rates include the lung, colon-rectal, prostate, and esophagus (CDC, 2005a). The number one site of cancer among Black men is the digestive system, with an incidence rate of 123.5 per 100,000 (Liao, Tucker, Okoro, Giles, & Harris, 2004). Black patients are less likely than White patients to undergo surgical resection (68% to 78%), even after controlling for age, comorbidity, and location and extent of tumor. Black patients are also more likely to die (2-year mortality rate of 40% vs. 33.5% in White patients) (Cooper, Yuan, Landefeld, & Rimm, 1996). Cancer of the prostate is more prevalent in Black men, and Black women have cervical cancer more than twice as often as do White women. When adjusted for social class, the Black-White differential falls by 60% but does not disappear (Millon-Underwood & Sander, 1990).

Although breast cancer survival has improved during the past 30 years, disparities in survival between Black and White women have not declined but remain sizable. In a historical cohort study, 906 patients were followed for a median of 10 years; 64 (24.9%) Black women died of breast cancer compared with 115 (18.3%) White women (Tammemagi, Nerenz, Neslund-Dudas, Feldkamp, & Nathanson, 2005). The study's authors said diabetes and hypertension were the two main contributors to Black women's lower rate of survival and stated that "control of comorbidity may be an important way of improving the survival of Black breast cancer patients and reducing racial disparity" (Tammemagi et al., 2005, p. 1772).

Cigarette smoking prevalence is higher among Black Americans, although Whites tend to smoke more cigarettes per day than do Blacks. Prevalence of smoking among White (38.3%) and Hispanic high school students (34%) is higher than among non-Hispanic

Black students (19.2%). Smoking tends to be more popular among White teen girls; in 1999, 40% of White high school females were current smokers compared with 32% of Hispanic and 19% of African American high school females (U.S. DHHS, 2001). Despite the fact that Blacks smoke 20% fewer cigarettes, they have a higher incidence of lung cancer (Magnus, 1991).

Whether a person gets cancer depends on exposure to cancer-causing substances, a family history of cancer, and other factors. Whether a person dies from cancer depends on the availability of screening, the stage at which the cancer is detected, and the type of treatment received. The latter are telltale markers of the quality and accessibility of health care, all of which reveal that Black Americans come up short.

Infant Mortality. Black babies are twice as likely as White babies to die before their first birthday (U.S. DHHS, 1990b). Infant mortality is used to compare the health and well-being of populations across and within countries. The United States ranked 28th in the world in infant mortality in 1998, with that ranking due in large part to disparities that exist among various racial and ethnic groups within the country, especially Black Americans (CDC-OMH, 2005b). Infant mortality rates, according to several studies, are higher for mothers with less than 12 years of schooling and lower for those with 16 or more years of schooling (Kleinman, Fingerhut, & Prager, 1990).

Only 61% of Black women receive prenatal care in the first trimester of pregnancy (U.S. DHHS, 1990b). Each dollar spent on prenatal care saves between $3 and $20 in medical expenses in the infant's first year of life (Gorman, 1991). The leading causes of infant death include congenital abnormalities, preterm/ low birth weight, sudden infant death syndrome, problems related to complications of pregnancy, and respiratory distress syndrome (CDC-OMH, 2005b). Birth weight is one of the most important predictors of an infant's survival chances; infant mortality rates are much higher for infants born at low birth weight (LBW, less than 2,500 g) or very low birth weight (VBLW, less than 1,500 g) than for heavier babies (Centers for Disease Control and Prevention, National Center for Health Statistics, 2005). There have been small reductions in the Black-White disparities in LBW and VLBW in the 1990s but this has been due primarily to the increase in these two categories among White women, rather than a reduction among Black women.

Teenage Pregnancy. Adolescent pregnancy is a major concern because of its social and economic consequences as much as its health effects. There are higher risks of infant mortality and LBW, especially for very young pregnant girls. But even greater risks indirectly threaten the health of both mothers and babies because of the patterns of poverty and low educational attainment that often become entrenched as a result of early childbearing. Actual rates of childbirth among Black teenagers have dropped since the 1960s; in 1994, the teen birthrate dropped slightly among Blacks, while it stayed the same among Whites (Planned Parenthood of Connecticut, 2005). One in five Black teenagers becomes pregnant each year (Planned Parenthood of Connecticut, 2005).

Obesity. Black women have a higher prevalence of obesity than do either White women or Black men; the proportion of Black women who are obese is 80% higher than the proportion of Black men (U.S. DHHS, 2001). In every age group above 20 years, 20% to 50% of Black women are overweight compared with 10% to 20% of White women (Magnus, 1991). The rate of obesity increases with age; among Black women in the 45- to 67-year age group,

60% are more than 20% above their ideal weights (Bowen, Tomoyasu, & Cause, 1991).

Bowen et al. (1991) attribute the weight problem of the population to three major risk factors, which they term the "triple threat": gender, race, and poverty. They contend that race and class play powerful but often-neglected roles in women's weight and in the perceptions and attitudes that accompany it. Magnus (1991) reports that studies have found that obesity is six times more common among poor women than among affluent women.

Ethnic differences probably are not due to anthropometric differences, genetic differences or differences in caloric intake between Black and White females. Williams (1992) postulates that differences in physical exercise may be an important contributor to obesity in Black females. Black women are more likely to be poor, to be single parents, and to reside in poor neighborhoods, making it difficult to find the facilities and opportunities to obtain physical exercise.

Bowen et al. (1991) suggest that obesity among poor Blacks may be due to an external locus of control. Poor people often perceive that they cannot control their lives or the events in their environments. This sense of powerlessness reflects the limited choices imposed by economics; money creates choices, and without it you have none.

The dietary contribution to obesity also must be considered. Although "soul food" is thought to be for Blacks only, this is a misconception. It is difficult to say who eats more of the so-called soul food—urban Blacks, rural Blacks, or their White counterparts. Bloch (1983) points out that the scraps of food and leftovers from the slave masters' tables were the origin of much of the soul food. It was not the native food of the Black community; rather, it had its roots in slavery, not in Africa. The diet of West Africa consists of mainly cereals, green vegetables, peas, beans, cassava, yams, and sweet potatoes. Slave masters in the United States, however, fed their slaves as little as possible of the cheapest food available, which most often was pork and dried corn. Slaves contrived to make edible meals from pigs' trotters, knuckles, tails, ears, snouts, necks, stomachs (hog maw), and intestines (chitterlings). They marinated and smothered these and other scraps with seasonings such as Louisiana hot sauce and served them with turnips and collard greens, black-eyed peas, and hot cornbread, dishes that today are know as soul food (Mutumbi, 1981).

In recent years, pigs' feet and chitterlings have been replaced in many Black households by smoked sugared ham, pork chops, and bar-becued ribs. Diets have expanded to include larger quantities of highly refined convenience foods. Frying and frequent use of pork and pork fats continue to contribute a high content of saturated fats to the diet, a factor associated with increased risk of cancer and heart disease (Guillory, 1987).

Lactose Intolerance. The National Institute of Diabetes and Digestive and Kidney Diseases (NDDKD) estimates that between 30 and 50 million Americans are lactose intolerant. Within this population, 75% of Black Americans and 90% of Asian and Native Americans are lactose intolerant (NDDKD, 2003). Interestingly, the majority of Blacks do not classify themselves as lactose intolerant (National Medical Association [NMA], 2004).

Lactose intolerance is the inability to digest significant amounts of lactose, the predominant sugar of milk. It is the result of a shortage of the enzyme lactase, normally produced by the cells that line the small intestine. Symptoms of lactose intolerance include nausea, cramps, bloating, gas, and diarrhea, which being about 30 minutes to 2 hours after eating or drinking foods contacting lactose. Symptoms can be controlled by careful attention to the diet, avoiding milk and milk products. Such restrictions, however, may prove difficult during pregnancy and lactation, as women may avoid milk and deprive themselves and their babies of needed nutrients.

The vast majority of Black Americans (86%) get only half the daily recommended amount of calcium, and only half eat one or more servings of dairy products a day (NMA, 2003). While some Blacks are lactose intolerant, other reasons they give include cultural and taste preferences. Calcium and other components of dairy products provide significant health benefits. "Three to four daily servings of low fat dairy products could assist in reduction of obesity and hypertension, and a reduction of several diseases that affect Black American, including heart disease and cancer" states NMA President Dr. Winston Price (NMA, 2004, p. 1).

Mental Health. Although Blacks more often are exposed to social conditions considered to be important antecedents of psychiatric disorders, they do not have higher rates of mental illness than do Whites (Williams, 1990a). According to the National Institute of Mental Health's Epidemiological Catchment Area Program studies, 14% of Black males had psychiatric disorders compared with 13% of White males (Williams, 1992). In addition, 27% of Black males in institutions had psychiatric disorders, compared with 26% of White males. Recently, there has been an increase in suicide rates among Black males that peak in the 25- to 34-year age group, whereas White male rates peak for those aged 65 years or more.

Williams (1990a) comments, "The overall evidence on Black mental health clearly indicates that there are important resources and strengths in the Black community that [are] protecting the community from the onslaught of pathogenic stressors" (p. 26). One of these important and neglected resources is probably Black churches. Renewed research attention should be given to the possible health-promoting functions of religious involvement.

Historically, the major diagnostic category of mentally ill Blacks was tertiary syphilis. The infamous Tuskegee study[1] corroborates this.

Tobacco. Tobacco use varies within and among racial/ethnic groups. Among adults, American Indians/Alaska Natives have the highest prevalence of tobacco use, and Black Americans and Southeast Asian men have a high prevalence of smoking (CDC, 1998). Among adolescents, cigarette smoking prevalence increased in the 1990s among Blacks and Hispanics after several years of substantial decline. This is particularly striking among Black youth, who had the greatest decline of the four racial/ethnic groups during the 1970s and 1980s (CDC, 1998). Smoking tends, however, to be more popular among White teen girls; the CDC found in 2003 that 27% of White high school females were current smokers compared with 11% of Black high school females (NCHS, 2005, p. 35).

Tobacco companies deny targeting youth with their marketing, but the figures belie this. To maintain current market size and profits, tobacco manufacturers must recruit approximately 4,000 new smokers each day to replace the 1,100 smokers who die and the 3,000 smokers who quit (Aghi, Asma, Yeong, & Vaithinathan, 2001).

No single factor determines patterns of tobacco use among racial/ethnic minority groups. The patterns are the result of an interaction of factors such as socioeconomic status, acculturation, stress, targeted advertising, price of tobacco products, and the capacity of communities to establish effective tobacco control initiatives (CDC, 1998).

Chemical Dependency. Chemical dependence, particularly the use of illegal drugs such as crack, marijuana, and methamphetamine, is a major threat to the Black community. Although Blacks constitute less than 13% of the U.S. population, in 1999 they accounted for 23% of admissions to publicly funded substance abuse treatment facilities (Minority Nurse, 2004). The dramatic impact of substance abuse is evidenced by increased crime, wanton violence, mental disorders, family disruptions, and social problems in school and on the job.

The impact of cocaine and methamphetamine abuse results in an unprecedented number of children being abused, neglected, or mistreated. Many parents seeking the next crack fix abandon their young children in the streets and hospitals. They sell food stamps and their children's clothes for drug money. Some even sell their children as prostitutes. Since the use of drugs dulls the parents' appetites, they have no desire or inclination to have food in the home. The neglected children eat what they can find and spend hours—sometimes days—alone. Some 6-year-olds have been found taking care of their younger brothers and sisters.

Both crack and methamphetamine addicts, more than with other drugs, are found among young mothers with small children, few child-rearing skills, and no spouses to share the load. In the extended family, even some of the grandparents are addicted. The rates of infant mortality, sudden infant death syndrome, child abuse, and HIV infection are significantly linked to maternal substance abuse, most often caused by crack/cocaine and methamphetamine but also by other illegal drugs and alcohol.

Violence, Homicide, and Intentional Injuries. Violence is a public health issue with an impact on quality of life. Violent behavior is committed disproportionately by young males (late teens to early 30s) situated in the lowest levels of socioeconomic status. They are more likely to be not only the perpetrators but also the victims of violence. Although there is an over-representation of Blacks (44% of all homicide victims are Black) and other non-Whites in U.S. violence statistics, Page et al. (1992) point out

that socioeconomic status is a better predictor of violence than is racial status.

Many Black children and adolescents grow up in poverty, which increases their exposure to and experience with violence. Thus, they are at risk for using or experiencing violence in their interpersonal relationships. In some neighborhoods, close to 25% of elementary and high school students have seen someone killed (Bell & Jenkins, 1990).

Bell and Jenkins (1990) note that when women kill their partners, the women often have been physically abused and are acting in self-defense. Black men are more likely than White men to be killed by spouses who are acting in self-defense. Approximately 1 in 19 Black males becomes a murder victim. By comparison, 1 in 124 Black females, 1 in 186 White males, and 1 in 606 White females become murder victims (Page et al., 1992).

Violence prevention should include family and school interventions designed to teach children and parents problem-solving skills for conflict resolution, anger management, communication skills, and substance abuse prevention (Page et al., 1992).

HIV/AIDS. Acquired Immunodeficiency Syndrome (AIDS), a communicable disease first identified in 1981, is caused by the human immunodeficiency virus (HIV) primarily transmitted through semen, vaginal fluid, and blood or breast milk of infected people. Individuals are often infected and infectious without knowledge of their HIV status, although tests are readily available to determine that status. The virus may lie dormant within the body, producing no symptoms, for up to 10 years, yet HIV-infected persons can be transmitting the virus to other individuals, usually through sexual intercourse (oral, vaginal, or anal) or through needle sharing among intravenous drug users.

At present, no vaccine is available to prevent the infection. Early treatment may delay progression to AIDS. The use of antiviral agents may also prevent the transmission of the virus from mothers to their unborn infants. Treatment with a combination of drugs can clear HIV from the blood of infected individuals for up to 1 year.

In the United States, the HIV/AIDS epidemic is a health crisis for Black Americans. In 2002, it was among the top three causes of death for Black men aged 25 to 54 years. It was the number one cause of death for Black women aged 25 to 34 years (CDC, 2006). Blacks account for 50% of the estimated 38,730 new HIV/AIDS diagnoses in the United States in the long-term, confidential name-based HIV reporting areas (CDC, 2006).

The primary mode of HIV transmission among Black men is sexual contact with other men, followed by heterosexual contact and injection drug use. The primary mode of transmission among Black women is heterosexual contact, followed by drug use (CDC, 2006). Of the estimated 145 infants infected with HIV, 105 (73%) were Black. Of the 48 children in the United States younger than 13 years of age who had a new diagnosis of AIDS, 29 were Black Americans. The 178,233 Blacks living with AIDS in the United States in 2006 account for 43% of all people living with AIDS in the United States (CDC, 2006).

Barriers to preventive efforts include poverty, inadequate health care, mistrust, lack of knowledge, and low educational levels. The daily struggle for survival may make it difficult to consider preventive measures for a disease that can take a decade to develop. The risk is compounded for those who must resort to prostitution to ensure a ready supply of crack, methamphetamine, or other drugs. Individuals who drink heavily or take drugs are more likely to engage in unprotected sex (U.S. DHHS, 1990a).

In 2003, the CDC announced a new initiative, Advancing HIV Prevention (AHP), to further reduce the incidence of HIV. It includes four strategies: (1) making HIV testing a routine part of medical care, (2) implementing new models for diagnosing HIV infections outside medical settings, (3) preventing new infections by working with HIV-infected persons and their partners, and (4) further decreasing perinatal HIV transmission (CDC, 2006).

Black churches are beginning to be more accepting of person with AIDS, although the belief that HIV is a divine indictment for a sinful life persists. Black churches, as do many White fundamentalist churches, preach sexual fidelity and a drug-free life as the only solution to the HIV problem.

NATIONAL GOALS: IMPLICATIONS FOR HEALTH PROMOTION AND DISEASE PREVENTION AMONG BLACK AMERICANS

Since 1980, the United States has been setting national goals by decades, the most recent being published in *Healthy People 2010* (U.S. DHHS, 2000). In 1990, the federal government established the Office of Minority Health to coordinate department efforts to reduce excess mortality and morbidity among Blacks and other minorities. This office publishes regular updates on progress toward the national goals. In addition, it established a nationwide hotline (800-444-6472) to sources of information, maintaining a database of organizations and volunteers to assist in local minority health programs.

Healthy People 2010 have two major goals, one of which is to eliminate health disparities among segments of the population, including differences that occur by gender, race or ethnicity, education or income, disability, geographic location, or sexual orientation (U.S. DHHS, 2000). The goal is to recognize that medical care alone will not eliminate the devastating impact of chronic disease, the rate of infant mortality, and the burden of homicide and violence. It lists 28 objectives for the nation, 25 of which specifically target Black Americans. Most of the objectives are based on the assumption that individuals can control their own destinies in significant ways. This assumption means that the Black community as a whole might not get to the promised land of *Healthy People 2010* because there exists a correlation between poor health and socioeconomic status.

Progress toward achieving the objectives of *Healthy People 2010* is being monitored by various studies during the 2000 to 2010 decade. In 2002, Blacks trailed Whites in at least four health indicators, including percentages of (1) persons above 65 years of age with health insurance (81% to 87% respectively), (2) adults above 65 years vaccinated against influenza (50% vs. 69%) and pneumococcal disease (37% vs. 60%), (3) women receiving prenatal care in the first trimester (75% vs. 89%), and (4) persons above 18 years who participated in regular moderate physical activity (25% vs. 35%) (CDC, 2005a). Regular update reports are available on the home page of the *Healthy People 2010* Web site.

Availability and Accessibility of Health Care and Resources

Individuals with a usual source of health care are more likely than those without a usual source of care to receive a variety of preventive health care services; 15% of the U.S. population lacks a usual source of health care. Young children and adults above 65 years of age are most likely to have a usual source of health care; adults aged 18 to 64 are least likely. Ninety-five percent of the children below age 17, however, now have a specific source of care due to the implementation of the Child Health Insurance Program in 1997. See Web site for State Children's Health Insurance Program, www.hhs.gov/every americaninsured?schip/

Access to health services, whether preventive, primary, or tertiary care, often depends on whether a person has health insurance. Eighty one percent of the Black population has health insurance, compared with 90% of the White population and 65% of the Hispanic population (NCHS, 2005, p. 29).

Comprehensive primary care services can reduce the severity of certain illnesses. Hospital admission rates for "ambulatory care-sensitive" conditions serves as an indicator of limited access to primary care or low-quality primary care. Substantial disparities in hospital admission rates for pediatric asthma and uncontrolled diabetes exist. Poor Black children are also at the highest risk for asthma-related morbidity (NCHS, 2005,p. 45).

Van Ryn, Burgess, Malat, and Griffin (2006) found that physicians recommend coronary artery bypass surgery (CABG) for Black men less often than they do for White men (21% compared with 40%, respectively); there was no difference in recommendations for Black women versus White women. The authors found that physicians apparently were making such decisions based on educational level and the desire for an active lifestyle, although an earlier study indicated that physicians consistently underestimated Black patients' education levels (Van Ryn & Burke 2000).

Of those undergoing dialysis for kidney disease, Whites are 33% more likely to get kidney transplants. Blacks who are hospitalized for pneumonia received less-intensive treatment than do Whites (Gorman, 1991).

Correcting the inequities in health care alone will not solve the health problems of Black Americans. Even those studies that find a positive impact for physician services note that the effect of medical care is small when compared with that of nonmedical variables (Williams & Collins, 1995). A reduction in cigarette smoking would do more to improve health than would an increase in medical expenditures. Goldman and Cook (1984) analyzed the decline in ischemic heart disease between 1968 and 1976. They found that changes in lifestyle saved more lives than did all medical interventions combined. Louis Sullivan, former Secretary of Health and Human Services, stated, "Stopping smoking, losing weight, and cutting down on alcohol consumption could eliminate up to 45% of deaths from cardiovascular disease, 23% of the deaths from cancer, and more than 50% of the disabling complications of diabetes" (quoted in Gorman, 1991, p. 52).

Caveats When Generalizing About Health and Black Americans

Stereotypes may be commonplace and convenient for conservation of thought, but they have no place in a health worker's practice. As this chapter shows, Black Americans have been shaped by 400 years of history, the forces of slavery, migration, and socioeconomic status. There are as great a number of differences within the Black American population group as among it and other population groups in the United States. Health professionals should remember the following caveats when working with individuals who consider themselves Black Americans:

- Not all Black Americans share the same history or culture; many are immigrants who may or may not identify with the term *African American.*
- Health beliefs and practices will vary between urban and rural Blacks and between countries of origin.
- Socioeconomic status has a greater impact on health status than does ethnicity.
- Lifestyle risk factors are more important predictors of disease than is ethnicity (e.g., intravenous drug use and HIV infection).
- Health promotion and health care programs need to be tailored to the identified needs of individuals whenever possible; health beliefs

and concerns can be elicited by asking individuals in a manner that demonstrates genuine care and concern.

CHAPTER SUMMARY

Black Americans, through their 400-year history in the United States, have a legacy that results in their suffering a disproportionate rate of disease, less access to and use of curative and preventive health care, and a mistrust of the health care system. Many continue to rely on self-care and ethnomedicine and on the extended family primarily or in parallel with scientific medical care.

Health beliefs and practices vary according to the degree of acculturation, country of origin, education level, socioeconomic level, and time of acquiring freedom historically. Recent immigrants are at an increased risk for chronic disease and injury, particularly those who lack fluency in English and are not conversant with the U.S. health care system. The health care practitioner should avail himself or herself of the information available from the literature and directly from patients and community members with whom the practitioner works in planning appropriate programs of health care and health promotion. The health practitioner should use community resources such as Black churches that are respected as an integral part of Black communities. The practitioner also should respond positively to the challenge to add to the body of knowledge about differences among subgroups by reporting, through case studies and other qualitative methods, the results of his or her observations and interactions with these members of American society.

Chapter 14, which follows, discusses several specific elements of the health promotion and disease prevention (HPDP) planning process unique to the Black American experience. These elements include planning frameworks, selected health issues, and cultural concerns. The authors also discuss, within a program planning context, the importance of in-depth target group needs assessment, appropriate selection of program design, and particular aspects of program implementation and evaluation. They offer tips based on their extensive experiences and make suggestions for more effective HPDP program design within the Black American populations.

DISCUSSION QUESTIONS AND ACTIVITIES

1. Explain how the traditional health beliefs of many Blacks (e.g., illness induced by malevolent spirits or demons, strongly adhered to folk remedies and potions) might conflict with that of their medical practitioner in terms of diagnosis, treatment, and follow-up?

2. How might their health belief system affect their health-seeking behaviors relevant to their participation in community health promotion and disease prevention activities?

3. Many Blacks feel disconnected from the traditional health care system. They feel disrespected and unfairly treated. How could you identify such feelings toward health care programs and caregivers? How would you as a health promotion planner obtain important needs assessment information from members of the Black community? What does it mean to be nonjudgmental and sensitive in these situations?

4. Black Americans have their own cultural traits and health profiles that could present challenges to practitioners who are unknowledgeable and unprepared to deal with these differences. List several ways you could assist others in your class or workplace to understand the importance of the Black patient's cultural beliefs and practices as these can improve the quality of health delivery.

5. Identify at least three stereotypes you believe others in your class or workplace share about the level of knowledge and attitudes toward health and wellness held by Black Americans. Create a case study for each specific stereotype identified and present this information for discussion at your next class or staff meeting.

6. Organize a survey team from members of your class. Visit, observe, and interview health providers in at least three health care facilities in your community where large numbers of Black Americans seek health care. As an exercise, (a) determine if a formal cultural competency training component is provided to all staff at those sites, (b) describe the range of cultural competency activities provided, and (c) if they are not provided, have your team prepare an outline for developing a cultural competency workshop at each site. Present your findings and recommendations at your next class.

NOTE

1. Jones's (1981) publication, *Bad Blood: The Tuskegee Syphilis Experiment—A Tragedy of Race and Medicine*, records the 40-year government-sponsored study of rural Black men with syphilis to monitor the venereal disease's long-term effects. Although 399 men were examined, they were never treated. Even after the discovery of penicillin during the 1940s, their symptoms were left unchecked. Although they received free physical examinations, free rides to and from the clinics, and burial stipends, they were deceived into thinking that they were receiving treatment. Nearly 100 of the men died from direct complications of the disease. The study was discontinued after public outcry in 1972.

REFERENCES

Adams, D. L. (1995). Cultural diversity and institutional inequity. In D. L. Adams (Ed.), *Health issues for women of color* (pp. 5–26). Thousand Oaks, CA: Sage.

Aday, L. A. (1993). *At risk in America: The health and health care needs of vulnerable populations in the United States.* San Francisco: Jossey-Bass.

Aghi, M., Asma, S., Yeong, C. C., & Vaithinathan, R. (2001). Initiation and maintenance of tobacco use. In J. M. Samet & S.-Y. Yoon (Eds.), *Women and the tobacco epidemic* (pp. 49–68). Geneva, Switzerland: World Health Organization. Retrieved September 16, 2007, from www.who.int/tobacco/media/en/Women Monograph.pdf

Airhihenbuwa, C. O., & Harrison, I. E. (1993). Traditional medicine in Africa: Past, present and future. In P. Conrad & E. Gallagher (Eds.), *Healing and health care in developing countries* (pp. 122–134). Philadelphia: Temple University Press.

American Cancer Society. (1989). *Cancer facts and figures.* New York: Author.

Bell, C., & Jenkins, E. (1990). Preventing black homicide. In J. Dewart (Ed.), *The state of Black America, 1990* (pp. 143–155). New York: National Urban League.

Bloch, B. (1983). Nursing care of black patients. In M.S. Orgue, B. Bloch, & L.S. Monrroy (Eds.), *Ethnic nursing care: A multi-cultural approach* (pp. 81–113). St. Louis, MO: C. V. Mosby.

Bowen, D. J., Tomoyasu, N., & Cause, A. M. (1991). The triple threat: A discussion of gender, class and race differences in weight. *Women & Health, 17,* 123–143.

Braithwaite, R. L., & Taylor, S. E. (Eds.). (1992). *Health issues in the black community.* San Francisco: Jossey-Bass.

Cabral, H., Fried, L. E., Levenson, S., Amaro, H., & Zuckerman, B. (1990). Foreign-born and U.S. born black women: Differences in health behaviors and birth outcomes. *American Journal of Public Health, 80,* 70–72.

Caplan, L. R. (1991). Cardiovascular disease and stroke in African-American and other racial minorities in the United States: Strokes in African-Americans. *American Health Association Scientific Statement: Special Report, 83,* 1469–1470.

Centers for Disease Control and Prevention. (1998). Tobacco use among U.S. racial/ethnic minority groups, African Americans, American Indians and Alaska Natives, Asian Americans and Pacific Islanders, Hispanics: A report of the Surgeon General (Executive Summary). *MMWR Recommendations and Reports, 47*(RR-18), 1–16.

Centers for Disease Control and Prevention. (2000). Update: Newborn screening for sickle cell disease: California, Illinois, and New York, 1998. *MMWR Weekly, 49*(32), 729–731.

Centers for Disease Control and Prevention. (2004). Reach 2010 surveillance for health status in minority communities: United States, 2001–2002. *MMWR Weekly Report, 53* (SS-6), 1–36.

Centers for Disease Control and Prevention. (2005a). Health disparities experienced by Black or African-Americans: United States. *MMWR Weekly, 54*(1), 1–3.

Centers for Disease Control and Prevention. (2005b). *National diabetes fact sheet United States, 2005.* Atlanta, GA: Author. Retrieved February 10, 2006, from www.cdc.gov/diabetes.

Centers for Disease Control and Prevention. (2005c). National Center for Chronic Disease Prevention and Health Promotion. *Cardiovascular health: Racial and ethnic disparities in stroke* (pp. 1–9). Atlanta, GA: Author. Retrieved February 10, 2006, from www.cdc.gov/cvh/maps/strokeeat las/03-section.htm

Centers for Disease Control and Prevention. (2006, February). HIV/AIDS among African-Americans. *CDC HIV/AIDS Fact Sheet,* 1–5.

Centers for Disease Control and Prevention, National Center for Health Statistics. (2005, January 24). Explaining the 2001–02 infant mortality increase: Data from the linked birth/infant death data set. *National Vital Statistics Reports, 53*(12), 1–22.

Centers for Disease Control and Prevention, Office of Minority Health. (2005a). *Eliminate disparities in diabetes.* Retrieved February 10, 2006, from www.cdc.gov/omhd/AMH/factsheets/ diabetes.htm

Centers for Disease Control and Prevention, Office of Minority Health. (2005b). *Eliminate disparities in infant mortality.* Retrieved February 10, 2006, from www.cdc.gov/omhd/AMH/factsheets/ infant.htm

Congress, E. P., & Lyons, B. P. (1992). Cultural differences in health beliefs: Implications for social work practice in health care settings. *Social Work in Health Care, 17*(3), 81–96.

Cooper, G. S., Yuan, Z., Landefeld, C. S., & Rimm, A. A. (1996). Surgery for colorectal cancer: Race-related differences in rates and survival among Medicare beneficiaries. *American Journal of Public Health, 86*, 582–586.

Coughlin, E. K. (1987, October 28). Scholars work to refine Africa-centered view of the life and history of black Americans. *Chronicle of Higher Education*, p. 32.

Flaskerud, J. H., & Rush, C. E. (1989). AIDS and traditional health beliefs and practices of black women. *Nursing Research, 38*, 210–215.

Goldman, L., & Cook, E. E. (1984). The decline in ischemic heart disease: An analysis of the comparative effects of medical interventions and changes in lifestyles. *Annals of Internal Medicine, 101*, 821–836.

Gorman, C. (1991, September 16). Why blacks die young. *Time*, p. 52.

Gregg, J., & Curry, R. H. (1994). Explanatory models for cancer among African-American women at two Atlanta neighborhood health centers: The implications for a cancer screening program. *Social Science Medicine, 39*, 519–526.

Guillory, J. (1987). Ethnic perspectives of cancer nursing: The black American. *Oncology Nursing Forum, 14*(3), 66–69.

Heckler, M. M. (1985). *Report of the Secretary's Task Force on Black and Minority Health: Vol. 1. Executive summary*. Washington, DC: Government Printing Office.

Institute of Medicine. (1988). *Homelessness, health and human needs*. Washington, DC: National Academy Press.

Jacques, G. (1976). Cultural health traditions: A black perspective. In M. E. Blanck & P. P. Paxton (Eds.), *Providing safe nursing care for ethnic people of color*. Norwalk, CT: Appleton-Century-Crofts.

Jones, J. H. (1981). *Bad blood: The Tuskegee syphilis experiment—a tragedy of race and medicine*. New York: Free Press.

Kleinman, J. C., Fingerhut, L. A., & Prager, K. K. (1990). Differences in infant mortality by race, nativity status, and other maternal characteristics. *American Journal of Disease of Children, 145*, 194–199.

Liao, Y., Tucker, P., Okoro, C. A., Giles, W. H., & Harris, V. B. (2004, August 27). *Reach 2010 surveillance for health status in minority communities—United States, 2001-2002* (Vol. 53/No. SS-6). Washington, DC: U.S. Department of Health and Human Services.

Livingstone, L. R., Levine, D. M., & Moore, R. D. (1991). Black-white differences in blood pressure: The role of social factors. *Ethnicity & Disease, 2*, 125–141.

Magnus, M. D. (1991). Cardiovascular health among African-Americans: A review of the health status, risk reduction and intervention strategies. *American Journal of Health Promotion, 5*, 282–290.

McBride, D. (1993). Black America: From community health care to crisis medicine. *Journal of Health Politics, Policy and Law, 18*, 319–334.

McCord, C., & Freeman, H. P. (1990). Excess mortality in Harlem. *New England Journal of Medicine, 322*, 173–177.

Million-Underwood, S., & Sander, E. (1990). Factors contributing to health promotion behaviors among African American men. *Nursing Oncology Forum, 17*, 707–712.

Minority Nurse. (2004, July 21). African Americans, Substance Abuse and Spirituality. *HCR ManorCare: The career and educational resource for the minority nursing profession Quarterly Newsletter*, pp. 1–6. Retrieved February 22, 2006, from www.minoritynurse.com

Mutumbi, D. (1981, July). African homeland. *East West Journal*, pp. 38–41.

National Center for Health Statistics. 2005. *Health, United States, 2005 with chartbook on trends in the health of Americans*. Hyattsville, MD: U.S. Government Printing Office.

National Institute of Diabetes and Digestive and Kidney Diseases. (2003, March). *Lactose intolerance* (NIH Publication No. 03-2751, pp. 1–9). Bethesda, MD: National Digestive Diseases Information Clearinghouse.

National Medical Association. (2004). *National Medical Association Report encourages 3–4 servings of dairy a day for all African*

Americans to reduce chronic disease risk [Press release]. pp. 1–2. Retrieved February 22, 2006, from www.nmanet.org/pr_120704.htm

Page, R. M., Kitchin-Becker, S., Solovan, D., Golec, T. L., & Hebert, D. L. (1992). Interpersonal violence: A priority issue for health education. *Journal of Health Education, 23,* 286–292.

Planned Parenthood of Connecticut, Inc. (2005). *Teen pregnancy.* © 2005, SIECUS, pp. 1–3. Retrieved February 10, 2006, from www.ppct .org/facts/research/teenpregnancy.shtml

Rich, C. (1976). Born with the veil: Black folklore in Louisiana. *Journal of American Folklore, 89,* 328–335.

Rotter, J. B. (1966). Generalized expectancies for internal versus external control of reinforcement. *Psychological Monographs, 80*(Whole No. 609).

Snow, L. E. (1974). Folk medical beliefs and their implications for care of patients. *Annals of Internal Medicine, 81,* 82–96.

Snow, L. E. (1978). Sorcerers, saints and charlatans: Black folk healers in urban America. *Culture, Medicine and Psychiatry, 2,* 69–106.

Snow, L. E. (1983). Traditional health beliefs and practices among lower class black Americans. *Western Journal of Medicine, 139,* 820–828.

Sowell, T. (1981). *Ethnic America: A history.* New York: HarperCollins.

Sowell, T. (1994). *Race and culture: A world view.* New York: HarperCollins.

Tammemagi, C. M., Nerenz, D., Neslund-Dudas, C., Feldkamp, C., & Nathanson, D. (2005). Comorbidity and survival disparities among black and white patients with breast cancer. *Journal of the American Medical Association, 294*(14), 1765–1772.

Thomas, S. B. (1992). Health status of the black community in the 21st century: A futuristic perspective for health education. *Journal of Health Education, 2,* 7–13.

U.S. Bureau of the Census. (1992). *The black population in the United States: March 1992.* Washington, DC: Government Printing Office.

U.S. Department of Energy, Biological and Environmental Research. (2005, May 5). Genetic disease profile: Sickle cell anemia. *Gene gateway: Exploring genes and genetic disorders. Human Genome Project Information.* Retrieved February 15, 2006, from www.ornl .gov/sci/techresources/Human_Genome

U.S. Department of Health and Human Services. (1990a). *Closing the gap: AIDS/HIV infection and minorities.* Washington, DC: Government Printing Office.

U.S. Department of Health and Human Services. (1990b). *Healthy People 2000.* Washington, DC: Government Printing Office.

U.S. Department of Health and Human Services. (1995). *Progress report for heart disease and stroke.* Washington, DC: Government Printing Office.

U.S. Department of Health and Human Services. (1996, May 3). Healthy people 2000 progress report for heart disease and stroke. *Morbidity and Mortality Weekly Report, 17.*

U.S. Department of Health and Human Services. 2000. *Healthy people 2010: With understanding and improving health and objectives for improving health.* (2nd ed.). 2 vol. Washington, DC: U.S. Goverment Printing Office.

Van Ryn, M., Burgess, D., Malat, J., & Griffin, J. (2006). Physicians' perceptions of patients' social and behavioral characteristics and race disparities in treatment recommendations for men with coronary artery disease. *American Journal of Public Health, 96*(2), 351–357.

Van Ryn, M., & Burke, J. (2000). The effect of patient race and socio-economic status on physicians' perceptions of patients. *Social Science Medicine, 50*(6), 813–828.

Webb, J. Y. (1971). Louisiana voodoo and superstitions related to health. *HSMHA Health Reports, 86,* 291–301.

Will, J. C., & Casper, M. (1996). The contribution of diabetes to early deaths from ischemic heart disease: U.S. gender and racial comparisons. *American Journal of Public Health, 86,* 576–579.

Williams, D. R. (1990a). Social structure and the health status of black males. *Challenge: A Journal of Research on Black Men, 1,* 25–46.

Williams, D. R. (1990b). Socioeconomic differentials in health: A review and redirection. *Social Psychological Quarterly, 53,* 81–89.

Williams, D. R. (1992). Black-white differences in blood pressure: The role of social factors. *Ethnicity & Disease, 2,* 125–141.

Williams, D. R. (1996). The health of the African American population. In S. Petrosa & R. Rhomboid (Eds.), *Origins and destinies: Immigration, race and ethnicity in America.* Belmont, CA: Wadsworth.

Williams, D. R., & Collins, C. (1995). U.S. socioeconomic and racial differences in health: Patterns and explanations. *Annual Review of Sociology, 21,* 349–386.

Williams, D. R., Lavizzo-Mourey, R., & Warren, R. C. (1994). The concept of race and health status in America. *Public Health Reports, 109,* 28–41.

14

Health Promotion and Disease Prevention Planning in African American Communities

MARY ASHLEY

MAYA HARRIS

Chapter Objectives

On completion of this chapter the health promotion student and practitioner will be able to

- Formulate an operational framework for health promotion and education programs for increasing access and services for members of African American communities

- Identify, emphasize, and differentiate between key aspects of program planning, program development, implementation, and evaluation of health promotion and education efforts

- Describe applications of health promotion planning and implementation intended for African American populations

- Identify and propose recommendations to assist with health promotion efforts for African Americans

- Identify and define the levels of change sought by programs at the health promotion and health education levels for increasing access and services to the African American communities

As health providers who have worked extensively in black communities, we aim to provide critical insight into health promotion and planning, which will assist professionals and nonprofessionals alike in accessing and serving African American communities. Not only do we draw on the literature, but this chapter is also informed by our own experiences and in-depth interviews of four health promoters who have worked in African American and other multicultural communities. The experiences and lessons learned of those in the field, along with literature, provide pertinent information about this important work of health promotion for African Americans. This chapter has been revised and updated from the first edition, especially with regard to expounding on the topics previously addressed and to introduce new concepts.

Health providers—in developing health promotion and disease prevention (HPDP) programs for African Americans—must research, understand, and appreciate the history and culture of black people in the United States. Relevant HPDP program planning must consider the history of institutionalized racism and discrimination directed toward African Americans with respect to health care. It is also essential that health providers understand the historic social, political, and economic conditions that affect access to health care among black people in the United States.

The early 20th century found most blacks living in the southern United States without any formalized system of health care. Many lived in substandard housing with poor sanitary conditions and meager nutritional resources. A number of blacks who migrated to the urban North found that their living conditions were somewhat better than in the South. However, poverty, substandard housing, inadequate education, and insufficient health care continued to be problematic (Iglehart & Becerra, 2000; T. S. Quinn, 1996). These multiple factors affected the health status of black Americans, and the

vestige of these conditions is still apparent in many black communities today.

In the 21st century, African Americans continue to lag behind many other U.S. population groups on virtually all health status indicators. The leading health disparities among blacks in America include diabetes, HIV/AIDS, cancer, heart disease, and stroke (Satcher & Pamies, 2006; U.S. Department of Health and Human Services, Office of Minority Health, n.d.). Other important public health issues that affect family and community health are homicide, unintentional injuries, infant mortality, and substance abuse (T. S. Quinn, 1996). A number of complex factors contribute to these poor health outcomes. Low-income African American communities are particularly affected by the lack of adequate health insurance and quality health care, high rates of unemployment, educational disparities, toxic and unsanitary environmental conditions, substandard housing, and limited access to nutritional foods.

Institutional and individual racism continues to be a major contributor to disparate health outcomes between black and white Americans. In addition, structural inequities and institutional racism in the health care system and health education infrastructures are ongoing issues (Byrd, 1990; Byrd & Clayton, 1993; Hirsch, 1991). Since early in the 20th century, many scholars agree that factors related to lifestyle, reduced access to health care resources, lack of health insurance, limited knowledge of HPDP behaviors and practices, increased exposure to environmental hazards and toxins, and certain genetic variables have also been vital contributors to disparate health issues among African Americans (DuBois, 1903; Haynes, 1975). Many of these problems are preventable.

Governmental systems have perpetuated behaviors that have compounded these issues and may contribute to mistrust and skepticism among African Americans, particularly regarding the use of health and social services. One famous example is the 40-year Tuskegee experiment, in which the U.S. government withheld medical treatment from nearly 400 black men infected with syphilis from 1932 to 1972 (Centers for Disease Control and Prevention [CDC], 2005; Office of Research Integrity, n.d.). While the governmental study was used for the purpose of advancing medical research, the experiment was a clear indication of the U.S. government's lack of value for the life of black Americans. In 2005, Hurricane Katrina devastated parts of New Orleans, Louisiana, and surrounding areas in Mississippi. The nation witnessed a 4-day public outcry for food, medical attention, public safety, and rescue. These issues create added barriers since African Americans may not seek services from systems that they do not feel a sense of trust in.

This chapter provides specific strategies to access and engage African American populations in HPDP planning given their complex history and culture in the United States. African Americans are not a homogeneous group. This chapter provides insight about HPDP planning with consideration of the great diversity within populations in general and the variation in attitudes, behaviors, and values regarding health and HPDP (Herring & Montgomery, 1996). However, when planning HPDP programs intended for black populations, the same tenets of program planning, program development, implementation, and evaluation apply. An approach such as the six stages of intervention mapping described by Bartholomew, Parcel, Kok, & Gottlieb (2006) can be used to systematically design and implement health promotion programs.

PROGRAM PLANNING

Planning of HPDP programs in African American communities is an important stage in the health promotion process. Thorough and efficient planning enables the health promoter to clearly articulate and achieve the project objectives, priorities, and desired outcomes for the intended population (Bartholomew et al., 2006; C. C. Clark, 2002; see also Chapter 7, this volume). Since, access to the African American community is key to program planning, the focus of this section is on relationship development, creation of a skilled planning team, and considerations when conducting a community asset and needs assessment.

Relationship Development and Community Access

Access to a designated community will depend on developing copious relationships with its members. Establishing viable connections will allow the health promoter to

- obtain an informal assessment of perceived community strengths, problems, and needs (these interactions will inform the needs assessment to follow);
- leverage preexisting relationships with community members who will be served through the health promotion program;
- identify people and organizations with whom to collaborate, expand available resources, and create opportunities for sustainability; and
- understand how the health promoter's observations intersect with those of members of the community.

Forging relationships and involving community members from the beginning and throughout the entire life of the program constitute a critical ingredient that can contribute to the overall success of the program. This includes developing relationships with both formal and informal leaders who are trusted members of the community. Some of the community leaders may not have formal titles or positions (in-depth interview, personal communication, April 13, 2006). For example, in one urban community, we found that the leadership was divided among three powerful black women. Failure to involve even one of them was tantamount to disaster. These women held informal positions, were highly respected, and had influence within the community. It is therefore important to know the community members who can effect change and cultivate working relationships with those change-agents (in-depth interview, personal communication, April 13, 2006).

A health promoter can conduct several activities to research and document information on influential leaders and organizations. Initial activities include Internet searches and a review of local media outlets (i.e., community newspapers, city and county governments, the local health department). While doing these searches, it is best to conduct the following ongoing activities:

- Compile a list of local community leaders and organizations.
- Specify the person/organization's role in the community.
- Highlight efforts that the person/organization has championed.
- Indicate potential linkages to the HPDP program being developed.
- Document contact information—that is, Web sites, mailing/e-mail addresses, phone numbers.

The list should include religious and civic leaders, local citizens groups, and community coalitions with a health focus. Nonhealth organizations are useful resources for identifying influential people (e.g., 100 Black Men, 100 Black Women, the Links, Eastern Star, the Masons, Urban Leagues). Historically, black colleges and universities within the community are helpful resources, along with other universities in the area. Both types of institutions often have black student groups and multicultural programs that address health and social services in local communities (e.g., black sororities and fraternities, black student unions, black student health organizations).

In addition to conducting research, visibility of the health promoter in the community is also important for access. The promoter may attend community gatherings such as health fairs, festivals, and church or other religious services. The promoter may engage in similar activities, where he or she may assist in championing the cause of the program or in developing relationships. For example, we interviewed a health promoter whose culture was different from the community she served. She attended community meetings when she began work at a health organization. The events lasted several hours and often ended at night. Her attendance remained consistent. Eventually, community members perceived her as genuine and sincere. The health promoter learned that she had to be consistent, patient, and committed before she was accepted into the community (in-depth interview, personal communication, February 11, 2006).

Access to African Americans in rural settings might be a bit more difficult. However, local ministers and other religious leaders have been successfully enlisted for health program support in rural areas, and the use of lay health advisers has been found to be very effective in delivering HPDP programs and services (Eng & Hatch, 1991). Identifying issues relevant to the organization might create increased access. The provider must realize that the organization might have different purposes and agendas, which may or may not include health. Assistance in achieving the goals for that organization might lead to cooperation in and assistance with health promotion efforts. Church size and the educational level of the minister have been identified as the strongest predictors of participation, with larger churches and ministers with higher education levels being more likely to participate in HPDP programs (S. C. Quinn, Billingsley, & Caldwell, 1994). The health promoter may have to be creative to access this population and leverage relationships with informal leaders including a church mother's board, a deacons committee, and assistant pastors (in-depth interview, personal communication, April 13, 2006).

Planning Team

Once the health promoter makes and cultivates the necessary contacts, a planning committee of 15 to 20 individuals should be formed. The committee can include program staff, skilled evaluators, content experts, and specific individuals to be served by the HPDP program. Diversity in the planning committee brings valuable knowledge and expertise to the group.

Keeping the group together and engaged in the planning process is essential. This ensures continuity and the critical involvement of those who will eventually use the services (Bartholomew et al., 2006). The health promoter will find that regular contact and meetings with group members from the community is one strategy that works especially well in fostering trust, friendship, and motivation to stay involved. Although conventional wisdom dictates that providers maintain a strictly professional relationship, experience in the field has demonstrated that interacting in the real-life events of individuals within the community is enriching for those involved and provides a glimpse, at a deeper level, into the barriers and incentives that motivate action within the community.

It is important that planning sessions are open to the public and held in an accessible and safe location. Churches, schools, and libraries are ideal locations in the community. Discussion on what it will take to plan and carry out the program should be addressed. Meetings should include an agenda to guide the discussions. At the conclusion of each meeting, action steps for planning committee members to perform should be identified. Those working on the action steps can provide an update at subsequent meetings. Members of the planning team will then have a better sense of the magnitude of the work that may be required of them.

Set boundaries. List priorities. Make compromises whenever necessary. An honest discussion of all these issues can help foster respect for the program staff, who have the responsibility of developing and implementing the program. The health promoter will need to be sensitive to the needs of planning team members because some will have their own vested interests, which they will hope to promote through their involvement in the planning efforts. Identifying these interests early on in the process can help minimize and/or bring into focus these interests and decide how they might be addressed to benefit all parties and the community in general during the actual planning process.

Community Asset and Needs Assessment

Many health promoters approach community service provision from a deficit model. This model identifies the problem as a beginning stage of the planning process. An African American health promoter elaborates, "The norm is to talk about the problem. Our approach is asset-based. What does the community already have?" (in-depth interview, personal communication, April 13, 2006). The assets and strengths within a community are just as important to identify as community problems or needs. An asset assessment is an observation of the physical and nonphysical resources within a community. This assessment is conducted by visiting a neighborhood to identify the resources in the area. The health promoter then documents the resources that she or he observes. A common form of charting includes geographic mapping of the resources. Through this process, the health promoter can chart the general proximity of a liquor store in relationship to a middle/high school, for example. Table 14.1 highlights the categories of community assets, specific types of resources, and observations that a health promoter might consider when conducting the assessment (also see Appendix A on p. 328).

As identified in Table 14.1, there are several types of resources for each category of service.

Table 14.1   Community Asset Assessment

Category	Resource Type	Observation
Transportation	Trains, subways, buses—e.g. stops and stations, taxi cabs Highway/freeway entrances and exits	Creates access to resources outside the neighborhood, including employment and health services
Community-based organizations	Community centers—e.g., senior, youth Religious organizations—e.g., churches, mosques Housing assistance, shelters, transitional governance bodies—e.g., city hall Food and clothing distribution centers	Assists with community coping skills, contributes to safety and survival and individual and family functioning
Health services	Neighborhood clinics, outpatient centers, emergency rooms Hospitals (public and private) Dialysis centers Mental health programs Mobile medical vans	Access to affordable health care and services; indications of prevalent health issues
Food and retail	Neighborhood ethnic food markets, large supermarkets, health food stores Fast-food restaurants Liquor stores Drug stores/pharmacies Manufacturing companies Locally owned businesses	Access to healthy foods; indication of nutrition practices and/or intervention opportunities; availability of community retail resources
Housing	Public/affordable housing Multi- and single-dwelling homes Apartment buildings Mixed-use housing	Coexistence of low-, moderate-, and high- income residents; insight on community living conditions
Education	Early-education centers—e.g., preschools, head starts Primary and secondary schools, district offices Adult schools—e.g., language and literacy Universities, colleges, technical/trade schools Public libraries	Access to educational resources; academic, skill, and trade development; community viability for competitive job market
Neighborhood conditions	Conditions of the following: streets, sidewalks, alleys, lawns, buildings—e.g., occupied or abandoned Murals, statues, and cultural art	Access to clean and safe physical environments as well as indications of blight; exhibits of community pride through murals and other art forms

Category	Resource Type	Observation
	Waste systems—e.g., garbage bins Parks and green space Power lines, creeks, power plants	
Information systems and media	Signs, billboards, advertisements Community newspapers Payphones/public phones Computer and Internet services	Community access to information, modes of communication, advertisement, and messaging
Social networks (formal and informal)	Community planning councils Local artists, oral historians Youth networks Parent support groups	Formal and informal leaders provide insight on community dynamics and power structures in the community

For example, the presence of health clinics and public hospitals in the neighborhood provides an indication of accessible health services. Asset mapping provides important insight about the community before the hands-on work begins. It also helps identify gaps or resources that are needed. The planning committee can validate the information gathered and can identify additional assets, community strengths, or observations that may have been missed by the health promoter. This process also provides deeper insight into what the community views as an asset. The health promoter can enhance this information in the needs assessment process to follow.

In addition to identifying the strengths within a community, health promoters must conduct an assessment to determine the wants, needs, and health problems that persist in the community. The needs assessment helps identify community members' perceptions of health and HPDP programs and services. The health promoter will need to have an assortment of strategies for involving residents in the needs assessment process and for collecting needs assessment data. The health promoter will have to determine whether certain topics are better explored through community forums, while surveys or in-person interviews might be more appropriate for other topics. Individuals from the community, the planning committee, and evaluation staff can help identify the best approach for needs assessment data collection.

Regardless of the strategy selected, any procedure or instrument used to collect needed data must be pilot tested with a small sample of the group that will be the focus of the assessment. The instrument must be appropriate and norm tested for the African American community to be served. In the experience of the authors, some standardized questionnaires are developed for the majority culture and often contain questions that have little meaning in the lives of the intended population. This became evident when reviewing a telephone survey instrument regarding breast health. Many of the questions needed restructuring for appropriate use in the African American community.

Cottrell et al. (1995) describes four major domains to facilitate the identification of community needs. These domains provide a guide to inform the development of a needs assessment instrument that takes into account historical, economic and political, traditional and cultural, and religious factors. These components are summarized in Table 14.2.

Table 14.2   Needs Assessment Considerations by Component

Component	Considerations
Historical information	Historical events, conflicts and concerns of the community—e.g., civil unrest
	Relationships with the government—e.g., community/police relations
	Demographic shifts in the community—e.g., migrations of populations
	Reputation and perceptions of health care providers and institutions in the community
Economic and political information	Socioeconomic status levels—e.g., low, middle, and upper-middle income
	Percentage of families receiving public assistance
	Educational levels of community residents
	Business ownership
	Identification of health services in the community
	Structure and involvement of local political representatives
	Organizations that successfully serve the community
Traditional and cultural context	Identification of how the intended population defines health, healing, and illness
	Common beliefs and health practices that carry over from previous generations—e.g., use of herbs and faith healers
	Use of nontraditional medicine
	Family structures in the community—e.g., strong matriarchal ties
	Role of women as formal and informal leaders
	Modes of communication of health information and usual source of health information
	Perceptions of major health problems based on various age and gender groups
	General beliefs about disease causation, prevention, and treatment
	Community member's experience with the existing health delivery system
Religious context	Levels and types of religious leaders
	Religious leader's involvement with health issues
	Roles of faith leaders in communities
	Community member's religious beliefs about faith and healing

SOURCE: Adapted from Cottrell et al. (1995).

The considerations for each domain help the planning team identify detailed factors that inform the content of needs assessment development and help shape the strategies for collecting needs assessment data.

Strategies for collecting needs assessment data will vary with the community and the health issues to be addressed. Suggested strategies that have been successfully used are community surveys (both self-administered and assisted questionnaires), focus groups, direct interviews, community forums, and collection of health services data. Needs assessment data collection should minimize the burden on community participants whenever possible. Participants completing the needs assessment should be compensated for their time and participation. This includes a financial stipend such as a check or gift card, grocery voucher, or other parting gifts. In the case of interviews or focus groups, the health promoter and planning team may provide transportation, child care for the participants, and dinner or refreshments. This is particularly important for working parents or participants with limited mobility. It is also important for community members to be considered partners in the needs assessment process (in-depth interview, personal communication, April 13, 2006). This may occur through community member feedback on the assessment questions and integration of the input in a revised document to the extent that it is feasible and relevant.

PROGRAM DEVELOPMENT

The health promoter and the planning team must consider a theoretical model or framework for the program to be developed. There are a number of possible theoretical models and frameworks available to the planner. Few HPDP programs use the strict models identified in the health promotion and education literature. Hochbaum, Sorenson, and Lorig (1992) observe that it might be difficult to apply some of the theories currently available but comment that they still can be useful guides for selecting or developing promising approaches to a given program. Frequently, the choice is to use a combination of theories that focus on both predicting change and measuring actual behavioral outcomes (N. M. Clark & McLeroy, 1995). Ryan and Heaney (1993) suggest a process for selecting a workable theory that begins by first knowing the specific intended population, the behaviors that are to be addressed, and the goals and objectives the program will try to address (Chapter 4, this volume). They also identify criteria for selecting a useful theory using questions such as the following:

- Does the theory complement and flow with the worldview of the intended group?
- Has the theory been tested on a population similar to the one to be served in the developing program?
- Has the theory been used in a program similar to the one being developed?
- Has the theory been successfully used in other programs with the intended population?
- Does the theory make sense to the health promoter?

Two theories that are similar in approach and are useful in addressing HPDP programs in African American communities are social learning theory and the theory of planned change. Social learning theory, which was renamed social cognitive theory by Bandura (1986), is concerned with the cognitive, environmental, and behavioral variables that help describe human behavior and learning. The application of this theory is discussed extensively by Ryan and Heaney (1993), who note three factors involved in the behavior change process that must be modified for a new behavior to be acquired, performed, and sustained over time. These are (1) having the necessary skills to perform the desired behavior, (2) believing that one is capable of carrying out the new behavior, and (3) believing that performing the desired behavior will result in a desired outcome. These three variables are especially important when addressing issues in the black community.

The Theory of Planned Behavior (Ajzen, 1991; Ajzen & Driver, 1991; Ajzen & Madden, 1986), which is an extension of the Theory of Reasoned Action (Fishbein, 1967), is discussed by Gielen and colleagues as a plausible theory for use in HPDP efforts (Gielen, Wilson, Faden, Wilson, & Harvilchuck, 1995) They note that the theory seeks to predict behavioral intention to actually carry out any given behavior on the basis of personal beliefs about performing the behavior, including evaluation of possible outcomes of the behavior;

attitudes toward the behavior; the influence of normative and subjective beliefs; motivations to comply with normative pressures; and perceived behavioral control, including barriers and resources necessary to perform the behavior (Gielen et al., 1995).

These models are valuable frameworks, not only for thinking about health behavior change in the African American community but also because they suggest areas for inclusion in the needs assessment process that can provide data on current knowledge, attitudes, and beliefs of the intended group. With this information, interventions can be structured that take into account the areas where deficits in particular may exist and where work needs to be done to facilitate new health-promoting behaviors within the intended group.

Once decisions are reached about a theoretical approach to a health issue or problem, the health promoter must revisit the dynamics of the planning team. The practitioner may need to maintain and/or perhaps expand the team's membership to ensure that all parties that have an interest in the outcome of the program or service are involved in the planning. The expansion may include specific subgroups of the African American population—for example, seniors, teenage parents, child care providers, HIV-positive women, and so on. Periodic reassessment of the quality of the core group with respect to whether it represents the diversity of the population the health promoter is serving will be necessary.

In addition to shaping the dynamics of the planning team, the health promoter and skilled evaluator can engage the committee in developing a conceptual theory of change for the program. A theory of change is a visual framework that outlines the desired outcome(s) of the program and the specific pathways or intermediate stages of change to bring about the outcome (Anderson, 2004). Each intervention and/or program activity should link back to a specific desired result. Engaging the committee in the development of a program theory

of change early in the planning process helps identify whether the interventions are realistic, doable, and appropriate given the program goals. It helps clarify the purpose of the program, the interventions, and the evaluation. It helps staff and stakeholders agree on the program and evaluation outcomes that can shape implementation and evaluation.

IMPLEMENTATION

Marin and his colleagues (1995) describe a set of criteria that should be considered when planning interventions for underserved population groups. They note that the interventions must be based on the cultural values of the intended group. They should reflect the subjective cultural characteristics and the behavioral preferences and expectations of the intended population. This speaks to the importance of including a cultural assessment as part of the overall needs assessment process carried out by the health promoter and the planning team. For example, accessibility to appropriate health services is an important consideration. The planner must be cognizant of the real and perceived barriers that may be preventing the intended group from participation in or use of existing services. There is the matter of competing priorities in the African American community, such as basic survival needs—that is, food, shelter, safety, child care, and employment. There may be cultural issues, such as apprehension to discussing personal or family needs with people who are not family members. Environmental factors such as lack of transportation and unsafe neighborhoods may affect the willingness of community members to participate in affordable health promotion programs such as walking or bicycling.

Lack of knowledge about health issues and prevention practices within the intended group is a major implementation consideration for those working in low-income African American communities. Some community residents may not believe that they are at risk of unfavorable outcomes because of their lifestyle practices. A major part of developing and improving a culture of health promotion in African American communities is instilling a sense of awareness about individual health risks. For example, in a series of focus groups conducted in southern California regarding breast and prostrate cancer, participants expressed a lack of knowledge about their risk for developing these diseases. This information coupled with needs assessment findings might suggest that a major emphasis should be placed on awareness of risks in conjunction with efforts to instruct on and promote screening and periodic checkups for specific health conditions.

It is important that all activities necessary to carry out the stated objectives of the program are thoroughly explored by planning team members, especially by those who represent the community being served. This can help identify issues that may have been missed or overlooked in the assessment phase and potential strategies that might be unrealistic for the community and population to be served by the program. The activities developed should directly link to the desired outcomes and objectives outlined in the programmatic theory of change. The activities should also relate to the behavior change models to ensure that there is continuity between the theory and the specific strategies that will be implemented. Program interventions and the activities associated with them must be carefully written to include what is to be done, by whom, how often, and where. As interventions are developed, they should be pilot tested with members of the community, using focus group processes or other procedures to ensure that the interventions are acceptable, understandable, and relevant to the intended population. This is particularly important with the use of educational materials developed for the mainstream culture, because these might not be culturally sensitive and appropriate for the intended population. The staff may need to find out whether the materials have been successfully used with a population similar to the black community to be served. The program may also locally develop culturally relevant and meaningful materials for the potential participants. The health promoter must take care that program-developed materials are clear and empirically relevant to the theory and program design.

In terms of recruitment and program delivery, the health promoter should consider nontraditional sites and captive audiences. One approach entails recruiting and/or implementing interventions in churches, Laundromats, nail shops, beauty salons, barber shops, family and class reunions, social clubs, and organizations. In-home strategies may also be useful, such as health parties, demonstrating nutrition practices such as cooking healthy foods and engaging family members in health promotion practices. The strategies should be cultivated by the planning team. Activities developed from an evidence base may be helpful, particularly for activities that yield positive outcomes with similar populations. Input from interested community members should also be considered as the activities are being developed. Observation in the field has revealed the difficulty of getting participants to attend multiple sessions of an intervention. Exploring ways to remove the barriers to participation may prove useful for the health promoter (e.g., providing incentives or transportation, or adjusting the time of day or week when the program is delivered).

EVALUATION

Evaluation is a critical component of HPDP programs. It is ongoing, begins early in the planning process, continues throughout each phase of the program, and may continue after the program ends. Evaluation assists program staff, participants, and stakeholders in understanding the value and worth of the health promotion effort (Thorogood & Coombes, 2004). It provides a basis for program planning (e.g., when developing the theory of change and constructing the needs assessment instruments and protocols). It provides information for program improvement and can help assess the impact of the program (Bartholomew et al., 2006).

The planning team, health promotion staff, and evaluators should work together to articulate the purpose of the evaluation and the questions to be answered. This can be viewed as a process of inquiry to address a range of topics such as

- how well the program functioned to meet its stated objectives,
- how well the staff performed in their program tasks,
- how much learning and behavior change occurred among participants from pre- to postprogram, and
- how much money was spent to achieve the desired outcomes (Dignan & Carr, 1987; Green & Kreuter, 2005).

The evaluation questions and priorities must align with the program design, the services to be provided, and the intended outcome of the program. Development of an evaluation plan can assist with clear identification of those connections.

The evaluation should also take into account stakeholders' specific needs and interests to the extent that it is feasible and appropriate to include them in the evaluation design. For example, it would be problematic if a program is designed to change health-seeking practices of its participants and key stakeholders want to evaluate whether participants are healthier because of participation in the program. Since the program was designed to address health-seeking practices, it would not be feasible to address the stakeholders' concern. The staff might have to modify the program to address the stakeholders' question if it is agreed on that the issue is critical enough for

that type of change. Another option is to communicate the purpose of the program and the questions that are appropriate and feasible to address given the program design.

In addition, Thorogood and Coombes (2004) note that programs may tend to measure outcomes that are easily quantifiable and provide less attention to outcomes that are not easily quantified. They suggest that multiple methods be used to evaluate different health interventions. This flexibility will allow the health promoter to collect both quantitative and qualitative data to identify whether and why relationships exist (Thorogood & Coombes, 2004). Use of multiple methods may also help the program staff manage evaluation costs, which can quickly become excessive. Developing an evaluation budget should be a priority for the program, and the evaluation activities must be relevant and within the budget.

Data collection can often be viewed as a cumbersome process that does not readily link to health program service delivery. It may take creativity to obtain buy-in from program participants and staff (e.g., provide incentives for participation). Program staff and participants may be more committed to the evaluation processes when they understand the purpose and uses of the data obtained. It is good practice to share data findings and modify the program based on evaluation results wherever appropriate and feasible.

APPLICATION OF HEALTH PROMOTION PLANNING IN AFRICAN AMERICAN COMMUNITIES

The following examples provide important considerations when implementing health promotion strategies in African American communities. The examples focus on two frequently cited problems in inner-city black communities: hypertension and HIV/AIDS among African American women.

Hypertension Intervention in an African American Community

In an effort to highlight some of the suggestions that have been made thus far, the following example is offered to illuminate some strategies that were successfully used for working with African American and other minority populations in the inner-city areas of Los Angeles. In the mid-1970s, at the Martin Luther King Jr. General Hospital, Drew Medical Center in Los Angeles, Mary Ashley and an editor of this book were involved in planning, implementing, and evaluating a health promotion program. The goal was to reduce the number of community residents who had uncontrolled hypertension. Information gathered at a local health fair revealed a low level of knowledge about hypertension in the community. Participants who received a blood pressure screening at the health fair were unaware of their blood pressure levels and of the impact of elevated blood pressure on health outcomes.

The program began to offer three components of service. The first component consisted of blood pressure screenings to captive audiences at every opportunity, including at community health fairs, in churches, during senior citizen programs, at community group meetings, in local schools and community colleges, and in the lobby of the hospital. On these occasions, individuals were offered screening and a simple questionnaire to further assess the knowledge level of the community with respect to hypertension. The results confirmed that knowledge levels were low and needed to be addressed. A three-pronged program using community residents as major partners in the development and implementation of a hypertension control program was implemented. To address the knowledge issues in the community, a preventive health education team was organized to include two community workers, health educators, allied health personnel, and a physician. The team's primary goal was to provide innovative

educational experiences about hypertension throughout the community and develop educational materials, songs, dance routines, lectures, and individual educational sessions to get the message out about hypertension.

The second component of the program focused on training and certifying a group of residents to conduct screening and educational sessions throughout the community. The staff were able to provide screening and individual/ group education to hundreds of individuals. In addition, they were responsible for identifying, referring, and following up with individuals regarding elevated blood pressure. Hospital and community clinical services were made available to participants.

The third aspect of the program was providing effective, accessible care to participants. To accomplish this goal, the team focused on the clinical setting, including staff attitudes and the actual physical environment of the hypertension clinic, which was established specifically to diagnose, treat, and track patients with hypertension. Trained community workers were assigned to conduct education in the clinic, which was transformed to create an atmosphere conducive to education. For example, the walls of the clinic were painted with scenes that depicted behaviors associated with control of hypertension, including proper meal planning with low salt/low fat diets, smoking cessation, exercise, stress management, medication adherence, and making regular doctor visits to the clinic. The scenes on the walls provided a complete visual outline of the concepts for controlling high blood pressure and were a reminder to patients at each visit of their responsibility in the treatment process. In addition, small-group discussion proved to be the most effective method of education in this setting. It allowed for participants to discuss their issues and receive suggestions on how to take better care of themselves. A trained health educator was always available to troubleshoot issues and provide accurate information to the participants.

This example suggests that the health promotion planner will need to consider multiple intervention strategies. This is particularly true of activities that have been successfully implemented in African American communities.

HIV/AIDS Intervention Among African American Women

In 2002, the leading cause of death among black women aged 25 to 34 was HIV/AIDS (CDC, 2006a). In 2003, the rate of new cases for black women was 20 times that of white women and 5 times greater than the rate for Hispanic/Latino women. The CDC (2006b) reported that in 2004, "the rate of AIDS diagnoses for African American women was approximately 23 times the rate for white women and 4 times the rate for Hispanic women" (p. 2).

In a study by Bogart and Thorburn (2005), they found that 50% of African Americans, regardless of age and income, believe that AIDS is a man-made disease. Many believe that it was designed by the government to decimate the black community. Even though HIV/AIDS is posing a major threat to African Americans, some still think that it is a gay white man's disease.

Views espoused by African Americans determine whether they access health services and embrace health promotion activities. Strategies to address the issue of HIV/AIDS in the black community therefore must be carefully considered. Aggressive educational activities have had an impact in the white gay community. However, those strategies have not been as successful in the black community. The situation for women is critical. The health promoter must ask why this condition exists. He or she must consider the cultural, social, economic, and religious values of the community.

Knowing the statistics, the health promoter must use innovative strategies to capture the attention of black women. A project titled

Sisters Informing Sisters About Topics on AIDS (SISTA) was developed by African American women to meet the needs of African American women. The project was a peer-led program to prevent HIV infection among young adult African American women. It is an educational strategy that has proven to be an effective tool among women in the black community.

This project is now being successfully implemented throughout the United States and is available through the CDC. Below is a description of the SISTA project being implemented in Los Angeles.

After attending the mandatory 3-day training in Alabama, the health promoter went back to Los Angeles enthusiastic and committed to implementing the program. She was given the box that contains suggestions for getting started and all the materials to implement the program, but she realized that getting started requires organizational support and commitment as well as access to a willing community. She took the following steps:

- Obtained a commitment from her organization to provide the time and resources that would be needed
- Developed relationships by meeting with other HIV/AIDS providers, going to community meetings, being visible at activities within the community
- Recruited potential participants at health fairs and any type of community event, making radio announcements, getting on the agenda of existing organizations, and making concerted efforts to recruit other women working in the community
- Educated and signed up women at events and organizations, responding to requests to make presentations at meetings within the community
- Surveyed the women to establish a convenient meeting place and time, exploring whether participants needed transportation and child care

Most of the women in the first program were middle class, educated, and recruited from existing organizations. The health promoter found that many individuals had the idea that AIDS was affecting poor uneducated women. More affluent women tended to feel they were safe. Because the program consisted of six 2-hour sessions and two follow-up sessions, getting a comfortable meeting space was very important. The sessions were scheduled for Saturday mornings in a room over a small tea and entertainment facility. The promoter was able to secure a commitment to provide lunch from the shop below because food can be a good incentive for participation.

Even though this group was composed of mostly professional women, the lack of sufficient information about HIV/AIDS was apparent. The program was successfully completed. The evaluations at the end of each 4- and 8-week follow-up session were very good, and members spoke openly of the commitment for change they were willing to make. The members also made new friends and made a commitment to help with the recruitment of clients and staff members with whom they worked.

CHAPTER SUMMARY

This chapter sought to describe program development strategies that can be helpful when working with African American communities. There is an urgent need to make HPDP programs and services more accessible to all segments of this population. There are and have been initiatives at all levels of government, universities, and the private sector to address and enhance HPDP efforts. Some of these have been quite successful, although major gaps still remain to be addressed in others. When starting to plan for HPDP programs in African American communities, consideration should be given to the following key issues.

- Research should be conducted by the health promoter to understand the history and culture of African Americans in the United States as well as identify the values, beliefs,

practices, and barriers one might encounter within the different segments of the population intended for intervention.

- There must be a willingness to understand the important aspects of black culture, such as language, traditional culture, religion, and social life, within the context of social history and racism.

- Health promoters must be willing to invest time and energy to make certain that there is a partnership with the community to ensure that community members are involved in every step of the planning, development, implementation, and evaluation of the program.

- The health promoter should have an in-depth knowledge of the perceived needs of the community to be served. This includes an understanding of the community's health beliefs and practices and how these affect the traditional biomedical model of health care delivery.

- The health promoter must be equipped with a variety of strategies for working in the African American community and be able to employ these effectively in all phases of program plan development.

- The health provider must provide comprehensive multifaceted intervention strategies that are culturally relevant to the community. HPDP programs and services, including the messages sent to the community about these, must be developed within the context of the lives of individuals and norms of the community in which they live.

- The health provider, planning team, and program staff must hold themselves accountable for measurable progress of the health promotion program, supported by a thorough and comprehensive evaluation.

- The health promoter must be able to garner the necessary support from local organizations, local and national politicians, and influential individuals within the community.

This list of recommendations is by no means exhaustive. It represents some salient points that have been covered in the body of this chapter. In spite of perceived insurmountable barriers, there are many people in the black community who are eager to learn and assist in improving health outcomes for themselves, their families, and their neighbors.

The next chapter presents a case study where the author tries to emphasize the points made in the overview and planning chapters. The study is concerned with the application of concepts and approaches for bridging the gap between theory and practice. They provide an opportunity for the student and the practitioner to get a "bird's-eye" view of some of the specific methods and techniques of HPDP program planning, application, and problem solving.

DISCUSSION QUESTIONS AND ACTIVITIES

Consider this scenario: Mortality and morbidity from type 2 diabetes, heart disease, and HIV/AIDS have been increasing for the past several years among African American population groups living in a large multicultural metropolitan community.

The local health jurisdiction, private providers, voluntary agencies, and community members are very concerned and want to reduce the number of deaths and illnesses drastically. Local government officials recognize that increased screening, referral, and treatment programs are critically needed for identifying problems. Limited monies are available for providing HIV/AIDS, diabetes, and heart disease *health promotion and education programs* to selected multicultural target groups. Select a specific African American target group in a specific geographical area in your community as a frame of reference to work from. Then, break up into planning teams, and consider the following questions relevant to needed health promotion and education programs designed to increase access and services to that target group:

- How would you involve those affected by the problem?
- How would you assess the needs of African American target groups in the community or target populations with regard to the aforementioned diseases?
- What specific health promotion and education program goals and objectives related to target group accessibility to education and treatment programs would be included in the plan?
- What issues of implementing your program(s) should you be aware of?

REFERENCES

Ajzen, I. (1991). The theory of planned behavior. *Organizational Behavior and Human Decision Processes, 50,* 179–211.

Ajzen, I., & Driver, B. L. (1991). Prediction of leisure participation from behavioral, normative, and control beliefs: An application of the theory of planned behavior. *Leisure Sciences, 13,* 185–204.

Ajzen, I., & Madden, T. J. (1986). Prediction of goal-directed behavior: Attitudes, intentions, and perceived behavioral control. *Journal of Experimental Social Psychology, 22,* 453–474.

Anderson, A. A. (2004). *Theory of change as a tool for strategic planning: A report on early experiences.* The Aspen Institute Roundtable on Community Change. Retrieved October 17, 2006, from www.theoryofchange.org/tocII_fina14.pdf

Bandura, A. (1986). *Social foundation of thought and action: A social cognitive theory.* Englewood Cliffs, NJ: Prentice Hall.

Bartholomew, K. L., Parcel, G. S., Kok, G., & Gottlieb, N. H. (2006). *Planning health promotion programs: An intervention mapping approach.* San Francisco: Jossey-Bass.

Bogart, L. M., & Thorburn, S. (2005). Are HIV/AIDS conspiracy beliefs a barrier to HIV prevention among African Americans? *Journal of Acquired Immune Deficiency Syndrome, 38(3),* 213.

Byrd, W. M. (1990). Race biology and health care: Reassessing a relationship. *Journal of Health Care for the Poor and Underserved, 1,* 278–292.

Byrd, W. M., & Clayton, L. A. (1993). The African American cancer crisis. Part 2: A prescription. *Journal of Health Care for the Poor and Underserved, 4,* 102–116.

Centers for Disease Control and Prevention. (2005, May 23). *Tuskegee syphilis study: A hard lesson learned.* Retrieved May 16, 2006, from www.cdc.gov/nchstp/od/tuskegee/time.htm

Centers for Disease Control and Prevention. (2006a, February). *HIV/AIDS fact sheet: HIV/AIDS among African Americans.* Retrieved November 1, 2006, from www.cdc.gov/hiv/topics/aa/resources/factsheets/pdf/aa.pdf

Centers for Disease Control and Prevention. (2006b, April). *HIV/AIDS fact sheet: HIV/AIDS among women.* Retrieved November 1, 2006, from www.cdc.gov/hiv/topics/women/resources/factsheets/pdf/women.pdf

Clark, C. C. (Ed.). (2002). *Health promotion in communities: Holistic and wellness approaches.* New York: Springer.

Clark, N. M., & McLeroy, K. R. (1995). Creating capacity through health education: What we know and what we don't. *Health Education Quarterly, 22,* 273–289.

Cottrell, M. A., Davis, W., Schlaff, A., Liburd, L., Orenstein, D., & Presley, C. L. (1995). *Promoting healthy lifestyle in inner-city minority communities.* Washington, DC: U.S. Department of Health and Human Services.

Dignan, M. B., & Carr, P. A. (1987). *Program planning for health education and health promotion.* Philadelphia: Lea & Febiger.

DuBois, W. E. B. (1903). *The souls of black folk: Essays and sketches.* Bend, OR: A. C. McClurg.

Eng, E., & Hatch, J. W. (1991). Networking between agencies: The lay health advisor model. *Human Services, 10,* 123–146.

Fishbein, M. (Ed.). (1967). *Readings in attitude theory and measurement.* New York: Wiley.

Gielen, A. C., Wilson, M. E. H., Faden, R. R., Wilson, L., & Harvilchuck, J. D. (1995). In home injury prevention practices for infants and toddlers: The role of parental beliefs, barriers and housing quality. *Health Education Quarterly, 22,* 85–95.

Green, L. W., & Kreuter, M. W. (2005). *Health program planning: An educational and ecological approach* (4th ed.). New York: McGraw-Hill.

Haynes, M. A. (1975). The gap in health status between black and white Americans. In R. A. Williams (Ed.), *Textbook of black related diseases.* New York: McGraw-Hill.

Herring, P., & Montgomery, S. (1996). Health beliefs, health values and prevention, health promotion activities of black and white women: A comparative study. *Journal of Wellness Perspectives, 12,* 188–197.

Hirsch, J. (1991). Race, genetics and scientific integrity. *Journal of Health Care for the Poor and Underserved, 2,* 331–334.

Hochbaum, G. M., Sorenson, J. R., & Lorig, K. (1992). Theories in health education practice. *Health Education Quarterly, 19,* 295–313.

Iglehart, A. P., & Becerra, R. M. (2000). *Social services and the ethnic community.* Prospect Heights, IL: Waveland Press.

Marin, G., Burhansstipanov, L., Connell, C. M., Gielen, A. C., Helitzer-Allen, D., Lorig, K., et al. (1995). A research agenda for health education among underserved populations. *Health Education Quarterly, 22,* 346–363.

Office of Research Integrity. (n.d.). In *Responsible conduct of research: Conflict of interest* (sec. 2.3, Clinical research: Tuskegee Study). Retrieved May 16, 2006, from http://ori.hhs.gov/education/products/columbia_wbt/rcr_conflicts/foundation/index.html

Quinn, S. C., Billingsley, A., & Caldwell, C. (1994). The characteristics of northern black churches and community outreach programs. *American Journal of Public Health, 84,* 575–579.

Quinn, T. S. (1996). The National Negro Health Week, 1991 to 1995: A descriptive account. *Journal of Wellness, 12*(4), 172–179.

Ryan, M. V., & Heaney, C. (1993). What's the use of theory? *Health Education Quarterly, 19,* 315–330.

Satcher, D., & Pamies, R. J. (Eds.). (2006). *Multicultural medicine and health disparities.* New York: McGraw-Hill.

Thorogood, M., & Coombes, Y. (Eds.). (2004). *Evaluating health promotion: Practice and methods* (2nd ed.). Oxford, UK: Oxford University Press.

U.S. Department of Health and Human Services: Office of Minority Health. (n.d.). Retrieved May 2, 2006, from www.omhrc.gov/templates/browse.aspx?lvl=2&lvlID=29

Appendix A

HEALTH PROMOTION AND DISEASE PREVENTION PLANNING IN AFRICAN AMERICAN COMMUNITIES

Guiding Questions to Assess Community Assets

What are the conditions of the streets, allies, and sidewalks?

What businesses are there in the community? How many?

What types of social service organizations are there in the community?

What medical resources/organizations are there in the community (e.g., dialysis centers, clinics, hospitals)?

What are the nonphysical assets that exist in the community?

What seem to be gaps in resources within the community?

How might health promotion efforts maximize the community assets?

How might health promotion efforts address the gaps within the community?

Guiding Needs Assessment Questions

Answer the following questions about the community that you plan to serve:

What subgroups within the community would it be critical to include in the needs assessment process (e.g., youth groups, senior women)?

What historical events have occurred in this community (i.e., civil unrest, community/police relations)?

What are the economic dynamics within the community (e.g., middle-class families juxtaposed with a community of families living in affordable housing developments)?

What mechanisms do community members use to obtain health information (e.g., local newspaper, word of mouth, YMCA, YWCA, Community Recreation Centers, Boys and Girls Clubs)?

What health-related issues are addressed in religious organizations within the community you are trying to serve? How might your health promotion efforts build on existing activities within the religious organization?

Appendix B

USEFUL WEB SITES

AIDS Healthcare Foundation, www.aidshealth.org

American Evaluation Association: Guiding Principles for Evaluators, www.eval.org/Publications/GuidingPrinciples.asp

The Body: The Complete HIV/AIDS Resource, www.thebody.com/african_american/411-resources.html

University of Kansas Community Tool Box, http://ctb.ku.edu/tools/en/sub_section_main_1020.htm

U.S. Department of Health and Human Services, Office of Minority Health: *National Standards for Culturally and Linguistically Appropriate Services in Health Care: Final Report*, www.omhrc.gov/assets/pdf/checked/finalreport.pdf

U.S. Department of Health and Human Services, Office of Minority Health: *National Standards for Culturally and Linguistically Appropriate Services (CLAS)*, www.omhrc.gov/templates/browse.aspx?lvl=2&lvlID=15

U.S. Department of Health and Human Services, Office of Minority Health: *What Is Cultural Competency?* www.omhrc.gov/templates/browse.aspx?lvl=2&lvlID=11

15

Promoting Health in African American Groups

Preventing HIV Among African American Female Adolescents

GINA M. WINGOOD

Chapter Objectives

On completion of this chapter, the health promotion student and practitioner will be able to

- Search, identify, and review pertinent professional literature relevant to increasing their knowledge about the epidemiology of HIV/AIDS among African American adolescent females

- Discuss and illustrate how the investigators in this case study chapter developed a theoretically derived and culturally congruent HIV/AIDS prevention curriculum for African American adolescent females

- Describe the evaluative methodology used by the investigators of this study for assessing the effectiveness of their HIV prevention intervention for African American adolescent females

INTRODUCTION

Adolescents and Sexually Transmitted Diseases: The Risk Is Real

The risk of acquiring a sexually transmitted disease (STD), including human immunodeficiency virus (HIV), is one of the most significant and immediate risks to the health and well-being of adolescents. While there has been marked progress in the development of HIV prevention interventions for adolescents, programs designed specifically for females, and more specifically for African American females, have lagged behind that of other at-risk adolescent populations. Despite recently reported declines in the percentage of school-age adolescents who are sexually active, the proportion of adolescents initiating sexual intercourse at younger ages has increased (Kahn et al., 2000; Meschke, Bartholomae, & Zentall, 2000), and the prevalence of sexual risk taking among adolescents in the United States remains high (Centers for Disease Control [CDC], 2002a). Specifically, a recent study found that while 47% of adolescents attending high school had ever had sexual intercourse, 14% reported four or more lifetime sexual partners (Grunbaum et al., 2004). Moreover, approximately one third of all adolescent males and one half of adolescent females attending high school reported not using a condom at last sexual intercourse (CDC, 2002a). Perhaps as a consequence, the incidence and prevalence of STDs among adolescents is exceptionally high.

In the United States, the risk of acquiring an STD is higher among teenagers than among adults (CDC, 2000). More recent investigations have reported that approximately one quarter of new STD cases, almost 4 million, are diagnosed in teenagers (CDC, 2000; National Institute of Allergy and Infectious Diseases, 1997). Even more alarming, recent estimates suggest that about one half of all new HIV infections occur in adolescents/ young adults under 25 years of age, and one quarter of new HIV infections occur among adolescents 21 years of age or younger (CDC, 2002b). The primary mode of HIV transmission among adolescents is sexual contact as opposed to other methods of acquisition (e.g., injection drug use with shared needles and syringes) (CDC, 2003).

The risk of adverse consequences associated with high-risk sexual behavior, such as STD/HIV infection, is not equally distributed among adolescents. Females are at particularly high risk for contracting STIs because they are physiologically more vulnerable to both viral and nonviral STIs, including HIV, and the effects of such STD infections are notably more problematic and costly (Bauer et al., 1991; Burk et al., 1996; Cates, 1999; CDC, 2004; Walsh & Irwin, 2002).

In addition to gender differences in STD prevalence rates, the risk of contracting STDs is substantially greater for African American adolescents (DiClemente & Crosby, 2003), as is the risk for HIV infection (DiClemente, 1990; Eng & Butler, 1997; National Institutes of Allergy and Infectious Diseases, 1997; Office of National AIDS Policy, 1996). For instance, African American adolescent females have higher infection rates of chlamydia and gonorrhea as compared with Caucasian adolescent females (CDC, 2001; Ellen, Aral, & Madger, 1998), with studies reporting that among females between 15 and 19 years of age, African Americans have almost seven times the rate of chlamydia when compared with Caucasian females (CDC, 2002c). African American adolescent females are also more likely than their similar-age white females to have AIDS (DiClemente, 1996). A large-scale seroepidemiologic study conducted among Job Corps applicants indicated that African American adolescent females had an HIV prevalence significantly higher relative to same-age white or Hispanic adolescent females (4.9 vs. 0.7 and 0.6 per 1,000, respectively) (Valleroy, MacKellar, Karon, Janssen, & Hayman, 1998). Among this population, those residing in urban areas in the southern United States experience an even greater risk of HIV acquisition (CDC, 2001).

Focus on STD/HIV Risk-Reduction Interventions for Adolescents: The Need Is Real

Not surprising given these statistics, the CDC and the Institute of Medicine have recommended that adolescents be targeted as a high-priority population for HIV prevention (Eng & Butler, 1997; Valleroy et al., 1998). In response to this call, multisession, small group interventions have been developed, and their efficacy demonstrated in altering theoretically important mediators associated with sexual risk behavior, such as partner communication and attitudes toward condom use (Boyer, Schafer, & Tschann, 1997; Coyle et al., 1999; Jemmott & Jemmott, 2000; Main et al., 1994) and on measurable behavioral outcomes, such as condom use (Jemmott, Jemmott, & Fong, 1998; Shain et al., 1999; Shrier et al., 2001; St. Lawrence et al., 1995; Stanton et al., 1996).

In spite of their demonstrated efficacy, the impact of the interventions is not always uniform across genders. In at least two of the aforementioned effective trials targeting African American adolescents the interventions were not tailored to be gender appropriate for young females and the programs were less effective for female participants in comparison with males (St. Lawrence et al., 1995; Stanton et al., 1996). One possible reason for these results is that males have direct control over condom use, whereas females have to negotiate with males to use condoms. Negotiating condom use is an often difficult skill, especially in light of gender roles, cultural norms, power imbalances, and age differences, often resulting in younger females having to negotiate safer sex behaviors with older male sexual partners.

Just as important as tailoring interventions to be gender appropriate, they also benefit from being tailored to the unique cultural background of the population being served. Mounting evidence indicates that a critical component for effective HIV intervention programs for adolescent females is that they thoroughly address the sexual and relational culture surrounding adolescent females' sexual decision making (Jemmott & Jemmott, 2000; Shain et al., 1999). In spite of this evidence, coupled with the fact that African American adolescent females are disproportionately affected by the HIV/STD epidemic, no intervention designed

specifically for this population has demonstrated efficacy in reducing HIV-associated risk behaviors (Ellen, 2003; Mullen, Ramirez, Strouse, Hedges, & Sogolow, 2002).

THE CURRENT STUDY: THE SiHLE INTERVENTION

In an attempt to address this health disparity, as well as to attend to some of the limitations in previous intervention studies, our research team recently developed and evaluated a theory-guided, culturally appropriate, and gender-tailored sexual risk reduction program for African American female adolescents, between 14 and 18 years of age, called SiHLE (Sistas Informing, Healing, Living, and Empowering). SiHLE was conceptualized by Drs. DiClemente and Wingood and is a modified version of an established and efficacious HIV intervention specifically for African American women (between 18 and 29 years of age) that has been adopted by the CDC in their *Compendium of HIV Prevention Programs With Demonstrated Evidence of Effectiveness* (DiClemente & Wingood, 1995).

Participants

The study was conducted from September 1995 to August 2002. From December 1996 through April 1999, recruiters screened 1,130 African American adolescent females seeking services at four community health agencies. Of these, 609 (53.9%) met the eligibility criteria. Eligibility criteria included being an African American female, between 14 and 18 years of age, reporting vaginal intercourse in the preceding 6 months, and providing written informed consent (parental consent was waived). Of those not eligible, nearly 93% were not sexually experienced. Thus, 522 adolescents agreed to participate in the study, completed baseline assessments, and were randomized to study conditions. Participants were compensated $25 for travel and child care to attend intervention sessions and complete assessments. The University of Alabama at Birmingham Institutional Review Board approved the study protocol prior to implementation.

Study Procedures

The study design was a randomized controlled trial. Participants were randomly assigned, using a computer-generated algorithm, to either the HIV intervention (SiHLE) or a general health promotion condition. The HIV intervention consisted of four, 4-hour interactive group sessions, implemented over consecutive Saturdays. Each session averaged 10 to 12 participants and was implemented by a trained African American female health educator and two African American female peer educators cofacilitated each condition. Peer educators were instrumental in modeling skills and creating group norms supportive of HIV prevention. To reduce the likelihood that the effects of the HIV prevention could be attributed to group interaction or Hawthorne effects, participants randomized to the general health promotion condition also received four, 4-hour interactive group sessions, two sessions emphasizing nutrition and two sessions emphasizing exercise, administered on consecutive Saturdays. Given the focus of this chapter, the content and activities of the general health promotion condition will not be discussed further.

HIV Intervention Condition: SiHLE

The aim of SiHLE, an acronym that stands for Sistas, Informing, Healing, Living, and Empowering, was to reduce the risk of HIV and STDs among sexually active African American adolescent females (DiClemente et al., 2004). Social Cognitive Theory (SCT) (Bandura, 1994) and the Theory of Gender and Power (Wingood & DiClemente, 2000) were complementary theoretical frameworks

guiding the design and implementation of the SiHLE intervention. SCT addresses both the psychosocial dynamics facilitating health behavior and the methods of promoting behavior change. Applying the gender-relevant theoretical framework of the Theory of Gender and Power was critical as it highlights HIV-related social processes prevalent in the lives of African American female adolescents, such as having older male sex partners, having violent dating partners, being stereotyped by the media, perceiving society as having a limited regard of African American teens, engaging in serial monogamy, experiencing peer pressure, and communicating nonassertively about safer sex. Ultimately, by creating an intervention for adolescent females grounded in both SCT and the Theory of Gender and Power we hoped to address more fully the processes that specifically impede young women's adoption of risk-promoting behaviors while teaching them multidimensional strategies to protect themselves from acquiring STDs and HIV (see Table 15.1 for details on how the theories were applied to the intervention).

By using theory mapping, intervention activities associated with constructs articulated in SCT and the Theory of Gender and Power were designed to address the social realities that are more prevalent among African American adolescents. To be effective, HIV prevention programs must be behavior specific and teach adolescents about safe and risky sexual practices as well as the outcomes associated with each practice. Effective programs must also teach adolescents critical skills, such as goal setting, recognizing stimuli that trigger unsafe behaviors, reinforcing positive behaviors, and effective communication skills, that are vital for relationship formation and negotiating safer sex (Bandura, 1992). Thus, all sessions were designed to be engaging with liberal use of interactive games, music, role-plays, and open discussions in an effort to be deemed effective intervention activities. Additionally,

Table 15.1 Mapping of Theory to the SiHLE Intervention Sessions

	Social Cognitive Theory	*Theory of Gender and Power*
Session 1	Provide an opportunity for goal setting Reinforce health-promoting thoughts and actions in the group	Address and challenge the societal norms that dictate appropriate emotional and sexual behavior for females Address factors that place women at an economic disadvantage
Session 2	Provide knowledge on condom use and correct misconceptions of risk-reduction practices Discuss positive outcomes of reducing risky sexual behavior Reinforce previous sessions message through discussion, problem solving, and decision making Promote norms supportive of reducing risky sexual behavior	Reaffirm personal self-worth and pride as it relates to gender and ethnicity
Session 3	Enhance emotion-coping responses by practicing communication skills in arousing situations Enhance self-efficacy through role plays Promote mastery through skills-learning activities Provide opportunities for decision making and problem solving	Create an atmosphere of normality surrounding women taking control over sexual health
Session 4	Enhance coping during emotion-arousing situations Consider multiple avenues to reduce risky sexual behavior	Breakdown societal and institutional structures that creates a power imbalance in relationships

the thematic focus of the intervention, "Stay Safe for Yourself, Your Family, and Your Community," was designed to promote a sense of solidarity and ethnic pride among participants and may have inspired them to modify risk behaviors for altruistic motives; by enhancing their health, they were also enhancing the health of their family and the broader African American community. Unlike many HIV/STD prevention interventions that focus only on cognitive decision making and social and technical competency skills, SiHLE also focused on developing relational skills and amplifying intrinsic motivation (altruism, pride, self-esteem, perceived value, and importance in the community) and mobilizing extrinsic motivators (peer normative influences from the group, modeling by the peer educator) to create an environment that enhanced adolescents' likelihood of adopting and, as important, sustaining preventive behaviors after participation in the intervention. Below, we describe, albeit briefly, each of the four sessions of SiHLE.

Session 1

The first session, titled *My Sistas . . . My Girls,* began with an icebreaker activity, which consisted of a fun game, to allow the group to become acquainted with one another. This activity was followed by providing vital information about the program, introducing the young ladies to the SiHLE motto, and establishing group ground rules. The goal of the first session was to foster sisterhood among young women through activities that promote discussion about African American adolescent topics. Throughout the session, the young women were encouraged to begin developing positive relationships within the group. It was important for the young women to feel a sense of camaraderie with each other as well as with the health educator and peer educator to help make the program a success. Working from the gender-relevant theoretical framework of the Theory of Gender and Power, the activities in session were created to highlight HIV-related social processes prevalent in the lives of African American female adolescents. Through the examination of poetry written by African American women, discussion of challenges and joys of being an African American female, exposure to artwork from African American women, identifying African American role models and prioritizing personal values participants were empowered to raise their expectations of what it is to be a woman cognizant of her sexuality regardless of how society may view them. Also following from the Theory of Gender and Power, other activities in the first session, such as stressing the importance of completing educational requirements, developing career goals, and writing effective professional resumes, were designed to be economically empowering. Table 15.2 provides a detailed overview of the specific activities employed in Session 1.

One activity that demonstrates how the message of sisterhood and self-pride was articulated and promoted in Session 1 is Activity F, *A Room Full of Sisters.*

A Room Full of Sisters (an excerpt) by Mona Lake Jones

A room full of sisters, like jewels in a crown

Vanilla, cinnamon, and dark chocolate brown . . .

Now picture yourself in the midst of this glory

As I describe the sisters who are part of this story.

They were wearing purples, royal blues, and all shades of reds

Some had elegant hats on their heads

With sparkling eyes and shiny lips

They moved through the room swaying their hips

Speaking with smiles on their African faces

Their joy and laughter filled all the spaces.

Peer Educator: Did Mona Lake Jones "reveal her pride in being a black woman in this poem? If so, how?

Mona Lake Jones described black women's outer beauty.

What were some of the descriptive phrases she used to describe black women's outer beauty?

" . . . *like jewels in a crown*"

" . . . *wearing purples, royal blues, and all shades of reds*"

" . . . *with sparkling eyes and shiny lips*"

How did she describe black women's inner beauty?

" . . . *Their beauty was in the values they revered*"

" . . . *loving and caring*"

Session 2

The goal of the second session, titled *It's My Body,* was to introduce the young women

Table 15.2   Themes and Activities in Session 1

	Theme	*Description*
Session 1: My sistas . . . my girls		
Activity A	Greeting and Icebreaker	Allows the group to introduce themselves to each person in the group by participating in a fun activity
Activity B	SiHLE Program Introduction	Discusses the name and objectives of the program
Activity C	Who Are SiHLE Sistas?	Introduces the SiHLE concept and fosters a sense of sisterhood
Activity D	The SiHLE Pact	Discusses the importance of young ladies participating in the workshops as an important step in their learning how to be a SiHLE Sista and also covers the SiHLE motto
Activity E	Young, Black, and Female	Encourages the SiHLE Sistas to think of positive characteristics that describe young black women by allowing the Sistas the opportunity to assert their self-worth and pride
Activity F	A Room Full of Sisters	Encourages the SiHLE Sistas to further discuss pride among young black women by describing the many shades of beauty that are so common among black women
Activity G	Strong Black Women	Encourages the SiHLE Sistas to recognize the importance of African American women as role models by identifying important women in their life and by learning about African American women important in shaping our history
Activity H	A Taste of Culture	Teaches the SiHLE Sistas about African American culture by making their own pictures using African American prints
Activity I	Values—What Matters Most?	Encourages the SiHLE Sistas to recognize their personal values and to assist them in understanding why it is important to first consider their personal values before they make a decision
Activity J	Thought Works	Promotes the participants' identification of their goals and dreams

to the risks related to STDs, especially HIV, and what this can mean to them. This workshop began with a review of the young women's values, goals, and dreams. Additionally, the girls were provided information about STDs and HIV, including a discussion of behaviors that put them at risk for the diseases, and how the diseases can affect their goals and dreams. Subsequently, correct condom skills were introduced as a means of lowering STD risk. The workshop ends with a review of STD/HIV information.

The majority of activities in this session focused on defining and discussing facts evolved around AIDS, STDs, and HIV prevention strategies, the discussion of situations and behaviors that may increase women's HIV risk (douching, having older partners, gang involvement, and sexually degrading media exposures). This information was imperative in providing adolescents with the knowledge to prevent infection. Table 15.3 provides a detailed overview of the specific activities employed in Session 2.

One activity that exemplifies how the message of protecting ones' self from STDs and HIV was integrated into Session 2 is Activity L, *Introducing OPRaH*.

Table 15.3   Themes and Activities in Session 2

	Theme	*Description*
Session 2: It's my body		
Activity A	Greeting and Icebreaker	Greets participants and reinforces group bonds
Activity B	Motto	Recites and reinforces the SiHLE motto
Activity C	Call Me Black Woman	Reinforces the concept that SiHLE Sistas are beautiful women with a strong rich heritage by reading and discussing poetry written by an African American artist
Activity D	Share Your Thought Works	Reviews the SiHLE Sistas personal values and future goals and reinforce their importance in decision making
Activity E	SiHLE Sistas Are Special!	Reinforces and reexamines concepts taught in Session 1
Activity F	Speaking of STDs . . .	Teaches SiHLE Sistas about STDs and how having an STD affects pregnancy
Activity G	Card Swap Game	Illustrates to the SiHLE Sistas how HIV is spread by heterosexual contact and injection drug use
Activity H	HIV/AIDS What Every SiHLE Woman Should Know	Educates the SiHLE Sistas about what AIDS is, myths about AIDS, and how to protect yourself from AIDS
Activity I	R U at Risk?	Informs the SiHLE Sistas about sexual behaviors that reduce their chance of getting STDs, including HIV
Activity J	Consider This . . . The Penetrating Question	Evaluates how getting an STD including HIV could change the SiHLE Sistas values and goals
Activity K	Takin' Care of You!	Introduces the concept of responsibility by having women state how they care for themselves
Activity L	Introducing OPRaH	Refines women's knowledge of HIV/STD prevention
Activity M	SiHLE Jeopardy	Refines women's knowledge about HIV/STD transmission and prevention

Peer Educator: OPRaH consists of

Four simple steps—Open, Pinch, Roll, and Hold!

O = Open the package and remove rolled condom without twisting, biting, or using your fingernails. This could damage the condom and allow fluid to leak out.

P = Pinch the tip of the condom to squeeze the air out, leaving 1/4 to 1/2 inch of extra space at the top.

R = Roll condom down on penis as soon as the penis is hard, before you start to make love.

a = and after sex is over . . .

H = Hold the condom at the rim or base while partner pulls out after ejaculation but before the penis goes soft. You could lose protection if the condom comes off inside you.

Session 3

The third session, titled *SiHLE Skills,* addressed resisting partner pressures to engage in unsafe sex. Often, it is difficult for young women to make healthy choices about sex when they are not assertive during sexual encounters especially if their partner plays the dominant role in those encounters. Young women must assertively convey their sexual intentions and possess the skills to negotiate safer sex to make choices for a healthier lifestyle. While males and females are both responsible for safer sex, the responsibility often falls on the female partner, because males do not always practice safer sex and young women bear the disproportionate burden of adverse health outcomes. Previous sessions focused on the fact that females can protect themselves from engaging in unsafe sex.

However, this session provided the young women with the skills to properly use condoms and refuse risky sex. Through role-plays, women also learned how to eroticize condom use to develop their positive attitudes toward using condoms and to enhance their male partner's acceptance of condom use. The group facilitators were especially crucial in this session as they created a norm as it relates to females putting condoms on their male partners. Additionally, this activity led into a group discussion on how a woman's ability to apply a condom tends to reduce their perceived barrier to using condoms for HIV/STD prevention. Role-plays were also used to model assertive communication. These role-plays were designed as a hierarchical gradient, first in nonsexual scenarios and then in progressively more sexual situations. As the women actively participated in role-plays focusing on assertive communication, they were able to increase their communicative self-efficacy as well as develop new strategies for handling emotions that often accompany difficult conversations with romantic partners. Facilitators provided positive reinforcing feedback for role-plays that used assertive communication and corrective feedback for role-plays that did not use assertive communication. They also provided positive reinforcing feedback for demonstrations of correct condom use. Table 15.4 provides a detailed overview of the specific activities employed in Session 3.

One activity that is highly representative of the strong emphasis on skill development throughout Session 3 is Activity I, *Talking the Talk.*

Peer Educator:

Scenario: Andre and Tijuana

Tijuana has been attending a woman's group called SiHLE. She has learned a lot about being a strong black woman who has a right to realize her dreams and goals. She

Table 15.4   Themes and Activities in Session 3

	Theme	*Description*
Session 3: SiHLE skills		
Activity A	Greeting and Icebreaker	Greet one another, reinforce the message of timeliness, and enhance group bonds
Activity B	Motto	Reads and reinforces the SiHLE motto
Activity C	Phenomenal Woman	Refines the SiHLE Sistas sense of beauty, self-worth, and pride
Activity D	Luv and Kisses	Enhances the SiHLE Sistas knowledge about what sexual behaviors place women at risk for HIV/STD infection
Activity E	What's in It for You	Increases the SiHLE Sistas knowledge about HIV/STD prevention
Activity F	Why Don't People Use Condoms?	Introduces the SiHLE Sistas to some common reasons why young women don't use condoms and to reintroduce the concept of sexual responsibility for using condoms
Activity G	KISS—Keep it Simple Sista!	Teaches the SiHLE Sistas a model to assist them in asking their sex partner(s) to use condoms
Activity H	Three Ways to Say It	Teaches the SiHLE Sistas to distinguish between passive, assertive, and aggressive communication styles
Activity I	Talking the Talk	Teaches the SiHLE Sistas the difference between passive, aggressive, and assertive communication styles by having them model in sexual scenarios, both verbally and through body language, these communication styles
Activity J	OPRaH "Rehearsal"	Teaches the SiHLE Sistas the steps for proper condom use
Activity K	Alcohol and Sex—Not a Good Mix	Teaches the SiHLE Sistas the importance of avoiding alcohol prior to and during sex
Activity L	Condom Consumer Report	Teaches the SiHLE Sistas the importance of examining the condom for safety, personal appeal, and ease of application
Activity M	Thought Works Assignment	Reviews the concepts taught in today's session

has learned an important way to stay healthy—a simple way to prevent STDs, HIV, and unplanned pregnancy. She has made the decision to use condoms EVERY time they have sex.

Role-play Tijuana's talk with Andre. Make sure that you use an assertive style of communication. Pay particular attention to both, your body language and your verbal language! Make sure they are clear, consistent, and unambiguous.

Session 4

The fourth session, titled *Relationship and Power*, was designed to encourage women to take ownership of their bodies by informing them that their partner's decisions and choices regarding their bodies should be second to their own decision and choice. The session commenced by distinguishing healthy from unhealthy relationships and defining the words *abuse* and *respect*. Adolescents were taught that the lack of recognition by other people is viewed as disrespectful and abusive. Subsequently, adolescents were taught coping skills to more effectively handle a verbally abusive or physically abusive partner. Participants were also taught coping skills to more effectively handle abuse that may occur as a consequence of introducing HIV/STD prevention practices (i.e., condom use) into the relationship. The majority of activities in the fourth session were designed to address and breakdown the power imbalance often present in sexual heterosexual dyadic relationships. Defining healthy and unhealthy relationships, discussing local community resources for participants who are in unhealthy relationships, and explaining the relationship between having an unhealthy partner, HIV/STD risk taking, and HIV/STD acquisition were all activities employed that enabled the participants to act on or to change their own relationships. Table 15.5 provides a detailed

overview of the specific activities employed in Session 4.

One activity that exemplifies the emphasis on relationships and power in Session 4 is Activity E, *What Do Healthy and Unhealthy Relationships Look Like?*

Peer Educator: When you are in a healthy relationship, it is easier to negotiate with your male partner to use a condom EVERY time you have sex. Let's look at why this is true.

First, let's talk about what a healthy relationship is. A group of SiHLE women like you were asked to describe a healthy relationship. The following characteristics and attributes are what they identified as important in a healthy relationship.

POWER is balanced

No one has an unfair advantage over the other

COMMUNICATION is good

Both partners talk and listen

RESPECT is real

For oneself and one another

TRUST is strong

Feeling safe both physically and emotionally with one another

When you are in an unhealthy relationship, it is more difficult to negotiate with your male partner to use a condom EVERY time you have sex. Let's look at why this is true. First, let's talk about and describe an unhealthy relationship.

POWER is not balanced

One partner has an unfair advantage over the other

Table 15.5   Themes and Activities in Session 4

	Theme	*Description*
Session 4: Relationship and Power		
Activity A	Greeting	Greet one another, reinforce and practice assertive communication skills
Activity B	Motto	Reads and reinforces the SiHLE motto
Activity C	Poem: Still I Rise	Enhances the self-confidence and pride among the SiHLE Sistas by reciting poetry written by African American women
Activity D	What Have We Learned?	Refines the women's knowledge about HIV/STD transmission and prevention
Activity E	What Do Healthy and Unhealthy Relationships Look Like?	Discusses the influence of power, communication, respect, and trust on relationships
Activity F	Pieces and Parts	Raises women's awareness about healthy and unhealthy relationships
Activity G	What Does Abuse Look Like?	Increases women's knowledge about verbal, emotional, physical, and sexual abuse
Activity H	The Power Pie	Discusses how imbalances of power within a relationship can make it difficult to practice safer sex
Activity I	Your Options	Discusses a woman's options for safety and counseling if she is concerned about her relationship
Activity J	Your Time to Shine	Refines and enhances the women's safer sex knowledge and safer relationship knowledge and skills by conducting role reversal activities
Activity K	Graduation	Acknowledges appreciation of the SiHLE Sistas for participating in the SiHLE program by giving them certificates of empowerment and having a graduation exercise

COMMUNICATION is not good

Both partners don't talk and listen to each other

RESPECT is not real

For oneself and one another

TRUST is not strong

Not feeling safe both, physically and emotionally, with one another

ASSESSING THE EFFICACY OF THE SIHLE INTERVENTION

To assess the effectiveness of the SiHLE HIV intervention on reducing risk-associated behaviors, data collection occurred at baseline (i.e., before the participants were randomly assigned to either the SiHLE intervention or a time-equivalent general health promotion comparison condition), as well as 6 and 12 months after participating in either the SiHLE or general health promotion intervention. At each assessment, data were obtained from four sources. First, participants completed a self-administered questionnaire assessing socio-demographics and psychosocial mediators of HIV-preventive behaviors. Subsequently, a trained African American female interviewer administered an interview assessing sexual behaviors. Next, the interviewer assessed participants' ability to correctly apply condoms using a direct observation of skills assessment protocol. Finally, participants provided two self-collected vaginal swab specimens that were analyzed for the presence of three STDs: chlamydia, trichomonasis, and gonorrhea.

Effects of the HIV Intervention

Relative to participants in the general health promotion condition, participants in the SiHLE intervention condition were more likely to report using condoms consistently in the 30 days preceding the 6-month assessment (Intervention = 75.3% vs. Comparison = 58.2%) and at the 12-month assessment (Intervention = 73.3% vs. Comparison = 56.5%). Likewise, participants in the SiHLE intervention were more likely to report using condoms consistently during the 6 months prior to the 6-month assessment (Intervention = 61.3% vs. Comparison = 42.6%) and the 12-month assessment (Intervention = 58.1% vs. Comparison = 45.3%). Additionally, participants in the SiHLE intervention were more likely to report using a condom at last vaginal sexual intercourse, less likely to self-report a pregnancy, and less likely to report having a new male sex partner in the 30 days prior to the follow-up assessments. Importantly, this was the first intervention to demonstrate effectiveness in reducing new chlamydia infections in the SiHLE intervention group participants over the entire 12-month follow-up period (see DiClemente et al., 2004, for a detailed description of the findings).

The SiHLE intervention also had strong effects on empirically and theoretically derived psychosocial mediators of HIV-preventive behaviors. In general, participants in the SiHLE intervention reported fewer perceived partner-related barriers to condom use, more favorable attitudes toward using condoms, more frequent discussions with male sex partners about HIV prevention, higher condom use self-efficacy scores, higher HIV prevention knowledge scores, and demonstrated greater proficiency in using condoms at the 6- and the 12-month assessments and over the entire 12-month period.

While other studies have shown that self-reported sexual risk behaviors can be reduced in adolescents, this is the first trial demonstrating that an HIV intervention can result in substantial reductions in sexual risk behaviors, including the acquisition of a new male sex partner, and markedly enhance theoretically important mediators and skills associated with HIV preventive behaviors among sexually experienced African American adolescent females. Given that STDs, particularly chlamydia, are prevalent among adolescents (Weinstock, Berman, & Cates, 2004) and facilitate HIV transmission (Fleming & Wasserheit, 1999; Wasserheit, 1992), even small reductions in incidence could result in considerable reductions in treatment costs as well as sizeable reductions in HIV morbidity (Bozzette et al., 2001) and their associated treatment costs (Chesson, Blandford, Gift, Tao, & Irwin, 2000). This is particularly important in light of findings from mathematical modeling studies suggesting that reductions in incident chlamydia infections may be one of the most promising surrogate markers for HIV incidence in prevention trials (Pinkerton & Layde, 2002).

CHAPTER SUMMARY

This chapter has highlighted the public health problem created by increased rates of STDs and HIV in adolescents, especially in African American adolescent females. This disproportionate burden necessitates the urgent design and implementation of gender- and culturally tailored STD/HIV risk-reduction interventions specifically targeting this particularly vulnerable subpopulation of adolescents. Thus, the main focus of the current chapter was to provide a detailed description of, to our knowledge, the only demonstrated effective HIV intervention specifically designed for sexually active African American adolescent females.

Several characteristics of the SiHLE program may have attributed to the efficacy of the intervention in reducing risk-associated behaviors in African American adolescent females. First, the utilization of SCT, which provided a theoretical framework for developing the skills training components of the SiHLE intervention, in addition to the Theory of Gender and Power, which was employed to address the role of contextual and sociocultural variables, such as gender, class, and ethnicity and their influence on adolescent females sexual behavior, was a successful combination that broadened the scope of the intervention beyond the individual.

Related to this, the efficacy of the SiHLE intervention may be attributable partly to the gender-tailored and culturally appropriate framework that highlighted the underlying social processes, such as the dyadic nature of sexual interactions, and relationship power and emotional commitment that may promote and reinforce risk behaviors. Conceptualizing HIV prevention within the broader context of a healthy relationship also marshaled new intervention strategies and offered new options for creating STD/HIV-preventive behavior change. Additionally, the thematic focus of the intervention, *"Stay Safe for Yourself, Your Family, and Your Community,"* was designed to promote a sense of solidarity and ethnic pride among participants, and may have inspired them to modify risk behaviors for altruistic motives; by enhancing their

health, they were also enhancing the health of their family and the broader African American community.

Finally, the role of the facilitator is vital to the overall success of the program, and ultimately the young ladies making healthy changes in their lives. Therefore, having the SiHLE intervention implemented by a trained and experienced African American female health educator and African American female peer educators as cofacilitators was likely a factor contributing to the efficacy of the intervention. Employing health educators and peer educators matched to the participants' gender and race was instrumental in modeling social and technical competency skills, and creating a group norm supportive of HIV/STD prevention.

In the current era of HIV prevention, there is a need to prioritize designing STD/HIV prevention programs for adolescents who are developmentally, culturally, and gender appropriate. As the SiHLE intervention illustrates, it is possible to develop programs that address contextual factors or conditions that confer significant vulnerability for young women's risk of HIV/STD (i.e., age, ethnicity, and risk behaviors). Encouragingly, empirical data suggest that the greater the specificity between the HIV prevention intervention and the contextual factors prevalent among a target population, the greater the likelihood the program will be effective in reducing HIV risk (Wingood & DiClemente, 2006). Combining the three aforementioned features (theoretical frameworks that expand the scope of the intervention to include broader contextual and social variables, specificity of content tailored to the gender and culture of the participants, and employing trained, matched-to-sample health educators to implement the intervention) in the SiHLE intervention, optimally enhanced the specificity between the HIV intervention and directly addressed, through diverse learning strategies, contextual factors that enhanced participants' risk for STDs and HIV. Undoubtedly, this targeted and tailored approached significantly contributed to the overall success of the SiHLE intervention.

In conclusion, as the need for effective STD/HIV risk-reduction interventions for adolescents remains high, we as clinicians, practitioners, and prevention researchers working with America's youth need to continue to strive to meet the needs of the population we serve. As suggested by this chapter, acknowledging that adolescents are not a homogeneous group, but rather a heterogeneous population, is a critical first step in designing effective risk-reduction interventions tailored for diverse at-risk adolescent subgroups.

DISCUSSION QUESTIONS

1. How was the SiHLE intervention designed to be culturally appropriate?

2. How was the intervention designed to address the theoretical constructs of the Theory of Gender and Power?

3. How was the intervention designed to address the theoretical constructs associated with SCT?

4. What epidemiologic data should be used for legitimately identifying and illustrating African American female adolescents' risk of HIV in your community?

5. Why are the findings of the SiHLE HIV prevention intervention important for public health practice?

REFERENCES

Bandura, A. (1992). A social cognitive approach to the exercise of control over AIDS infection. In R. J. DiClemente (Ed.), *Adolescents and AIDS: A generation in jeopardy* (pp. 89–116). Newbury Park, CA: Sage.

Bandura, A. (1994). Social cognitive theory and exercise of control over HIV infections. In R. J. DiClemente & J. Petersons (Eds.), *Preventing AIDS: Theories and methods of behavioral interventions* (pp. 25–29). New York: Plenum Press.

Bauer, H. M., Ting, Y., Greer, C. E., Chambers, J. C., Tashiro, C. J., Chimera, J., et al. (1991). Genital human papillomavirus infection in female university students as determined by a PCR-based method. *Journal of the American Medical Association, 265*(4), 472–477.

Boyer, C. B., Shafer, M., & Tschann, J. M. (1997). Evaluation of a knowledge-and-cognitive-behavioral skills-building intervention to prevent STDs and HIV infection in high school students. *Adolescence, 32*(125), 25–42.

Bozzette, S. A., Joyce, G., McCaffrey, D. F., Leibowitz, A. A., Morton, S. C., Berry, S. H., et al. (2001). Expenditures for the care of HIV-infected patients in the era of highly active antiretroviral therapy. *New England Journal of Medicine, 344*(11), 817–823.

Burk, R., Ho, G., Beardsley, L., Lempa, M., Peters, M., & Bierman, R. (1996). Sexual behavior and partner characteristics are the predominant factors for genital human papillomavirus infection in young women. *Journal of Infectious Diseases, 174*(4) 679–689.

Cates, W. (1999). Estimates of the incidence and prevalence of sexually transmitted diseases in the United States. *Sexually Transmitted Diseases, 26*(4), s2–s7.

Centers for Disease Control and Prevention. (2000). *Tracking the hidden epidemics: Trends in STDs in the United States.* Atlanta, GA: U.S. Department of Health and Human Services, Public Health Service.

Centers for Disease Control and Prevention. (2001). *Sexually transmitted disease surveillance, 2000.* Atlanta, GA: U.S. Department of Health and Human Services.

Centers for Disease Control and Prevention. (2002a). Trends in sexual risk behaviors among high school students—United States, 1991–2001. *Morbidity and Mortality Weekly Report, 51,* 856–862.

Centers for Disease Control and Prevention. (2002b). *Young people at risk: HIV/AIDS among America's youth.* Retrieved November 16, 2004, from www.cdc.gov/hiv/pubs/facts/youth.htm

Centers for Disease Control and Prevention. (2002c). *Sexually transmitted disease surveillance, 2001.* Atlanta, GA: U.S. Department of Health and Human Services.

Centers for Disease Control and Prevention. (2003, July 8). *Young people at risk: HIV/AIDS among America's youth* [Fact sheet]. Atlanta, GA: CDC-NCHSTP-Divisions of HIV/AIDS Prevention.

Centers for Disease Control and Prevention. (2004). Chlamydia screening among sexually active young female enrollees of health plans—United States, 1999–2001. *Morbidity and Mortality Weekly Report, 53,* 983–985.

Chesson, H. W., Blandford, J. M., Gift, T. L., Tao, G., & Irwin, K. L. (2000). The estimated direct medical cost of sexually transmitted diseases among American youth, 2000. *Perspectives on Sexual and Reproductive Health, 36,* 11–19.

Coyle, K., Basen-Engquist, K., Kirby, D., Parcel, G., Banspach, S., Harrist, R., et al. (1999). Short-term impact of safer choices: A multicomponent, school-based HIV, other STD, and pregnancy prevention program. *Journal of School Health, 69*(5), 181–188.

DiClemente, R. J. (1990). The emergence of adolescents as a risk group for human immunodeficiency virus infection. *Journal of Adolescent Research, 5,* 7–17.

DiClemente, R. J. (1996). Adolescents at-risk for acquired immune deficiency syndrome: Epidemiology of AIDS, HIV prevalence and HIV incidence. In S. Oskamp & S. Thompson (Eds.), *Understanding and preventing HIV risk behavior* (pp. 13–30). Thousand Oaks, CA: Sage.

DiClemente, R. J., & Crosby, R. A. (2003). Sexually transmitted diseases among adolescents: Risk factors, antecedents, and prevention strategies. In G. R. Adams & M. Berzonsky (Eds.), *The Blackwell handbook of adolescence* (pp. 573–605). Oxford, UK: Blackwell.

DiClemente, R. J., & Wingood, G. M. (1995). A randomized controlled trail of an HIV sexual risk-reduction intervention for young African-American women. *Journal of the American Medical Association, 274,* 1271–1276.

DiClemente, R. J., Wingood, G. M., Harrington, K. F., Lang, D. F., Davies, S. L., Hook, E. W., et al. (2004). Efficacy of an HIV prevention intervention for African American adolescent girls: A randomized controlled trial. *Journal of the American Medical Association, 292*(2), 171–179.

Ellen, J. M. (2003). The next generation of HIV prevention for adolescent females in the United States: Linking behavioral and epidemiological sciences to reduce incidence of HIV. *Journal of Urban Health, 80,* 40–49.

Ellen, J., Aral, S., & Madger, L. (1998). Do differences in sexual behaviors account for the racial/ethnic differences in adolescents' self-reported history of a sexually transmitted disease? *Sexually Transmitted Diseases, 25,* 125–129.

Eng, T., & Butler W. (Eds.). (1997). *The hidden epidemic: Confronting sexually transmitted diseases.* Washington, DC: National Academy Press.

Fleming, D. T., & Wasserheit, J. N. (1999). From epidemiological synergy to public health policy and practice: The contribution of other sexually transmitted diseases to sexual transmission of HIV infection. *Sexually Transmitted Infections, 75,* 3–17.

Grunbaum, J., Kann, L., Kinchen, S., Ross, J., Hawkins, J., Lowry, R., et al. (2004). Youth risk behavior surveillance—United States (2003). *Morbidity and Mortality Weekly Report, 53,* 1–95.

Jemmott, J. B., & Jemmott, L. S. (2000). HIV behavioral interventions for adolescents in community settings. In J. L. Peterson & R. J. DiClemente (Eds.), *Handbook of HIV prevention* (pp. 103–128). New York: Plenum Press.

Jemmott, J. B., III, Jemmott, L. S., & Fong, G. T. (1998). Abstinence and safer sex HIV risk-reduction interventions for African American adolescents: A randomized controlled trial. *Journal of the American Medical Association, 279,* 1529–1536.

Kahn, L., Kinchen, S., Williams, B., Ross, J. G., Lowry, R., Grunbaum, J. A., et al. (2000). Youth risk behavior surveillance—United States. *Morbidity and Mortality Weekly Report, 49*(SS–05), 1–96.

Main, D. S., Iverson, D. C., McGloin, J., Banspach, S. W., Collins, J. L., Rugg, D. L. et al. (1994). Preventing HIV infection among adolescents: Evaluation of a school-based education program. *Preventive Medicine, 23,* 409–417.

Meschke, S., Bartholomae, S., & Zentall, S. (2000). Adolescent sexuality and parent-adolescent processes: Promoting health teen choices. *Family Relations, 49,* 143–154.

Mullen, P. D., Ramirez, G., Strouse, D., Hedges, L. V., & Sogolow, E. (2002). Meta-analysis of the effects of behavioral HIV prevention interventions on the sexual risk behavior of sexually experienced adolescents in controlled studies in the United States. *Journal of Acquired Immune Deficiency Syndromes, 30,* S94–S105.

National Institute of Allergy and Infectious Diseases. (1997). *Sexually transmitted diseases statistics.* Washington, DC: U.S. Department of Health and Human Services.

Office of National AIDS Policy. (1996). *Youth and HIV/AIDS: An American agenda.* Washington, DC: Author.

Pinkerton, S. D., & Layde, P. M. (2002). Using sexually transmitted disease incidence as a surrogate marker for HIV incidence in prevention trial. *Sexually Transmitted Diseases, 29,* 298–307.

Shain, R. N., Piper, J. M., Newton, E. R., Perdue, S. T., Ramos, R., Chapion, J. D., et al. (1999). A randomized, controlled trial of a behavioral intervention to prevent sexually transmitted disease among minority women. *New England Journal of Medicine, 320*(2), 93–100.

Shrier, L. A., Ancheta, R., Goodman, E., Chiou, V. M., Lyden, M. R., & Emans, S. J. (2001). Randomized controlled trial of a safer sex intervention for high-risk adolescent girls. *Archives of Pediatrics and Adolescent Medicine, 155*(1), 73–79.

St. Lawrence, J. S., Brasfield, T. L., Jefferson, K. W., Alleyne, E., O'Bannon, R. E. I., & Shirley, A. (1995). Cognitive-behavioral intervention to reduce African American adolescents' risk for HIV infection. *Journal of Consulting and Clinical Psychology, 63*(2), 221–237.

Stanton, B. F., Li, X., Ricardo, I., Galbraith, J., Feigelman, S., & Kaljee, L. (1996). A randomized, controlled effectiveness trial of an AIDS prevention program for low-income African American youths. *Archives of Pediatrics and Adolescent Medicine, 150,* 363–372.

Valleroy, L., MacKellar, D., Karon, J., Janssen, R., & Hayman, C. (1998). HIV infection in disadvantaged out-of school youth: Prevalence for US Job Corps entrants, 1990 through 1996. *Journal of Acquired Immune Deficiency Syndromes and Human Retrovirology, 19,* 67–73.

Walsh, C., & Irwin, K. (2002). Combating the silent Chlamydia epidemic. *Contemporary OB/GYN, 47*(4), 90–98.

Wasserheit, J. N. (1992). Epidemiological synergy: Interrelationship between human immunodeficiency virus infection and other sexually transmitted diseases. *Sexually Transmitted Diseases, 19,* 61–77.

Weinstock, H., Berman, S., & Cates, W. (2004). Sexually transmitted diseases in American youth: Incidence and prevalence estimates. *Perspectives on Sexual and Reproductive Health, 36,* 6–10.

Wingood, G. M., & DiClemente, R. J. (2000). Application of the theory of gender and power to examine HIV related exposures, risk factors and effective interventions for women. *Health Education and Behavior, 27,* 313–347.

Wingood, G. M., & DiClemente, R. J. (2006). Enhancing diffusion of HIV interventions: Development of a suite of effective HIV prevention programs for women. *AIDS Education and Prevention, 18*(Suppl. A), 161–171.

16

Tips for Working With Black American Populations

ROBERT M. HUFF

MICHAEL V. KLINE

The term *African American* often is used to label black populations that represent a wide diversity of ethnic and cultural backgrounds. Many of these peoples do not perceive or identify themselves as African American. That is, they may identify with Haitian, British, Brazilian, or any number of other cultural or ethnic groups (Hopp & Herring, 1999). As Hopp and Herring also observed, new immigrants who have not acculturated into the mainstream culture of the United States might not identify with American-born blacks, nor will they necessarily identify with those who are descended from the slaves who were brought into the United States early in its history. Thus, it is important to recognize that, like other cultural groups described in this book, one cannot conveniently place everyone into the one broad category of "African American" without first noting that this is being done with the knowledge that the term is not necessarily an accurate representation of the group being discussed. The caveat to the reader is to determine the particular term(s) the target group uses to describe itself and how that group's cultural characteristics, including its history, immigration patterns, acculturation and assimilation levels, socioeconomic status, and generational and other related factors, are similar to or different from those of the mainstream culture before launching into a major needs assessment and other planning activities.

This brief "tips" chapter draws from the three preceding chapters (i.e., Chapters 13–15) as well as from a number of other sources (Chapters 1 and 2, this volume; Hopp & Herring, 1999; Locks & Boateng, 1996; Willis, 1992) and is only a beginning list of suggestions and recommendations for working with this large and very diverse group of people.

CULTURAL COMPETENCE

Anyone involved in the delivery of health promotion and disease prevention (HPDP) programs and services needs to develop cultural competence and sensitivity to the differences between themselves and the multicultural group with which they will be working. This is no less true for those working with groups broadly classified as "African American," "black," or any other term reflecting this particular population grouping. Thus, the health promoter is encouraged to consider the following suggestions related to cultural competence:

- Research the history of the target group to be involved in the HPDP program or service and seek to become familiar with its members' cultural values, beliefs, and ways of life as a people living in the United States.
- Remember that there is a great diversity of backgrounds and countries of origin for this population group and that this also means there is likely to be a significant diversity of beliefs and practices different from those of the individuals planning the HPDP intervention or service.
- Examine your own perceptions, stereotypes, and prejudices toward the target group and be willing to suspend judgments, where they exist, in favor of learning who these people really are instead of who you might think they are. This is one of the most important steps you can take toward cultural competence and sensitivity.
- Take the time to make multiple visits to the community where the target group lives. Talk with community leaders and members, visit important sites within the community, eat at local restaurants, attend local events, and otherwise become familiar with the community's way of life.
- Seek to establish early and continuing support from the community for any HPDP programs and services that are to be offered.
- Recognize that there is a healthy suspicion in some black communities about programs and services coming from existing health institutions both inside and outside the community. This might be the result of having a history with institutions that sought to offer intervention programs and services, research projects, or other types of programs and services that did not continue after the funding ran out and everyone left.
- Be aware that just because an individual from an institution or agency might be of the same ethnic group as the community, it does not necessarily guarantee that person entry into or trust from the community. Having been trained outside the community might place that person into an outsider frame, and the individual will need to demonstrate his or her sincerity and true interest in helping the community deal with its particular needs and concerns.

HEALTH BELIEFS AND PRACTICES

There are a wide variety of health beliefs and practices that characterize this broad multicultural population group, and the need to assess what these beliefs and practices are early in the intervention planning process cannot be stressed enough. The health promoter is encouraged once again to review the history of the target group, speak to the formal and informal leaders in the community about their perceptions of the health beliefs and practices of the community, and work to suspend their judgments about these. Not doing so might lead to conflict and to a failure of the program or service to achieve the goals and objectives it has set for and with the community. Thus, the health promoter should consider the following tips:

- Identify and seek to understand the explanatory models that the individuals within the community use to make sense of and deal with threats to their personal health and well-being.
- Expect that there will be a variety of explanatory models that are employed across this broad multicultural population group, ranging from very traditional folk health beliefs and practices to those reflective of the current biomedical model.

- Where differences exist between the explanatory models of the target group and your explanatory models, make efforts to ameliorate or otherwise find ways to work within these different frames of reference and perception.
- Consider becoming more familiar with traditional healing practices where these are prevalent in the community, because this may provide opportunities to bring beneficial practices into the biomedical framework while also modifying those practices that can potentially be harmful.
- Be aware that variations in health beliefs and practices can be attributed to a variety of variables, including socioeconomic status, education, area of residence, access to health care services, health insurance, and other related factors.
- Recognize that the use of traditional folk healing practices can be linked to a number of factors, including ease of access to traditional healers and medicines within the community, their cultural acceptability, and their expense (which often is far less than what is charged in the Western biomedical system).
- Remember that traditional folk healers sometimes are the first and only health practitioners used by low-income blacks for all the reasons that have been cited earlier in this discussion.
- Remember that traditional explanations for illness and disease often fall into two general categories: *natural causes* (including cold, stress, and improper eating or lack of moderation in one's daily life) and *unnatural causes* (resulting from witchcraft practices including voodoo, hoodoo, bad spirits, and other works of the devil).
- Be aware that, in general, the Western biomedical system is highly respected and used for serious medical problems, although folk healing traditions also may be employed.

PROGRAM PLANNING CONSIDERATIONS

Program planning for HPDP is a systematic, all-encompassing process whose aim is to create highly effective, well-structured and implemented

interventions for promoting change of health-damaging behaviors to more positive health-promoting behaviors within individuals, small groups, communities, and the larger society (Chapter 7, this volume). Keeping in mind the basic program-planning considerations espoused by the many contributors to this book, the following suggestions and recommendations also should be considered by the health promoter:

- The community must be involved in every aspect of the program-planning process, from needs assessment through evaluation.
- It is very important to begin developing positive alliances with the leadership of the community as you consider developing HPDP programs and services for the community.
- Be sure that HPDP programs and services reflect the values, beliefs, and interests of the community in which they are targeted.
- Review all previous HPDP program efforts in the community to identify potential community resources and assets, interventions that have been found to enhance or impede the successful adaptation of programs in the community, and any other factors that might play a role in the new program or service to be developed.
- Be sure that the goals, objectives, and interventions of the HPDP program or service reflect the felt needs of the target group. Where community needs and interests do not meet this criterion, consider developing strategies to increase awareness of those less well-known issues that might exist prior to launching a full-blown program that is not considered important by the community.
- Be aware that the employment of an indigenous model for planning and carrying out an HPDP program or service in the community has been found to be an extremely effective approach for delivering high-quality programs to the community.

NEEDS ASSESSMENT CONSIDERATIONS

Well-designed and conducted needs assessment processes can provide a strong baseline for understanding the health and other social needs of a community. The process should be rigorous and should consider not only the usual targets of assessment (i.e., morbidity and mortality rates, demographics) but also the cultural factors that can affect the successful implementation of an HPDP program or service. The reader is encouraged to review the Cultural Assessment Framework presented in Chapter 6 (this volume) as well as the following suggestions as he or she prepares assessment instruments and methodologies:

- Be aware that no matter what planning model is employed, it is essential that a cultural assessment be included with the other data gathered in the baseline study of the target group.
- Needs assessment instruments need to reflect the linguistic, literacy, and cultural symbols and values of the community.
- Standardized needs assessment instruments designed for the mainstream culture often have little meaning in black communities. Thus, instruments will need to be shaped to reflect the community in which they are to be administered.
- Consider including acculturation measures in the community assessment process.
- Where possible, seek to involve community members in identifying key informants who can speak to the real and felt needs of the community, including the resources that might be available in the community to support HPDP activities.
- Be aware that key informants may not always know what the issues are in the community or might be operating with their own agendas in mind. Thus, always seek to triangulate the data that are gathered from those who are involved as key informants, using focus group data and other data gathered as a part of the baseline assessment of the community.
- Be sure to include assessment of the media resources and channels that are used by members of the community, because these might play an important role in the marketing of the program or service developed by community representatives and yourself.

- Recognize that the PRECEDE model can be a useful framework for identifying and describing health behaviors with respect to their predisposing, enabling, and reinforcing factors and can help point the way toward the design of interventions that accurately target the factors most amenable to change.
- Seek to involve community members in the actual conduct of needs assessment activities, because this can help foster involvement and ownership of the program or service to be developed.
- Be sure that assessment and evaluation efforts reflect the needs, interests, and values of the stakeholders within the community.

INTERVENTION CONSIDERATIONS

The design of well-planned and culturally appropriate interventions is critical to the success of any HPDP program or service offered in a community. *Cultural tailoring* encourages the planner to design intervention strategies, methods, and materials to the specific cultural characteristics of the target group and should be an integral component of the design process (Pasick, D'Onofrio, & Otero-Sabogal, 1996). With these ideas in mind, the health promoter also might wish to consider the following additional comments and suggestions as they begin the intervention phase of his or her work:

- Recognize that "one size fits all" is not a useful approach to intervention design. A program needs to be tailored to the target group for which it is intended.
- Be aware that the most effective HPDP interventions are built on the community's strengths, resources, and assets, all of which serve to foster community ownership and involvement with the HPDP program or service being developed.
- Be aware that intervention design needs to include significant involvement from the target group whose members will be the recipients of the program or service.
- Linguistic, literacy, gender relevance, and other cultural factors must be considered in

the design of the intervention to be carried out in the community.

- Recognize that using captive audiences and unconventional sites for an HPDP program or service can be a highly effective approach to reaching the community. These might include laundromats, social clubs, hair and nail salons, home parties, family reunions, and other locations and events likely to draw community members.

- Churches often have been used as sites for conducting HPDP programs, but you should be aware that these sites are not always the easiest to involve in HPDP efforts because many of them have their own causes, which may or may not have a health focus.

- If you are designing educational sessions for the community, then be aware that it is often difficult to get community members to attend such sessions, especially if they are multiple sessions. Taking the intervention to the community rather than having the community come to the intervention might be much more effective.

- Be aware that the use of peer educators from the community has been found to be a very effective method for delivering HPDP programs or services to the community.

- Intervention design should be theory based because these types of intervention designs have been found to be much more effective than those without that type of foundation.

- Consider the learning styles of the target group when designing interventions and seek to incorporate educational approaches that reflect these ways of learning within the target population.

- Development of educational materials must reflect the relevant cultural values, themes, and literacy levels of the target group for which they are intended.

- Recognize that developing partnerships with the local media can be an effective way in which to disseminate information about the HPDP program or service being planned and offered to the community.

- Seek to develop interventions that focus on positive health changes rather than those with negative or fear-arousing consequences.

EVALUATION CONSIDERATIONS

Evaluation is at the heart of all well-conceived HPDP programs and must be among the first considerations when planning an HPDP program or service. It begins with formative assessments to establish baseline information for building a program and continues through process, impact, and outcome evaluation to measure the success of the program or service in achieving its identified objectives. For this reason, the health promoter is encouraged to consider the following recommendations:

- Seek to develop evaluation strategies, methods, and instruments that reflect an understanding of current theory and practice in the evaluation and research literature.

- Recognize that evaluation and assessment are processes that frequently are difficult to gain support for, even in the most sophisticated of groups. Thus, an effort to explain the underlying assumptions governing these processes and the methods and anticipated outcomes of assessment and evaluation activities can serve to strengthen support and involvement of the community and planning group in these most important of activities.

- Be aware that providing evaluation and assessment training for the community can help foster support for and empower the community to become more actively involved in data collection efforts related to assessment and evaluation activities.

- Evaluation and assessment measures should be culturally relevant and tailored to the linguistic and educational capabilities of the target group.

- Evaluation must consider the needs and interests of stakeholders in both the community and the agency providing the HPDP program or service.

- Evaluation processes must include the participation of the community, and the criteria for evaluation should be sought from the community because its members are the ones who know what is important to them.

- Recognize that HPDP program participants might have limited test-taking skills or abilities. Thus, efforts to design evaluation methods should reflect these potentialities by seeking approaches that are within the relevant experiences of the target group whenever possible.

- Be sure to design evaluation and assessment reporting and feedback mechanisms to ensure that the target community is regularly made aware of how well the program is functioning to improve the health issues or problems for which it was designed.

The next section of the book considers the American Indian and Alaska Native population groups. This section includes three chapters followed by a customized "tips" chapter. The first chapter in this section presents an overview devoted to understanding this special population from a variety of perspectives and includes terms used to define the subgroups within the broader population, historical and demographic characteristics, immigration patterns, health and disease issues and concerns, and health beliefs and practices. The second chapter of the section is concerned with how to assess, plan, implement, and evaluate programs for American Indian/Alaska Native groups, including tips, models, and suggestions for more effective program design. The third chapter in this section presents a case study to emphasize points made in the overview and planning chapters. This section begins with Chapter 17.

REFERENCES

Hopp, J. W., & Herring, P. (1999). Promoting health among Black American populations: An overview. In R. M. Huff & M. V. Kline (Eds.), *Promoting health in multicultural populations* (pp. 201–221). Thousand Oaks, CA: Sage.

Locks, S., & Boateng, L. (1996). Black/African Americans. In J. G. Lipson, S. L. Dibble, & P. A. Minarik (Eds.), *Culture and nursing care: A pocket guide* (pp. 37–43). San Francisco: UCSF Nursing Press.

Pasick, R. J., D'Onofrio, C. N., & Otero-Sabogal, R. (1996). Similarities and differences across cultures: Questions to inform a third generation for health promotion research. *Health Education Quarterly*, 23(Suppl.), S142–S161.

Willis, W. (1992). Families with African American roots. In E. W. Lynch & M. J. Hanson (Eds.), *Developing cross-cultural competence: A guide to working with young children and their families* (pp. 121–150). Baltimore: Paul H. Brookes.

PART IV

American Indian and Alaska Native Populations

17

Health and Disease of American Indian and Alaska Native Populations

An Overview

FELICIA SCHANCHE HODGE

SARA RODRIGUEZ'G

CHRISTOPHER ELLIOTT HODGE

Chapter Objectives

On completion of this chapter, the health promotion student and practitioner will be able to

- Discuss the issues that make the search for a single name to describe Native peoples in North America a problem

- Discuss at least three sociodemographic issues that affect American Indian and Alaska Native (AI/AN) communities

- Describe the three most prevalent health issues and their associated health-damaging behaviors affecting AI/AN communities today

- List and discuss at least three barriers to health promotion and disease prevention (HPDP) in AI/AN communities

This chapter provides an overview of American Indian and Alaska Native (AI/AN) populations for those who are interested in the broad brushstroke of issues, concerns, and basic understandings of the terminology, geographic diversity, historical perspectives, as well as health and disease issues. Such an overview provides a much needed basic grounding in the status of AI/AN that is necessary for research, education, program planning, and development.

A variety of terms have been used interchangeably for Native North Americans such as *Indian, American Indian, Native, aborigine, indigenous people, First Nation, First People,* and *First American.* The search for a single name, however, has not been successful. In the United States, the term *Native American* has been used but has fallen out of favor recently because anyone born in North or South America may claim to be a Native American. The term *American Indian* currently is in favor despite its misnomer; *Indian* still carries the stigma of being bestowed on tribal groups by European explorers in search of the Indian subcontinent of Asia. As such, the term fails to define the origin status of pre-Columbian American peoples. That the Inuit, Yupik, and Aleut peoples of Alaska consider themselves distinct from other indigenous North American peoples compromises the term *American Indian* even further, as these groups of Alaskan peoples do not wish to be called *Indian.* Thus, when generalizations of the entire group are necessary, it is preferred to use the term *American Indian* and *Alaska Native.*

Native peoples in the United States do not form a single ethnic group, and they always have resisted a homogeneous definition. They are better understood as thousands of distinct communities and cultures. Many AI/AN peoples have distinct languages, religious beliefs, ceremonies, and sociopolitical organizations. Characterizing this diverse array of cultures and peoples with one inclusive name reduces any effort to assess cultural development specific to time and place, encouraging common misunderstandings based on preconceived assumptions. In recognizing them by their specific tribal or community identities such as Apache, Hopi, or Cherokee, these peoples are distinguished from others in ways that they

themselves always have preferred. These tribal names usually mean "the people" or "the real people," in reference to themselves as set apart from the rest of the world. Such identifications more accurately capture the unique and varied tribal and cultural distinctions found among AI/AN peoples.

Culture areas, such as the sub-Arctic and the Southwest, are used to describe geographical areas in which several American Indian nations live and share a similar ecological environment and, hence, similar methods of food production, such as hunting and gathering or horticulture. Nevertheless, within a specific culture area, there may be several very different cultures and a multiplicity of languages and dialects—an example is in the Southwest, where the Navajo speak an Athabascan language and whereas the Zuni speak a Penntian language. Culture areas have been used by anthropologists primarily to reconstruct how Indians lived prior to Western contact after the year 1500. However, the manner in which AI/AN live today is more determined by political and economic relations with the United States than by the ecological environments of the precontact period. For example, Alaska and California are listed as separate cultural areas rather than as part of the sub-Arctic and West Coast because of their unique histories and relations with non-Indians. The following list of culture areas not only draws on the basic anthropological culture areas but also takes into account the people who live in the culture area; their cultural, social, and political histories; and major contemporary issues.

DIVERSITY OF SUBGROUPS

Northeastern Indians

The culture area defined as the Northeast is noted for its relative degree of cultural cohesiveness despite its wide variety of environmental and ecological conditions. The demographic settlement of contemporary Indian tribes in the Northeast is the result of intensified struggles for land brought about by the arrival of European settlers. Tribal displacement resulting from such struggle during the 16th and 17th centuries contributed to an unending cycle of dislocation and decline in Indian populations resulting from infectious diseases contracted from European immigrants. Continual contact with European explorers and settlers from 1497 onward had made it increasingly difficult for the Iroquois and Algonquian tribes to maintain land holdings and traditional means of support, that is, horticulture and hunting.

The culture area in the Northeast, then, is determined not only by Indian subjection to colonial law but also to changing economic environments such as the decline of the fur trade in the mid-19th century. Having had to abandon a subsistence economy for one based on trade, northeastern tribes had no alternative but to sell lands to meet their need for manufactured goods once those markets failed. Whereas coastal Indians such as the Algonquian found themselves subject to English colonial law in the 17th century, tribes such as the Iroquois were emulated by late-18th-century white Americans for their spirit of democracy and liberty. American Indian political custom, as such, played a constructive role in the very formation of the early American government as the colonies sought their independence from Britain.

Despite the peaceful assimilation of the Algonquian Indians into colonial coastal communities and the subsequent role the Iroquois fulfilled in forging the early American nation, American Indians suffered from both the loss of tribal lands and their vulnerability to European diseases throughout the 19th century. The reservation became the final refuge for those who had survived the processes of social and economic isolation well into the 20th century.

Southeastern Indians

The major tribes of the American Southeast are the Catawba, the Cherokee, the Creek, the Chickasaw, the Choctaw, and the Seminole. Their common territory is bounded by the Atlantic Ocean, the Gulf of Mexico, the Trinity River in present-day Texas, and the Ohio River. Southeastern Indian tribes share a widespread traditional culture known as Mississippian, a term referring to practices associated with the construction of ceremonial mounds central to the village and its cultivated fields of corn, beans, and squash.

Southeastern peoples shared a balanced economy centering on agriculture and supported by hunting wildlife. Such a subsistence-level economy had been kept in balance by spiritual beliefs and ritual practice. For example, hunting never exceeded actual food requirements, and killing itself was preceded by prayer to animal spirits. Excessive slaughter was commonly forbidden among tribal groups.

The spiritual values common to the Southeastern tribes center on the spirit of balance and harmony with other humans, the natural world, and the spirit world. All things had spirits, either good or evil, and success in life depended on the careful cultivation of these spirits. Just as European settlement uprooted the balance of American Indians in the Northeast, tribal cultures of the Southeast suffered widespread disruption of traditional life over the course of three centuries beginning in the years 1540 and 1541. A new economy, based on trade for profit, usurped and replaced a traditional subsistence economy, sending tribal life into disarray. American Indians were ill prepared to incorporate commercialism based on product and profit into a spiritual tradition that had evolved on need-based hunting and self-sufficient agriculture.

Despite the upheaval caused by such foreign intervention, subsequent loss of tribal lands, widespread migrations westward, the emergence of mixed-blood families, and the collapse of traditional village life, the tribes of the Southeast have been remarkably resilient in surviving four centuries of change. For many of the Native peoples living in the Southeast today, the past 20 years have been a period of marked population growth for both urban- and rural-dwelling Indians (O'Donnell, 1994).

Southwestern Indians

Southwestern Indian culture is the product of a coherent cultural network dating back to the Aztecs. Early Indian settlements centered around agricultural communities defined by an architecture of multistory buildings and large ceremonial centers. The major peoples of this area include the Hopi, the Pueblo, and the Athabascan-speaking Navajo and Apache, who migrated south from the sub-Arctic region sometime around the 13th century. The nomadic Apache people mixed with agriculture-based village peoples such as the Navajo. The interchange of cultural heritage engendered new ceremonial and performance forms such as ritual dance. New and complex themes emerged, underlying traditional creation myths previously held sacred in the region.

The Spanish intervention in the early 16th century brought tight control of village peoples and widespread suppression of traditional cultural practices. American Indians faced hardships such as forced labor, military conscription, and compulsory religious conversion. Southwestern tribes such as the Navajo, the Apache, and the Ute—hunting and gathering peoples—resisted intervention by defending themselves with military power at their disposal. The emigration of the Comanche people into New Mexico from their Shoshoni homeland complicated the cultural dynamics of the region. By the mid-18th century, they were the dominant bison-hunting people of the southern Plains and the Southwest. Their trade dominance grew in influence as they soon controlled the horse and

gun trade, selling to the Spanish themselves. Intertribal warfare was on the rise during this period, with the Comanche often allied with the Spanish in battles against the Apache and the Navajo. By the mid-1800s, the U.S. military entered the region, meeting strong opposition from Indian tribes collectively, particularly the Apache.

The modern southwestern Indian region, then, brings together the Apache, the Hopi, the Navajo, and the Pueblo people of New Mexico. Each culture offers distinct contributions to the area. The Navajo nation, as the largest group within the area (as well as within the entire United States), possesses the potential for significant consolidation of political power given its size. The Hopi and the Pueblo peoples have been known throughout the centuries for their talents in the narrative and visual arts. The Pueblo have produced many well-known artists, novelists, poets, scholars, and painters among their people. The southwestern culture area remains a vital center for the transmission of American Indian culture.

Northern Plains Indians

Despite a long history of economic and political forces amassed to destroy Plains culture, tribal communities have maintained their integrity and have endured into the late 20th century. The tribes now associated with the High Plains had in fact migrated to the area from points farther east. Migration took place during the colonial period after 1650 as European settlement expansion forced many Indians westward.

Tribes such as the Cheyenne were among those forced westward into the Northern Plains as Iroquois expansion after 1650 pushed southern Canadian peoples and tribes in the Great Lakes region out of their lands. By the 1700s, the Cheyenne had occupied North Dakota and were subsisting on the cultivation of corn, the use of horses, and the hunting of buffalo.

Although the common non-Indian perception of Indian culture evokes an image of the nomadic Indian hunter/warrior, such a stereotype is at odds with American Indian history in the centuries preceding the rapid expansion of colonial settlements. Before the 1700s, most Indians in the East were farmers, living without horses. Nevertheless, Plains culture survived and advanced for two centuries until U.S. military forces "pacified" the Plains Indians, confining survivors to reservations. By the late 1870s, U.S. hunters had virtually slaughtered the large herds of buffalo, and without adequate buffalo supplies as a major food source, the Plains Indian culture was no longer possible.

Contemporary reservation life is the product of flexibility and endurance. The Plains Indians have absorbed western settlement without abandoning their cultural practices. Traditional practices such as powwows, tribal fairs, sun dances, sweat ceremonies, and naming rituals have survived the historical process of colonization and expansion into Indian lands. Tribes such as the Crow, the Sioux, and the Cheyenne remain alive and well, despite the widespread poverty and isolation that characterizes life on the Northern Plains reservations (Clow, 1994).

Northwest Coast Indians

The Northwest Coast is bounded by southeastern Alaska, western portions of British Columbia, and the states of Washington and Oregon. The cultures of the area have remained defiantly unique, despite the forces of demographic change beginning in the late 18th century. Tribal economies depended heavily on salmon and cedar as Indians worked in both the Pacific Ocean and the forests of the Pacific Northwest.

Scholars reconstructing these early cultures see evidence that tribes worked both as traders and as farmers. Tribes such as the Tlingit were fishermen, whereas the Haida of southeast Alaska are better known for their woodworking

skills and the craft of totemic art. A third group, the Tsimshian, sometimes are collectively known as the *northern matrilineal tribes* because of their distinctive form of social organization. Scattered among these major groups are dozens of distinct tribes and bands residing in southwest mainland British Columbia, southeast Vancouver Island, and much of western Washington. Linguistic diversity typifies the area, with several bands of such diverse tribes residing along the Oregon Coast and inland in the Willamette River Valley.

It is perhaps this combination of linguistic and cultural diversity that has enabled tribes of this area to participate in American and Canadian society without having lost their unique traditional roots. As Native communities in Alaska, British Columbia, Washington, and Oregon begin to assert their sovereignty as a means to develop economically and politically, they will continue to bring about positive change in a culturally sensitive manner (Boxberger, 1994).

Alaska Natives

There are four major indigenous groups in Alaska: the Aleut, the Eskimo (Yupik and Inuit), the coastal Tlingit and Haida, and the Athabascan. The Aleut people occupied small villages scattered throughout the Aleutian Islands, whereas the Eskimo peoples resided in an environment that spans mountain ranges, deep fjords, tundra, and flat coastal lowlands of the Arctic province. Yupik and Inuit peoples are "central-based wanderers" who spent part of the year moving from place to place while spending the other months as stationary settlers. The Tlingit, Haida, and Tsimshian occupied southeastern Alaska. The northern Athabascan people occupied a vast territory that extended through most of interior Alaska, bordered by the Arctic to the north and the temperate forests to the south.

Alaska Native culture has survived the adverse impact of competing colonial forces vying for

Native lands. Whereas the Russians' hostile colonial enterprise occupied much of the 18th century, American colonialists seeking economic reward sought to legislate laws in favor of white settlements through most of the 19th century. As in other North American indigenous cultures, a subsistence economy was central to the lives of most Alaska Natives. Unlike their European American counterparts, these peoples have managed to retain subsistence economic models well into the 20th century. Many Natives also consider themselves first and foremost hunters and fishermen. There is also evidence that subsistence economies are not only resilient but even growing in certain villages.

Tribal sovereignty is at the core of Alaska Native tribal government. Villages often maintain a right to self-rule, forming their own governments. Alaska Natives believe in exercising their local power to provide for self-sufficient village economies throughout the area (Maas, 1994).

Oklahoma Indians

Today, as in the past, Oklahoma is the home of the largest number of Indian tribes and peoples within the United States. A total of 38 federally recognized Indian nations continue to exercise their sovereign tribal status within Oklahoma. The great majority of these tribes are not indigenous to Oklahoma; rather, they were "resettled" in the state, most involuntarily, under the 19th-century federal Indian removal policy. Driven out of the South on what historians call "the Trail of Tears," tens of thousands of Indians from the Five Civilized Tribes—the Choctaw, the Chickasaw, the Creek, the Cherokee, and the Seminole— perished on forced marches that were often conducted in the dead of winter. Prior to the American Civil War, other tribes, including the Quapaw, the Seneca, and the Shawnee, also were removed to what is now Oklahoma.

Indian tribes in Oklahoma have worked to maintain their own sovereign governments from precontact through forced removal and the bitter betrayal of statehood up to the present. The Five Civilized Tribes achieved a level of literacy and economic prosperity exceeding that of many other states by the mid-19th century.

Today, Oklahoma's Indian population reflects demographics with great diversity in its large numbers. The current generation of Oklahoma's Indians is producing children who are combinations such as Choctaw-Ponca-Cheyenne-Delaware and Cherokee-Osage-Omaha-Creek-Apache. Contemporary Okalahoma tribes seem to be undergoing a revived interest in old ways and an increased pride in Indian identity (R. Strickland, 1994).

Indians of the Plateau, Great Basin, and Rocky Mountains

The Indian peoples of this area continue to live in their ancestral homes. The boundaries of this region span a distance between the states of Washington and Utah and from California to Wyoming. Given such a wide expanse of geographical distance, there is great variety in the cultural and economic systems of the region's tribes. Some cultures have remained intact over the past three centuries; all the tribes enjoy a rich oral tradition about their origins, and tribal elders consider the stories to be both literature and history.

Today, tribes such as the Shoshoni and the Bannock have made the transition to the realities of a modern American economy. They often are employed in ranching, farming, and small business. They have their own agricultural enterprise and construction businesses. Most important is the 20,000-acre irrigation project that the tribe operates, providing water to Indians and non-Indians alike. Other tribes have made strides in education and economic self-determination. The Warm Springs of Oregon and the Yakima people of Washington are active in both of these areas, with major investments in the local lumber and utility industries. The Yakima have been successful in maintaining their own spiritual beliefs and promoting their own economic self-determination.

The Indians of this region are composed of a diverse group of cultures. Although they have suffered tremendous losses to the forces of European colonial expansion, they, like so many other tribal groups from other geographical areas, have survived. Since the 1960s, the tribes have asserted themselves with greater force, offering tribally managed education, health, and economic development programs. This type of innovative spirit, which has served them so well in the past, will be a source of strength in the coming century, as the Indians of this culture area continue on the road toward reclamation and reconstruction of traditional tribal sovereignty (Trafzer, 1994).

California Indians

The Native people of California, like almost all AI/AN tribes, believe that they originated in North America. Traditional origin stories tell of a creator or creators whose awesome powers brought forth the physical universe and all plant and animal life. This cultural centrism created the precedent that tribal territories were sacred and intimately connected to the divine intentions of the Creator. Consequently, land, place, and sacred sites all had a tie to the Creation and to traditional events that were the major events and symbols in Indian history.

The Native Californian worldview centered on seeking balance between the physical and spiritual well-being at both the extended family and tribal levels. Such a balance is based on the idea of reciprocity. Just as the individual or village would bring forth an offering to the spirit world, humans would in turn expect a favorable relationship with the spirit engaged. In addition, reciprocity formed the basis of economic relationships among individuals, extended families, and neighboring villages.

Such a worldview was brutally tested during the Spanish colonization of California. The Spanish Empire's plan was to reduce the numerous free and independent Native hunting and collecting villages and societies into a mass of peon laborers via the mission system. Survival for California Indians remained difficult well into the late 19th century. Mission life was unbearable, and death through the transmission of European diseases took a devastating toll on the Indian population. Some tribes and village populations had virtually disappeared from the face of the earth. Those Indians who survived the ravaging effects of infectious diseases were then confronted with violence from white settlers and the U.S. military throughout the 19th century.

Faced with the threat of complete extinction, California Indians have fought through the numerous legal channels made sparingly available to them since the early 1900s. Since that time, the California Indian population has grown to more than 200,000. Although it will take far longer than a century to reclaim what had been lost to a relentless series of policies designed specifically to destroy Indian culture and tribal life, much is now in the process of changing. Although issues such as poverty and health still threaten Indians going into the next century, many tribes are reclaiming the strength found in original identity, as they look through the specter of their recent past, to reclaim that spirit of reciprocity governing the world of their ancestors (Castillo, 1994).

HISTORICAL PERSPECTIVES: A BRIEF OVERVIEW OF AI/AN HISTORY IN NORTH AMERICA

When European explorers first stepped ashore on North American soil, they encountered a wide variety of American Indian cultures that had existed in every region of the continent for thousands of years. North America was not a "vacant" continent as early European explorers had believed. To the contrary, some of the regions first touched by Europeans were in fact the homelands of the continent's most complex cultures. In the southeastern United States, tribal societies developed hereditary leadership, long-distance trading networks, and elaborate systems for obtaining and displaying wealth. With the arrival of Europeans in North America, many fully developed Indian cultures suffered catastrophic collapse. European diseases, warfare, and the social disruptions caused by loss of resources forever changed the people of this continent, but it did not destroy them. American Indians found many ways of adapting to change.

By the 1450s, many American Indian civilizations had risen and disappeared. During the years before Columbus's arrival, Indians were developing rich and diverse cultures and were engaging in agricultural development, cultivating uniquely American crops such as corn, tomatoes, potatoes, green beans, squash, pumpkins, and tobacco. They were living in teepees, Quonsets, longhouses, A-frames, pueblos, hogans, sod huts, or other types of dwellings. During this time, American Indians also were gaining considerable knowledge about medicine and astronomy and were developing a wide variety of music, art, and literature. Historians estimate that the American Indian population numbered between 1 and 2 million when Columbus landed in 1492. In a letter to the Queen of Spain, Columbus called these Natives a race of hardy people (Brown, 1970, p. 1). Early physicians, traders, and explorers remarked about the extraordinarily good health of the Natives, noting that Native peoples were clean, good looking, without apparent illness, and peaceful (Brown, 1970). With the arrival of the Europeans came the epidemic of diseases that killed hundreds of thousands of Indians. At the turn of this century, Native Indians were reduced to a paltry 200,000. More than 200 (out of an estimated 700) tribes became extinct. American Indians were ill prepared to fight off the diseases and illnesses brought over with the early settlers. Unlike the Europeans, who had built up a natural immunity through prior exposure, Indians had no natural immunity to smallpox, measles, tuberculosis, or typhoid. Indian people lived in small communities with clean water, sanitation, and healthy food that were free from the diseases that were so widespread in the European countries.

Today, the American Indians have increased to the numbers reported 500 years ago and have organized themselves into social and political groups concerned over the health and social welfare of their members. Meanwhile, the U.S. federal policy toward Indians has had a significant influence on the development of the Indian social and political groups. The history of American Indian federal policies can be roughly divided into four major periods since 1880.

1880–1932, Assimilation and incorporation. During this period, the policy of the federal government was to "civilize" Indians and incorporate them into mainstream society. Boarding schools were built as a means to educate Indian youths in the ways of white people. Mechanism to educate, assimilate, and incorporate the Indian population into the larger social order was the policy driving the federal policies during this timeframe.

1933–1945, Indirect rule. The federal government had a major role in reorganizing Indian social and political groups. Traditional Indian leadership was reorganized into counsels that adopted Western rules and structures.

1946–1960, Termination. A serious termination policy proved to be significantly damaging to tribes as wholesale "termination" of tribes took effect. This resulted in loss of services, Indian "status," and Indian land. The intent was to end the "Indian problem" by ending the federal government's special responsibility to the tribes.

1961–1990s, Economic development and self-determination. This period marks tribal reemergence as AI/AN develop new models for economic sufficiency. This process provides the financial means for reclaiming a level of self-determination widespread among pre-Columbian American peoples. Tribes and tribal groups initiate steps to take over major aspects of federal programs and services such as medical care services, boarding schools, and tribal colleges (Young & Kim, 1993, p. 7). The 1960s marked a major turning point in U.S. Indian policy. By the mid-1960s, the threat of termination of Indian tribes and reservations had subsided, and new government programs were introduced. These new programs were aimed at eliminating poverty throughout the United States. Many Indian reservations and tribal governments benefited from these newly developed programs. These federal government policies redirected their services, thus allowing reservation-based tribal governments more control over local administration of governmental programs. Self-governance and management of community services on reservations, historically managed by the Bureau of Indian Affairs since the 1880s, became the theme of the new U.S. Indian policy. This policy, called "self-determination," characterized most of the period from 1965 to the present and became the policy for Indian affairs for the foreseeable future. Through the 1960s and 1970s, reservation-based tribal governments received considerable federal funding to support community needs such as housing, health, community action, and education. During the 1980s, federal funding available to Indians declined, and inflation made the smaller level of funding worth even less.

The 1980s, however, increasingly saw Indian communities work to gain more control over reservation governments, reservation industry and mineral resources, education and other reservation institutions that were generally managed through the Bureau of Indian Affairs. With the passage of Public Laws 93-638 and 94-437, as well as more recent administrative processes providing for "self-governance" and "self-determination," the funding base for the Indian health care delivery system has shifted more toward the desires of tribal entities. This has contributed to the reduction of the Indian Health Service (IHS) staff and program offices, in favor of tribal development and management of the health and social welfare services. In the future, it is anticipated that most Indian reservation communities will work toward furthering the goals of cultural and political self-determination.

SOCIODEMOGRAPHIC CHARACTERISTICS OF AI/AN POPULATIONS

The U.S. census reports 2.47 million American Indians, Eskimos, and Aleuts residing in the United States, representing 0.8% of the U.S. population (U.S. Department of Commerce, 2001), the smallest racial minority in the United States. There are more than 562 federally recognized tribes and more than 100 state and nonfederally recognized tribes and bands (U.S. Department of the Interior, 2002). The federal government recognizes 310 reservations, 217 Alaska Native villages, 12 Alaska Native regional corporations, 50 American Indian trust lands, and 17 tribal jurisdiction statistical areas. Most reservations are clustered in 35 states, primarily in the western half of the United States. Approximately, one half of the American Indian population lives in the West, with the remainder residing primarily in the South (29%), Midwest (17%), and Northeast (6%) (U.S. Census Bureau, 1990).

The American Indians of today can be described as the poorest, least educated, and most neglected minority group in the United States. Identified problems include a pattern of poverty, social problems, and health disparity unparalleled among major ethnic groups.

Nationally, American Indians have one of the youngest populations comparatively. According to the 2000 census, 25.7% of the general population was younger than 18 years, and 12.4% was older than 65 years (U.S. Census Bureau, 2000a). The median age for Indians was 28 years, compared with 35.3 years for all U.S. races (U.S. Census Bureau, 2000a). The characteristics of the younger population residing in the Indian community may account for the high Indian birthrate. The American Indian live birthrate of 28.1 per 1,000 for the period 1989 to 1990 was 68% higher than the rate of 16.7 per 1,000 for all U.S. races during that period (IHS, 1990).

The social and economic profile of American Indians indicates that the Indian population differs substantially from U.S. residents in general. The Indian population is younger, with larger families that are more likely to be maintained by adult females. American Indians are less likely to have a higher education and more likely to be unemployed. Median income is lower, and Indian families have higher rates of poverty. Data from the 2000 census report the following statistics: 20.9% of Indian households are headed by females; 70.9% of American Indians aged 25 years or older completed high school degrees or higher, compared with 80.4% of all U.S. races; American Indians were less than half as likely to earn a bachelor's degree (7.6% vs. 15.5%); 7.5% of Indian males were unemployed, compared with 3.7% for all U.S. races; the median income for Indian households in 1999 was $30,599, which was below national median income of $41,994; and in all age categories over the age of 16 years (except those aged over 75 years), American Indians ranked higher in reported percentage below poverty level than did any other ethnic group (U.S. Census Bureau, 2000b, 2000c).

One of the most difficult problems affecting the American Indian community is the high school dropout rate. Data from the 2000 census report that among persons aged 25 years or over, approximately 29.1% had not finished high school and that, of these, 11.1% had less than a ninth-grade education (U.S. Census Bureau, 2000b). In the Indian foster care system, 45% of the school-age children are in special education or individual education programs (Division of General Pediatrics and Adolescent Health, 1992).

ACCULTURATION, INTEGRATION, AND GROWTH OF AI/AN POPULATIONS IN THE UNITED STATES

The multiplicity of tribes within the United States is further complicated by the increasing migration of AI/AN to urban areas. More than 50% of AI/AN reside in large metropolitan areas. This migration pattern has brought about new concerns for Native people. Migration to the city brings isolation because the urban environment lacks the network of family and community support found in the rural reservation/rancheria/village areas. Urban Indians tend to live dispersed within the larger population in the city, thus losing important support systems. Life in large metropolitan areas often can be somewhat bleak and stressful. More than half of urban Indians sampled in a research study (Hodge, Fredericks, & Kipnis, 1996) did not have enough money for food, clothing, housing, and other necessities of life. They also reported more fears about the safety of their neighborhoods and having been the victims of theft more frequently than Indians living in rural areas. Furthermore, urban Indians were more likely to be unemployed, with 54% having been out of work for 1 month or more in the previous 3 months. Overall, urban Indians reported being more transient and having higher smoking rates, higher unemployment, less social support systems, and more "hassles" than did American Indians in the rural sites or reservations sampled. For more than 500 years, American Indians have been forced to assimilate into larger society, resulting in threat to, and loss of culture and ethnic identity. Long-term isolation from reservations and traditional homelands may contribute to the breakdown of social support systems among urban Indians.

The early reports on Indians in the city tended to create a generalized composite view of urban life for Indians. Today, it is counter-productive to talk about "the urban Indian" in the singular because the adjustment patterns, recreational behavior, and employment and educational expectations vary as much as the people classified as AI/AN. The urban Indian, like the rural or reservation-based Indian, does not fit neatly into one unified category. Rather, any effort to construct a composite American Indian is undercut by the multiple levels of adjustment experienced by numerous and differing groups of American Indians within a variety of urban environments.

Most of the past research has targeted urban Indians deemed first-generation Bureau of Indian Affairs–supported groups relocated during the 1950s and 1960s. Today, there is a generation of urban-dwelling Indians who have never seen their reservations, spoken their native tongues, or listened to their tribal elders. They are the urban Indians born in San Francisco, Los Angeles, Denver, or Anchorage—reared away from their traditional roots.

In the city, being Indian is tied to participating in the life of the Indian community. This aspect of life, more than anything else, identifies someone as Indian because it is a public statement of belonging, commitment, and pride. Even though the urban Indian has a community—a social network of other Indians—this sense of community differs dramatically from prescriptive cultural formation. Urban life has undone traditional tribal identity for some American Indians, posing a new set of challenges for the reclamation and nurturing of Indian tradition within the postmodern world.

HEALTH AND DISEASE AMONG AI/AN

An Overview of the Issues

The health status of American Indians is at a critical stage. Whereas Indians once died of acute infections such as smallpox, measles, and diphtheria, today they die of chronic diseases such as alcoholism, heart disease, cancer, and diabetes. The federal IHS reports that American Indians continue to present with extremely high disease rates for common, easily treatable illness and health problems. The two leading causes of death among American Indians are cardiovascular disease (CVD) and cancer (Centers for Disease Control [CDC], 2003a). Although American Indians reported very low CVD rates in past years, today CVD is the leading cause of death among American Indians (American Heart Association, 2003; Ellis & Campos-Outcalt, 1994).

The prevalence of CVD among American Indians has steadily increased over the years and is today more than double that of the general population (Galloway, 2004; Howard et al., 1999). CV-related mortality rates (strokes) in 2004 are slightly more prevalent in Indian females (35.1%) than males (35.09%) (American Heart Association, 2008).

Reports of rising cancer rates, especially cancers found in American Indian women, such as cervical cancer, are alarming. Unfortunately, cervical cancer survival rates are poorer than that reported for other populations. Breast cancer is reported to be the second leading cause of death for American Indian women followed by cervical cancer (Edwards, 2001).

Other diseases that are linked to high-risk behaviors are diabetes, lung diseases (from smoking), and alcoholism. AI/AN are reported to have 2.6 times more likelihood of a diabetes diagnosis than non-Hispanic whites of a similar age (CDC, 2003c). A recent CDC report states that "The majority of health behaviors and status measures for American Indians were more likely than other respondents or other racial/ethnic groups to be at increased risk" (CDC, 2003c, p. 1). Other health problems associated with health-risk behaviors include obesity, smoking, substance abuse, and poor nutrition. Indeed, the Behavioral Risk Factor Surveillance System (CDC, 2003a) survey reports that many of these health problems are chronic in nature and are linked to risk behaviors.

The CDC also reports that AI/AN suffer disproportionately from depression, substance abuse, and domestic violence (CDC, 2003a). American Indians have the highest rates of alcoholism and face higher rates of liver cancer and cirrhosis than the general U.S. population (U.S. Department of Health and Human Services [DHHS], 2003). A study of domestic violence within a southwest tribe reported that 53% of women aged 18 to 59 years, and 28% of women aged 50 years and older reported physical abuse at least once by their intimate partner (Robin, Chester, Rasmussen, Jaranson, & Goldman, 1997). It is interesting to note that these rates are significantly higher than those reported for U.S. women in all ethnic categories. Studies of suicide (Strickland, 1997) indicate that rates are increasing and factors related with American Indian adolescent suicide included depression, substance abuse, and family violence. A study by Strickland, Walsh, and Cooper (2006) reported that suicide risk and depression among youth in the Northwest were linked to intergenerational pain, fractured families, community prejudice, and lack of employment.

American Indians are more likely to die in accidents than are those in the general U.S. population. The American Indian accident rate for the period 1990 to 1991 was higher for all ages relative to the general population. For Indian youths (aged 1 to 14 years), the rate was twice as high (23.5 vs. 12.4 per 100,000). Deaths of American Indian youths are caused by violent accidents and injury, accounting for 75% of the total deaths (CDC, 2003b). For Indian children and youth, the accident death rate was more than twice as high. For Indian adults, the death rate from accidents was 3.3 times higher. And for older Indians (aged 45 to 64 years), the rate was 232.3 per 100,000 versus 226.2 per 100,000 (CDC, 2003b).

Type 2 diabetes is one of the leading causes of outpatient visits for the adult age group at IHS facilities. The age-adjusted prevalence of diabetes among adult Indians was reported by the IHS to be 16.3% (IHS, 2007) The rates of type 2 diabetes have been documented to range from 33% to 72% for those aged 45 to 74 years. Alarmingly, the prevalence rate rises to 50% for those aged 55 to 75 years. This is quite high as compared with the U.S. rate of 5.5% within this same age group (IHS, 1984). The risk factors for type 2 diabetes include obesity and hypertension (both of which continue to rise rapidly in American Indian populations).

In 1995, the Indian alcohol mortality was five times the rate for all other U.S. races combined (37.2 vs. 6.8 per 100,000) (U.S. DHHS, 1995). Fetal alcohol syndrome was 33 times higher among Indians than among non-Indians.

A study of American Indian adults in northern California found a depressive symptomology case rate (using the Center for Epidemiologic Studies—Depression scale) of 41%, which is almost triple the U.S. general population rate of 16%. Women scored higher than men, unemployed scored higher than employed, and age exhibited a curvilinear effect, with higher rates found in late adolescence and early adulthood (Hodge & Kipnis, 1996).

Behavioral Impact on Health Status

Today, American Indians are dying from chronic diseases that are largely attributed to environmental conditions and behavioral patterns. Acculturation and assimilation have contributed to the adoption of unhealthy behavioral patterns and habits such as smoking, drinking alcohol, and injuries and accidents. Behavioral influences have resulted in poverty, illness, and increased social disruption.

The prevalence of smoking among American Indians is twice the rate of that reported for the general population (Hodge et al., 1995; U.S. DHHS, CDC, National Center for Chronic

Disease Prevention & Heath Promotion, Office on Smoking and Health, 1998). Among racial and ethnic groups, the prevalence of smoking was found to be highest among American Indians (40.4%), followed by African Americans (25.7%), whites (27.4%), Hispanics (23.1%), and Asians/Pacific Islanders (16.2%). For Indian adolescents, smoking rates are also the highest, exceeding 50%. Studies have documented high smoking rates in the Northern Plains region (Bachman et al., 1991). Hodge (2002) found extremely high smoking rates among the Rosebud Sioux (73%) and Winnebago (62%) in South Dakota and Nebraska, respectively. Several other studies have also reported high smoking rates among Northern Plains and Western tribes. For example, a study of 668 non-urban Indians in Ontario (McIntyre & Shah, 1986) reported that 56.4% smoked while 37.4% of these smoked on a daily basis.

Very little evaluation and scientific research has been conducted to examine successful smoking cessation methods among American Indians. Over the past 20 years, there has been a national effort to decrease dependence on tobacco products. Although public health efforts directed at reducing the prevalence of smoking have been somewhat successful among the general population, the rate of decline in tobacco use has varied among diverse sociodemographically defined groups, such as American Indians (Hodge, 1995).

The historical importance of tobacco to American Indian culture is multidimensional. The role of tobacco in religious and ceremonial practices has been complicated by its economic importance for the American Indian population. As a cash crop, tobacco has provided economic security for American Indians for generations. In the traditional usage, tobacco is a gift of the earth. It is used as a spiritual communicator and as a cleansing agent. Tobacco is given as a gift to healers and often is used in healing ceremonies. Tobacco also has become one of the few sources of economic stability in otherwise poor rural reservation areas. Small vendors (e.g., smoke shops) are able to make a living by selling tax-free tobacco products on Indian lands. The economic incentive in areas where unemployment is high presents a barrier to smoking cessation and control now that it is clear that smoking presents an undeniable health hazard for Indians and non-Indians alike.

Alcoholism among American Indians has reached epidemic proportions and has been described as the number one health problem among Indians. The federal government reports that the Indian alcoholism death rate is more than five times greater than that reported for all U.S. races (U.S. DHHS, 1995). Of the 10 leading causes of death for AI/AN, four are alcohol related. The death rate from cirrhosis is five times higher among AI/AN between 2 and 44 years of age than for the general population. At least 80% of homicides, suicides, and motor vehicle accidents in the American Indian population are alcohol related. Cigarette smoking combined with alcohol usage place American Indians at risk for throat cancer and neoplasms of the pharynx. They also contribute to accidents, home fires, and violence.

Accidents and violence, often a consequence of alcohol or substance abuse, accounted for 21% of all Indian deaths during the period 1990 to 1992, almost three times the national figure. Accidents and violence also are a leading cause of inpatient and outpatient care for Indians (U.S. DHHS, 1992). The IHS has determined that 75% of all accidental deaths to American Indians are alcohol related.

Impact of Environmental Contamination on Health Status

Health status is a function of a variety of factors such as behavior, environment, heredity, and health services. Of these, the poisoning of the environment is an irreversible harm that will threaten generations of American Indians.

In the late 19th and early 20th centuries, gold, timber, minerals, and water were mined, harvested, and harnessed in the West. Many

Indian reservations were found to be rich in minerals highly sought by non-Indians. Little thought was given to environmental consequences, which resulted in extensive damage to land, posing a new threat to Indian health. For instance, arsenic used in mining camps contaminated the water. Logging disrupted the game supply and damaged the land; dams erected on rivers for electrical power changed the course of water to downstream sites and halted the annual migration of fish. Newer riches were sought from the land. Uranium mining on the Navajo reservation left many Indians with a new disease—cancer and radiation poisoning.

Development of reservation resources has brought environmental concerns that mirror those of the United States as a whole. For instance, trace metal content in the teeth of postindustrial Hopi are similar to that found in California suburban residents showing contamination from heavy metals. Indian reservations are on federal land and, as such, often are near toxic waste dumps. Contaminated water supplies, contaminated soil, and even diminished air quality are now more commonplace on reservation sites. It is not too surprising that presently there is an increase of cancers and other health problems related to the environmental contamination of Indian lands.

Four of the five leading causes of hospitalization at IHS facilities (respiratory illness, digestive system diseases, injuries and poisoning, and circulatory ailments) have potential environmental causes, and three of the five leading causes of outpatient visits (respiratory diseases, nervous system and sense organ ailments, and endocrine, nutrition, and metabolic disorders) might have environmental linkages.

Many of these elevated disease risks are due to poverty, excessive use of alcohol and tobacco, lack of health care services, and high risk-taking behavior (Grandbois, 2005; Valway, Kileen, Paisano, & Ortiz, 1991). In addition, individuals engaged in occupations such as uranium mining have elevated risks of chronic lung diseases, silicosis, lung cancer, and other radiation-related malignancies because of the lack of disposal facilities, hazardous wastes from mining, agriculture, and petroleum extraction that have contaminated many Indian lands in the western states of Utah, Arizona, New Mexico, California, and Washington, where Indian lands carry higher concentrations of industrial toxins (U.S. DHHS, 1992). This has led to the contamination of air, water, and soil and to despoliation of sacred grounds. In addition, this contamination has affected certain agricultural products such as berries and the reeds and willows used in traditional basket weaving. Forest trails and rural roadsides often are sprayed with weed-retarding chemicals and other highly toxic pesticides, thus affecting potential agriculture used for food or crafts.

Urban Indian residents consequently share a frightening environmental legacy with poor inner-city communities: high exposure to lead-based paints, air pollution, noise, unsanitary plumbing, and exposure to urban toxic and industrial wastes. These environmental impacts are not the only changes affecting Indian health. Stress caused from unemployment and relocation to large cities has created new problems. Indians have found themselves in large metropolitan areas where they were unaccustomed to "city living." They no longer could hunt, fish, or grow their food; a self-sufficient subsistence lifestyle had become a way of the past. Their family members were too far away to visit. Bad habits acquired in their new neighborhoods contributed to poor health: cigarette smoking, poor nutrition, alcoholism, and dysfunctional families added to the stress.

Overview of the IHS

AI/AN have a special relationship with the federal government with regard to their medical care. Indians living on or near their reservations are eligible for medical services at IHS facilities. Although IHS services are not limited to reservation-based Indians, IHS clinical facilities usually are found on or near reservations and receive most of the federal funds allocated for Indian health.

The U.S. Department of Health and Human Services, primarily through the IHS of the Public Health Service, is responsible for providing health and medical services to AI/AN. The Indian Self-Determination and Education Assistance Act of 1975 (amended in 1988, 1990, and 1994) gave Indian tribes the capability of contracting directly with the IHS for the management and control of their own health programs. These contracted programs are commonly referred to as "638 contracts." Thus, the Self-Determination and Education Assistance Act enabled Indians to become more actively involved in determining their health care for the first time. Access to health care and health insurance is the lowest out of all minority populations in the United States. Only 62% of AI/AN under the age of 65 years are covered under some type of medical insurance and have adequate health services (National Health Interview Survey [NHIS], CDC, NCHS, 1997).

Currently, the IHS program consists of both IHS and tribally operated hospitals, clinics, and health centers as well as its Contract Health Services component. Services are coordinated through regional administrative units called IHS area offices. IHS facilities and Indian-operated clinics are able to enter into contracts with outside facilities and physicians to provide services needed.

The operation of the IHS health service delivery system is managed through local administrative units called *service units.* A service unit is the basic health organization of a geographical area served by the IHS program. These are defined areas, usually centered on a single federal reservation in the continental United States or a population concentrated in Alaska. The service units are grouped into larger cultural-demographic-geographic management jurisdictions that are administered by IHS area offices.

The American Indian experience with regard to risk factors is both alarming and disgraceful. Serious behavioral and social problems, leading to injuries and early death, are well-known. Suicide rates are rising, and deaths due to homicide, accidents, and injuries are leading causes of Indian mortality. Newer threats to Indian health such as cancer, diabetes, nutritional diseases, and other illnesses due to changing behavioral and to environmental contaminants are on the rise. These behavioral problems have become epidemic and contribute heavily to death and disease. They must become priority areas to control if the *Healthy People 2010* objectives are to be reached.

BARRIERS TO HEALTH PROMOTION AND DISEASE PREVENTION IN AI/AN POPULATIONS

There are several significant barriers to Indian health care. These can be identified as (a) cultural barriers, (b) system barriers, and (c) financial barriers. Over the years, American Indians have been forced to assimilate rapidly into mainstream society with consequent deterioration of culture and ethnic identity. American Indian youths, in particular, are strongly affected by the adverse conditions affecting their family units. High mobility of long-standing urban residents and reservation-based new arrivals to urban areas, disintegration of the family unit, high unemployment rates, and serious behavioral and emotional problems of adults add to the situation.

A significant portion of the American Indian population receives health care services from the IHS, a part of the federal Public Health Service. Health services to Indians actually began in the Department of War as an attempt to control the spread of epidemics to military post personnel and their families. The IHS was designed primarily for Indians residing on reservation lands. Today, however, with more than 50% of Indians residing in large metropolitan areas, access to health services is limited. The health care delivery system has developed into a dual system in which a "cradle-to-grave" system is operating in rural reservation sites and a limited, piecemeal system is operating in several urban sites.

CHAPTER SUMMARY

Some 500 years ago, the Native peoples of North America roamed this vast continent. Their subsistence economy, which depended on nature and the land, was physically and spiritually healthy. Some tribes became farmers and grew corn and squash; others were hunters and gatherers following the seasons. Game animals were stalked, and physical exercise was a way of life. Diseases caused by poor nutrition, such as heart disease, diabetes, high blood pressure, and obesity, were unknown.

The relentless processes of acculturation and assimilation brought about by the economic forces of urbanization and industrialization is troublesome. Today, many Indians no longer fish and stalk game animals; they cannot hunt buffalo because the buffalo are gone—exterminated by the settlers. Salmon fishing in the Northwest has been restricted due to the barriers placed by the dams. Cities have been erected over traditional sites. Herbs and healing medicines have been plowed under the ground or paved over for highways. Nuclear plants, toxic waste dumps, and contaminated waste have infected reservation lands with pollutants.

Since the arrival of European settlers, the American Indian population has survived policies of genocide, cultural assimilation, and social disruption. None of these destructive forces, however, has carried the potential threat to land, livelihood, and future generations as

has the current contamination and toxic damage to Indian lands. The answer to controlling or eliminating this contamination might lie in educating Indians to the extent and enormity of the threat to tribal lands.

Chapter 18, which follows, discusses several specific elements of the HPDP planning process unique to the AI/AN experiences. These elements include planning frameworks, selected health issues, and cultural concerns. The authors also discuss, within a program-planning context, the importance of in-depth target group needs assessment, appropriate selection of program design, and particular aspects of program implementation and evaluation. They offer tips based on their extensive experiences and make suggestions for more effective HPDP program design within the AI/AN populations.

DISCUSSION QUESTIONS AND ACTIVITIES

The magnitude of health problems confronting American Indians, ranging from the emotional and psychological to the physiological, presents a formidable challenge to health educators. Working in small groups, please discuss the following questions and share your answers with the rest of your class.

1. What is the key to responding to these health problems?

2. If health care providers are educated to better understand the unique historical context of Native peoples, would the provision of health services result in substantive changes in the health and social welfare of our First Americans? How might this be?

REFERENCES

American Heart Association. (2003). *Heart disease and stroke statistics—2004 update*. Dallas, TX: Author.

Bachman, J. G., Wallace, J. M., Jr., O'Malley, P. M., Johnston, L. D., Kurth, C. L., & Neighbors, H. W. (1991). Racial/ethnic differences in smoking, drinking, and illicit drug use among American high school seniors, 1976–89. *American Journal of Public Health, 81*(3), 372–377.

Boxberger, D. (1994). Northwest Coast Indians. In D. Champagne (Ed.), *The Native North American Almanac* (2nd ed., p. 315). Detroit, MI: Gale Research.

Brown, D. (1970). *Bury my heart at wounded knee: An Indian history of the American West.* New York: Holt, Rinehart & Winston.

Castillo, E. (1994). California Indians. In D. Champagne (Ed.), *The Native North American Almanac* (2nd ed., pp. 360–361). Detroit, MI: Gale Research.

Centers for Disease Control. (2003a). Findings from the Behavioral Risk Factor Surveillance System, 1997–2000. *Morbidity and Mortality Weekly Report Surveillance Summaries, 8*(52), 1–13, SS07.

Centers for Disease Control. (2003b). Injury mortality among American Indian and Alaska Native children and youth, 1989–1998. *Morbidity and Mortality Weekly Report, 52*(30), 697–701.

Centers for Disease Control. (2003c). *Trends in diabetes, prevalence among American Indians and Alaska Native children, adolescents, and young adults—1990*–1998 (Diabetes Publications and Products). Atlanta, GA: Author.

Clow, R. (1994). Northern Plains Indians. In D. Champagne (Ed.), *The Native North American Almanac* (2nd ed., pp. 305–308). Detroit, MI: Gale Research.

Division of General Pediatrics and Adolescent Health. (1992). *The state of Native American youth health.* Minneapolis: University of Minnesota.

Edwards, B. (2001). *A national perspective on cancer surveillance and measuring health disparities.* American Indian/Alaska Native Leadership Initiative Biennial Conference: Changing Patterns of Cancer Care in Native Communities, Scottsdale, AZ.

Ellis, J. L., & Campos-Outcalt, D. (1994). Cardiovascular disease risk factors in Native Americans: A literature review. *American Journal of Preventive Medicine, 10*(5), 295–307.

Galloway, J. M. (2004). Cardiovascular prevention activities within Indian health: A status report. *The Indian Health Service Primary Care Provider, 29*(2), 27–28.

Grandbois, D. (2005). Stigma of mental illness among American Indian and Alaska Native nations: Historical and contemporary perspectives. *Issues in Mental Health, 26*(10), 1001–1024.

Hodge, F. S. (1995). Tobacco control leadership in American Indian communities. In K. Slama (Ed.), *Tobacco and health* (pp. 275–278). New York: Plenum Press.

Hodge, F. S. (2002). *Diabetes wellness: A report of a four-year research study of diabetes and American Indians on the Winnebago, Pine Ridge, Rosebud, and Yankton Sioux Reservations.* Berkeley, CA/Minneapolis, MN: Center for American Indian Research and Education.

Hodge, F. S., Cummings, S. R., Fredericks, L., Kipnis, P., Williams, M., & Teehee, K. (1995). Prevalence of smoking among adult American Indian clinic users in northern California. *Preventive Medicine, 24*, 441–446.

Hodge, F., Fredericks, L., & Kipnis, P. (1996). Urban-rural contrasts, patient and smoking patterns in northern California American Indian clinics. *Cancer, 78*, 1623–1628.

Hodge, F. S., & Kipnis, P. (1996). Demoralization: A useful concept for case management with Native Americans. In P. Manoleas (Ed.), *The cross-cultural practice of clinical case management in mental health* (pp. 79–98). New York: Haworth Press.

Howard, B., Lee, E., Cowan, L., Dereveneux, R., Galloway, J., Go, O., et al. (1999). The rising tide of cardiovascular disease in Native Americans: The Strong Heart Study. *Circulation, 99*, 238–239.

Indian Health Service. (1984). *IHS chart series book, June 1984.* Washington, DC: Government Printing Office, U.S. Department of Health and Human Services.

Indian Health Service. (1990). *Trends in Indian health: 1990.* Rockville, MD: Author.

Maas, D. (1994). Alaska Natives. In D. Champagne (Ed.), *The Native North American Almanac* (2nd ed., p. 326). Detroit, MI: Gale Research.

McIntyre, L., & Shah, C. (1986). Prevalence of hypertension, obesity and smoking in three Indian communities in Northwestern Ontario. *Canadian Medical Association Journal, 134,* 345–349.

National Health Interview Survey (NHIS), CDC, NCHS, 1997. Retrieved December 27, 2007, from http://www.cdc.gov/nhis.htm

O'Donnell, J. (1994). Southeastern Indians. In D. Champagne (Ed.), *The Native North American Almanac* (2nd ed., p. 287). Detroit, MI: Gale Research.

Robin, R. W., Chester, B., Rasmussen, J. K., Jaranson, J. M., & Goldman, D. (1997). Factors influencing utilization of mental health and substance abuse services by American Indian men and women. *Psychiatric Services,* 48(6), 826–834.

Strickland, R. (1994). Oklahoma Indians. In D. Champagne (Ed.), *The Native North American Almanac* (2nd ed., pp. 333–334). Detroit, MI: Gale Research.

Strickland, C. J. (1997). Suicide among American Indian, Alaska Native, and Canadian Aboriginal Youth: Advancing the research agenda. *International Journal of Mental Health, 25*(4), 11–32.

Strickland, C. J., Walsh, E., & Cooper, M. (2006). Healing fractured families: Parents and elder perspectives on the impact of colonialization and youth suicide prevention in a Pacific Northwest Indian tribe. *Journal of Transcultural Nursing, 17*(1), 5–12.

Trafzer, C. E. (1994). Indians of the Plateau, Great Basin, and Rocky Mountains. In D. Champagne (Ed.), *The Native North American Almanac* (2nd ed., pp. 347–348). Detroit, MI: Gale Research.

U.S. Census Bureau. (1990). *We, the First Americans, September 1993.* Retrieved January 1, 2008, from www.census.gov/apsd/wepeople/we-5.pdf (p. 2).

U.S. Census Bureau. (2000a). DP-1. *Profile of general demographic characteristics: 2000.* Retrieved January 1, 2008, from http://factfinder.census .gov/servlet/QTTable?_bm=y&-geo_id= 01000US&-qr_name=DEC_2000_SF2_U_ DP1&-ds_name=DEC_2000_SF2_U &-reg=DEC_2000_SF2_U_DP1:001|006 &-_lang=en&-redoLog=false&-format=&- CONTEXT=qt

U.S. Census Bureau. (2000b). *DP-2. Profile of selected social characteristics: 2000.* Retrieved January 1, 2008, from http://factfinder .census.gov/servlet/QTTable?_bm= y&-geo_id=01000US&-qr_name=DEC_ 2000_SF4_U_DP3&-qr_name=DEC_2000_ SF4_U_DP2&-qr_name=DEC_2000_ SF4_U_QTP19&-qr_name=DEC_2000_SF4_ U_QTP26&reg=DEC_2000_SF4_U_DP2:001| 006;DEC_2000_SF4_U_DP3:001;DEC_ 2000_SF4_U_QTP19:001;DEC_2000_SF4_ U_ QTP26:001&-ds_name=DEC_2000_SF4_ U&-_lang=en&-redoLog=true&-format= &-CONTEXT=qt

U.S. Census Bureau. (2002c). *DP-3. Profile of selected economic characteristics: 2000.* Retrieved January 1, 2008, from http://fact finder.census.gov/servlet/QTTable?_bm=y &-reg=DEC_2000_SFAIAN_DP2:001|01A; DEC_2000_SFAIAN_DP3:001|01A;DEC_200 0_SFAIAN_DP4:001|01A;&-qr_name= DEC_2000_SFAIAN_DP3&-qr_name=DEC_ 2000_SFAIAN_DP4&-qr_name=DEC_2000_ SFAIAN_DP2&-ds_name=DEC_2000_SFA- IAN&-TABLE_NAMEX=&-ci_type=T &-CONTEXT=qt&-redoLog=false &-charIterations=01A&-_caller=geoselect &-geo_id=01000US&-geo_id=NBSP &-format=&-_lang=en

U.S. Department of Health and Human Services. (1992). *Trends in Indian health.* Rockville, MD: Indian Health Service.

U.S. Department of Health and Human Services. (1993). *Regional differences in Indian health.* Rockville, MD: Indian Health Service.

U.S. Department of Health and Human Services. (1995). *Regional differences in Indian health (charts).* Rockville, MD: Indian Health Service.

U.S. Department of Health and Human Services. (2007). *Indian Health Service, diabetes in American Indians and Alaska Natives: Facts at-a-glance.* Rockville, MD: Department of Health and Human Services, Indian Health Service.

U.S. Department of Health and Human Services, CDC, National Center for Chronic Disease Prevention & Health Promotion, Office on

Smoking and Health. (1998). *Tobacco use among U.S. racial/ethnic minorities groups—African Americans, American Indians and Alaska Natives, Asian Americans and Pacific Islanders, and Hispanics: A report of the surgeon general*. Atlanta, GA: Author.

U.S. Department of the Interior. (2002, July 12). *Part IV, Department of the Interior: Bureau of Indian Affairs; Indian entities recognized and eligible to receive services from the United States Bureau of Indian Affairs; Notice* (Vol. 67, No. 134). Retrieved January 1, 2008, from www.census.gov/publicinfo/www/FRN02.pdf

Valway, S., Kileen, M., Paisano, T., & Ortiz, E. (1991). *Cancer mortality among Native Americans in the United States: Regional differences in Indian health, 1984–1987*. Rockville, MD: Indian Health Service.

Young, I. S., & Kim, E. C. (1993). *American mosaic: Selected readings on American multicultural heritage*. Englewood Cliffs, NJ: Prentice Hall.

18

Assessment, Program Planning, and Evaluation in Indian Country

Toward a Postcolonial Practice of Indigenous Planning

BONNIE M. DURAN

TED JOJOLA

NATHANIA T. TSOSIE

NINA WALLERSTEIN

Chapter Objectives

On completion of this chapter, the health promotion student and practitioner will be able to

- Understand and discuss at least three issues related to assessment, program planning, and evaluation in "Indian Country"

- Describe epidemiological data sources for American Indian/Alaska Native (AI/AN) communities

- Discuss community-based participatory approaches to public health work in AI/AN communities

- Discuss at least two issues related to community control over evaluation and research and potential steps that can be taken in a community approval process

- Identify tools for logic models and theory operationalization in program planning in AI/AN communities

This chapter discusses the pleasures and challenges of conducting public health needs assessment, program planning and implementation, and evaluation in "Indian Country."[1] It begins with a discussion of potentially unconscious elements of the practitioner's conceptual framework and the multiple functions and outcomes of health promotion and disease prevention (HPDP) efforts. It then outlines standard public health approaches to needs assessment, indigenous planning and implementation, and evaluation and specific nuances of that work in Indian Country. So long as Native American and Alaska Native communities suffer disproportionately from disease, trauma, and other social problems, HPDP efforts will be indispensable.

The authors support a postcolonial indigenous planning approach to work in Native communities (Duran & Duran, 1995; Jojola, 2001). This approach is inherently interdisciplinary. It uses the latest that public health and other social science disciplines have to offer in assessment, planning, and evaluation while anchoring HPDP efforts within Native American control and in their community worldview. In addition to improving health status, an inherent aim of many Native American–controlled HPDP efforts is to empower people and transform ethnocentric social structures and social science. In this sense, they are founded on the principles of social justice, cultural revitalization, and Indigenous sovereignty.

Constructing a Workable Conceptual Framework

Conceptual frameworks typically include the theory of etiology and theory of change for the health issues or problems for which interventions are planned. More fundamentally, conceptual frameworks include, among other things, our assumptions about target populations, motivations for wanting to work with specific groups, and ideas about the roles professionals and community representatives

assume in that work. It is useful to make conceptual frameworks explicit (an exercise in self-reflection) when working in environments that might be organized by worldviews, historical experiences, and principles that are different from our own (Marcus & Fischer, 1986).

Successful working relationships between Native American communities and health professionals depend on overcoming misconceptions and clarifying assumptions about both Native peoples[2] and public health practice. For example, popular culture beliefs about Native people's homogeneity are misguided. A crucial step in liberating Native subjectivities from the straitjacket of binary oppositions (white/Indian, Native person/public health worker) is gaining an understanding of the diversity of Native communities and perspectives (Fleming, 1992; Prakash, 1995). In 1492, more cultural and linguistic diversity existed on this continent than could be found in all Europe. The differences among tribes still account for 50% of American cultural diversity (Berkhofer, 1979; Hodgkenson, 1990). Native heterogeneity is marked by differences in language, normative beliefs and behavior, gender roles, spiritual practices, migration, social class, economic opportunity, openness to other cultures, religion, and history, among other differences. Presently, there are 569 federally recognized tribes. They are among other tribal communities that include state-recognized tribes in the process of petitioning for federal recognition and innumerable urban-Indian groups. In 2000, it was estimated that of the 4.1 million people (1.5% of total U.S. population) that reported themselves as AI/AN, 57% of all persons who identified as American Indian[3] lived in metropolitan areas as defined by the U.S. Census.

In addition to differences between tribes, differences among tribal members and groups are significant. It is inaccurate to assume that all members of one tribe or Native community share opinions about matters such as the role of government, tradition, spirituality, and economic development. Like all communities in the postmodern social context, AI/AN groups can be factionalized. For example, individuals in impoverished communities where social service funds are an important source of revenue are often stratified by access to federal and other public resources (Ong, 1987).

Community-Based Participatory Approaches

Attitudes toward outsiders vary among Native American groups. Social research and interventions in Indian Country have left many participants feeling exploited and mistrustful (Duran & Duran, 1995; Manson, Garroutte, Goins, & Henderson, 2004; Oberly & Macedo, 2004; Wallerstein, Duran, Minkler, & Foley, 2005; Warne, 2006). The issue of Euro-Americans and other non-Indians working in communities of color, therefore, is a common concern of Natives and others. In some situations, even Native "intellectuals" who have been trained in the West have been regarded as problematic because of their alignment with class and cultural interests and values outside the traditional community (Noe et al., 2007).

Understanding the motivation for wanting to work in ethnic communities different from one's own is an important focus of professional reflection. A research assistant, for example, told one author that she wanted to work with Native Americans to voice their concerns to people in power. The author's response was to ask her whether her anthropology education included a course in ventriloquism. Can any research or researcher hope to speak authentically of the experience of the "other"? This thorny problem is partially addressed through participatory and collaborative public health practice and through efforts of historically marginalized groups to increase public health practice capacities of their own. It is fully addressed as one principle tenant of indigenous planning where practitioners are told directly that indigenous voices

need no translation and that they must be allowed to take their rightful roles as enablers and empowerers (Jojola, 2001).

The ideal situation for the public health practitioner wanting to work with Native peoples is to be contracted by or to work directly under the supervision of the tribe or Native community agency. Because this is not how all public health projects are initiated, many tribes and urban groups have established policies that give their communities more control over outside research and evaluation. The tribal or agency institutional review board or health board is gaining popularity as a way to control the amount and type of research and programs conducted on reservations or in Indian agencies. Tribal council or board approval is, at the very least, always required to begin any intervention work (Manson et al., 2004).

Community-based participatory research and approaches (CBPR/CBPA) have emerged in the past decade, though their exploration and use have been part of social psychology in the United States since the 1940s and part of more radical social sciences and their transformation agenda in Latin America, Africa, and Asia since the 1970s (Trickett & Espino, 2004; Wallerstein & Duran, 2003). Defined by the Kellogg Foundation (2001), CBPA is a "collaborative approach to research that equitably involves all partners in the research process and recognizes the unique strengths that each brings. CBPA begins with a research topic of importance to the community with the aim of combining knowledge and action for social change to improve community health and eliminate health disparities" (Minkler & Wallerstein, 2003, p. 4). CBPA is not a method per se and can engage both qualitative and quantitative strategies. The distinction of CBPA is that it challenges the traditional roles of expert and community to examine the roles of power, participation (who is included and who excluded), potential impact of racism (Chavez, Duran, Baker, Avila, & Wallerstein,

2003), and who is leading the knowledge creation agenda. CBPA partnerships therefore become involved in the development of collaborative principles that address these issues (Green, 1995; Israel, Eng, Schulz, & Parker, 2005; Schulz et al., 1998). In addition to being concerned with collaborative development of the intervention design, outcome measures, target population, evaluation data collection, and analysis, CBPA strategies can embrace the question of the added dimension of participation in the intervention process and outcome. How do participatory processes change the intervention and evaluation itself? What might be the added value of participatory processes to the health enhancement of the tribal community?

There is now recognition that politics and science are inextricably linked. Fundamental to this position is the acknowledgment that HPDP efforts are enacted by people, embodied as we all are by multiple subject positions—ethnicity, gender, class, sexual orientation, religion, and so forth. The recipients or audiences of HPDP efforts are likewise situated and may desire projects for different reasons—cultural, spiritual, political, economic, medical, and bureaucratic, among others.

Apart from dealing with health problems, tribal and community leaders often see HPDP funds as economic development opportunities or educational pipeline opportunities. Cultural integration and community building are other important outcomes of HPDP projects (Minkler & Wallerstein, 1997). Social and cultural activities and relationships constitute Native American communities as such and inscribe meaning to identity. Central to this identity is the community's worldview and the values associated with territory, land tenure, and stewardship. It represents a philosophical construction of humankind's relationship to the natural world and is demarcated by territories that balance human's social and health needs with an ecologically viable and sustainable lifestyle. Implementing efforts that are rooted in cultural and spiritual tradition helps

reestablish tribal and family social networks as well as forms of social control that were lost largely through government efforts to diminish Native land base and eradicate Indian language and culture (O'Brien, 1989).

CLASSIC NEEDS ASSESSMENT AND ISSUES PARTICULAR TO NATIVE COMMUNITIES

Classic needs assessment describes health and social service requirements in a geographic or social area and then estimates the relative importance of those needs in the context of available resources (Siegel, Attkission, & Carson, 1987). Needs assessment is an integral component of a cyclical public health core functions framework in which assessment informs policy that guides assurance activities.

Needs Assessment Process Issues

Within Native communities, increasing local capacity to conduct assessments and assuaging historical mistrust are important goals. Developing an inclusive and empowering process, therefore, requires attention to and planning of the procedures of assessment. The public health practitioner who has trained and worked within formal organizations is often oriented toward outcomes rather than process and, therefore, is less attuned to issues of process.

Empowering processes include oversight power by community leaders and an opportunity for community members to voice their satisfaction, concerns, and complaints about health assessment and subsequent services. Health care programs still run by Indian Health Services (IHS), for example, work closely with tribal health boards in defining and addressing health needs and projects in their regions. In this case, tribal health boards have an informal approval authority on the yearly strategic plans of the IHS. Reservation-based town hall meetings provide an opportunity for the dissemination of epidemiological data on health status as well as giving time for dialogue about the needs and quality of services from a community perspective. Community input must be designed into the process, regardless of whether or not people immediately take advantage of the opportunity to speak. Patience is the real mark of commitment in Native communities.

Although processes can be designed to improve community control and participation, the practitioner should not be discouraged or surprised if he or she encounters resistance to his or her efforts. Regarding the degree to which colonial structures share similarities, Scott (1990) asserts, "They will, other things equal, elicit reactions and patterns of resistance that are also broadly comparable" (p. xi). Scott identifies four types of political discourse produced by historically marginalized groups:

1. Public discourse: official ideology of relations between oppressed and oppressor that takes as its basis the flattering self-image of elites

2. Hidden transcript: subordinates gathering outside the gaze of power and constructing a sharply critical political and cultural discourse

3. Coded counter hegemonic discourse: subordinate groups making use of disguise and anonymity to find an avenue for the veiled expression of hidden transcripts within public discourse

4. Open defiance: a public refusal to comply with words, gestures, or other signs of normative compliance; a public announcement of the intention to engage in conflict

A public unveiling of "hidden transcripts" resulting in community conflict is a sign that disenfranchised groups are realizing and exercising their inherent power. Building an ally base from within the community, developing cross-cultural communication skills, and cultivating sensitivity to the historical bases of conflict and mistrust are ways to prevent or lessen conflicts. If the HPDP practitioner is confident of his or her cross-cultural competence (which is ideally based on successful experience with a multitude of ethnic groups different from the practitioner's own rather than on classroom success), then not taking the conflict personally is an important attitudinal approach. Time, commitment, knowledge, and sensitivity will be recognized by tribal leaders and will be rewarded with trust.

Another important indigenous planning tenant is to acknowledge that tribal communities are not "the minority." The territories of indigenous people are characterized by a social and cultural geography where the *outsider* or non-Native is often the minority. Indigenous communities and their lands may seem small by comparison with the dominant surrounding society, but within its borders, outsiders may appear nonexistent. The postmodern discourse indicates that as long as indigenous communities continue to unconsciously ply the notion that their power is insolvent because they are demographic majorities, the collective will continue to be marginalized and made to appear invisible and insignificant.

Compiling Existing Data

A standard element of needs assessment includes the compilation and synthesis of existing social indicator, epidemiological, and health service data. Although health service utilization data have their limitations in capturing population health status, the national office of the IHS periodically compiles and synthesizes data on morbidity and mortality. Two publications, *Trends in Indian Country* and *Regional Differences in Indian Health* are excellent starting points for understanding the distribution of disease and trauma in IHS serviced tribes. State health departments also routinely collect data on AI/AN health status. The National Institutes of Health have funded epidemiologic studies of chronic mental and physical illness in "Indian Country" and many journal articles report the results of those studies. Another excellent source for tribal population data and government reports is the American Indian and Alaska Native U.S. Census Web site.

On a regional level, IHS, tribal, and state health department offices compile and synthesize data for smaller geographic locations. In New Mexico, for example, health service utilization data are available for small tribal areas and, in some cases, for reservation towns. Unfortunately, to our knowledge, no one is currently collecting widespread health services outcome data. Fairly accurate denominators (i.e., total population numbers needed to calculate rates) are available from the national census or tribal census. Given a known denominator, RE-AIM (reach, efficacy/effectiveness, adoption, implementation, and maintenance, see www.re-aim.org) is a useful framework to conceptualize implementation of evidence-based approaches in Indian Country (Glasgow & Emmons, 2007). Federal regulations allow the IHS to conduct population health surveys, but probability sample surveys involve a more complex approval process as described above. The Navajo Health and Nutrition Examination Survey (NHANES) is an example of the type of health and behavioral survey that may be available by IHS area office or tribe (C. Percy, personal communication, January 25, 1996).

Regional business associations are useful sources of data on urban Indian communities. These entities often compile census and market data by ethnicity. Information about education and poverty levels, household makeup, and other social indicators is available for free or for a small fee. The Bureau of Indian Affairs regional offices and tribal economic development offices have comparable data for rural or reservation residents.

Some states, working alone or with the tribes and IHS, are beginning to oversample Native population in their Behavioral Risk Factor Surveys. State vital statistics offices also provide Native birth and death records, including demographics and community of residence. Tribal health departments have conducted or sponsored community health surveys and needs assessments; and Tribal health departments are crucial sources of survey data, needs assessment data, and most important, collaboration.

Primary Data Collection

In comprehensive needs assessments, population-based community surveys are important sources of information about the community's perceptions of capacities and needs. Client utilization data capture information about a specific segment of the community, whereas population surveys provide access to sections of the population that might not, for a variety of reasons, use existing public resources. Community surveys are best undertaken either under the direction of or in conjunction with tribal health departments, tribal councils, or urban health or social service agencies. Although tribal governments may have a membership enrollment or housing office, it is important to note that they may not have or maintain current rosters of households actually living on their reservation. In addition, population data on tribal members may be considered proprietary by the tribe. As stated earlier, many tribes and Indian organizations have an internal institutional review board process that governs all research activities.

Developing a realistic sampling frame requires collaboration with individuals very knowledgeable about Native residence and social network patterns. Although random or probability sampling is the most rigorous approach, this type of sampling for Native communities is problematic in both rural and urban areas. In most urban areas, the cost of probability sampling is prohibitive. Native researchers and others, however, have uncovered important patterns and insights about health-related needs, behavior, and attitudes by using purposive, convenience, and quota sampling (Evans-Campbell, Lindhorst, Huang, & Walters, 2006; Walters, Evans-Campbell, Simoni, Ronquillo, & Bhuyan, 2006).

Key Informants in Indian Country

Key informants are important sources of information about community health status, community concerns, and health-related behavioral patterns, attitudes, and beliefs (Siegel et al., 1987). In the standard approach, key informants include personnel from social and health service agencies, elderly centers, schools, economic development endeavors, police and fire departments, and the like. Long-term community residents not in an official capacity are also a meaningful source of community knowledge. In Native communities, it is important to include information from cultural, spiritual, and political leaders. Each reservation community may have a person or family teaching cultural arts such as singing, drumming, dancing, and regalia design. Spiritual people and their helpers, medicine women and men, sweat lodge leaders, "road men," sobriety group leaders, and other religious or spiritual workers not only provide insight into assessment efforts but also support and provide legitimacy for the health practitioner's work. Cultural protocol is an important daily aspect of social life.

Often, there are advocacy groups working on salient community issues such as environmental, educational, and economic development concerns. These individuals illuminate the current political climate and help identify "natural helpers," people who, because of some characteristic that is highly valued in the culture, are influential and respected. Youth are another important source of information, particularly about the way in which they are influenced and affected by the variety of adolescent subcultural trends. Research in eastern California found that many Native adolescents identified highly with the vibrant Latino culture in the area and claimed Latino ethnicity on school-based surveys.

Talking to many types of individuals provides insight into community capacities and needs. If the forums or interviews are thorough, then the health practitioner probably will uncover differences of opinion about key community issues; he or she should be prepared to hear some venting or challenging of one's role. It is important not to be seen as taking sides or as supporting any position on these issues until the assessment is complete. Although it is impossible to be "disembodied" or totally neutral in any assessment, it is necessary to try and minimize perceptions of working for any particular community political group or contingent.

Tying It All Together: Postcolonial Convergent Analysis

In a rational policy model, the distribution of resources depends on the relative importance, costs, and benefits of addressing any particular health problem compared with all others (Siegel et al., 1987). The postcolonial, self-determined, or empowerment approach that is adopted by many tribes and Native communities, however, also determines value from the perspective of community stakeholders and traditional values. An important principle of this approach is that Native community values, beliefs, and knowledge are valid and integral to the process of valuing (Duran & Duran, 1995). This point is significant in the tenants of indigenous planning where a standard cost-benefit analysis is necessary, but it not sufficient for determining community needs or program priorities.

Having identified and prioritized those problems that are affecting a particular community (and subpopulations of that community) the most, and having chosen appropriate etiological theories and thus targets of change, program planning proceeds toward devising interventions with a specific goal, a specific target, and measurable outcome objectives in mind. As with assessment efforts, program planning in Native communities is a collaborative effort that actively involves key leaders and members of the target population.

Key Components of Indigenous Health Promotion: Community Capacity Building and Cultural Revitalization

In addition to the CBPR approaches discussed above, community capacity building is an important component of successful indigenous HPDP efforts. Community capacity has been defined as "the characteristics of communities that affect their ability to identify, mobilize, and address social and public health problems" (Goodman et al., 1998). Community capacity has been articulated as having multiple dimensions: active participation, leadership, rich support networks, skills, ability to bring in resources, critical reflection, sense of community, understanding of history, articulation of values, and access to power (Goodman et al., 1998). Definitions of community capacity overlap with related concepts, such as "community competence," "social capital," and "empowerment." In the first operationalization of social capital/community capacity for tribal communities, Mignone (2003) working with Canadian First Nations peoples, has identified specific tribal bonding social capital measures, as well as bridging and linking measures (the ability of tribes to interact well with outside governments and entities, and tribal members to interact outside reservation life). These dimensions of community capacity and social capital open the door to examining organizational leadership and policy measures within the socioecologic framework, such as assessment of program commitment and resources for prevention, leadership involvement with community-defined problems, and systemwide ability to support children and families. These dimensions of community

capacity may be important to monitor and measure to ensure longstanding benefit to Native communities.

The social ecologic model (McLeroy, Bibeau, Steckler, & Glanz, 1988) is a useful framework for developing a theory of etiology for Native social problems and is culturally congruent with many AI/AN cultural and social beliefs. This approach, emphasizing determinants in the intrapersonal, interpersonal, institutional, community, and public policy spheres is consistent with indigenous theories of etiology that often include social and historical determinants of health and social problems. Using the ecological perspective enables one to recognize that Native peoples are not always the appropriate targets of change. This recognition is important for workers in Native communities where "commonsense" etiological understanding often includes the effects of historical processes, colonization, racism, cultural hegemony, poverty, and other outcomes of unequal power relations. It also acknowledges the fact that community change requires collective action.

The Logic Model

In Step 1 (see Table 18.1), problem identification, the planner makes succinct statements about measurable intervention aims across ecological domains—reduce alcohol and drug use, decrease obesity rates, reduce unprotected sexual activity, increase screening behavior, and so on. The factors most mutable and most significant are targeted for change. This information is garnered from existing epidemiological and other research about the correlates of problems and from experience at the local level about the antecedents to problems.

In Step 2, the assumptions and literature that support the problem identification are delineated. For each of the problems or risk factors, there is an assumption that the factor is related to the current or subsequent problem. In Step 3, program objectives are

Table 18.1   Logic Model for Alcohol, Tobacco, and Other Drug Prevention for a Specific Subpopulation of American Indian Youths

Level	Problem Identification	Assumptions and Literature	Project Objectives	Program Strategies	Anticipated Outcomes
Individual	Lack of sobriety skills; poor positive Native ethnic group identification	Experience of prevention workers (Trimble, Padilla, & Bell, 1987)	Reduce ATOD use; increase sobriety and coping skills; increase positive cultural identification	12-week sobriety skills curriculum; 12-week Native cultural education curriculum	Increased coping and sobriety skills; increase bicultural competency
Peer	Lack of peer support for nonuse	Experience of prevention workers (Trimble et al., 1987)	Create ATOD nonusing support/peer groups	Peer-managed self-control; Native American youth groups	Nonusing peer groups; perceptions of peer use decreased
School	Lack of commitment to school; low teacher expectations of Native youths; hostile environment	Parents and community leaders unhappy with what they perceive as racism in the schools	Reduce school-based racism; increase cultural competency of teacher	Community organizing; competency training of school staff; enforced school policy against racist activities	School mission includes honoring diversity; increase cultural competency; higher teacher expectations of Native youths
Community	Lack of clear-cut sanctions against use	Experience of prevention workers (Trimble et al., 1987)	Increase community sanction against use by youths	Community organizing to change tribal council policies	Tribal policy concerning ATOD at community events, buildings

NOTE: ATOD = alcohol, tobacco, and other drugs.

selected. The planner takes the problem statement and turns it into an action statement indicating what needs to be done to alleviate the problem or condition or to promote the protective factor. Each objective should specify a single measurable quantifiable result and should be accomplishable with existing resources and within the program time frame. In Step 4, program strategies for achieving the objectives should always be based on culturally appropriate theories of change. For example, in Table 18.1, the sobriety, coping, and bicultural skills curriculum is based on principles of Social Learning Theory and principles of cultural revitalization. In Step 5, anticipated outcomes assist the evaluation process by clearly delineating the results of the program. This step identifies the outcome indexes that the planner needs to determine whether his or her intervention was effective in fulfilling its objectives.

Operationalizing Theory

Subsequent to developing a causal theory, change theories help explain and delineate how those factors identified in disease and illness causality are best manipulated. Change theory is "operationalized" in the context of the practitioner's health problem and target population (Stanton, Black, Engle, & Pelto, 1992). Operationalization involves four steps: (a) defining components of the theory or model, (b) translating the component for the targeted behavior within the culture, (c) determining options for intervention design, and (d) determining content of intervention. Table 18.2 illustrates the first steps in this task using Social Cognitive Theory for an alcohol, tobacco, and other drugs (ATOD) prevention program with high-risk youths in one reservation population. This type of joint activity with community partners brings experience and wisdom to bear on the problem and encourages communities and agencies to implement and maintain the intervention.

Translation and Implementation

The past decade has seen tremendous growth in theories and approaches to program implementation though the science is just beginning. Often, situated within larger discussions of adaptation and dissemination of evidence-based HPDP (Fixsen, Naoom, Blase, Friedman, & Wallace, 2005) and

external validity of health services innovations (Glasgow & Emmons, 2007), the focus on implementation bridges science and services.

There are no reported implementation studies in Indian Country. Given the dearth of culturally supported evidence, one approach to implementation is to follow the advice provided by the recent "best practices" findings. Well-designed implementation plans can be used to improve programs and services at the practitioner, organization, and national level. Fixen et al. (2005) identify the implementation framework as (a) the Source, (b) the Communications link, and (c) the Destination. The source concerns the key intervention and implementation components and "packaging." In Indian Country, trust for the intervention itself may be determined by how components align with traditional community values and norms and, in some cases, by the relationship between the originating institution and the community. For example, an innovation imported from another tribe or Native agency may be better received than an intervention directly from a university-based randomized controlled trial. The communication link refers to the *purveyors* of a new intervention or services, credible consultants who help ready the Destination and provide training, coaching, and feedback to staff in departments and agencies within larger institutions. The Destination is the department or agency that has achieved a level of readiness to implement the new program and is resourced to provide the administrative, evaluative, training, and couching support needed to sustain the intervention. To ensure success, the Destination organization agrees to undergo the changes necessary to implement the evidence-based program and also agrees to develop the functions to sustain the program/practice by installing the core implementation components. The feedback from Purveyors to Destination includes information about the fidelity of the program and the core implementation elements.

Table 18.2 Operationalization of Social Cognitive Theory to Alcohol, Tobacco, and Other Drug Prevention Among Indian Youths

Define Theory Components	Cultural Interpretation	Determine Options for Intervention	Determine Content of Intervention
Behavioral capacity	Drinking alleviates stress or anger Fun involves drinking	Increase level of sobriety and coping skills Increase ATOD-free recreational activities	Adopt 12-week curriculum in intervention in youth groups
Expectations	Drinking is part of Indian social life Nonusing will isolate youths from Indian peer group No role for Indians in mainstream culture Success in school means acting "white"	Cultural education about history of ATOD in Indian Country Parental and teacher training to increase expectations of youths	8-hour teacher cultural competency training 8-hour parenting training Attend four local cultural events as part of intervention Develop Indian academic club at school with support from Native professionals
Self-efficacy	Youths doubt their ability to resist peer pressure Low self-esteem and self-efficacy due to racism and internalized oppression	Develop nonusing peer groups Reinstitute initiation rituals for youths	Native American youth societies in each town Weekly age- and gender-specific support groups in each town Skill-building workshops
Observational learning	There is a cadre of anti-drinking leaders in the community National Indian sobriety movement activities (e.g., National Association of Native American Adult Children of Alcoholics, Wellness Conference) High level of substance abuse among adults	Exposure to role models Exposure to consequences of excessive drinking	Attend one Indian men's and one Indian women's wellness conference Invite sobriety movement leaders to three community education events Invite Indian Alcoholics Anonymous speakers to two events
Reinforcement	There are more reasons to drink than not to drink	Increase community supports for ATOD-free behavior Develop tribal acknowledgements of success	Youth appointments to tribal council Youth "whip" persons at powwows Develop youth sobriety drum/dancing group Chance school and tribal policy

NOTE: ATOD = alcohol, tobacco, and other drugs.

The core implementation components or drivers are as follows:

- Selection of a site that is ready (as described in Destination above)
- Selection of key implementation staff at local sites
- Training local implementation staff in coaching/consulting, evaluating, facilitative systems, and administrative support skills
- Consulting and coaching implementation staff as they practice their newly acquired skills
- Evaluating implementation staff performance at the provider, agency, and systems levels
- Administratively supporting the implementation staff to enact organizational changes
- Facilitating systems innovations to ensure favorable structural conditions for change

A key issue in the implementation of evidence-based approaches in tribal and urban Indian organization's is resources. IHS and federal funds to tribes are allocated at 40% to 60% "level of need" (U.S. Commission on Civil Rights, 2003). Since the cost of basic services is not fully covered, lack of resources precludes systems and clinical innovations that call for staff time and other resources. It is crucial, therefore, that any new program or service innovation comes with its own resources for program and implementation of core components.

EVALUATION IN NATIVE COMMUNITIES

Program evaluations of HPDP efforts in Indian Country are undertaken for a variety of purposes and, by nature of the heterogeneity of Indian life, in a variety of contexts. Evaluations conducted by tribal health programs and local IHS offices frequently have incremental program improvement as a key outcome, whereas demonstration and research projects funded by the federal government or national foundations usually focus on causal modeling, health service outcomes, and discovery The theory of social program evaluation has progressed significantly during the past 10 years and warrants consideration here as the range of appropriate approaches for Indian Country are considered. Articulating the assumptions of various approaches allows us to conscientiously determine the best fit for the goals of Native communities.

Evaluation Theory Overview

Shadish, Cook, and Leviton (1991) have developed a useful three-stage topology of evaluation theory based on each stage's approach to five fundamental issues: (1) social programming, (2) knowledge construction, (3) valuing, (4) knowledge use, and (5) evaluation practice.

Stage 1 theory asserts that the purpose of evaluation is to determine causal relationships in an investigation of social problems. Positivistic methods are the only acceptable methodology. Experimental design, valid instrumentation, and bias control are key evaluative principles. Viewing evaluations as objective science, this approach urges practitioners to keep their distance from program stakeholders, advocates, and detractors. The lack of direct fit between social interventions and social problem amelioration, combined with the difficulty of applying strict experimental methods to Native communities, will for the most part, preclude this evaluative approach.

The pragmatist approach of Stage 2 theory focuses on the manner in which evaluative information is used to design and modify social interventions and on the uses and perspectives of various stakeholders. This approach is consistent with the methods and processes of CBPR. Stage 2 evaluation theory emphasis is on the utility of knowledge and case studies, ethnographies, and other qualitative approaches where all are acceptable. In contrast to the distance approach of the Stage 1 theorist, evaluation practice involves close contact with program plans and implementation.

Stage 3 theory retains the belief in rigorous methodology and the search for ultimate truth about program effectiveness while stressing the importance of descriptive knowledge and contextual fit. Stage 3 theorist prescribes the use of rigorously evaluated mixed qualitative/ quantitative demonstration projects that explore theoretical explanation and causal mediating processes.

Use of evaluation results in Indian Country often depends on the placement of the evaluator. With these theoretical considerations in mind, the selection of a relevant evaluation approach in Native communities depends on (a) an identification of community partners, (b) the potential uses of the produced knowledge, (c) the epistemological framework of the Native community, and (d) the values that will guide the assessment of program merit. Social science now recognizes that these concepts are culturally specific and not universal paradigms (Bernstein, 1988; Derrida, 1980; Foucault, 1972, 1973, 1980; Habermas, 1988; Lyotard, 1984; Marcus & Fischer, 1986; Said, 1993). Programs and evaluations aspiring to postcolonial or empowerment practice must therefore be founded on Native worldviews to make real their overall capacity for self-determination.

Managing the Evaluation

Evaluations are often contracted out to public health or other social science specialists. Management of the evaluation begins by developing a contract that defines resources, staffing, qualifications, timing, and other issues that are specific to the project and locale. A primary concern is the adequacy of program resources for evaluation. A rigorous and thorough evaluation may consume up to 30% of the total project costs and, likewise, a high percentage of program staff time. The division of labor between the evaluation and the program staff is outlined before any activities begin. Program staff are routinely charged with collecting data from their participants and activities. The program director or manager is charged with governing the evaluation tasks of the program staff and ensuring that all staff-related data are collected and stored for use or review by the evaluator. Program administrators and the evaluator choose or develop the instruments, and the evaluator analyzes and reports process and outcome findings. Evaluation staff or other neutral parties administer instruments and satisfaction surveys. An adequate schedule for on-site visits and monitoring should be part of the contract. In the first 12 or 18 months of new projects, evaluation reports may be required more frequently, and evaluation visits may be required as well. A clear plan for regular meetings and a format to obtain and use process evaluation feedback are important contract items (DeJung, 1991).

Developing an Evaluation Protocol

Once these issues are considered and decisions have been made about how to proceed, the steps or components of the evaluation are delineated. A standard approach is to develop an evaluation protocol (Green & Lewis, 1986). This document is a detailed blueprint (20 to 25 pages) for evaluation practice and may include the following sections:

1. Significance of the problem addressed by the program

2. Description of the program

3. Program impact theory or model: the rationale that justifies the claim that the program will remedy the problem (the logic model is useful here)

4. Program objectives and measures

5. Evaluative research design, dimension to be evaluated (process and outcome), and methodological strategy to be used

6. Participant selection criteria

7. Data collection procedures

8. Methods and example of analysis

9. Anticipated use of results and implications for policy and practice

10. References

The evaluator working with community partners has the primary responsibility for developing the protocol.

Process Evaluation

The process evaluation answers questions about the program's fit and implementation within the community's current context, program staffing, and the feedback mechanisms to improve or redesign the intervention. Some possible implementation questions include the staff's ability to articulate goals and objectives; a description and judgment about the quality of each intervention; the adequacy of dosage to individual clients; adequacy of documentation to record dosage and participant involvement; frequency of staff and management meetings; the cultural, age, and gender appropriateness of any curriculum or manuals used; ratio of staff to participants; staff prior experience, training, and current competency; and adequacy of staff and/or participant supervision (Green & Lewis, 1986). Evaluators should schedule ongoing observations of interventions to evaluate content, participant receptiveness, and staff competency.

Differing characteristics of universal versus selected interventions are a concern in some Native communities (Offord, 2000). In youth programs particularly, stigmatization might be attached to either inclusion or exclusion, depending on the popularity of the HPDP effort and the intervention focus. In one example, youth who used any amount of alcohol or drugs were excluded from a primary ATOD prevention project. This created a perception that the project was labeling families

as good or bad, and a division in the community ensued. This rule, and the project's rigid confidentiality regulation, created animosity and suspicion from those families excluded from participation in the program. In the process of changing norms and improving social capital, some level of community upheaval can be expected.

Client record-keeping systems are important not only to ensure intervention quality but also for funding reporting requirements. Process evaluation questions related to record keeping might include a review of standardized forms related to client confidentiality (particularly with computerized systems), release of information to other agencies or parents, documentation of group and individual contacts with participants, and community events records. Client confidentiality is crucial in bounded Indian communities, particularly when data are collected on sensitive issues such as ATOD use and sexual activity. Parental and community desires to know about interventions, and participants must be weighed against individual and family rights to privacy and fear of rumor and gossip. Fear of breach of confidentiality is a major barrier to prevention and treatment services (Duran et al., 2005).

Monitoring the stability of administrative systems is an important consideration in the interpretation of HPDP outcomes. Because of generally low pay and the amount and severity of "life events" experienced by Native families, high staff turnover even for administrative positions may be common. Formal staff orientations and training plans help keep the program running at optimal levels in the event of staff turnover. Appropriate evaluation questions for administrative systems might include the plans for staff development and training; board, other staff, and higher administrative support; a review of personnel and grievance procedures; staff credentialing and certification; and the adequacy of secretarial support.

Process evaluation activities should include an examination of facilities. Program environs affect participation both culturally and physically. Adequate space for meetings, training, and events attracts community members and maintains staff morale. Assigning space that can be secured for confidential reports or documents should also be planned.

A review of community linkages is an important focus for process evaluation. A formalized memorandum of agreement and procedures should be established between agencies that exchange referrals. Other community issues for process evaluation include the staff's understanding of community linkages, delegation of responsibility to maintain and initiate contacts, and the availability of other agency resources for the HPDP client population.

Outcome Evaluation

In addition to the philosophical choices outlined here, the rigor and design of the outcome evaluation, in many cases, depends on funders' requirements. Evaluations conducted internally are by definition less rigorous and usually do not entail comparison or control groups. Nonexperimental designs such as the one-shot case study, the one-group pretest/posttest design, and the static-group design are common methods for internal outcome evaluation (Campbell & Stanley, 1963). Qualitative methods such as case study, participant observation (Greene, 1994; Yack, 1991) and rapid ethnographic assessment (Murray, Tapson, Turbull, McCullum, & Little, 1994) have been successfully used to provide thick description of program activities and outcomes. Qualitative methods are particularly useful when more information is needed about the population at risk, the determinants of the health problems under question, and/or their risk and protective factors.

The use of standardized valid instruments is a concern for Native American populations, as with other populations of color. Some instruments, fortunately, are normed for Native populations. The Tri-Ethnic Center at the University of Colorado, the Native American and Alaska Native Center for Mental Health Research at the University of Colorado at Denver, and the Indigenous Wellness Research Institute at the University of Washington have produced valid and reliable mental health and cultural identification measures, as have other Native-specific research endeavors. A viable alternative to developing new outcome measures is to contract with one of the Native American Public Health Consultant groups. Some of these organizations not only supply prevention-related instruments but also statistically analyze the data and provide detailed reports for a reasonable price.

Report Writing and Dissemination of Results

The evaluation staff has responsibility for process and outcome evaluation reports to funders. Refereed journal articles are the customary way in which program and evaluation knowledge is circulated to the professional community. In instances where the information may be considered proprietary, the authorship of any journal articles or other papers on the intervention should be discussed in advance with the appropriate tribal authorities. Consistent with the tenets of CBPR, project staff contributing to the intervention and evaluation should be included in authorship of journal articles and presentations.

Journal articles do not routinely reach a significant Native audience. Video documentaries or other video reports of intervention projects and outcomes are beginning to become popular in Indian Country (Rhine & Pierce, 1995). Video documentaries are an excellent medium in which to circulate knowledge about interventions, and their results directly to Indian Country and are also a significant source of community pride.

CHAPTER SUMMARY

This chapter has reviewed important issues and identified key resources in needs assessment, program planning, and evaluation in Indian Country. So long as Native communities suffer disproportionately from disease, trauma, and other social problems, HPDP efforts are indispensable. Conducting these efforts affords multiple pleasures and challenges for all health professionals as well as multiple outcomes. HPDP programs accomplish cultural revitalization, empowerment, and self-reflection; increase local capacity; and raise health consciousness and status. The authors support a postcolonial, indigenous planning approach to work in Native communities. This approach is inherently multidisciplinary. It uses the latest that public health and other social science disciplines have to offer in assessment, planning, and evaluation while anchoring HPDP efforts within the distinctive cultural worldviews and value systems of the Native communities.

The authors advocate more CBPR approaches to community-based assessment, planning, and evaluation for Indian Country. Although the prevention field has made great strides during the past decades, not enough is known about root causes of health problems or strategies for effective amelioration. Much of the work of the National Institutes of Health and the Centers for Disease Control and Prevention, unfortunately, is still far removed from the realities of life on the reservation or in urban Native communities. However, this does not preclude tribes and communities from building their own local capacity and using their own trained people to solve health problems. We need more expert Indians, rather than Indian experts (B. Pigman, personal communitcation, July 25, 2006). Native wisdom and methods of knowledge production need to be accepted by mainstream social science not only because they enhance translation efforts and participation but also because

in our changing society we are all enriched by diversity.

The next chapter presents a case study in which the author tries to emphasize points made in the overview and planning chapters. The study is concerned with the application of concepts and approaches for bridging the gap between theory and practice. They provide an opportunity for the student and practitioner to get a "bird's-eye" view of some of the specific methods and techniques of HPDP program planning, application, and problem solving.

NOTES

1. In this chapter, Indian Country refers not only to the standard definition of land within a reservation and land outside the reservation that is owned by tribal members or the tribe and held in trust by the federal government (O'Brien, 1989) but also to urban community-based organizations and corporate enterprises that are Native run and operated primarily for the benefit of Native peoples.

2. In this chapter, the term *Native* or indigenous peoples includes American Indians and Alaska Natives as well as other tribal groups whose homelands are ancestral to the Americas.

3. The U.S. Census 2000 definition of American Indian/Alaska Native (AI/AN) includes two totals; one for "AI/AN alone" and another for AI/AN in combination with other races.

4. An example is the Navajo Area Office.

DISCUSSION QUESTIONS AND ACTIVITIES

1. In small groups identify some important key stakeholders in public health assessment, planning, and evaluation among AI/AN communities and describe some important cultural and political considerations when working with these groups. Share your discussions with the rest of the class.

2. Using data sources mentioned in this chapter and the socioecologic framework develop a risk and protective factor table

for diabetes as a health problem in any AI/AN community of your choice.

3. Outline the components of an evaluation protocol you would use for the diabetes health problem identified in #2 above and the evaluation approval and consultation process you would use to create and implement your evaluation activities.

REFERENCES

American Heart Association (2008). *Statistical fact sheet—populations 2008 update*. New York: American Heart Association.

Berkhofer, R. (1979). *The white man's Indian*. New York: Vintage Books.

Bernstein, R. (1988). *Beyond objectivism and relativism: Science, hermeneutics, and praxis*. Philadelphia: University of Pennsylvania Press.

Campbell, T., & Stanley, J. C. (1963). *Experimental and quasi-experimental designs for research*. Boston: Houghton Mifflin.

Chavez, V., Duran, B., Baker, Q., Avila, M., & Wallerstein, N. (2003). The dance of race and privilege in community based participatory research. In M. Minkler & N. Wallerstein (Eds.), *Community based participatory research for health* (pp. 81–97). San Francisco: Jossey-Bass.

DeJung, J. (1991). *Evaluation guidelines*. Paper presented at the New CSAT Grantees Workshop, Washington, DC.

Derrida, J. (1980). *Of grammatology*. Baltimore: Johns Hopkins University Press.

Duran, B., & Duran, E. (1995). *Native American postcolonial psychology*. Albany: State University of New York Press.

Duran, B., Oetzel, J., Lucero, J., Jiang, Y., Novins, D. K., Manson, S., et al. (2005). Obstacles for rural American Indians seeking alcohol, drug, or mental health treatment. *Journal of Consulting and Clinical Psychology, 73*(5), 819–829.

Evans-Campbell, T., Lindhorst, T., Huang, B., & Walters, K. L. (2006). Interpersonal violence in the lives of urban American Indian and Alaska Native women: Implications for health, mental health, and help-seeking. *American Journal of Public Health, 96*(8), 1416–1422.

Fixsen, D. L., Naoom, S. F., Blase, K. A., Friedman, R. M., & Wallace, F. (2005). *Implementation research: A synthesis of the literature*. Tampa: University of South Florida, Louis de la Parte Florida Mental Health Institute, The National Implementation Research Network.

Fleming, C. M. (1992). American Indians and Alaska Natives: Changing societies past and present. In M. A. Orlandi (Ed.), *Cultural competence for evaluators* (Publication No. [ADM] 92-1884) (pp. 147–171). Washington, DC: U.S. Department of Health and Human Services, Office of Substance Abuse Prevention.

Foucault, M. (1972). *The archeology of knowledge* (A. Sheridan, Trans.). New York: Pantheon Books.

Foucault, M. (1973). *The order of things: An archeology of the human sciences* (A. Sheridan, Trans.). New York: Vintage/ Random House.

Foucault, M. (1980). *Power/knowledge: Selected interviews and other writings 1972–1977*. New York: Pantheon Books.

Glasgow, R. E., & Emmons, K. M. (2007). How can we increase translation of research into practice? Types of evidence needed. *Annual Review of Public Health, 28*, 413–433.

Goodman, R. M., Speers, M. A., McLeroy, K., Fawcett, S., Kegler, M., Parker, E., et al. (1998). Identifying and defining the dimensions of community capacity to provide a basis for measurement. *Health Education & Behavior, 25*(3), 258–278.

Green, L., & Lewis, E. (1986). *Measurement and evaluation in health education and health promotion*. Mountain View, CA: Mayfield.

Green, L. W. (1995). Who will qualify to fill positions in health promotion? *Canadian Journal of Public Health, 86*(1), 7–9.

Greene, J. C. (1994). Qualitative program evaluation: Practice and promise. In N. Denzin & Y. Lincoln (Eds.), *Handbook of qualitative research* (pp. 530–544). Thousand Oaks, CA: Sage.

Habermas, J. (1988). *On the logic of the social sciences*. Cambridge, MA: MIT Press.

Hodgkenson, H. (1990). *The demographics of American Indians: One percent of the people, fifty percent of the diversity*. Washington, DC: Center for Demographic Policy Institute of Medicine.

Israel, B. A., Eng, E., Schulz, A. J., & Parker, E. A. (Eds.). (2005). *Methods in community-based participatory research for health* (1st ed.). San Francisco: Jossey-Bass.

Jojola, T. (2001). Indigenous planning and resource management. In R. Clow & I. Sutton (Eds.), *Trusteeship in change: Toward tribal autonomy in resource management* (pp. 303–314). Boulder: University Press of Colorado.

Lyotard, J. (1984). *The postmodern condition: A report on knowledge.* Minneapolis: University of Minnesota Press.

Manson, S. M., Garroutte, E., Goins, R. T., & Henderson, P. N. (2004). Access, relevance, and control in the research process: Lessons from Indian Country. *Journal of Aging and Health, 16*(5 Suppl.), 58S–77S.

Marcus, G., & Fischer, M. (1986). *Anthropology as cultural critique: An experimental moment in the human sciences.* Chicago: University of Chicago Press.

McLeroy, K., Bibeau, D., Steckler, A., & Glanz, K. (1988). An ecological perspective on health promotion programs. *Health Education Quarterly, 15,* 351–377.

Mignone, J. (2003). *Measuring social capital: A guide for first nations communities.* Winnipeg, Manitoba, Canada: University of Manitoba, Human Ecology, Department of Family Social Sciences.

Minkler, M., & Wallerstein, N. (1997). Improving health through community organization and community building. In K. Glanz, E. Lewis, & B. Rimer (Eds.), *Health behavior and health education* (2nd ed., pp. 403–424). San Francisco: Jossey-Bass.

Minkler, M., & Wallerstein, N. (Eds.). (2003). *Community based participatory research for health.* San Francisco: Jossey-Bass.

Murray, S., Tapson, L., Turbull, L., McCullum, J., & Little, A. (1994). Listening to local voices: Adapting rapid appraisal to assess health and social needs in general practice. *British Journal of Medicine, 308,* 698–700.

Noe, T. D., Manson, S. M., Croy, C., McGough, H., Henderson, J. A., & Buchwald, D. S. (2007). The influence of community-based participatory research principles on the likelihood of participation in health research in American Indian communities. *Ethnicity & Disease, 17*(1 Suppl. 1), S6–S14.

O'Brien, S. (1989). *American Indian tribal governments.* Norman: University of Oklahoma Press.

Oberly, J., & Macedo, J. (2004). The R word in Indian Country: Culturally appropriate commercial tobacco-use research strategies. *Health Promotion Practice, 5*(4), 355–361.

Offord, D. R. (2000). Selection of levels of prevention. *Addictive Behaviors, 25*(6), 833–842.

Ong, A. (1987). *Spirits of resistance and capitalist discipline.* Albany: State University of New York Press.

Prakash, G. (1995). Postcolonial criticism and Indian histiography. In L. Nicholson & S. Seidman (Eds.), *Social postmodernism: Beyond identity politics* (pp. 87–100). Cambridge, UK: Cambridge University Press.

Rhine, G., (Writer) & Pierce, C. (Producer). (1995). *The red road to sobriety* [Motion picture]. United States: Kifaru Productions.

Said, E. (1993). *Culture and imperialism.* New York: Knopf.

Schulz, A. J., Parker, E. A., Israel, B. A., Becker, A. B., Maciak, B. J., & Hollis, R. (1998). Conducting a participatory community-based survey for a community health intervention on Detroit's east side. *Journal of Public Health and Management Practices, 4*(2), 10–24.

Scott, J. (1990). *Domination and the art of resistance.* New Haven, CT: Yale University Press.

Shadish, W. R., Jr., Cook, T. D., & Leviton, L. C. (1991). *Foundations of program evaluation: Theories practice.* Newbury Park, CA: Sage.

Siegel, L. M., Attkission, C., & Carson, L. (1987). Need identification and program planning in the community context. In E. Cox, J. Erlish, J. Rothman, & J. Tropman (Eds.), *Strategies of community organization* (pp. 229–265). Itasca, IL: E. E. Peacock.

Stanton, B., Black, R., Engle, P., & Pelto, G. (1992). Theory-driven behavioural intervention research for the control of diarrheal diseases. *Social Science & Medicine, 35,* 1405–1420.

Trickett, E. J., & Espino, S. L. (2004). Collaboration and social inquiry: Multiple meanings of a construct and its role in creating useful and valid knowledge. *American Journal of Community Psychology, 34*(1/2), 1–69.

Trimble, J., Padilla, A., & Bell, C. (1987). *Drug abuse among ethnic minorities* (No. [ADM] 87-1474). Washington, DC: National Institute on Drug Abuse.

U.S. Commission on Civil Rights. (2003). *A quiet crisis: Federal funding and unmet needs in Indian Country*. Washington, DC: U.S. Commission on Civil Rights.

Wallerstein, N., & Duran, B. (2003). The conceptual, historical and practical roots of community based participatory research and related participatory traditions. In M. Minkler & N. Wallerstein (Eds.), *Community based participatory research for health* (pp. 27–52). San Francisco: Jossey-Bass.

Wallerstein, N., Duran, B., Minkler, M., & Foley, K. (2005). Developing and maintaining partnerships with communities. In B. Israel (Ed.), *Methods for conducting community-based participatory research for health* (pp. 31–51). San Francisco: Jossey-Bass.

Walters, K. L., Evans-Campbell, T., Simoni, J. M., Ronquillo, T., & Bhuyan, R. (2006). "My spirit in my heart": Identity experiences and challenges among American Indian two-spirit women. *Journal of Lesbian Studies, 10*(1/2), 125–149.

Warne, D. (2006). Research and educational approaches to reducing health disparities among American Indians and Alaska Natives. *Journal of Transcultural Nursing, 17*(3), 266–271.

Yack, D. (1991). The use and value of qualitative methods in health research in developing countries. *Social Science & Medicine, 35,* 603–612.

19

Developing and Implementing Health Care Programs for American Indians and Alaska Natives

A Case Study

FELICIA SCHANCHE HODGE

CHRISTOPHER ELLIOTT HODGE

BETTY GEISHIRT CANTRELL

Chapter Objectives

On completion of this chapter, the health promotion student and practitioner will be able to

- List the steps that would be necessary in planning, implementing, and evaluating a health education or health promotion program for an American Indian/ Alaska Native (AI/AN) community

- Identify and discuss at least two intervention approaches that can be used for HPDP programming in AI/AN communities

This chapter describes the steps taken in developing and implementing a health care program for American Indians and Alaska Natives. A case study reporting on a diabetes research project conducted among four Northern Plains tribes describes real-life experiences encountered by the researcher team. The collaborative effort in the development and implementation of the program requires a multipronged approach on several levels.

Considering the developmental phase, having a good working relationship with the community, knowledge of the population in terms of illness beliefs, cultural constructs of wellness and illness, and tribal priorities and communication styles is essential. With regard to the implementation phase, understanding the community's social capital, cultural ways of negotiation, and historical context of health care and political environments is needed to ensure competent delivery of health care services.

Given that there are over 562 separate and distinct American Indian tribes and Alaska Native groups and villages in the United States, and given that many of these groups maintain their traditional healing ceremonies, illness beliefs, languages, and practices, designing programs that will easily be accepted and adopted within the targeted group is a challenging goal. In spite of the numerous tribes and Native groups in North America, there exist many similarities and base concepts that can be drawn on to develop and implement health care programs. These include values such as the importance of family and community, respect, sharing, and harmony with nature. These values are preserved in the tradition of oral storytelling, which provides the history, values, and lessons learned for present and future generations.

BACKGROUND

Type 2 diabetes was first documented among American Indians in 1945. Since then, diabetes has reached epidemic proportions and is a significant health concern among American Indians throughout North America (Bullock, 2001). There are reports indicating diabetes prevalence rates of 30% to 40% or higher in several Native communities (Lee et al., 1995). Indeed, other researchers (Burrows, Engelgau, Geiss, & Acton, 2000) note that the prevalence of type 2 diabetes among American Indians in the state of Arizona is the highest in the world. The U.S. Department of Health and Human Services

and Indian Health Services (2003) reports that American Indians have a 249% greater chance of dying from diabetes than any other ethnic group in the United States. These and other reports have led many tribes to voice a concern over this evolving epidemic, which has also reached Indian children (Story et al., 1999). Tribes are finding out that diabetes damages many organs in the body, including the kidneys, which can lead to a life dependent on dialysis or a kidney transplant. The long-term damage to the eyes and vascular system can result in blindness, strokes, heart attacks, and peripheral artery disease. Damage to these organs at an early age may not only reduce the quality of life but will also surely affect longevity.

It is important to note that obesity, sedentary lifestyles, and poor eating habits are risk factors associated with type 2 diabetes. American Indians and Alaska Natives have extremely high rates of obesity. The lack of exercise and sedentary lifestyles are well documented in this population. Poor eating habits are areas needing clarification and documentation. Knowledge levels, attitudes about diabetes, and treatment compliance are important factors to consider in the planning phase.

The very high incidence of obesity among American Indians is a serious occurrence, resulting in increased incidence of chronic diseases, such as diabetes, cancer, coronary heart disease, and hypertension. The problem of obesity has prompted an outcry from various American Indian groups, who have expressed concern about the quality of the Food Distribution Program on Indian Reservations (FDPIR) (U.S. Department of Agriculture [USDA], 1990, 1991) since use of this program is high. For many years, food items supplied by the commodity food program have been high in fat and sugar. However, an evaluation of the FDPIR concluded that it provides an acceptable, and often preferred, alternative to food stamps for many Indian families (USDA, 1990). And although the availability and desirability of different food commodities were evaluated, their nutritional value in the diet was not evaluated.

DIABETES WELLNESS PROJECT

The Diabetes Wellness Project was formed from an initial contact and request from Native health care leaders from the Northern Plains tribes. Years of epidemiological reports highlighted the continued increase in the prevalence of diabetes in that region. What was lacking was an appropriate, culturally sensitive intervention that would address the problem of diabetes. Following several meetings between university researchers and leading tribal health care representatives and providers, a plan of action was identified to conduct a research project that would gather information from those who were most affected by diabetes (individuals and their families) and to design and test an intervention that would be based on culturally appropriate methods and approaches.

Project Leadership. The Diabetes Wellness Project was led by a team approach employing community participatory methods. The participating tribal councils held ultimate authority in approving or disapproving all aspects of the study. Each tribe was required to approve the proposed research design and approach. Additionally, each tribe provided a certified resolution of support and approval for the submission of the proposal to the federal funding agency. Final study results were likewise reviewed and approved by each participating tribe, culminating in resolutions of acceptance of the study's findings.

The principal investigator provided scientific direction and overall supervision for the design, implementation, and evaluation of the intervention. Collaborating investigators included Indian and non-Indian research scientists with expertise in various areas of diabetes research, culture competency, statistical

methodology, and intervention design. Staff included local facilitators and educators led by the head field project director, a member of one of the local tribes. The field staff consisted of local residents who were members of one of the four participating tribes, had diabetes, or had a close member of their family with diabetes. These field staff were employed to assist in the gathering of data and the coordination of the intervention sessions.

Site Selection. Four large reservations in South Dakota and Nebraska were selected to participate in the study. These sites were the Pine Ridge, Rosebud, and Yankton reservations, all located in the lower part of the state of South Dakota. The fourth site was the Winnebago reservation, located in the upper part of the state of Nebraska. These sites had access to a health care clinic and were within driving distance from each other and to local health care facilities such as an Indian hospital and mental and social service programs. The selection of these four reservation sites was based on the interest of the tribes in participating, their geographic location in close proximity to each other, their potential for recruiting individuals with diabetes or at risk for diabetes, and their relative cultural cluster. And because previous research suggests that the majority of rural American Indians use the local Indian clinic services for their health care, local Indian clinics were selected as a focal point to identify and access the population in this study.

Participant Selection. Adult American Indians with a diagnosis of type 2 diabetes or at risk of developing diabetes were recruited to participate in the study. The criteria for inclusion in the study were being American Indian, 18 years of age and older, and a resident of the reservations targeted in this study.

Institutional Review Boards' Approvals. Protection for human subjects' approval was obtained from the institutional review boards (IRB) at the University of California at San Francisco, University of Minnesota, Aberdeen Area Indian Health Service (IHS), and the Little Priest College, holder of the Winnebago IRB. Written consents were obtained from each participant following a careful introduction and review of the purpose of the study and the potential risks and benefits of participating in the study. Each participant was told that participation was voluntary and that they could quit participating at any time. Also, they were told of the expectation of their participation in the study should they decide to join the project. It was also explained that confidentiality of any and all information that participants imparted would be maintained through nondisclosure of any participant identifiers (e.g., a code is used instead of the participant's name).

PROJECT PHASES

The Diabetes Wellness Project consists of three major phases (1) focus groups, (2) a randomized intervention trial, and (3) an evaluation of the project.

In the first phase, community-based focus groups were held to define the meaning and the cultural context of *diabetes*. The focus groups allowed the researchers to investigate the culturally based practices of participating tribes. Cultural strengths were identified, which would be helpful in the development of a culturally appropriate health promotion model. This information then guided the development of the intervention phase of the project. The tools necessary to implement and test the intervention were designed during this phase. This task included the development of a "talking circle" diabetes curriculum, pre- and posttest surveys, associated anthropometric measures, and chart reviews.

The second phase of the project involved the implementation of a randomized intervention trial to reduce the prevalence of diabetes. The four reservation sites were randomly assigned to the intervention or control group. The intervention group (two sites) implemented the project, which consisted of a series of educational workshops, or talking circles, on the topic of diabetes prevention and control. The remaining two sites (control group) were provided regular health care services. A pre- and a posttest were administered to the groups to evaluate the impact of the intervention. Trained staff conducted medical chart reviews to note any change in the health status of participants.

The talking circle intervention involved implementation of the model health education program, which incorporated several significant strategies, such as the use of story sharing as an educational and cultural tool, the use of a culturally based setting of intergroup communication, and traditional Western health education materials. Participants came to a weekly session, which lasted approximately 2 hours, for a total of 12 sessions. Incentives were provided at each of the sessions along with a meal, which included traditional buffalo meat.

The final part of the project consisted of analysis of the findings and evaluation of the project. The data that were collected were entered into a computer-based statistical program. Statistical runs generated information on the demographics, changes in participant behavior, level of knowledge gained, and changes in attitudes. Results of the study were first presented to each of the tribal council for their review and approval. Discussions on the intervention impact, replication of the program, and unforeseen outcomes were topics generally discussed at collaborating meetings.

USE OF CULTURALLY APPROPRIATE INTERVENTIONS

One way to provide relevant prevention materials is to incorporate culturally based practices into current health education efforts. To accomplish this, the Diabetes Wellness Project used storytelling via the talking circles to identify American Indian culturally based concepts of health and wellness. The project recruited and trained local American Indian facilitators to assist in recruiting local participants to be a part of the study. The facilitators assisted in coordination, recruitment efforts, and administering of surveys. Guidance was also received from American Indian advisors on artwork and the use of appropriate language for written materials. This information proved invaluable in the development of the diabetes curriculum used in the project intervention.

Significant time and effort was expended to ensure that the project was culturally significant and that the staff and researchers proceeded in a culturally appropriate manner. The sessions were held at agreeable sites, food was provided, sufficient information was provided, and time was allotted so that participants had time to understand the project and the intervention process. The tribal councils were provided information at the beginning, midway, and at the end of the project. Resolutions of support were provided by the tribal councils of each of the four tribes to show their support and to document the success of the project.

Staff at the local clinics, hospitals, and tribal programs was provided general information on the project so that they would be aware of the research taking place. A final lay report was provided to the tribal councils and shared with the staff on the findings of the study, prior to any professional publication.

The use of stories in an intervention program is an excellent way of providing health education material to American Indians because stories often provide a cultural index for both appropriate and inappropriate behaviors. The characters in American Indian stories present positive as well as negative examples. Participants learn of ways to keep healthy, the manner in which cultural practice provides

support, and proper protocol and action. The positive characters fit harmoniously into their surroundings; the negative characters break the rules and make life difficult for themselves and everyone else. The stories provide a wonderful format for the "lesson of the day" discussion in a nonthreatening and entertaining manner. The process of storytelling compels persons to draw their own conclusions based on the discussions. They move with their own thinking, adopting the information.

FOCUS GROUPS

During the initial developmental phase of the Diabetes Wellness Project, a series of focus groups were employed to gather information on lifestyles, attitudes, and knowledge about diabetes and its risk factors. Two focus groups per reservation were held—designed by the joint leadership of the research project to provide preliminary information in the initial stages of the research project.

The understanding of the community in terms of illness beliefs, cultural constructs of wellness and illness, and tribal priorities and communication styles was elucidated during the focus groups. Literary documentation, historical documents, and discussions with tribal leaders provided information on the community's social capital, cultural ways of negotiation, power struggles, historical context of health care, and political environments

Composed of adult members of the Oglala, Rosebud, Yankton, and Winnebago tribes, the focus groups became the initial recruiting tool for the research study and served as the basic information-sharing tool between the researchers and the community. Focus groups can be a valuable tool in planning and designing new programs. For this reason, focus groups were the primary source of information gathering for program planning and decision making during the first 2 years of the project.

A meal was served at each focus group in accordance with American Indian tradition to share food at a gathering. Potential partici-pants were informed that the general informa-tion would be used in developing the culturally appropriate intervention to be used in the research project. All focus groups sessions were tape-recorded, transcribed, and analyzed for content analysis. Focus group transcripts were coded for the construction of themes and explanatory models.

The focus groups provided information on the beliefs and eating patterns of the Sioux and Winnebago tribes, at the targeted reservation sites for the research project. An American Indian facilitator led all the groups to gather this valuable information. Some participants made their comments in their native language. These comments were translated so that all the information was accessible for the intervention-planning process. The information proved invaluable in selecting the areas for inclusion in the curriculum, designing the educational approach, and deciding on the recruitment and retention methodology for the study.

INCORPORATING THE CULTURE IN THE INTERVENTION: TALKING CIRCLES

The talking circle is a well-known method of intragroup communication in many American Indian communities. It is commonly composed of about 10 to 15 members, sitting in a circle, meeting to share information, support each other, and solve problems. Often, following an opening session story and presentation of the education materials, a talking stick is passed around the circle of participants signifying individual control of the floor. While speak-ing, each participant has total control of the floor without fear of interruption.

The format of the talking circle allows each participant to discuss his or her opinions, con-cerns, or needs in relation to the topic in an acceptable manner. Participation in the talking circle is expected to increase the participants' personal strengths and guide them toward

greater input and discussion surrounding the core topic.

The circle method transcends tribal bound-aries, as the stories emphasize values that are significant to all Indian tribes. Such a cultural approach to conducting a focus group is read-ily applicable to all tribes, as the use of talking circles to relay important messages and pro-vide positive direction and feedback is a com-mon tradition among tribes. The circle method is an easily adaptable method of communica-tion that has been successful in many situa-tions. The use of the talking circle provides a culturally sensitive base for the presentation of health education material.

The project facilitator was responsible for recruiting adults to participate in the circles. Each circle session began a health message, which connected the central idea of the story with an important health concept. The facilita-tor then began leading a discussion on a specific topic from the curriculum. The curriculum was designed to incorporate diabetes knowl-edge items (nutrition, exercise, etc.) with tradi-tional concepts of wellness.

The intervention sites ran five consecutive 16-week circles. The control sites met twice in the same 16-week period. Both the control and the intervention sites administered the pretest questionnaire at the first session. The interven-tion sites conducted weekly meetings for the next 10 weeks. The control sites did not meet during those intervening weeks. Then, the intervention and control sites met at the 16th week and repeated the self-administered ques-tionnaire and the dietary recalls. This cycle was repeated until all sites had the required number of participants.

Each facilitator was asked to keep a jour-nal. Journals were to be used to make notes about outreach efforts to recruit participants, and efforts were made to publicize the circles to the community. Journals were to be used to record what happened during each session of the circles and to comment on problems and questions that arose during and throughout the program. They were also used to record the facilitator's feelings and impressions about the sessions. The journal also provided documentation of how much time was spent on specific duties such as reading and preparing for the session, preparing refreshments for the sessions, and recruiting and retaining participants.

The intervention sites facilitators were also asked to audiotape each session. The objective for audiotaping was to document how the sessions were conducted and how the participants were responding to the project and to assist the research staff in monitoring the project.

Each facilitator was responsible for recruiting 10 to 12 individuals to each of their circle sessions. Outreach and recruitment efforts were intensive, requiring many phone calls and in-person contacts. Facilitators also attended powwows and other social functions to recruit participants. The facilitator's position in the community was essential for successful recruitment and retention.

All intervention sites successfully completed a minimum of 40 to 50 participants during the implementation phase. Each intervention site reported very good retention of the participants during the individual circles.

RECRUITING AND HIRING FACILITATORS FOR THE TALKING CIRCLES

Job descriptions and recruitment flyers were sent to each of the four intervention sites. Clinic directors/staff assisted in the recruitment and hiring process. Four female American Indian facilitators were subsequently hired to lead the talking circles. Each facilitator had previous training or experience in leading and organizing group sessions and working with Indian people from their communities.

The facilitators were trained by the principal investigator and coinvestigators at the Porcupine Clinic on the Pine Ridge (Oglala)

reservation. An initial 2-day training brought the facilitators together for the first time. They were trained in several key areas, such as (1) how to run a talking circle and (2) how to use the curriculum to facilitate discussions and learning experiences for diabetes prevention and education and study key points. The facilitators were given a protocol guide as a reference. It included instructions for administering all aspects of the circles.

A booster training was held between the first and second circles. This brought the facilitators together to share experiences/problems and solutions with the research team and with each other. Each facilitator submitted his or her first circle evaluation addressed at the booster training.

RESEARCH DESIGN

The project research design was a randomized pre- and posttest design. Clinics were randomly assigned to the intervention (talking circles) and the control group. Within each group, individuals completed the pretest at the time they were recruited. The pretest was completed only after the study had been explained and informed consent given. Following this step, the survey was administered. Anthropology tests consisting of weight, height, and BMI measures were given. At the end of the intervention sessions (3 months), the posttest was completed. Individuals in the comparison condition did not receive an intervention. Instead, they were given an informational booklet and received standard medical care. Following the intervention phase, the control group was offered and provided the materials and one talking circle session per clinic site.

EXAMPLE OF A TALKING CIRCLE

The following example of a moderator's guide will facilitate the start-up, momentum, and wrap-up of a talking circle:

"Hello and welcome. I want to warmly welcome you and thank you for coming today to this talking circle session. My name is _____ and I am working on a project for American Indians. Let me introduce to you other staff members: _____. This project has many members who function as advisers, committee members, consultants, and others who are working together to help American Indian communities manage their diabetes—such as eating habits, exercise, and weight control.

Our purpose today is to provide information from individuals who are either at risk of diabetes or have diabetes in order to find the best ways of providing a diabetes program for American Indian communities. To do this, we need guidance on several areas of the issue. We need to know the following:

1. What are the communication patterns for community members with diabetes or at risk for diabetes as they talk with their health care providers?

2. What are the images/artwork that must be used in the educational materials?

3. What are the materials that you feel should be used?

4. What diabetes prevention approaches work for you and your community?

We thank you for your time and involvement in this project. You have been invited to participate in this session as we think you can tell us about what you and others experienced, your belief, and the story of your diabetes experience. After introductions and preliminary questions, we will conduct a talking circle to begin our discussion. Please remember that there is no right or wrong answer. We value your feedback, and you are free to pass the talking stick at any time you wish to postpone your comments.

Also, we have some refreshments for you, so please feel free to help yourself at the nearby table. We will then join in a talking circle.

Let's get back together in a circle so we can begin. The core questions that we are addressing are _____.

We will pass this talking stick around in a circle, and each person will have an opportunity to talk. The ground rules for these sessions are as follows [hand our ground rules sheet]:

1. Respect each member's comments by allowing each person to talk—all participants are allowed time to include their words as a part of the focus group

2. All members are encouraged to participate as much as possible.

3. Please talk one at a time so that we are able to capture your input.

4. No discussion or response is right or wrong.

5. Negative as well as positive responses are acceptable.

6. Participants can choose not to answer a question, as participation is voluntary.

7. All members are to keep focused on the topic, as veering off to other topics takes up time and lessens the momentum.

My role is as the talking circle moderator—so I will be asking the questions and listening closely for the responses. Your responses are important. We have set up a tape recorder, and I am asking for your permission to tape-record the talking circle. The other staff will take accurate minutes. Should you wish to have the tape turned off at any time, please ask me, and I will switch the machine off for that portion of time.

All of the responses and feedback that you give today will be summarized in a report—we will not use any individual name or directly quote you without your prior written permission. All that you say today will be held in the strictest confidence—your name is not be used or listed in any report (verbal or written). The tapes will be shredded after they are recorded, and no individual or personal information will be used. We will summarize what you have said and provide a group report.

We also need to have your agreement to not discuss any comments or information that you have heard during this talking circle. Do I have your agreement that all that is said will be held in your confidence? Good.

Perhaps we can take a few minutes for the group to introduce themselves. [Give about 35 minutes in total for each to say what he or she wishes.]

Our first topic for discussion is _____. Tell me, how do you feel, what is your opinion, and so on.

Following saturation of the discussion, move to the next question or topic.]

At the end of the talking circle, ask the group, Are there any more comments, anything else that needs to be brought out, or have we missed anything?]

Thank you all for participating and contributing to this talking circle. Should you wish to contact me for any reason, please contact me at this address (pass our business cards).

Please accept this small incentive for your contribution today, and please feel free to help yourself to the refreshments.

A copy of the report will be provided to you, so I will be following up with you to make sure that you get your copy.

Thank you again."

CURRICULUM DEVELOPMENT

The curriculum was administered in 12 weekly sessions (meeting once a week for approximately 2 hours for 3 months) addressing three basic topic areas:

1. *A healthy lifestyle* (what is a healthy lifestyle, what it includes, how it is achieved; the importance of balance; nutrition; exercise; regular health-screening exams; mental health; and the value of each individual to his or her family and the Indian community)

2. *Diet/nutrition* (what is a healthy diet; the importance of nutrition, diet, and health; nutrients; the food pyramid; reading food labels; cooking for health; how to prepare and cook foods that are healthy for the family; how to choose the best foods when eating out; and the value and importance of Native foods)

3. *Type 2 diabetes* (understanding diabetes and what you should know about it; the warning signs; the importance of diet and exercise and the healthy approach to both; nutrition and weight management; what food exchange means, and the importance of adherence to treatment)

The format of the talking circle allowed each participant to discuss his or her fears, concerns, or needs in relation to the health topic in an acceptable manner. Each participant was given the opportunity to discuss diabetes and to ask questions. We postulated that participation in the talking circle would increase the participants' personal strengths and guide them toward greater sense of control over decision making with regard to health-seeking behavior. We expected that giving and receiving help within the circle would increase emotional support within the group and reduce fatalistic attitudes.

There were three major educational products developed for this project: the talking circle curriculum, the diabetes video, and the diabetes cookbook.

1. *Curriculum:* The curriculum was the main teaching tool for the facilitators, both in their training and in facilitating the talking circle sessions. The curriculum chapter sequence was designed to take the facilitators and participants from basic concepts in health and diabetes in the first three sessions to specific topics in nutrition, exercise, and so on in the middle sessions and finally to applications of these in the final chapters on prevention and control. American Indian stories were inserted at the beginning of each session of the curriculum. Health messages connected

the story to health values. Copies of the stories were distributed to each participant and read aloud to begin each circle session.

A comprehensive guide for administering the talking circles was developed by the research staff. It contained detailed information on how to organize and run a talking circle. Administrative tasks were outlined, and resources were provided for additional information.

2. *Video:* A 20-minute film was produced titled *Diabetes: Notes.* This film introduces the project and provides information to the viewer on diabetes among American Indians. It provided a visual representation of the way a talking circle can open up the discussion of diabetes in a supportive atmosphere. It also describes how a talking circle can be set up in other communities and clinics, thus providing valuable information on how to organize a talking circle. Each of the participants was provided a copy of the film. At the conclusion of the study, each participating clinic was also provided with a copy of the film.

3. *Cookbook:* A cookbook, *American Indian Traditional Meals,* and stories associated with these were developed for the talking circle intervention. Traditional stories were collected from a review of the tribal storytellers. These stories were selected based on their authenticity, health message, and relevance to American Indians. The cookbook was published and presented to each of the participants.

Because there is a dearth of educational materials and knowledge that educators can use when developing health care programs for American Indians and Alaska Natives, it is important that researchers document their experiences, sharing what works and what does not work with Native communities and researchers working in these communities.

STUDY FINDINGS

The project findings were reported in two formats. First, a "layman's" report was generated

for each of the tribal council and community members from the four reservation sites. Following a brief time period for review, the research team obtained a resolution of agreement and acceptance of the findings. An oral report was subsequently provided to each tribal council at a regularly scheduled meeting. This allowed for open discussion and provided for a question-and-answer period. It also provided the opportunity to discuss the need for additional studies on smoking, obesity, and depression, topics that are of concern to the tribes.

The second group of publishable reports is being formatted for peer-reviewed journals. The study findings to be reported include the cultural constructs of illness (diabetes), barriers to care (fatalism), and the impact of the talking circle model on self-help behaviors surrounding improvement of diet and exercise.

Often the management of disease is so embedded with beliefs, prior experiences, and self-held perceptions that it colors the trajectory of the illness to the extent that treatment is less effective. The prevention and management of chronic illness require a full range of inputs, from the patient, the provider, and the community, that can support, inform, and treat those illnesses that have a strong cultural influence. Over time, investigation into these cultural constructs can aid in the overall management of a disease such as diabetes among American Indians.

CHAPTER SUMMARY

The talking circle model is an effective method for researchers, educators, and planners who are interested in improving the health and wellness of American Indian communities. The talking circle model has been a traditional mechanism for imparting knowledge and facilitating communication in most American Indian tribes. In the Diabetes Wellness circles project, American Indian story sharing, which emphasized the value of prevention, was coupled with the health education material and presented to the participants in the talking circles by trained Native facilitators. The participants now perceive their health as something they have more control over. They were reminded of their ability to make lifestyle choices and, with the information and group support provided through these talking circles, may be empowered to change their eating and fitness habits and to achieve healthier lifestyles.

The development, implementation, and evaluation of the Diabetes Wellness Project indicated the importance of culture in all phases of the project. Understanding and using the cultural context of illness, wellness, and social capital provides for successful outcomes. The use of the talking circle method as a means of communication and education proved to be significant in changing attitudes and improving knowledge and intragroup discussions. These discussions often led to better understanding and adoption of healthy behaviors, a desired goal of the project.

DISCUSSION QUESTIONS AND ACTIVITIES

1. As an outside class activity, either individual or in small groups, design, implement, analyze, and report results in class of a short survey focused on the perceptions of illness that people with chronic disease have.

2. How does the construct of illness influence the self-efficacy of treatment, prevention, and control of any disease?

3. If minority groups have a sense of fatalism regarding the control of a disease, is this related to their culture in terms of illness beliefs, and if so, is it amenable to change through a group exercise incorporating self-directed steps to manage the disease? How so?

REFERENCES

Bullock, A. (2001). *Connection of stress/trauma to diabetes and the insulin resistance syndrome.* Unpublished manuscript.

Burrows, N. R., Engelgau, M. M., Geiss, L. S., & Acton, K. J. (2000). Prevalence of diabetes among Native Americans and Alaska Natives, 1990–1997. *Diabetes Care, 23*(12), 1786–1790.

Lee, E. T., Oopik, A. J., Howard, B. V., Yeh, J., Savage, P. J., Go, O., et al. (1995). Diabetes and impaired glucose tolerance in three American Indian populations aged 45–74 years. Diabetes Care, *18*(5), 599–610.

Story, M., Evans, M., Fabsitz, R. R., Clay, T. E., Holy, R. B., & Broussard, B. (1999). The epidemic of obesity in American Indian communities and the need for childhood obesity-prevention programs. *American Journal of Clinical Nutrition, 69*(Suppl.), 747S–754S.

U.S. Department of Agriculture, Food and Nutrition Service. (1990). *Evaluation of the food distribution program on Indian reservations.* Alexandria, VA: Author.

U.S. Department of Agriculture, Food and Nutrition Service. (1991). *The food distribution program on Indian reservations (FDPIR).* Food Program Facts. Alexandria, VA: Author.

U.S. Department of Health and Human Services, Public Health Service, Indian Health Service. (2003). *Trends in Indian health 1998–99.* Retrieved March 8, 2008, from http://www.ihs.gov/publicinfo/publication/trends98/trends98.asp

20

Tips for Working With American Indian and Alaska Native Populations

ROBERT M. HUFF

MICHAEL V. KLINE

There are a variety of terms that are often used interchangeably when speaking or writing about American Indian or Alaska Native (AI/AN) population groups. Kramer (1996) has observed that Native peoples use their tribal name when referring to themselves but seem to prefer the use of the term *American Indian* over *Native American* when referring to all tribal groups. Thus, when working with (AI/AN) populations it would be advisable to determine what term(s) are preferred by the group or individual you are working with. It will also be important to recognize the diversity of cultural beliefs and practices that characterize the many distinct tribal communities living in North America. This brief chapter will seek to bring forth a few tips for working with (AI/AN) populations in health promotion and disease prevention (HPDP) activities. These recommendations have been culled from the preceding three chapters as well as a number of other sources (Duran & Duran, 1999; Fredericks, Collins,

& Hodge, 1999; Hodge & Fredericks, 1999; Huff & Kline, 1999; Joe & Malach, 1992; Kramer, 1996) and are offered as a starting point for consideration when engaging in HPDP activities with (AI/ANs).

CULTURAL COMPETENCE

As noted in Chapter 1 of this text, the need for health promoters to become culturally competent and sensitive to multicultural diversity is a critical skill to develop when working with any multicultural group. The tips given below may help begin that process. The health promoters should do the following:

- Seek to learn the history of the AI/AN population group with whom they are working.
- Become familiar with the cultural values, beliefs, and ways of life of the people with whom they are working.
- Seek to incorporate the cultural beliefs, values, and traditions of the AI/AN group they are working with in the design, implementation,

and evaluation of the HPDP program that is being developed; this can begin by including representatives of the target group in all phases of the program-planning process.

- Remember that every AI/AN group will have its own unique traditions and patterns of life; these may be very different from that of the agency or individual with the responsibility for the HPDP project, and thus, it will be critical, on one hand, to examine one's own values, beliefs, and biases as these relate to those of the target group and, on the other, to work toward suspending one's own issues to enter the culture of the target group with the respect and sensitivity to which they are entitled.

- Take the time to make multiple visits to the community where the target group resides, to talk with tribal leaders and members, to attend local events that are open to the public, and to otherwise seek to become familiar with the community's life ways.

- Seek to develop early and continuing support from the community for any HPDP programs and services that are to be offered.

- Remember that among AI/AN groups there is likely to be a range of acculturation levels from the very traditional to the fully acculturated; therefore, assess before making planning decisions to ensure that all members of the target group will benefit from the interventions planned.

- Seek to incorporate traditional values, beliefs, and life ways into the design of educational materials while respecting differences among tribal groups.

- Seek to incorporate appropriate cultural visuals, directions, instructions, and culturally appropriate translators when providing HPDP services to AI/AN populations.

- Become familiar with acceptable and appropriate verbal and nonverbal communication patterns for the tribal group(s) to whom HPDP services are being provided.

- Become familiar with traditional values and practices related to gender, touching, religion, food preferences, and other related cultural differences, because a failure to do so can lead to a failure of the program or service to achieve its desired aims.

- Respect tribal sovereignty when working with AI/AN population groups, because not doing so may result in resistance or the collapse of support for programs being planned; building community capacity to problem solve means respecting and learning to work from within rather than from outside the tribal group.

HEALTH BELIEFS AND PRACTICES

There are a variety of health beliefs and practices among the many diverse AI/AN tribal groups in North America. Thus, it is critical to develop some understanding and sensitivity to this diversity and to develop the flexibility to work within the traditional health practices of the AI/AN group you are seeking to provide services to. Thus, the health promoters should do the following:

- Identify and seek to understand the explanatory model(s) that the individuals within the community use to make sense of and deal with threats to their personal health and well-being (Huff & Yasharpour, Chapter 2, this volume).

- Expect that there will be a range of explanatory models that are employed across this broad multicultural population group, ranging from very traditional health beliefs and practices to those that are more reflective of the Western biomedical model.

- Where differences exist between the explanatory models of the target group and those of the health promoter, efforts should be made to ameliorate or otherwise find ways to work within these different frames of reference and perception.

- Remember that traditional ceremonies are still practiced that seek to promote balance and well-being among AI/AN tribal groups; thus, the health promoter is encouraged to become familiar with these ceremonies and other health practices as they may provide opportunities to merge beneficial practices into the biomedical model and thereby extend the range of potential healing and health promoting practices into the community.

- Remember that traditional healers, medicine men, herbal remedies and medicine are still very important in many urban and rural areas.
- Consider that modesty, taboos, and traditional healing practices must be respected when providing HPDP services and programs.
- Consider consulting with and involving spiritual, cultural, and traditional healers within the community when beginning the program-planning process.
- Seek to involve traditional healers where appropriate in the delivery of HPDP programs and services.
- Remember that *respect* is a strong central value of all AI/AN cultures; thus, treating everyone with kindness, equality, and goodness is very important.
- Remember that cultural sensitivity is an important value held by AI/AN peoples; thus, the health promoter must be open to and willing to accept and work within other worldviews and interaction styles.

PROGRAM-PLANNING CONSIDERATIONS

It has been stressed in many places throughout this text that program planning is a comprehensive and critically important process if one is to design and carry out high quality and successful HPDP programs and services. In Chapter 7, this volume, Kline has observed that it does not necessarily matter what planning model one uses as long as the basic elements of the planning process are involved including adequate needs assessment, objective setting, appropriate and culturally sensitive intervention planning, and evaluation to measure the efficacy of the program or service to meet its specified objectives. With this in mind, the health promoter is encouraged to identify and use a planning model and to consider the following suggestions and recommendations as they begin the planning process:

- Successful working relationships among AI/AN communities and those seeking to work with them are dependent on clarifying assumptions and overcoming misconceptions about AI/AN peoples and public health practice.
- Many AI/AN peoples feel exploited and mistrustful of Westerners. Thus, patience, sensitivity, and respect will be important components of any HPDP effort. You must build credibility by working *from within* the tribal group rather than *from outside* the group. This will help build community capacity and foster a more trusting relationship.
- The ideal working relationship for the health promoter is one in which they are working directly under the supervision of the tribe or Native community agency.
- The community should be involved in all aspects of the program-planning process from needs assessment through evaluation.
- Tribal leaders often see HPDP and other outside funding as economic and employment opportunities for their tribe. It will be important to keep this in mind when considering staffing and other manpower needs of the HPDP program.
- Review all previous HPDP program efforts in the community to identify potential community resources and assets, interventions that have been found to enhance or impede the successful adaptation of programs in the community, and any other factors that might play a role in the new program or service to be developed.
- Be sure that the goals, objectives, and interventions of the HPDP program or service reflect the felt needs of the target group. Where community needs and interests are not in agreement with those of the health promoter, seek ways to balance the needs of all concerned parties prior to launching a full-blown program or service.
- Above all things, be sure that HPDP programs and services reflect the values, beliefs, and interests of the community in which they are targeted.

NEEDS ASSESSMENT CONSIDERATIONS

Carefully crafted needs assessment instruments and methodologies are critical to establishing accurate baseline data about a community's health needs and interests. The process must be rigorous and include not only the more usual information that is gathered (i.e., morbidity and mortality rates, demographics) but also the cultural factors that can influence the successful implementation of a HPDP program or service. Thus, the health promoter is encouraged to review the cultural assessment framework presented in Chapter 6 (Huff & Kline, this volume) as well as to consider the following additional suggestions:

- Be aware that no matter what planning model is used for program development, it is essential to include a cultural assessment as part of the baseline data gathered about the target group.
- Needs assessment instruments will need to reflect the linguistic, literacy, and cultural symbols and values of the community.
- Standardized needs assessment instruments designed for the mainstream culture often have little meaning for those who are not fully acculturated and assimilated into the mainstream. Thus, instruments will need to be shaped to reflect the community in which they are to be administered.
- Providing opportunities for Native communities to conduct their own needs assessments can help build community capacity by empowering the community to become more involved in defining and solving their own health and social problems.
- If conducting a community survey, these are best undertaken with the support and direction of the tribal health department.
- Remember to include key informants, such as political, spiritual, and cultural leaders in the community needs assessment process.
- Be aware that key informant information should be triangulated with other data from the assessment process to ensure that all the needs of the community are identified and considered as program-planning efforts go forward.
- Be sure to include assessment of media resources and channels including informal channels of communication and information sharing that are used within the community. These may play a significant role in the

marketing of the HPDP program or service when these are ready to go online.
- The PRECEDE model can be a useful framework for identifying and describing health behaviors with respect to their predisposing, enabling, and reinforcing factors and help frame the new knowledge, attitudes, and behaviors that will be the targets of intervention in the community.
- Focus groups can provide a useful way to assess knowledge, attitudes, and health behaviors of AI/AN peoples.
- Be sure that assessment and evaluation efforts reflect the needs, interests, and values of the stakeholders within the community.

INTERVENTION CONSIDERATIONS

Well-planned and appropriate interventions are key to the success of any HPDP program or service. This will involve tailoring interventions to the particular cultural characteristics of the target group (Pasick, D'Onofrio, & Otero-Sabogal, 1996). That is, employing themes, values, and other important features of the culture in the intervention process. Therefore, the health promoter is urged to consider the following recommendations when planning their program interventions:

- *One size fits all* is not a useful approach to intervention design. Programs must be tailored to each individual target group.
- Effective HPDP interventions build on the strengths, resources, and assets of the community. Seek to identify and involve these in the intervention design and implementation process.
- Linguistic, literacy, gender relevance, and other cultural factors must be considered in the design of the intervention(s) to be implemented in the community.
- The development of a culturally appropriate educational intervention requires consideration of available resources and the inclusion of important cultural themes of the target group.
- Educational materials must be culturally appropriate and set within the context of the AI/AN culture for which they are being

designed. Remember, AI/AN tribal groups are very diverse and reflect different ways of looking at and relating to the world in which they live.

- As much as possible, educational materials should also reflect the learning styles and cultural values of the population for which they are being designed. This will require that these elements be included in the needs assessment process.
- The use of talking circles in conjunction with the use of tribal stories has been found to be a very useful and culturally appropriate educational intervention for AI/AN populations.
- Storytelling is a culturally appropriate educational technique because it uses an insider approach rather than working from outside the cultural milieu.
- Always assess the cultural appropriateness of any pictures, models, dolls, or other educational materials prior to their inclusion in the program as some materials may make the target group uncomfortable.
- Employing and training tribal members to facilitate educational programs is a valuable approach for facilitating implementation of HPDP programs in AI/AN communities.
- Intervention design should employ relevant theory to support design efforts.
- Seek to develop interventions that focus on positive health changes rather than those with negative or fear-arousing consequences.

EVALUATION CONSIDERATIONS

Evaluation is at the heart of all HPDP programs and services as this process provides validation for the activities that have been carried out, points to where the program or service can be improved, and lays the groundwork for ongoing support from funding agencies and the community itself. Health promoters should consider the following suggestions when planning their evaluation activities.

- Seek to develop evaluation strategies, methods, and instruments that reflect an understanding of current theory and practice in the evaluation and research literature.
- Support for evaluation of HPDP programs for Native communities will be dependent on the needs of the stakeholders, the potential use(s) of the knowledge to be gained, how the target group views and uses knowledge, and the values that have been used to guide program assessment.
- Evaluation and assessment are processes that are often difficult to gain support for even from the most sophisticated of groups. Thus, efforts to explain the underlying assumptions governing these processes as well as the methods and anticipated outcomes from these activities can help make explicit what is often unclear to those inexperienced with evaluation and assessment activities.
- Evaluation and assessment measures should be culturally relevant and tailored to the linguistic and educational capabilities of the target group. Thus, efforts to involve the community in identifying evaluation criteria that are important and meaningful to them are highly suggested.
- Evaluators should recognize that HPDP program participants may have limited test-taking abilities or skills. Thus, efforts to design evaluation methods should consider how best to measure participant gains from the program using approaches that are familiar, acceptable, and of interest to the community.
- Providing evaluation and assessment training for tribal members who are to be involved in program assessment, implementation, and evaluation activities can help promote input and support for these efforts.
- Wherever possible, provide opportunities for staff members from the community to be actively involved in all aspects of the program evaluation process.
- Be sure to design evaluation and assessment reporting and feedback mechanisms into the program to ensure that the community is made regularly aware of how well the program or service is functioning to improve the health issue or problem for which it was designed.

REFERENCES

Duran, B., & Duran, E. (1999). Assessment, program planning and evaluation in Indian Country:

Towards a postcolonial practice. In R. M. Huff & M. V. Kline (Eds), *Promoting health in multicultural populations: A handbook for practitioners* (pp. 292–311). Thousand Oaks, CA: Sage.

Fredericks, L., Collins, C., & Hodge, F. S. (1999). Traditional approaches to health care among American Indians and Alaska Natives: A case study. In R. M. Huff & M. V. Kline (Eds), *Promoting health in multicultural populations: A handbook for practitioners* (pp. 313–326). Thousand Oaks, CA: Sage.

Hodge, F. S., & Fredericks, L. (1999). American Indian and Alaska Native populations in the United States. In R. M. Huff & M. V. Kline (Eds), *Promoting health in multicultural populations: A handbook for practitioners* (pp. 269–290). Thousand Oaks, CA: Sage.

Huff, R. M., & Kline, M. V. (1999). Health promotion in the context of culture. In R. M. Huff & M. V. Kline (Eds), *Promoting health in multicultural populations: A handbook for practitioners* (pp. 3–22). Thousand Oaks, CA: Sage.

Joe, J. R., & Malach, R. S. (1992). Families with Native American Roots. In E. W. Lynch & M. J. Hanson (Eds.), *Developing cross-cultural competence: A guide for working with young children and their families* (pp. 127–164). Baltimore: Paul H. Brookes.

Kramer, J. (1996). American Indians. In J. G. Lipson, S. L. Dibble, & P. A. Minarik (Eds), *Culture and nursing care: A pocket guide* (pp. 11–22). San Francisco: UCSF Nursing Press.

Pasick, R. J., D'Onofrio, C. N., & Otero-Sabogal, R. (1996). Similarities and differences across cultures: Questions to inform a third generation for health promotion research. *Health Education Quarterly, 23* (Suppl.), S142–S161.

PART V

Asian American Populations

21

Asian American Health and Disease

An Overview

MARJORIE KAGAWA-SINGER

JUNG HEE HAN

Chapter Objectives

On completion of this chapter, the health promotion student and practitioner will be able to

- Explain how the diversity among Asian Americans affects health outcomes

- Provide general and brief background information to help students and practitioners become more familiar with a few of the many ethnic subgroups of Asian Americans

- Describe how culture affects both focus and design of health promotion and health education efforts in the Asian American populations

- Illustrate why combining the heterogeneous Asian American groups into one aggregated population is misleading for both practice and the scientific study of this population

AUTHORS' NOTE: Special thanks are given to Amy Zhou for her invaluable assistance in the literature searches and preparation of this manuscript. We would also like to thank John Tan, MPH, MA, and Annalyn Valdez, MPH, for their assistance with the Cambodian and Filipino sections of this chapter.

Asian Americans (AAs) constitute the fastest growing group in the United States, yet health promotion in this population is severely hampered by its invisibility in the U.S. population. Several factors contribute to this oversight: (1) the erroneous assumption that this is a "small" population with good overall health and therefore does not warrant extra attention, (2) the paucity of data about the status of health in this population and, importantly, its constituent subgroups to counter the myth that AAs are all healthy, (3) the invisibility of the population, and (4) the extreme diversity within the category AAs. Health professionals will be better able to develop effective strategies to promote and maintain the health of members of these AA groups if they were better informed about the social, historical, and cultural backgrounds and current status of these populations. This chapter will address each of the four factors that contribute to the lack of knowledge and health information about AAs.

The term *Asian American* is an ethnic gloss that aggregates over 50 highly diverse national groups and hundreds of different ethnic groups, each with very different languages, beliefs, cultures, and, importantly, epidemiological patterns of health outcomes. Generalizations about this group, as a whole, are not valid and are, therefore, dangerous. The health status of members of this population reflects wide between- and within-group differences, due to factors such as **culture**, immigration status, education, English language capacity, socioeconomic standing, age, and length of time in the United States, that predict significant variations in risk for morbidity and mortality. The lack of valid, **disaggregated**, subpopulation-based data on the various AA groups for most diseases hamper health promotion efforts.

Despite the inter- and intragroup variability, however, some broad similarities exist among the AA cultures, such as religions, traditional healing systems, and health care decision-making processes, yet specific ethnic group data are essential, and individual variation is paramount. This chapter provides general background information for researchers and practitioners to critically assess the existing literature on AAs, and presents available data, but due to the usual aggregation with Pacific Islanders, even AA data alone are often not possible, and the designation *AA/PI* will denote these statistics.

WHO ARE ASIAN AMERICANS?

The federal Office of Management and Budget defines an Asian American as a person having origins in any of the original peoples of the Far East, Southeast Asia, or the Indian subcontinent, including, for example, Cambodia, China, India, Japan, Korea, Malaysia, Pakistan, the Philippine Islands, Thailand, and Vietnam (Federal Register, 1997). More than 50 to 60 different countries are represented, with more than 100 different languages and multiple dialects spoken by those aggregated within the single category of AA (see Table 21.1).

Two major factors impede health promotion in this population. First, the heterogeneity in national origin, religion, socioeconomic status, education, and immigration history of each of the groups in the United States over the past 250 to 300 years influences their health promoting knowledge, beliefs, and practices, as well as learning needs and styles, and affects their health status, health risks, and health outcomes. Second, the myth of the **model minority** holds that AAs enjoy exceptionally good physical and mental health, because they are socioeconomically secure and well educated: that is, AAs are all healthy, wealthy, and wise. This erroneous perception is misleading at best and at worst, stereotyping. The history of the model minority myth stems from the Civil Rights era when the government created the term to counter the civil rights

Table 21.1   Asian Origins

Asian Americans: Persons "having origins in any of the original peoples of the Far East, Southeast Asia, or the Indian subcontinent."[a]			
Far East ("Asia")	*Southeast Asia*		*Indian Subcontinent ("South Asians")*
Chinese	Burmese[b]	Laotian	Asian Indian
Iwo-Jiman	Bornean	Malayan	Bangladeshi
Japanese	Cambodian	Mien	Bhutanese
Korean	Javanese	Mogolian	Maldives
Mongolian	Hmong	Nepali[b]	Nepali[b]
Okinawan	Indochinese	Pilipino/Filipino	Pakistani
Taiwanese	Indonesian	Singaporean	Sri Lankan
Tibetan[b,c]	Javanese	Vietnamese	Afghanistani[2]
		Thai	Burmese/Myanmar[b]
			Tibetan[b,c]

SOURCES: South Asian Public Health Association (SAPHA, 2002); U.S. Census Bureau (2000, 2004c); Congressional Research Service, Library of Congress (2005).

a. U.S. Census definition.

b. These groups are sometimes included in a broader definition of South Asian or Southeast Asian; although they are not always identified as being of "Asian origin."

c. Although the People's Republic of China claims sovereignty over the Tibetan people, Tibet maintains its independence as a government-in-exile. Officially, the U.S. government considers Tibet to be part of China. However, Tibet's exiled spiritual leader, the Dalai Lama, has many supporters in the United States and the Congress, and Tibet's political status remains controversial in the United States.

advocates who claimed that the government structure was holding down people of color. The intent was to create dissension, resentment, and division between the civil rights groups and AAs (Kim, 1999). Then, the 1985 Heckler Report on Black and Minority Health from the Department of Health and Human Services stated, "The Asian Pacific Islander minority *in aggregate* [italics added] is healthier than all racial/ethnic groups in the United States including whites" (Heckler, 1985, p. 81), which reinforced the model minority myth, resulting in the exclusion of AAs as an underserved, underrepresented minority group, and thus, no attention or resources have been allocated for AAs. AAs continue to bear the consequences of this myth through the lack of research funding and lack of financial support for the education of AA researchers as "underrepresented and underserved" minorities, especially in the behavioral and social sciences. Between 1986 and 2000, the federal government funded 150,369 grants, of which only 0.2% (342) were related to Asian American or

Pacific Islander health, and of the 10 million Medline papers published between 1966 and 2000, only 0.01% (1,499) reported any data on this population (Ghosh, 2003), resulting in misleading health statistics about the AA population and the lack of effort to correct this situation.

Methodological barriers also exist. Few national and state reports contain information on AAs, because the sample sizes of state and national surveys are often too small for analysis and are, therefore, often dropped from the reports. In addition, only a few surveys disaggregate this highly diverse population into its ethnic subgroups, masking those at highest risk, because the numbers are averaged across the multiple AA subgroups (Srinivasan & Guillermo, 2000). Language is also a barrier: The surveys are administered only in English and sometimes in Spanish. Therefore, more than 65% of the AA population is not represented;

and last, data by race/ethnicity classification often have a high rate of error (Mays, Ponce, Washington, & Cochran, 2003). The following demographic comparisons must be taken with some caution since limited English-speaking AAs may not be represented at all, and their circumstances are usually much more challenging.

DEMOGRAPHICS AFFECTING HEALTH ACCESS

AAs constitute 4.4% or about 13 million of the total U.S. population and are projected to reach 4.6% or 14.3 million by 2010, and more than 11% or 36 million by 2050 (see Table 21.2). The majority of the current AA population growth is from new immigration, with 61% of the population consisting of first-generation immigrants (U.S. Census Bureau, 2004a, 2004b).

Table 21.2   The Asian Population: 2000

Race/Ethnicity	Number	Percentage of Total U.S. Population
Total Population	281,421,906	100.0
Asian alone or in combination with one or more other races	11,898,828	4.2
Asian alone	10,242,998	3.6
Asian in combination with one or more other races	1,655,830	0.6
Asian, White	868,395	0.3
Asian, some other race	249,108	0.1
Asian, Native Hawaiian and Other Pacific Islander	138,802	—
Asian, Black or African American	106,782	—
All other combinations including Asian	292,743	0.1

SOURCE: U.S. Census Bureau (2002a).

NOTE: Dash indicates that percentage rounds to 0.0.

The six largest AA populations in the United States are Chinese, Filipino, Asian Indian, Korean, Vietnamese, and Japanese, and AAs also have a significant "more-than-one-race" proportion (U.S. Census Bureau, 2002b) (see Figure 21.1). The population of Asian alone or in combination increased by 5 million or 72% during the 1990 to 2000 decade (Barnes & Bennett, 2002).

More than 82% of all reported mixed race AAs are in four combinations: "Asian and white" 52%, "Asian and some other race" 15%, "Asian and Native Hawaiian and other Pacific Islander" 8.4%, and "Asian and black or African American" 6.4% (Barnes & Bennett, 2002). The variations are significant, because ethnicity affects health beliefs and practices and how researchers and practitioners classify individuals ethnically affects

research outcomes and practice interventions. Unless this classification is correct, the likelihood of error in the assumptions about the validity of the data or the effectiveness of the intervention will be compromised (Kagawa-Singer, 2006; Mays et al., 2003).

About 75% of all AAs are represented in just 10 states (California, New York, Hawaii, Texas, New Jersey, Illinois, Washington, Florida, Virginia, Massachusetts) compared with 47% of the total population, with one half of AAs living in the West (49%), and over half (51%) living in just three states, California, New York, and Hawaii, with California having the largest population (4.2 million) (see Table 21.3). Almost all (95%) AAs are urban and live in metropolitan cities, with the largest concentration in coastal and/or urban counties (Barnes & Bennett, 2002).

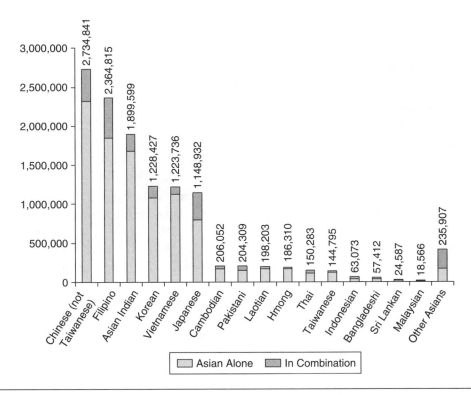

Figure 21.1   Selected Asian Groups (2000 Census Alone and in Combination)

SOURCE: U.S. Census Bureau (2002b).

Table 21.3   U.S. States With the Largest Asian American and Pacific Islander (Inclusive) Populations

U.S. States	Actual Census/% Total State Population
California[a]	4,155,685/12.3
New York	1,169,200/6.2
Hawaii[a]	703,232/58.0
Texas	644,193/3.1
New Jersey	524,356/6.2
Illinois	473,649/3.8
Washington[a]	395,741/6.7
Florida	333,013/2.1
Virginia	304,559/4.3
Massachusetts	264,814/4.2

SOURCE: Barnes and Bennett (2002).

NOTE: Actual census/% total state population in rank order.

a. Three states with the highest proportion of Asian and Pacific Island populations.

BIMODAL DISTRIBUTION

The aggregated data for AAs support the model minority myth, but a more informed look at the data quickly dispels the myth. AAs are the only group for which a **bimodal distribution** exists for the major health indicators: income, education, and insurance status (see Figure 21.2). AAs are overrepresented at the high socioeconomic status tail while being overrepresented in the extremely poor as well. Both ends of the curve, however, are at risk for health disease, and often from different sources and different diseases.

As can be seen from the following demographic indicators on income, education, English language capacity, and insurance status, the populations at highest risk for poor health access and utilization become apparent. The Southeast Asians are the most disadvantaged groups. This brief overview will provide the reader with a sense of the diversity that must be considered when working with the AA population.

Income

The median household income for AAs was $51,205 in 1999, which is higher than any other racial/ethnic group (U.S. Census Bureau, 2001). One third of households have incomes of $75,000 or more, and one fifth have incomes less than $25,000 (U.S. Census Bureau, 2001). Notably, however, most AA families have more than one wage earner within the household. In 60% of families, both the husband and wife work, and in 20% of families, there are three or more wage earners (Centers for Disease Prevention and Control [CDC], 1994). Although the overall household income is comparable with non-Hispanic whites, with multiple wage earners, the AA per capita income is actually lower compared with

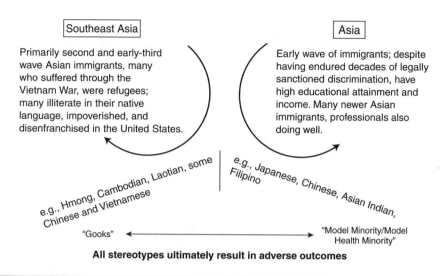

Figure 21.2 The Bimodal Distribution of Asian American Demographics
SOURCE: Adapted from Ong (2000).

NOTE: The term *bipolar distribution* in the original title has been changed to *bimodal distribution*.

non-Hispanic whites. In addition, more than 60% of AAs are first-generation immigrants. Many still send money to their families in their home countries, leaving even less money available for discretionary health care costs in the United States.

The poverty rate shown in Figure 21.3 for AAs was 10.8% in 2000, down from 12.5% in 1998 (U.S. Census Bureau, 2001). The rate is lower than that of the total population at 11.3%, but still higher compared with 7.5% for non-Hispanic whites (U.S. Census Bureau, 2003). Although the current rate is the lowest measured for the AA/PI population, the Census reveals many variations between groups. Poverty rates were highest for Hmong (37.8%), Cambodians (29.3%), and Laotians (18.5%) and lowest for Japanese (9.7%) and Filipino Americans (6.3%) (U.S. Census Bureau, 2004c).

Education

Educational attainment appears high for AA/PIs as a whole, but again, subgroup variations are significant. For instance, Japanese, Chinese, and Korean Americans who came to the United States prior to 1965 are educated, but after the first wave in 1975, refugees, especially from Southeast Asia, come with little education. Only 31% Hmong have high school diplomas compared with 88% of Japanese Americans.

About 40% of AAs 25 years and older have bachelor degrees, compared with only 6% of Southeast Asian immigrants (U.S. Census Bureau, 2000). In addition, AAs also have the largest percentage of individuals with no formal education (Lin-Fu, 1993). For instance, 6% of AA women have no education compared with 2% of the total female population.

Insurance Status

The rate of uninsured for AAs was 16.8%, and for non-Hispanic whites, Hispanic, and African Americans, the rates were 11.3%, 32.7%, and 19.7%, respectively (U.S. Census Bureau, 2005). Again, however, rates of insurance have wide variations as depicted in Figure 21.4. Korean Americans have the highest rate of uninsurance (34%) of all ethnic groups, and Japanese Americans have among the lowest (13%). AAs who have been in the

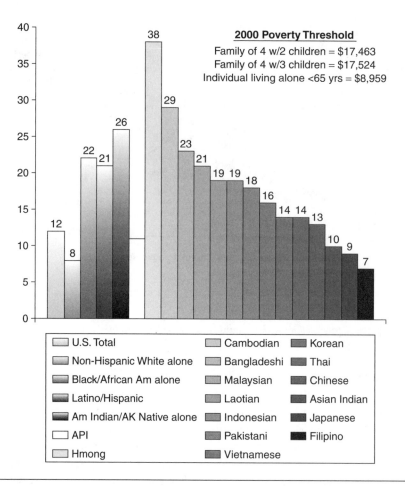

Figure 21.3   U.S. Poverty Rates, 2000

SOURCES: Percentage of U.S. totals by race/ethnicity from Dalaker (2001); selected Asian populations from Asian and Pacific Islander American Health Forum (APIAHF, 2004) and Asian American Justice Center and Asian Pacific American Legal Center (2006).

NOTE: Am Indian = American Indian; AK Native alone = Alaska Native alone; API = Asian/Pacific Islander.

United States for three or more generations have the lowest rate of uninsured of all at 8%.

AA elders have the lowest health care coverage by private insurance of all ethnic groups (National Center for Health Statistics, 1998). The actual rates may be even lower because the survey was administered in English only, and a large proportion of AA elderly are limited English speaking. AA elderly also have the highest proportion of Medicaid coverage or other public assistance in the United States. The recent Medicare Part D negatively affects the dual-covered Medicare-Medicaid population the most, thus disproportionately (Asian and

Pacific Islander American Health Forum [API-AHF], 2003) and adversely affecting AA elders.

Insurance is also one proxy for health care access. Statistics show that 8.2% of AA children compared with 3.0% of non-Hispanic whites, and 18% of AA adults compared with 10.8% of non-Hispanic whites are without a usual source of health care (National Center for Health Statistics, 2003).

Language

More than 100 languages and multiple dialects are spoken among AAs. Seven of the

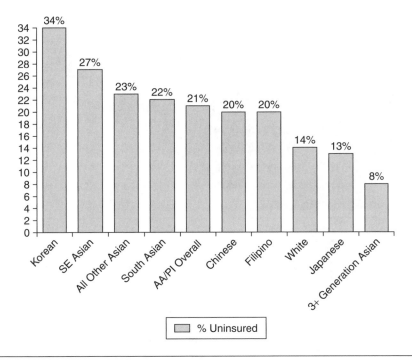

Figure 21.4   Uninsured Rates for Asian Americans (1997)

SOURCE: E. R. Brown, Ojeda, Wyn, and Levan (2000).

10 most frequently spoken languages in the United States are Asian: Chinese, Tagalog, Vietnamese, Korean, Hindi, Urdu, and Gujarati. Importantly, about one third of AAs have limited English-speaking ability, also known as being **limited English proficient (LEP)**. As shown in Figure 21.5, 61% of Vietnamese, 58% of Hmong, and 53% of Cambodians, and almost 50% of six other groups are unable to speak English well. LEP has been shown to negatively affect the quality of encounters with health practitioners, and health literacy significantly affects one's ability to understand health information. Thus, LEP AAs are significantly less able to benefit from mainstream health education and health promotion messages, interventions, and health services.

Length of Time in the United States

The length of time and history of each AA group in the United States is highly varied, creating varying patterns of disease incidence and prevalence both across and within each group (see Figure 21.6). An individual's familiarity with the U.S. health care structure varies accordingly and differentially influences their health status, beliefs, attitudes, and practices. Migration studies show that the longer the AAs live in the United States, the closer their disease patterns mirror those of the host country and change from those of their native countries. For example, group members exhibit more chronic diseases than infectious diseases as are characteristics of newer AA immigrants (CDC, 1994; U.S. Census Bureau, 2000). The first wave of AAs began in the 1700s with seafarers and students. The second wave consisted primarily of male laborers. The Chinese began arriving in the 1840s, and the Japanese, Filipinos, and Koreans in the late 1800s. The major influx of immigrants came after 1965, as the third wave, with the passage of the Immigration and Nationality Act (Hart-Cellar Act), which removed racial quotas on immigration. This wave is a mix of professionals, family members, and refugees.

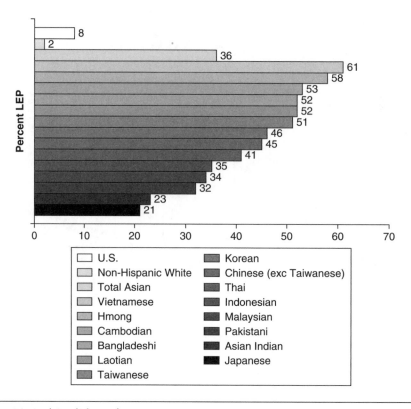

Figure 21.5   Limited English Proficient (LEP) Asian Americans Percentage of Population, 2000
SOURCES: Adapted from APIAHF (2005).

The groups who have been educated in the United States, resided in the United States the longest, and are citizens tend to have higher economic and education status and, concomitantly, better overall health status (CDC, 1994).

The circumstances for **immigration** also affect health outcomes. Immigrants usually come for better opportunities (the **"pull" factor**), but a significant proportion of immigrants have come to escape social and political oppression and genocide (e.g., Southeast Asians) (the **"push" factor**). Thus, the reasons for immigration, and therefore, who immigrated and when, also affect every demographic indicator as well as general health status.

Age Distribution

Age is also bimodally distributed. As primarily new immigrants, AAs are quite young and the percentage of children below 18 years is larger than other ethnic groups. Yet, the elderly comprise the largest and fastest growing group of all ethnic populations. From 1979 to 1981, overall life expectancy for AAs at birth was 81.9 years versus 73.9 years for the general U.S. population (Gardner, 1994). Data for women from 1980 show life expectancy for Chinese to be 86.1 years, for Japanese 84.5 years, and for Filipinas 81.5 years, compared with 79.5 years for women of all races/ethnicities (National Center for Health Statistics, 2000).

This characteristic means that the disease incidence and prevalence data must be adjusted for age in order to give a true picture of the disease burden in this population, and many of the chronic diseases of older adults have not yet appeared in the AA population. Yet, all indications show that the burden of

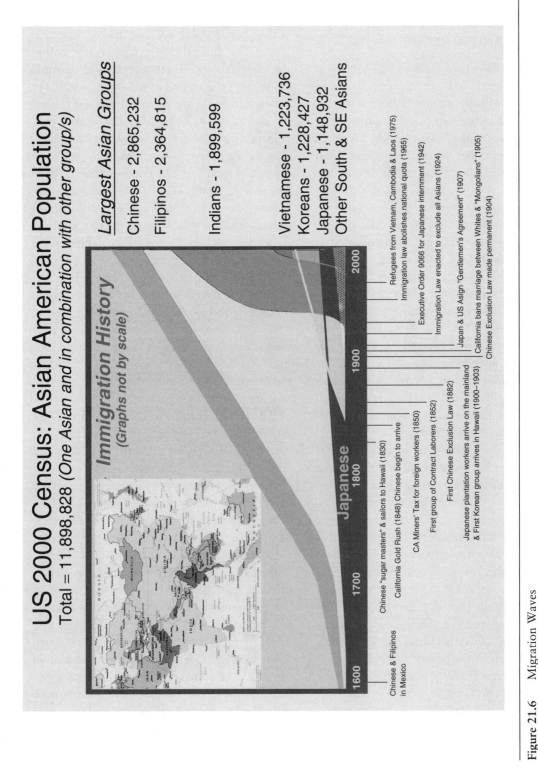

Figure 21.6 Migration Waves

SOURCE: Modified from slide by Snehendu Kar – Population data from US 2000 Census – Historical data from Sucheng Chan (1991), *Asian Americans: An Interpretive History*. Twayne Publishers, Boston.

chronic diseases is significant and, most notably, growing.

CULTURE AND HERITAGE

The Western biomedical model and European American lifestyle are not the only ways to ensure health. Protective and health-promoting beliefs and practices of Asian cultures also expand our understanding of healthy lifestyles. *Culture* is a term that is vaguely conceptualized and inaccurately used in health promotion research and practice. Most often it is glossed erroneously as synonymous with race or as a catchall, monolithic term to describe people who are phenotypically similar and assumed to have the same beliefs, values, and behaviors. Misuse of the concept of culture results in stereotypical, not scientific, thinking. Less than 5% to 10% of diseases are genetically caused. The remaining 90% to 95% are due to lifestyle/environmental factors. Thus, if health practitioners attended to the influence of the multidimensional nature of culture on health behavior, the likelihood of successful outreach and education programs might increase significantly (Kagawa-Singer, 2001).

There is no such thing as a single AA culture, but some commonalities exist. These commonalities are very broad generalizations and only serve as guidelines, not stereotypes. The category of AA is federally noted to be a social/political construct for government tracking of resource allocations. For health promotion, the consequences of the political nature of the racial/ethnic designations must be differentiated from any genetic basis and must be recognized in a social-ecologic framework (Fellin, 2001; McElroy & Townsend, 1996). *To scientifically tailor health promotion programs effectively and efficiently with AAs, we must disaggregate the groups according to their particular culture, experiences pre- and postimmigration, generation variations, and social-historical contexts.*

All cultures are designed to ensure the health and well-being of their members and provide a valued and meaningful way of life within a particular ecologic niche (Kagawa-Singer & Chung, 1994). Within any group, the physical, social, emotional, and spiritual health and the means to maintain, regain, or attain well-being are culturally defined (Foster & Anderson, 1978). Notably, the lifestyle (i.e., cultural) patterns and value system characteristic of each group—such as diet, marriage rules, and means of livelihood—influence gene expression, health status, and disease prevalence. The health system of every culture defines what health is for its members, determines the etiology of diseases, establishes the parameters within which and how distress is defined and signaled, and prescribes the appropriate means to treat the disorder, both medically and socially (Sargent & Johnson, 1996). Culture also prescribes appropriate means to ensure safety, to communicate caring, and to provide social support for its members. Thus, an understanding of the role of culture is fundamental to health promotion.

The multiple dimensions of culture are woven into an integrated whole fabric. The metaphor of weaving is useful to understand cultural variations. The technique of weaving is universal, but the patterns that emerge from each group are culturally identifiable. The symbols and metaphors used in the weavings, as in "material culture," express the ethos of each culture and the place of the individual within that cosmos. The two functions of culture are analogous to the warp and woof or the perpendicularly woven threads of a tapestry: the integrative and the prescriptive. The integrative function provides individuals with the beliefs and values that provide meaning in life and a sense of identity, and the prescriptions are the rules for behavior that support an individual's sense of self-worth and maintain group function and welfare. Specific, discrete beliefs and behaviors are like the threads in the tapestry. A single thread of one cultural tapestry can be taken out and compared across cultural groups for its inherent characteristics (such as postpartum rituals), but the usefulness and integrity of the thread as representative of the entire tapestry cannot be judged unless seen within the pattern of the entire cultural fabric within which such behaviors were meant to function across the life course. Taken out of context, a single thread, like a belief or behavior, may be misinterpreted or even disregarded as unnecessary or maladaptive, especially if evaluated against a standard appropriate for another culture.

In one study that compared the emotional responses of Japanese Americans and European Americans to cancer, the responses were found to be equally strong, but quite culturally identifiable. The idiom of strength for the Japanese Americans was of endurance—to bear the distress by bending when necessary: The metaphor was of bamboo. In comparison, the European Americans used the idiom of fighting an external enemy by not bending: The metaphor was of oak. Moreover, gender differences modified the responses considerably. The Japanese American women and the European American men were more similar, and experienced more distress, than the Japanese American men and the European American women, who were both able to draw on their social support networks more readily and accept the dependent role more easily. The use of each mode of coping was adaptive for the appropriate cultural group and likely maladaptive if used by the other (Kagawa-Singer, 1988).

The AA category is highly heterogeneous among as well as within each group, but as noted, each individual may hold varying levels of acculturation and assimilation to his or her group and the host group that will indicate differential expressions of cultural beliefs and practices and underscore the need for assessment of individual variation both within and between cultural groups and families. Varying levels of acculturation, assimilation, age, education, income, family structure, gender, wealth, foreign-versus U.S.-born status, and immigrant status all modify the degree to which one's cultural group membership may influence health practices and health status. In a multicultural society such as the United States, each cultural group is contemporaneously undergoing modifications and mixtures that render it different from the cultural group of origin and uniquely American. Lack of accountability for these differences perpetuates stereotypical evaluations and diverts the attention from accurately assessing the strengths of and potential conflicts with individual behavior compared with racial stereotypes.

Individuality and the values of autonomy form the basis of Western bioethics and the fundamental value on which our society and the health care system is based. Professionals are educated to provide care based on these values and how society expects recipients of care to respond within the system (Surbone, 2006). This Western European and U.S. belief system, however, is not universal. Without understanding the fundamental nature of culture and the integrity of differing belief systems, the risk of conflict and its negative impact on health promotion efforts is inevitable.

ASIAN AMERICAN CULTURES

Traditional Asian cultures are based on a belief system different from the ethos of the dominant European American culture. Individuality is subsumed under group welfare. One's decisions and actions are conducted with keen awareness of its impact on significant others. Thus, autonomy is considered selfish. Respect for hierarchy is acknowledged as the appropriate way to conduct interpersonal interactions—older over younger, male over female, and physician over patient. To counter this arrangement with an egalitarian approach is considered disrespectful and dishonorable to not only oneself, but, in the concept of "face" in Asian cultures, a reflection on one's entire family and upbringing (Zane, 2002).

Therefore, cultural etiquette of communication is quite different from the dominant Western mode of direct verbalization of thoughts and opinions. Direct communication, in most Asian cultures, is considered uncouth and inconsiderate. Thus, traditional Asian-based communication tends to be tangential and best offered in a hypothetical third-person manner (Carrese & Rhodes, 1995). These traits often cause great ethical and legal consternation for U.S.-trained health practitioners (Kagawa-Singer & Blackhall, 2001).

These differences emanate from different worldviews of how people and the life forces interact. Much of the variation is embedded in the religious and spiritual ethos of the Asian cultures and the fundamental belief that the mind and body are interconnected in one system. This view also underlies the difficulty that recent immigrants and more traditional AAs have with the U.S. division of the mind and body into physical health medicine and mental health with psychiatry and counseling—usually as two different service systems. Most Asian cultures view mental health services as only for the "crazy." Emotional distress due to life circumstances is felt to be normal and expressed through the body that is somatopsychic, which is not psychosomatic (Kawanishi, 1992). Outreach and education efforts designed in the Western model will not be effective.

A few of the commonalities in AA cultures affecting health outcomes are as follows:

- Belief that the mind and body are interconnected as one system.
- Questioning authority disrupts the hierarchy of respectful interpersonal behavior.
- Decision making is conducted as a group or by a designated decision maker, who is not

necessarily the patient. Hierarchy of authority within a family is followed and usually male dominated.

- Harmony is primary in interpersonal relationships rather than defining one's individuality separate from the others (intimacy). Therefore, little of one's inner feelings are commonly expressed—love or animosity.
- Disclosure is titrated according to level of trust. Ascribed authority is given respect hierarchically, but earned respect requires trust. Behaviors speak more truthfully than words. Integrity is demonstrated over time, not inherent.

Religion and Spirituality

The healing practices are based within the major religions of this population that either have their roots in or are strongly influenced by Buddhism, Confucianism, Taoism, and Animism. These religions all have a strong inner locus of control and preventive health focus. The major eastern traditions in healing, such as Ayurveda (East Asian medical system based on Hindu philosophy) or traditional Chinese medicine, can be traced back over several millennia, and have the basic belief that the mind, body, spirit, and universal forces function as an integrated system. Balance among these systems is health, and imbalance results in illness. This integrated worldview produces an awkward interface with the more mechanistic approach of Western biomedicine, which separates physical from mental health and leaves spirituality on the periphery.

HISTORY OF THE MAJOR SUBGROUPS OF ASIAN AMERICANS

A brief history of only the six largest groups and the more recent Southeast Asian groups will be covered (Chinese, Filipino, Korean, South Asian, Japanese, Vietnamese, Lao, Cambodian, and Hmong Americans), and a very brief overview of only the most common health conditions is presented to illustrate the differences among these groups and the danger in combining them statistically or in practice, for they are unique populations. The conduct of accurate and valid research and the design of effective interventions will be more likely if these differences are understood and incorporated into the community and individual assessments.

Immigration plays a key role in understanding the diversity within the AA community. The three major waves of AA immigration characterize the demographic differences in the Asian population (see Figure 21.6). Prior to the 1965 Immigration Act, AAs comprised only 1% of the U.S. population. This small population consisted primarily of fairly acculturated Chinese, Japanese, South Asian, and Filipino Americans. Between 1965 and 1990, the AA population grew in triple digits each decade and increased to 48% from 1990 to 2000. The influx of new immigrants has changed the demographics of each of the more established groups as well as brought in a number of new ethnic groups.

Chinese Americans (2,734,841 Chinese Alone or in Combination)

Chinese Americans began immigrating to the United States in the 1840s. Each generation has had very different experiences due to their home country variations and, importantly, the social climate in the United States at the time. Several discriminatory laws and policies, such as the 1882 Exclusion Act and the 1924 Immigration Act, were passed, targeting the Chinese in the late 1800s and early 1900s, to exclude them from jobs, citizenship, education, and health care (Yang, 2005). The Exclusion Act and its extensions, including antimiscegenation laws, special taxes, housing, and employment discrimination, essentially stopped immigration of the Chinese and forced them into Chinatown ghettos. The 1924 Immigration Act completely restricted Chinese and Japanese immigration to the United States until immigration restrictions

eased after World War II, allowing 150 Chinese per year to enter the United States.

The 1965 Immigration law removed all national quotas and led to the massive shift in immigration for Asians. Almost 60% of the Chinese American population is foreign born, but originate from different countries with different cultures: Taiwan, China, India, Vietnam, Cambodia, Thailand, and Africa as well. This diversity has dramatically changed the demographics and Chinese culture in the United States. Mandarin and Cantonese are the major languages, but several hundred dialects and languages are also spoken by many of the Chinese Americans.

Traditional Chinese medicine revolves around the concept of the balance of the opposite universal forces of nature of Yin/Yang (Yin represents darkness, cold, and emptiness, whereas Yang represents light and fullness, positivity, and warmth). Interventional practices exist, but the primary focus is on *preventive* lifestyle practices to promote and maintain health, such as diet, attitude, and behavior modifications (Louie, 1985). Traditional practices may be used initially, in conjunction with, or after Western biomedicine.

Filipino Americans (2,364,815 Filipinos Alone or in Combination)

The first Filipino settlers established permanent residence in Louisiana in 1763. Although Filipinos gradually arrived in the United States as migrant laborers, the largest migration of Filipinos occurred after 1965, seeking family reunification, better employment, and better futures for their children. Many of these immigrants were skilled laborers and professionals, such as nurses, teachers, doctors, or engineers.

The majority of Filipinos in the United States are immigrants or second generation, but are very acculturated. The American colonialism in the Philippines since the Spanish American War (1898) created a strong U.S. influence that continues today, despite its independence in 1946. With more than 7,100 islands, Filipinos speak more than 43 languages and 87 dialects, with 8 primary languages (Ilocano, Tagalog, Cebuano, Hiligaynon, Bicolano, Waray-Waray, Pampangan, and Pangasinan). Yet, most immigrants speak English well since English continues to be taught in schools in the Philippines.

Filipino Americans have a syncretic belief system of illness and disease that combines indigenous (more Malay) concepts with Spanish Catholicism and Western biomedicine. Their system also stresses disease and illness, which come from imbalance in spirit or morals, similar to the idea of hot/cold, but also the concept of retribution because of moral transgressions. They may turn to traditional healers or "hilots" first, depending on their education, income, and access to care. They also rely heavily on religious beliefs during illness (Frank-Stromberg & Olsen, 1993; Okamura & Agbayani, 1991).

Family involvement and respect for elders is essential to many Filipinos. The advice and opinions of family members and elders is often sought before seeking any medical treatment (Ordonez & Gandeza, 2004). Decisions are generally made by the eldest in the family, especially in caring for aging parents. The eldest child generally makes the decisions, though the duties and responsibilities are delegated among siblings. The link between the decision-making process and respect for those in authority is key for Filipinos. Many will not question doctors, and obtaining a second opinion is rarely done. Doing so would be viewed as an embarrassment for both parties and an insult to the wisdom of the physician.

Japanese Americans (1,148,932 Japanese Alone or in Combination)

Japanese American immigration began in the mid-1880s, and, since relatively few immigrants have come to the United States since World War II, are proportionately the most

acculturated of all the AA subgroups. However, their social-political history in the United States has affected their health behaviors and status differently than other AA groups.

The Japanese Americans are the only group to differentiate and "name" their generations in the United States. Male laborers began emigrating from Japan in around 1880, constituting the first, or Issei, generation. In 1907, the U.S. government instituted the Gentlemen's Agreement that restricted immigration from Japan. In 1924, the Immigration Act was passed, completely stopping immigration from Japan and thus, isolating the Japanese American community from their homeland. With the Alien Land Laws at the time, Japanese in America were not allowed to own property or become naturalized citizens. Japanese born in American, the second, or Nisei, generation, were fully American citizens, but they were not allowed to attend public schools. During World War II, Executive Order 9066 was issued. This was the first and only time that the United States incarcerated its citizens. More than 120,000 Japanese Americans (all Japanese Americans living on the West Coast, including the citizens) were sent to concentration camps around the country for the duration of the War. New immigrants (post World War II) comprise about one third (33%) of the Japanese American population—the lowest percentage of all the AA groups.

Traditional Japanese culture also follows the concept of balance in their health practices (Kanpo medicine in Japan) to promote, prevent, and manage health problems (Ishida & Inouye, 1995). Many continue to use traditional practices in conjunction with Western biomedicine.

Traditionally, the family assumes the responsibility for health, and the physicians are expected to be caring and solicitous. Families are expected to be involved in patient care to help relieve anxiety and provide physical/emotional support (Ishida & Inouye, 1995), and to be directly involved in discussions with their physicians. Many also practice Buddhism, which teaches the principle of avoiding verbalizing one's emotions (Ishida & Inouye, 1995) and respecting the hierarchy of education and profession. Thus, they may not question physicians about their treatment even if the treatment goes against their wishes or they do not understand the rationale. They assume health care professionals will only provide the care that is best for them as patients (Kagawa-Singer, Wellisch, & Durvasula, 1997).

Korean Americans (1,228,427 Koreans Alone or in Combination)

Only a few thousand Koreans lived in the United States before 1965 (Uba, 1994). Most Korean Americans (71%) arrived after 1965, contributing to the third wave of the AA migration. They immigrated as intact families, or sponsored family members to immigrate, and came to seek better standards of living and education for their children.

About 75% to 85% of Korean Americans in the United States are Christians compared with only about 25% of the population in Korea, which is significant socially and culturally (Lai & Arguelles, 2003). In the United States, the Korean church acts as an important source of information as well as religious and social support. Even for Christian Koreans, however, the Chinese philosophies of Confucianism, Taoism, and Buddhism remain influential (Kim et al., 1999; Pang, 1988). Many Korean Americans believe that in order to stay healthy, mind and body must be in balance and the mind must be at peace (Leininger, 1995). They also use traditional healing methods, such as acupuncture and herbal medicine, oftentimes in conjunction with Western medicine.

The educational training of many of the immigrant Koreans is above high school, and many are professionals. Their education, however, does not translate equally in the United States, and many are also not fluent in English. As entrepreneurs, therefore, they open small, self-owned and run businesses, and, thus, cannot

afford insurance. Consequently, the Korean Americans are the least insured of all ethnic groups (E. R. Brown, Lavarreda, Rice, Kincheloe, & Gatchell, 2005).

Medical and health care beliefs, practices, and decision making are similar to the other AA groups, and because of the large proportion of Christians among the Koreans, the support system for the individuals usually include their pastors and congregations.

Vietnamese and Other Southeast Asian Americans (1,223,736 Vietnamese; 198,203 Laotian; 150,283 Thai Alone or in Combination)

The Southeast Asian (SEA) population in the United States consists of several different national and multiple ethnic groups. The primary groups came from Vietnam, Laos, and Cambodia, and more recently, Thailand (see Table 21.1 for a listing of the other nationalities). The Vietnamese, Lao, Hmong, and Cambodians came as political refugees and also arrived in three waves. Each of the waves was composed of different socioeconomic groups. Their status as refugees sets them apart from the Asian immigrants, who came voluntarily, and their health status reflects these differences.

The first wave consisted of about 130,000 SEA refugees, primarily Vietnamese, who were resettled in the United States at the end of Vietnam War in 1975. The Vietnamese refugees were mainly urban and educated, more familiar with the Western cultures, and able to establish a social and economic infrastructure here in the United States, unlike the subsequent SEA refugees. The second wave was the largest group from Vietnam and began to arrive in about 1978. These refugees were called the "boat people," since many escaped from their homelands in desperation in makeshift boats overloaded to capacity and often traveled the seas without food or water (Uba, 1994). These individuals tended to be less educated and from the rural areas. The

Lao, Hmong, and Mien escaped Laos into Thailand usually by foot and often spent many years in the refugee camps in Thailand. The third wave began around 1982 and was composed primarily of those in the SEA refugee camps around the world. The most recent immigrants are the Thais, most of whom have come as sojourners or immigrants for a better life and are not classified as refugees.

The Vietnamese are the largest population from Southeast Asia, and have become well established in many areas of the country. Due to the variations in waves of immigration, however, the socioeconomic status of this population ranges from the very educated to the illiterate and non-English speaking. More than a third of the population is in poverty.

Folk treatments for self-care practices are still widely used, such as coining and cupping, but as with other groups, Western medicine is recognized as extremely effective and used as well. The choice of treatment is made by the supposed etiology of the disorder, as well as the economics of the family.

Almost a third to a half of Vietnamese refugees are Catholic compared with 10% in Vietnam (Gall, 1998), but the majority of Vietnamese in Vietnam and in the United States are Buddhist (Lai & Arguelles, 2003).

Hmong (186,310 Hmong Alone or in Combination)

The Hmong in the United States are primarily from the highlands of Laos and arrived after the fall of Saigon and Laos to Communist forces in 1975. The Hmong had aided and fought with American forces during the conflict and as a result were subject to retribution and annihilation in Laos. The major areas of residence are St. Paul, Minnesota, and Fresno and Sacramento, California.

The Hmong are a very strong and independent people, and many of the second-generation Hmong, raised or born in the United States, have become educated and successful as

business people, politicians, lawyers, and a growing number of doctors. The latter is essential. In 2000, there were only four Hmong doctors in the nation.

The more traditional Hmong are very wary of Western medicine, for their health system is completely different from that of biomedicine, integrating animism and, for many, Christianity (Muecke, 1983). The book *The Spirit Catches You and You Fall Down* (Fadiman, 1997) describes the clash between the health belief systems of Western biomedicine and a Hmong family with an infant with epilepsy and is now widely used in medical schools to teach cross-cultural health care, because it illustrates that the family and the health care practitioners live in very different worlds—both valid but at odds.

A study conducted by Tanjasiri and colleagues (2001) with the Hmong for breast cancer education, however, was successful. They worked with the community to develop information that was presented in a culturally consonant manner. The women had less than 2 years of formal education, but they tailored the information and delivery for their level of understanding, and they were motivated to obtain mammograms (Tanjasiri et al., 2001).

Cambodians (206,052 Cambodians Alone or in Combination)

Key to the lives of Cambodians living in the United States today is the legacy of the "Killing Fields" or the genocide wrought by the Pol Pot regime in the late 1970s of more than 3 million citizens, half the population of Cambodia. The current U.S. population consists of mainly those who experienced the Khmer Rouge savagery directly or their children. As such, mental and physical health care are important issues for the community. Many of the atrocities witnessed have created emotional and physical wounds that will never heal, and their needs remain great. Thus, due to the emotional trauma as well as the demographic composition of the refugees, Cambodians have one of the highest rates of poverty and mental illness of all ethnic groups (Marshall, Schell, Elliott, Berthold, & Chun, 2005).

Within the Cambodian community, Khmer, Cantonese, Mandarin, Teo Chew, and other regional dialects are spoken. Health practices are a combination of traditional practices, and these are based, again, on the concept of balance and total lifestyle integration of body, mind, and souls for health.

Cambodians also believe in spirits that can cause sickness coming from evil spells or soul loss. Traditional healers, "Kru Khmer," treat emotional and physical conditions thought to be caused by malevolent spirits and reestablish the balance necessary for health (Kemp, 1985).

South Asians (1,899,599 Asian Indians; 204,309 Pakistanis; 57,412 Bangladeshis; 24,587 Sri Lankans, Alone or in Combination)

South Asians refer to Asians from Afghanistan, Bangladesh, Bhutan, Burma/ Myanmar, India, the Maldives, Nepal, Pakistan, Tibet, and Sri Lanka. Within India itself, there are 15 official languages (not dialects) with distinct cultures, religions, and histories. South Asians practice all the major religions of the world, with all variations of Hinduism combined for the dominant religion. About 65% of Asian Indian Americans are Hindus (vs. 80% in India), and Sikhs and Christians are overrepresented in United States compared with their representation in India (Lai & Arguelles, 2003). India has also the second largest Muslim population in the world. Pakistanis and other South Asians comprise 25% of the 6 million Muslims in the United States (Lai & Arguelles, 2003).

South Asians are quite invisible socially, politically, and geographically as a community in the United States. Most South Asians came after the 1965 Immigration Act reform and are highly educated professionals and fluent in English. More recent immigrants, however, do not speak English as well and are not economically self-reliant. More than 25% of Asian Indians have limited English proficiency (South Asian Public Health Association [SAPHA] 2002).

Due to their invisibility, few health data exist on this population. The number one cause of mortality in this population, however, is heart disease.

HEALTH AND DISEASE PATTERNS

Mortality trends are often used to evaluate the overall health status of groups. The mortality rates show that AAs had the lowest death rate compared with other racial/ethnic groups in the United States, with a lower mortality rate (299.5 deaths per 100,000 population for AAs) than non-Hispanic whites (997.5 deaths per 100,000 population) (see Table 21.4). Yet, these data are again misleading due to either aggregation of the diverse groups, errors in the data due to misclassification (Hahn, 1992), or incomplete data (National Center for Health Statistics, 1999). Adjustments that must be made in assessing death rates are age-adjusted rates, since more than 65% of the AAs are immigrants and, thus, it is a young population; adjustment for undercount of this population in the Census, thereby skewing the denominator for calculation of rates; and third, the "salmon" effect. Many elderly AAs are here to help care for their grandchildren, while the parents work long hours and often multiple jobs. If these elders become critically ill, they will often return to their homelands and, therefore, not appear in the U.S. vital statistics (Elo & Preston, 1997).

Table 21.5 shows the five leading causes of death in the United States in 2002 for AAs.

Cancer

AAs are the only ethnic group for whom cancer is the number one cause of death for both men and women (Anderson & Smith,

Table 21.4   Death Rates[a] for the United States in 2002

	Asian American	Non-Hispanic White	All Races
Mortality rate	299.5	997.5	847.3
Mortality rate for males	331.4	983.9	846.6
Mortality rate for females	269.7	1,010.6	848.0

SOURCE: Anderson and Smith (2005).

a. Rates per 100,000 population.

Table 21.5   Percentage of Total Deaths Among AA/PIs as a Group and for Men and Women for the Five Leading Causes of Death for All Ages in the United States (2002 and 2004)

All AA/PIs, All Ages	%	Men	%	Women	%
1. Cancers diseases	26.1	1. Cardiovascular	27.0	1. Cancers	26.9
2. Cardiovascular diseases	26.0	2. Cancers	25.4	2. Cardiovascular diseases	25.0
3. Cerebrovascular diseases	9.2	3. Cerebrovascular diseases	7.8	3. Cerebrovascular diseases	10.8
4. Accidents	4.9	4. Accidents	5.7	4. Diabetes II	4.0
5. Diabetes II	3.5	5. Diabetes II	3.2	5. Accidents	3.9

SOURCES: Anderson and Smith (2005); American Cancer Society (2004).

2005). The percentage of total deaths for all AA/PIs is 26.1% compared with 22.8% for all races and 23.1% for white, non-Hispanics (Anderson & Smith, 2005).

AAs suffer from cancer in the same major cancer sites as all U.S. ethnic groups, such as lung, breast, prostate, and colorectal cancer, but these rates are increasing and changing (Prehn et al., 1999). For example, in China, the top five sites for cancer for males make up about 69% of the cancers and are, in order, lung (26%), stomach (20%), liver (12%), esophagus (6%), and colon (5%). In Hong Kong, the total is 59%, and the sites are lung (24%), liver (11%), nasopharynx (9%), colon (8%), and stomach (7%). Among Chinese in America, however, the total is 57%, and the sites are lung (18%), prostate (16%), colon (10%), liver (8%), and rectum (5%) (Prehn et al., 1999). These variations show that even within the same genetic pool, sites and rates of cancer vary considerably. These variations will be explored further in the section on health behaviors.

Several unique cancer sites predominate in the AA population as well. As noted, liver cancer is not only a significant site for Chinese but also for all AA groups. More than 75% of all chronic hepatitis carriers around the world are in those of Asian descent. Hepatitis B infection is the primary cause of liver cancer. The incidence of liver cancer in Chinese, Filipino, Japanese, Korean, and Vietnamese populations are 1.7 to 11.3 times higher than rates among white Americans.

Stomach cancer is a major site for AAs as well. Korean men experience the highest rate of stomach cancer of all racial/ethnic groups, with a fivefold increased rate of stomach cancer over white American men.

Lung cancer is the second leading cause of cancer among Asian males and third among women (U.S. Department of Health and Human Services, 1998). According to the National Cancer Institute's data system, Surveillance Epidemiology and End Results (SEER), incidence data, between 1988 and 1992, lung cancer was the most frequently diagnosed cancer among Korean men, and lung cancer rates for Southeast Asians were 18% higher than among white Americans. Cervical cancer incidence rates are five times higher among Vietnamese American women and more than four times higher among other Southeast Asian women than white women (Chen, Diamant, Kagawa-Singer, Pourat, & Wold, 2004).

Notably, while all other racial/ethnic groups showed significant declines, rates of breast cancer are increasing for AAs (Chu & Chu, 2005), and Southeast Asian women have cervical cancer rates three to five times that of other ethnic groups. Yet, AA women have the lowest screening rates for mammogram exams and Pap smears of all ethnic groups (Chen et al., 2004; Kagawa-Singer & Pourat, 2000).

Heart Disease

Heart disease accounts for 26% of total deaths for AAs. Risk factors related to heart disease include hypertension, high blood cholesterol, diabetes, obesity, smoking, and lack of physical activity, all of which are significant health problems for all AAs, but South

Asian Americans have the worst rates of coronary artery disease of all AAs: four times higher than whites (Office of Prevention Education and Control, 2000).

Ethnic differences in coronary calcification, a sign of subclinical coronary heart disease, are also influenced by acculturation and socioeconomic factors (Roux et al., 2005). According to this study, the mean body mass index (BMI) of U.S.-born Chinese Americans was significantly higher and the probability of calcification higher than non-U.S.-born Chinese Americans. Notably, the number of years in the United States is associated with the probability of calcification.

More than 73% of Japanese men ages 71 to 93 have high blood pressure (American Heart Association, 2004). The management of hypertension in AAs requires attention because there is a gap in knowledge that makes AA/PIs less likely to be aware of this "silent killer" (Office of Prevention Education and Control, 2000). Even for those treated, ethnic differences exists in response to antihypertensive drugs (Hui & Pasic, 1997).

High cholesterol indicates a buildup of excessive cholesterol that can narrow the arteries. Japanese men and women were found to have the highest mean cholesterol levels and the group "other Asians," the lowest (Klatsky & Armstrong, 1991). Data from 1999 showed that only 62.7% of AAs had their blood cholesterol level checked within the past 2 years, compared with 70.8% of the entire U.S. population and 73.1% of non-Hispanic white (D. W. Brown, Giles, Greenlund, & Croft, 2001).

Cerebrovascular Disease

Cerebrovascular disease accounts for 9.2% of total deaths in AAs with a relative risk for stroke, which is 1.3 times higher than non-Hispanic whites for ages 35 to 54 and 1.4 for 55 to 64 (Ayala et al., 2001). With better knowledge about healthier diets and lifestyles and access to care and treatment, however, the age-adjusted annual incidence rate (per 1,000) in Japanese American men has declined markedly, from 5.1 to 2.4 for total stroke, from 3.5 to 1.9 for thromboembolic stroke, and from 1.1 to 0.6 for hemorrhagic stroke (American Heart Association, 2004). The 2003 overall preliminary underlying death rate for stroke was 54.3. The 2002 stroke death rate for Asian/Pacific Islanders was 50.8 for males and 45.4 for females (National Center for Health Statistics, 2004).

Hypertension is also a risk factor for heart and kidney diseases as well as stroke. AA males, as a group, have higher mortality rates due to stroke than white males (Office of Prevention Education and Control, 2000). The proportion of all (hemorrhagic plus ischemic) acute cerebrovascular events that comprised hemorrhagic stroke was disparate among the ethnic groups: whites = 14.2% (223/1,579), Asians = 31.6% (42/133), Chinese = 24.6% (16/65), Japanese = 44.4% (8/18), and Filipino = 37.0% (17/46). The specific risks of stroke in Filipinos and in Japanese Americans mandate emphasis on preventive measures such as smoking cessation programs and aggressive lowering of hypertension in these groups (Klatsky et al., 2005).

Unintentional Injuries

Traffic accidents and pedestrian injury are leading causes of unintentional injury-related deaths. Recent immigrants are particularly at risk from such accidents because many have never attended driver education classes or completely understand traffic safety laws. Motor vehicle collisions were the major cause of death for AAs ages 15 to 54 (California Highway Patrol [CHP], 2006). In addition, illegal street racing has been an increasing trend for AA youth. Because traffic accidents are a key safety issue for the AA population and there are currently no traffic safety programs in California to address this, the CHP has recently launched Asian Pacific Islander Community Outreach, a program with the goal of reducing the number of Asian surnamed drivers and victims involved in traffic-related collisions. CHP officers of Asian ancestry or those who are bilingual and bicultural will organize community events, give traffic safety presentations, and serve as role models (CHP, 2006).

Drinking

AAs have a high percentage of alcohol consumption and misdemeanor and felony DUIs. The rates of DUIs have been steadily increasing, including a 56.3% increase in DUI arrests and a 26.4% increase of collisions involving fatality or injuries since 2002. Thus, alcohol consumption is a key issue that has a significant impact on AA unintentional injury-related deaths as well as their overall health.

AA/PIs, in general, habitually drink more per day than any other racial/ethnic group. Since data on AA/PIs are often aggregated or classified under "other," data for each ethnic group on actual levels of impaired driving are scarce. Korean immigrants, however, have the highest level of weekly alcohol consumption with an average of 7.5 drinks per week (J. M. Brown, Council, Penne, & Gfroerer, 2005). In addition, the culture of "hard core" drinking is especially striking within the Korean American community. Vietnamese immigrants have the second highest alcohol consumption rate with an average of 5.1 drinks per week, followed by Filipino and Japanese immigrants at 4.6 and 3.5 drinks per week (J. M. Brown et al., 2005). Multiracial AA adolescents have much higher alcohol consumption than monoracial AAs. They are twice as likely to drink and three times as likely to get drunk on a regular basis (Udry, 2003). DUI rates are also higher among multiracial AAs. Caetano and McGrath (2005) show how, among multiracial men (AA/PI and non-AA/PI), lifetime DUI rates (22.5%) and 12-month DUI arrest rates (5%) are higher than any other racial/ethnic group. Excessive alcohol consumption can also be a risk factor for hypertension and stroke.

Pedestrian injury is another important factor for unintentional injuries. For children ages

5 to 14, this is the second leading cause of unintentional injury-related death for all ethnic groups and accounts for 18% of fatalities for elderly 70 years and older (Ernst & McCann, 2002). Although there is a general lack of data on pedestrian fatality, there are indications that ethnic and racial minorities are overrepresented in pedestrian deaths (National Highway Transportation Safety Administration, 2001).

Pedestrian safety is also a major focus for AAs because the majority is urban and many live in inner cities. One study successfully addressed the high rate of pedestrian accidents through city council efforts to have traffic signal lights installed and extensive community outreach and in-language education efforts (Liou & Hirota, 2005).

In general, children are at risk for unintentional injury-related deaths, which include motor vehicle accidents, pedestrian, bicyclists, drowning, fire and burns, airway obstruction injury (choking and suffocation), unintentional firearm injuries, falls, and poisoning (SafeKids, 2006). Drowning is the leading cause of unintentional injury-related death for AA/PI children ages 1 to 14. Injury rates vary with age, gender, race/ethnicity, and socioeconomic status, with younger, poor, and male children suffering disproportionately. AA/PI children below 14 years have the lowest unintentional injury death rate (an incidence of 111 in 2001), the rate having declined 52% from 1987 to 2000 (SafeKids, 2006).

Diabetes

Type 2 diabetes is two to five times higher for AAs than non-Hispanic whites, placing diabetes as the fourth leading cause of death. The prevalence of diagnosed cases of diabetes increased threefold between 1990 and 1998, noting that the incidence of diabetes is rising much faster among the AAs (10% to 20%) than among the Caucasian American population (2.5% to 5%) (Joslin Diabetes Center, 2002).

The percentage of total deaths for AAs from diabetes is 3.5%, compared with 3.0% for all races and 2.6% for non-Hispanic whites. Women have a higher percentage of death from diabetes than men, with 4.0% compared with 3.2% (Anderson & Smith, 2005).

The rates of diabetes in Asia are around 3% to 5%. The influence of acculturation to Western lifestyle shows an inverse association between diabetes and traditional Asian lifestyles (Huang et al., 1996).

One of the major indicators for risk of diabetes is BMI, a BMI of 25 to 29.9 being overweight and a BMI greater than 30 being obese, and the risk of diabetes increases at a BMI of 25 or greater. For AAs, however, the BMI is not a valid indicator of risk for diabetes (Weisell, 2002), because diabetes occurs at BMI levels around 23 or 24 (Diabetes in Control, 2005). A more predictive indicator for AAs (and others) is the higher proportion of visceral fat.

Suicide and Mental Health

Overall rates of suicide are included among the prevalent diseases in the AA community because the overall percentage of deaths is higher (1.7%) than non-Hispanic whites (1.3%) (Anderson & Smith, 2005). Chinese American women have the highest rate of suicide of all ethnic groups (Anderson & Smith, 2005). These statistics indicate that the mental health needs of the AA community are significant, and again, a major unmet need (Sue, 1994). Many of the high levels of risky behaviors noted above, such as smoking, drinking, and addictive gambling, may be indications of emotional distress and unmet mental health needs for AAs.

HEALTH BEHAVIORS

In this section, data on the major behaviors targeted with general health promotion activities are covered for AAs. Lifestyle changes appear to be the major factor in disease pattern changes, and culture is a major determinant of lifestyle. Cultures are not static, especially as immigrants begin adopting a Westernized lifestyle and lose the protective factors of their traditional native lifestyles with diet, physical activity, and environmental constraints and toxins. Little information is provided, however, on the protective factors among the AA groups that could prevent the negative changes occurring in their lifestyles (Harrison et al., 2005) as well as education on healthier lifestyles overall.

Physical Activity

The CDC (2004) reports that 28.9% of AA/PI adults report no leisure or physical activity in the past 30 days. In the 1999 Behavioral Risk Factor Surveillance System in Hawaii, the physical activity level for Caucasians in Hawaii was approximately 32%, whereas for all the Asian American and Pacific Islander groups, the range of activity was 30% for part-Hawaiians to 21% for Chinese. The CDC (2000) reports that AAs overall have the highest rate of physical inactivity. Almost 29% reported no leisure or physical activity in the past 30 days. In California, 40% Vietnamese American males and 50% females were not exercising, compared with 24% men and 28% women in the general population, and 31% of Korean Americans respondents did not exercise, compared with 21% of the total Californian population.

Diet

Diet is a major factor in the changing patterns of disease for AA immigrants, whether it is due to availability of tasty foods or the desire to acculturate. Those who adopt more Western foods, which are much higher in fat, cholesterol, and calories than traditional Asian foods, on a regular basis tend to develop disease profiles that resemble those of the dominant U.S. society.

The Westernized diet appears to be the "common denominator" of the major chronic diseases: Unhealthy diets and increased obesity leads to higher rates of diabetes, cardiovascular disease, and cancer. Traditional Asian diets are high in complex carbohydrates, fruits, and vegetables and low in saturated fat and calories. As they Westernize, these health-protective diets are replaced with diets high in simple carbohydrates and animal meats replacing fish for protein (Kagawa-Singer, 2004; Kagawa-Singer & Ong, 2005). Notably, however, AAs also reduce or eliminate the higher risk behaviors that caused other diseases not as prevalent in the United States such as highly salted and pickled foods that cause stomach cancer and nasopharyngeal cancer. These diseases, more prevalent in Asia, are significantly lower among AA in the United States.

Obesity

Self-reported height and weight data from the 2001 California Health Interview Survey show that 42% of AA/PI men and 22% of AA/PI women were overweight or obese compared with 63% of men and 45% of women in the overall population. Weight gain, however, is rising for the AA community. More than half (55%) of men and 42% of women reported significant weight gain (>20 pounds) since the age of 18 years (Mirzadehgan, Harrison, & DiSogra, 2004). AA/PI youth have the fastest rise in obesity among all ethnic groups in California, increasing from 7% to 15% from 1994 to 2003 (California Department of Health Services, 2004), and another study shows that 20.6% of all AA adolescents were obese (Popkin & Udry, 1998). Again, important variations within the AA subpopulations exist: The Chinese (15.3%) and Filipino (18.5%) samples showed substantially lower obesity than non-Hispanic whites, but AA adolescents born in the United States are more than twice as likely to be obese as are first-generation residents of the 50 states (Popkin & Udry, 1998).

Although overall overweight/obesity rates are lower for AA/PIs than the general population, they suffer greater health risks even at slightly overweight levels. For instance, as noted above, the greater tendency for visceral fat in AA/PIs leads to increased risk for diabetes and cardiovascular disease than any other racial/ethnic group (Harrison et al., 2005).

Smoking

AAs have the highest rates of smoking of all ethnic groups. Smoking rates in Asia for men are significantly higher than in the United States, and recent immigrants/refugees bring these practices with them. The smoking rates for AA men range from 26.0% in South Asian men in New York City in 2001 to 54.5% in Chinese Vietnamese in San Diego County, California in 1985 (Lew & Tanjasiri, 2003). AA women, however, experience the opposite pattern. Smoking rates are very low in Asian countries (~2% to 5%), but are rising rapidly in the United States, as they become more acculturated (5% to 12%). The rates for Korean, Filipino, South Asian, Japanese, Chinese, and Vietnamese American young women between the ages of 18 and 24 were 9.4%, 11.0%, 8.9%, 6.3%, 11.2%, and 7.5%, respectively (Tang, Shimizu, & Chen, 2005). For women between the ages of 25 and 34, these rates are even higher, at 26.3%, 20.5%, 37.6%, 13.3%, 19.0%, and 18.5%, respectively (Tang et al., 2005).

Immunizations

The carrier rate of hepatitis B in the United States is 0.2% for all ethnicities, but 10% to 14% for AAs. Hepatitis B is a serious illness, and is also the leading cause of liver cirrhosis and liver cancer (Sung, 1990). The first successful vaccine against cancer was for hepatitis B. The policy in the United States is to immunize all neonates at birth, but with the large proportion of immigrants who come as families,

these children and adults missed immunization and need to be screened and immunized (Immunization Action Council, 2004). AA children were found to have low hepatitis B vaccination rates despite national vaccination guidelines and availability (Lai & Arguelles, 2003).

One study that tested refugees/immigrants found that 14% had chronic hepatitis B and could infect others. About 50% had sufficient antibodies to be immune, and about one third had never had hepatitis B and should be vaccinated. Among the different subgroups, the infection rates varied considerably. The rate for Hmong was 18%, Chinese 11%, Vietnamese 7.6%, Korean 6%, Filipino 4%, and Japanese 1.9% (Au, Tso, & Chin, 1997).

The vaccination rates for influenza in elderly AAs again vary by ethnicity. In one study in Hawaii and California, 65% of non-Hispanic whites received the influenza vaccine as did Japanese Americans, but only 50% of Filipinos obtained the vaccination (Chen, Fox, Stockdale, Kagawa-Singer, & Cantrell, 2006).

CHAPTER SUMMARY

Cultural beliefs and practices affect not only the biological risk factors for disease but also the existential and experiential meaning of particular diseases. How individuals weigh the costs and benefits of screening, early detection, treatment, and rehabilitation are culturally as well as individually determined. Therefore, incorporating an assessment of the cultural meaning of the disease as well as risky behavior into the study of ethnic differences in incidence and mortality rates would provide more accurate information on the AA population. This more focused and specific information would, in turn, affect health promotion efforts and each stage of health care, such as decisions to seek care, choice of treatments, and degree of adherence to treatment protocols.

More than 60% of the AA population are first-generation immigrants, many of whom do not have adequate health insurance. They also face language barriers that prevent them from adequately accessing and utilizing care. Bilingual/bicultural medical and health services are required to eliminate these barriers (President's Advisory Commission on Asian Americans and Pacific Islanders, 2003).

Most new immigrants are unfamiliar with the structure of the U.S. medical establishment. The "system" has little logic in how the body is compartmentalized for medical care and how access is designed. Even for educated individuals from other countries, the appointment system and the division of departments of medicine by organ system is considered illogical. Many ethnic-specific AA community programs provide health care navigation programs, but too few of these services exist to adequately serve this large and diverse population. Inclusion of these structural variables in reporting the health status of any of the AA groups would significantly increase the validity and usefulness of the findings.

To promote the health of AAs, health professionals should address the following challenges:

1. Health professionals should have knowledge of the cultural differences that are salient for effective and respectful cross-cultural communication.

2. Surveys and assessments must be conducted in language to be able to represent the majority of AAs.

3. Community-Based Participatory Research (CBPR) is an important framework to use for studies to ensure better representativeness of the sample population and improve validity of data.
   a. No one can be culturally expert in all AA cultures, but one can become culturally skilled enough to know how to ask better questions and to know one's limitations working in a culture different than one's own.
   b. Partnering with cultural experts will provide greater likelihood that the efforts will be effective and efficacious.

4. Provide culturally competent health education and promotion messages for the Asian American population. Many of these communities also believe the model minority myth.

A great deal more data are required on the subgroups of AAs. This chapter provides an introduction to the population and the health issues confronting both the community as well as health care practitioners due to the paucity of data to the contrary.

Chapter 22, which follows, discusses several specific elements of the HPDP planning process unique to AAs. These elements include planning frameworks, selected health issues, and cultural concerns. The authors also discuss, within a program planning context, the importance of in-depth target group needs assessment, appropriate selection of program design, and particular aspects of program implementation and evaluation. They offer tips based on their extensive experiences, and make suggestions for more effective HPDP program design within the AA populations.

DISCUSSION QUESTIONS AND ACTIVITIES

1. How does the diversity among Asian Americans affect health outcomes?

2. What steps might students and practitioners take to become more familiar with the particular ethnic groups?

3. What implications do cultural differences have for health promotion and health education?

4. How might we go about making the necessary adjustments?

5. Develop a case study around one disease that might compare and contrast two Asian American ethnic groups to demonstrate differences and similarities in the meaning of the disease, the traditional and allopathic medical means to treat the disease, and the potential effects on the family as well as on adherence to the treatment regimen (e.g., diabetes).

GLOSSARY TERMS AND DEFINITIONS

Asian Americans (AA)—*Asian* refers to those having origins in any of the original peoples of the Far East, Southeast Asia, or the Indian subcontinent, including, for example, Cambodia, China, India, Japan, Korea, Malaysia, Pakistan, the Philippine Islands, Thailand, and Vietnam (Reeves & Bennett, 2003).

Culture—1. Culture is the environment in which all life occurs. The functions of culture are to ensure the survival and well-being of its members and provide the reason for being (Baer, Clark, & Peterson, 1998). 2. A nested system of beliefs, values, lifestyles, religion, ecologic and technical resources and constraints that create a worldview for its members and proscribes a way of life, and way of being (Kagawa-Singer, 1996).

Disaggregate—To separate into component parts, for example, to separate the heterogeneous Asian American and Pacific Islander group into specific ethnicities—Chinese, Filipino, Japanese, Korean, Vietnamese, Hmong, Cambodian, and South Asian American—so that ethnic-specific characteristics and data can be collected and vulnerable populations identified.

Model minority—An ethnic group that has successfully assimilated to the American culture, achieved the "American Dream" by being socioeconomically secure and well educated, is characterized by hard work and patience, and serves as an example that other minority groups should follow.

Bimodal distribution—1. In statistics, a bimodal distribution is a distribution with two different peaks. 2. The bimodal distribution is characteristic of Asian American and Pacific Islanders: One end of the spectrum is overrepresented with individuals who are successful and achieve high levels of education, good jobs, and decent salaries, while the other end is overrepresented with those among the nation's most disadvantaged and impoverished, including many with a history of having suffered through decades of war, imprisonment, and even torture (Shinagawa, 2002).

Limited English proficient (LEP)—Individuals who do not speak English as their primary language and who have a limited ability to read, speak, write, or understand English can be limited English proficient, or "LEP." These individuals may be entitled language assistance with respect to a particular type or service, benefit, or encounter.

Immigration—To enter into a new country for permanent residence.

"Pull" factor—In migration, a positive social or ecological condition in one area that draws people living in another area to move there.

"Push" factor—In migration, a negative social or ecological condition in one area that drives people living there to leave for another area.

WEB SITES FOR ADDITIONAL INFORMATION

MedlinePlus, National Library of Medicine, www.nlm.nih.gov/medlineplus/asianamerican health.html

MedlinePlus is the National Library of Medicine's Web site for free consumer health information, providing a selective list of authoritative health information resources from the National Institutes of Health (NIH) and other organizations. It includes more than 700 health topics; generic, brand name prescription and over-the-counter drugs; an illustrated medical encyclopedia; medical dictionary; clinical research studies; and directories that include locations and credentials of doctors, dentists, and hospitals.

Asian Pacific Islander Cancer Education Materials (APICEM), www.cancer.org/docroot/ ASN/ASN_0.asp

The materials on this Web site have been created and translated through a cooperative effort between the American Cancer Society, research groups, and community-based organizations through AANCART and the National Cancer Institute (NCI) to provide health professionals with downloadable information about cancer in several Asian languages. The Asian Pacific Islander Cancer Education Materials Web portal can also be used to find links to materials from other organizations in Asian or Pacific Islander languages.

Asian American Populations, Office of Minority Health, www.cdc.gov/omh/Populations/AsianAm/AsianAm.htm

The Office of Minority Health coordinates White House Executive Orders and HHS Departmental Initiatives, supports Cooperative Agreements for research and professional development, reports on the health status of racial/ethnic minorities in the United States, and initiates strategic partnerships with governmental as well as national and regional organizations. This Web site provides links to newsletters, reports, and other sites with information on Asian American populations, as well as other racial/ethnic groups.

Selected Patient Information Resources in Asian Languages (SPIRAL), www.library.tufts.edu/hsl/spiral

SPIRAL is a joint initiative of the South Cove Community Health Center and Tufts University Hirsh Health Sciences Library and is supported by a grant from the New England Region of the National Network of Libraries of Medicine. The site provides health information for consumers in several languages, including Khmer/Cambodian, Chinese, Hmong, Korean, Lao, Thai, and Vietnamese.

EthnoMed, http://ethnomed.org

The EthnoMed site contains information about cultural beliefs, medical issues, and other related issues pertinent to the health care of recent immigrants to Seattle or the United States, many of whom are refugees fleeing war-torn parts of the world. The site also provides patient education materials on various health topics in different languages, including Amharic, Khmer/Cambodian, Chinese, English, Oromo, Russian, Somali, Spanish, Tigrean, and Vietnamese.

Healthfinder, U.S. Department of Health and Human Services, www.healthfinder.gov/justforyou

This Web site provides health information in English, as well as Chinese, Hmong, Khmer, Korean, Laotian, Samoan, Thai, Tongan, Vietnamese, and other languages.

Asian American Network for Cancer Awareness, Research, and Training (AANCART), www.aancart.org

The AANCART is a cooperative agreement between the National Cancer Institute (NCI) and the University of California, Davis. It is the first ever national cancer awareness research and training infrastructure intended to address Asian American concerns. AANCART seeks to build partnerships to increase cancer awareness, to promote greater accrual of AAs in clinical studies, to increase training opportunities for AAs, and to develop pilot programs in five targeted regions: Sacramento, Los Angeles, San Francisco, Honolulu, and Seattle.

Asian and Pacific Islander American Health Forum (APIAHF), www.apiahf.org

The APIAHF, founded in 1986, is a national advocacy organization dedicated to promoting policy, program, and research efforts to improve the health and well-being of AA/PI communities. APIAHF advocates on health issues of significance to AA/PI communities, conducts community-based technical assistance and training, provides health and U.S. Census data analysis and information dissemination, and convenes regional and national conferences on AA/PI health.

Association of Asian Pacific Community Health Organizations (AAPCHO), www.aapcho.org

The AAPCHO, formed in 1987, is a national association representing community health organizations dedicated to promoting advocacy, collaboration, and leadership that improves the health status and access of AAs, Native Hawaiians, and Pacific Islanders. This Web site provides links to data pertaining to AA/PI health and community health centers, information on national programs that address AA/PI health issues, a host of health education and resource materials for AA/PIs, fact sheets and maps detailing locations of medically underserved AA/PIs, and information on current legislative efforts and bills affecting health care service delivery for this population.

Asian Health, Charles Kemp, www3.baylor
.edu/~Charles_Kemp/asian_health.html

Charles Kemp, nursing faculty at Baylor
University, has put together a resource of cultural and health issues of Asian immigrants.

Healthy People 2010, Minority Populations
Gateway, http://hp2010.nhlbihin.net/minority/
asn_frameset.htm

The HP 2010 Asian American and Pacific
Islander Gateway of the National Heart,
Lung, and Blood Institute includes publication
highlights, NHLBI projects, and resources.

The 24 Languages Project, http://library.med
.utah.edu/24languages

The 24 Languages Project is a project of
the Spencer S. Eccles Health Sciences Library,
in partnership with the Utah Department of
Health, the Immunization Action Coalition,
AAPCHO, and many others to improve access
to health materials in multiple languages. This
Web site provides electronic access to more
than 200 health education brochures in 24
different languages.

Reducing Health Disparities in Asian American
and Pacific Islander Populations, The Provider's
Guide to Quality and Culture, Management
Sciences for Health, http://erc.msh.org/aapi/
index.html

Reducing Health Disparities in Asian
American and Pacific Islander Populations
is a section in The Provider's Guide to Quality
and Culture that aims to improve clinical outcomes among AA/PI populations. Please note
that within AA/PI populations, there is great
variation in disease patterns, communication
styles, beliefs, and health practices.

REFERENCES

American Cancer Society. (2004). *Cancer facts and figures 2004*. Atlanta, GA: Author.

American Heart Association. (2004). *Asian/Pacific Islanders and cardiovascular diseases: Statistics*. Dallas, TX: Author.

Anderson, R. N., & Smith, B. L. (2005). *Deaths: Leading causes for 2002* (National Vital Statistics Reports, Vol. 53, No. 17). Hyattsville, MD: National Center for Health Statistics.

Asian American Justice Center & Asian Pacific American Legal Center. (2006). *A community of contrasts: Asian Americans and Pacific Islanders in the United States*. Washington, DC: Author.

Asian and Pacific Islander American Health Forum. (2003). *Legislation threatens Medicare*. Retrieved August 18, 2006, from www .apiahf.org/policy/healthaccess/20040123pr_ Medicare_legislative_threat.htm

Asian and Pacific Islander American Health Forum. (2004). *API Center for Census Information and Services*. Retrieved November 30, 2006, from www.apiahf.org/programs/accis/index.htm

Asian and Pacific Islander American Health Forum. (2005). *Diverse communities, diverse experiences: The status of Asian Americans and Pacific Islanders in the U.S. (A review of six economic indicators and their impact on health)*. Washington, DC: Author.

Au, L., Tso, A., & Chin, K. (1997). Asian-American adolescent immigrants: The New York City schools experience. *Journal of School Health, 67*(7), 277–279.

Ayala, C., Greenlund, K. J., Croft, J. B., Keenan, N. L., Donehoo, R. S., Giles, W. H., et al. (2001). Racial/ethnic disparities in mortality by stroke subtype in the United States, 1995–1998. *American Journal of Epidemiology, 154*(11), 1057–1063.

Baer, R. D., Clark, L., & Peterson, C. (1998). Folk illnesses. In S. Loue (Ed.), *Handbook of immigrant health* (pp. 183–202). New York: Plenum Press.

Barnes, J. S., & Bennett, C. E. (2002, February). *The Asian population: 2000*. Washington, DC: U.S. Census Bureau.

Brown, D. W., Giles, W. H., Greenlund, K. J., & Croft, J. B. (2001). Disparities in cholesterol screening: Falling short of a national health objective. *Preventive Medicine, 33*, 517–522.

Brown, E. R., Lavarreda, S. A., Rice, T., Kincheloe, J. R., & Gatchell, M. S. (2005). *The state of health insurance in California: Findings from the 2003 California Health Interview Survey*. Los Angeles: UCLA Center for Health Policy Research.

Brown, E. R., Ojeda, V. D., Wyn, R., & Levan, R. (2000). *Racial and ethnic disparities in access* to *health insurance and health care.* Los Angeles: UCLA Center for Health Policy Research.

Brown, J. M., Council, C. L., Penne, M. A., & Gfroerer, J. C. (2005). *Immigrants and substance use: Findings from the 1999–2001 National Surveys on Drug Use and Health* (DHHS Publication No. SMA 04–3909, Analytic Series A-23). Rockville, MD: Substance Abuse and Mental Health Services Administration, Office of Applied Studies.

Caetano, R., & McGrath, C. (2005). Driving under the influence (DUI) among U.S. ethnic groups. *Accident Analysis and Prevention, 37*(2), 217–224.

California Department of Health Services. (2004, May 5, 2004). *Table 18C. 2003 Pediatric Nutrition Surveillance, California, Summary of trends in growth and anemia indicators by race/ethnicity.* Retrieved August 8, 2006, from www.dhs.ca.gov/pcfh/cms/onlinearchive/pdf/chdp/informationnotices/2004/chdpin04c/table18c.pdf

California Highway Patrol. (2006). *Asian Pacific Islander community outreach.* Retrieved August 7, 2006, from www.chp.ca.gov/community/html/ochats.html

Carrese, J. A., & Rhodes, L. A. (1995). Western bioethics on the Navajo reservation: Benefit or harm? *Journal of the American Medical Association, 274*(10), 826–829.

Centers for Disease Control and Prevention. (1994). Chronic disease in minority populations. *Morbidity and Mortality Weekly Report, 43*(48), 894–899. Atlanta, GA: U.S. Department of Health and Human Services, Public Health Service.

Centers for Disease Control and Prevention. (2000). State-specific prevalence of selected health behaviors, by race and ethnicity: Behavioral risk factor surveillance system, 1997. *Morbidity and Mortality Weekly Report, 49*(SS-2), 1–68.

Centers for Disease Control and Prevention. (2004). *Morbidity and Mortality Weekly Report* (ISSN: 0149–2195). Washington, DC: Author.

Chen, J., Diamant, A. L., Kagawa-Singer, M., Pourat, N., & Wold, C. (2004). Disaggregating Asian and Pacific Islander women to assess cancer screening. *American Journal of Preventive Medicine, 27,* 1–6.

Chen, J. Y., Fox, S. A., Stockdale, S. E., Kagawa-Singer, M., & Cantrell, C. (2006). Health disparities and prevention: Racial-ethnic barriers to flu vaccinations. *Journal of Community Health, 32,* 5–20.

Chu, K. C., & Chu, K. T. (2005). 1999–2001 Cancer mortality rates for Asian and Pacific Islander ethnic groups with comparisons to their 1988–1992 rates. *Cancer, 104*(12 Suppl.), 2989–2998.

Congressional Research Service, Library of Congress. (2005, May 6). *CRS report for Congress* (RL32804). Washington, DC: Author.

Dalaker, J. (2001). *Poverty in the United States: 2000* (No. Series P60-214). Washington, DC: U.S. Census Bureau.

Diabetes in Control. *Asian Americans face higher diabetes risk and not being screened.* Findings presented at a Diabetes symposium at the Joslin Diabetes Center in Boston, April, 2005.

Elo, I. T., & Preston, S. H. (1997). Racial and ethnic differences in mortality at older ages. In L. Martin & B. Soldo (Eds.), *Racial and ethnic differences in the health of older Americans* (pp. 10–42). Washington, DC: National Academy Press.

Ernst, M., & McCann, B. (2002). *Mean streets 2002: Surface Transportation Policy Project.* Retrieved August 7, 2006, from www.transact.org/PDFs/ms2002/MeanStreets2002.pdf

Fadiman, A. (1997). *The spirit catches you and you fall down: A Hmong child, her American doctors, and the collision of two cultures* (1st ed.). New York: Farrar, Straus & Giroux.

Federal Register. (1997). *Standards for maintaining, collecting, and presenting federal data on race and ethnicity* (FR Doc. 97–28653). Washington, DC: Office of the Federal Register, National Archives and Records Administration.

Fellin, P. (2001). Understanding American communities. In J. Rothman, J. Erlich, & J. Tropman (Eds.), *Strategies of community intervention* (5th ed., pp. 118–133). Itasca, IL: Peacock.

Foster, G., & Anderson, B. (1978). *Medical anthropology.* New York: Wiley.

Frank-Stromberg, M., & Olsen, S. J. (1993). *Cancer prevention in minority populations:*

Cultural implication for health care professionals. St. Louis: Mosby.

Gall, T. L. (1998). *Worldmark encyclopedia of culture and daily life: Vol. 2. Americas*. Cleveland, OH: Eastword Publications Development.

Gardner, R. W. (1994). Mortality. In N. W. S. Zane, D. T. Takeuchi, & K. N. J. Young (Eds.), *Confronting critical health issues of Asian and Pacific Islander Americans* (pp. 67–77). Thousand Oaks, CA: Sage.

Ghosh, C. (2003). Healthy People 2010 and Asian Americans/Pacific Islanders: Defining a baseline of information. *American Journal of Public Health, 93*(12), 2093–2098.

Hahn, R. (1992). The state of federal health statistics on racial and ethnic groups. *Journal of the American Medical Association, 267*(2), 268–271.

Harrison, G. G., Marjorie Kagawa-Singer, M., Foerster, S. B., Lee, H., Kim, L. P., Nguyen, T. U., et al. (2005). *Seizing the moment: California's opportunity to prevent nutrition-related health disparities in low-income Asian American populations*. Atlanta, GA: American Cancer Society.

Heckler, M. (1985). *Report of the Secretary's Task Force on black and minority health*. Washington, DC: U.S. Department of Health and Human Services.

Huang, B., Rodriguez, B. L., Burchfiel, C. M., Chyou, P.-H., Curb, J. D., & Yano, K. (1996). Acculturation and prevalence of diabetes among Japanese-American men in Hawaii. *American Journal of Epidemiology, 144*(7), 674–681.

Hui, K. K., & Pasic, J. (1997). Outcome of hypertension management in Asian Americans. *Archives of Internal Medicine, 157*, 1345–1348.

Immunization Action Council. (2004). *Hepatitis B information for Asian and Pacific Islander Americans* (Item #P4190). St. Paul, MN: Author.

Ishida, D., & Inouye, J. (1995). Japanese Americans. In J. N. Ginger & R. E. Davidhizar (Eds.), *Transcultural nursing: Assessment and interventions* (2nd ed., pp. 317–344). St. Louis, MO: Mosby.

Joslin Diabetes Center. (2002). Asian American Diabetes Fund. *Asian American Diabetes Fund Newsletter, 1*, 4.

Kagawa-Singer, M. (1988). *Bamboo and oak: Differences in adaptation to cancer between Japanese-American and Anglo-American patients*. Unpublished doctoral dissertation, University of California, Los Angeles.

Kagawa-Singer, M. (1996). Cultural systems related to cancer. In R. McCorkle, M. Grant, M. Frank-Stromberg, & S. B. Baird (Eds.), *Cancer nursing: A comprehensive textbook* (2nd ed., pp. 38–52). Philadelphia: W. B. Saunders.

Kagawa-Singer, M. (2001). From genes to social science: Impact of the simplistic interpretation of race, ethnicity, and culture on cancer outcome. *Cancer, 91*(S1), 226–232.

Kagawa-Singer, M. (2004). Asian American health. In N. B. Anderson & I. Kawachi (Eds.), *Encyclopedia of health and behavior* (Vol. 1). Thousand Oaks, CA: Sage.

Kagawa-Singer, M. (2006). Population science is science only if you know the population. *Journal of Cancer Education, 21*(1, Suppl.), S22–S31.

Kagawa-Singer, M., & Blackhall, L. J. (2001). Negotiating cross-cultural issues at the end of life: "You got to go where he lives." *Journal of the American Medical Association, 286*(23), 2993–3001.

Kagawa-Singer, M., & Chung, R. (1994). A paradigm for culturally based care for minority populations. *Journal of Community Psychology, 22*(2), 192–208.

Kagawa-Singer, M., & Ong, P. M. (2005). The road ahead: Barriers and paths to improving AAPI health. *AAPI Nexus, 3*(1), vii–xv.

Kagawa-Singer, M., & Pourat, N. (2000). Asian American and Pacific Islander breast and cervical carcinoma screening rates and Healthy People 2000 objectives. *Cancer, 89*(3), 696–705.

Kagawa-Singer, M., Wellisch, D. K., & Durvasula, R. (1997). Impact of breast cancer on Asian American and Anglo American women. *Culture, Medicine and Psychiatry, 21*(4), 449–480.

Kawanishi, Y. (1992). Somatization of Asians: An artifact of Western medicalization? *Transcultural Psychiatric Research Review, 29*, 5–36.

Kemp, C. (1985). Cambodian refugee health care beliefs and practices. *Journal of Community Health Nursing, 2*, 41–52.

Kim, C. J. (1999). The racial triangulation of Asian Americans. *Politics & Society, 27*(1), 105–138.

Kim, K., Yu, E. S., Chen, E. H., Kim, J., Kaufman, M., & Purkiss, J. (1999). Cervical cancer screening knowledge and practices among Korean-American women. *Cancer Nursing, 22*(4), 297–302.

Klatsky, A. L., & Armstrong, M. A. (1991). Cardiovascular risk factors among Asian Americans living in northern California. *American Journal of Public Health, 81,* 1423–1428.

Klatsky, A. L., Friedman, G. D., Sidney, S., Kipp, H., Kubo, A., & Armstrong, M. A. (2005). Risk of hemorrhagic stroke in Asian American ethnic groups. *Neuroepidemiology, 25,* 26–31.

Lai, E., & Arguelles, D. (2003). *The new face of Asian Pacific America: Numbers, diversity, and change in the 21st century.* Los Angeles: UCLA Asian American Studies Center Press.

Leininger, M. (1995). Southeast and Eastern Asians and cultural care. In M. Leininger (Ed.), *Transcultural nursing: Concepts, theories, research and practices* (2nd ed., pp. 535–558). New York: McGraw-Hill.

Lew, R., & Tanjasiri, S. P. (2003). Slowing the epidemic of tobacco use among Asian Americans and Pacific Islanders. *American Journal of Public Health, 93*(5), 764–768.

Lin-Fu, J. S. (1993). Asian and Pacific Islander Americans: An overview of demographic characteristics and health care issues. *Asian American and Pacific Islander Journal of Health, 1*(1), 20–36.

Liou, J., & Hirota, S. (2005). From pedestrian safety to environmental justice: The evolution of a Chinatown community campaign. *AAPI Nexus, 3*(1), 1–12.

Louie, K. B. (1985). Providing health care to Chinese clients. *Topics in Clinical Nursing, 7*(3), 18–25.

Marshall, G. N., Schell, T. L., Elliott, M. N., Berthold, S. M., & Chun, C. A. (2005). Mental health of Cambodian refugees 2 decades after resettlement in the United States. *Journal of the American Medical Association, 294*(5), 571–579.

Mays, V., Ponce, N. A., Washington, D. L., & Cochran, S. D. (2003). Classification of race and ethnicity: implications for public health. *Annual Review of Public Health, 24,* 83–110.

McElroy, A., & Townsend, P. K. (1996). *Medical anthropology in ecological perspective* (4th ed.). Boulder, CO: Westview Press.

Mirzadehgan, P., Harrison, G., & DiSogra, C. (2004). *California adults as obese as the nation and still gaining weight.* Health Policy Fact Sheet. Los Angeles: UCLA Center for Health Policy Research.

Muecke, M. A. (1983). Caring for Southeast Asian refugee patients in the USA. *American Journal of Public Health, 73*(4), 431–438.

National Center for Health Statistics. (1998). *Health, United States, 1998 with socioeconomic status and health chartbook* (Table 134 (PHS) 98–1232). Hyattsville, MD: U.S. Department of Health and Human Services, Centers for Disease Control and Prevention, National Center for Health Statistics.

National Center for Health Statistics. (1999). *Health, United States, 1999, with health and aging chartbook* ((PHS) 99–1232–1). Hyattsville, MD: U.S. Department of Health and Human Services, Centers for Disease Control and Prevention, National Center for Health Statistics.

National Center for Health Statistics. (2000). *Health, United States, 2000 with adolescent health chartbook* ((PHS) 2000–1232–1). Hyattsville, MD: U.S. Department of Health and Human Services, Centers for Disease Control and Prevention, National Center for Health Statistics.

National Center for Health Statistics. (2003). *Summary health statistics for U.S. children: National Health Interview Survey, 2003.* Hyattsville, MD: U.S. Department of Health and Human Services, Centers for Disease Control and Prevention, National Center for Health Statistics.

National Center for Health Statistics. (2004). *Health, United States, 2004, with chartbook on trends in the health of Americans* (2004–1232). Hyattsville, MD: U.S. Department of Health and Human Services, Centers for Disease Control and Prevention, National Center for Health Statistics.

National Highway Transportation Safety Administration. (2001). *Traffic safety facts 2001.* Retrieved August 7, 2006, from www-nrd.nhtsa.dot.gov/pdf/nrd-30/NCSA/TSF2001/2001pedestrian.pdf

Office of Prevention Education and Control. (2000). *Addressing cardiovascular health in Asian Americans and Pacific Islanders* (NIH Publication No. 00–3647). Bethesda, MD: National Institutes of Health, National Heart, Lung, and Blood Institute.

Okamura, J., & Agbayani, A. (1991). *Philippines culture, Filipinos, values, Philippine beliefs.* Retrieved August 7, 2006, from www.livingin thephilippines.com/values.html

Ong, P. M. (2000). *The state of Asian Pacific America: Transforming race relations.* Los Angeles: LEAP Asian Pacific American Public Policy Institute and UCLA Asian American Studies Center.

Ordonez, R. V., & Gandeza, N. (2004). Integrating traditional beliefs and modern medicine: Filipino nurses' health beliefs, behaviors, and practices. *Home Health Care Management & Practice, 17*(1), 22–27.

Pang, C. (1988). The Koreans. In N. Palafox & A. Warren (Eds.), *Cross-cultural caring: A handbook for healthcare professionals in Hawaii* (pp. 136–154). Honolulu, HI: Transcultural Health Forum.

Popkin, B. M., & Udry, J. R. (1998). Adolescent obesity increases significantly in second and third generation U.S. immigrants: The National Longitudinal Study of Adolescent Health. *Journal of Nutrition, 128*(4), 701–706.

Prehn, A., Lin, S., Clarke, C., Packel, L., Lum, R., & Lui, S. (1999). *Cancer incidence in Chinese, Japanese and Filipinos in the US and Asia 1988–1992.* Union City, CA: Northern California Cancer Center.

President's Advisory Commission on Asian Americans and Pacific Islanders, a White House Initiative. (2003). *Update of Commission activities 2002–2003.* Washington, DC: Author.

Reeves, T., & Bennett, C. (2003). *The Asian and Pacific Islander population in the United States: March 2002. Current population reports* (No. P20-540). Washington, DC: U.S. Census Bureau.

Roux, A. V. D., Detrano, R., Jackson, S., Jacobs, D. R., Schreiner, P. J., Shea, S., et al. (2005). Acculturation and socioeconomic position as predictors of coronary calcification in a multiethnic sample. *Circulation, 112,* 1557–1565.

SafeKids. (2006). *Fact sheet: Asian American and Pacific Islander (AAPI) alcohol use.* Retrieved August 7, 2006, from www.usa.safekids.org/tier3_cd.cfm?content_item_id=10390&folder_id=300

Sargent, C. F., & Johnson, T. M. (Eds.). (1996). *Handbook of medical anthropology: Contemporary theory and method* (Rev. ed.). Westport, CT: Praeger.

Shinagawa, S. M. (2002, November/December). Swept under the "oriental" rug: How Asian American stereotypes and cultural differences lead to inferior care. *Breast Cancer Action Newsletter, 74.*

South Asian Public Health Association. (2002). *A brown paper: The health of South Asians in the United States.* Retrieved July 27, 2006, 2006, from www.sapha.net/exec-sum.pdf

Srinivasan, S., & Guillermo, T. (2000). Toward improved health: Disaggregating Asian American and Native Hawaiian/Pacific Islander data. *American Journal of Public Health, 90*(11), 1731–1734.

Sue, S. (1994). Mental health. In N. Zane, D. T. Takeuchi, & K. N. J. Young (Eds.), *Confronting critical health issues of Asian and Pacific Islander Americans.* Thousand Oaks, CA: Sage.

Sung, J. L. (1990). Hepatitis B virus eradication strategy for Asia. The Asian Regional Study Group. *Vaccine, 8*(Suppl.), S81–S85.

Surbone, A. (2006, July 8–12, 2006). *Truth telling and ethical issues: An overview.* Paper presented at the UICC World Cancer Congress, Washington, DC.

Tang, H., Shimizu, R., & Chen, M. S. (2005). English language proficiency and smoking prevalence among California's Asian Americans. *Cancer, 104*(12 Suppl.), 2982–2988.

Tanjasiri, S. P., Kagawa-Singer, M., Foo, M. A., Chao, M., Linayao-Putman, I., Lor, Y. C., et al. (2001). Breast cancer screening among Hmong women in California. *Journal of Cancer Education, 16*(1), 50–54.

Uba, L. (1994). *Asian Americans: Personality patterns, identity, and mental health.* New York: Guilford Press.

Udry, J. R. (2003). Adolescent health: Health and behavior risks of adolescents with mixed-race identity. *American Journal of Public Health, 93*(11), 1865–1870.

U.S. Census Bureau. (2000). *Census Bureau facts for features: Asian Pacific American Heritage Month: May 1–31*. Retrieved 1 November, 2000, from www.census.gov/Press-Release/www/2000/cb00ff05.html

U.S. Census Bureau. (2001). *U.S. Census 2000: Overview of race and Hispanic origin* (Census Brief). Washington, DC: Author.

U.S. Census Bureau (2002a). *Census 2000 Summary File 1 (SF 1)*. Retrieved November 30, 2006, from http://factfinder .census.gov/servlet/DatasetMainPageServlet?_ lang=en

U.S. Census Bureau. (2002b). *The Asian population: 2000*. Retrieved August 31, 2005, from www .census.gov/prod/2002pubs/c2kbr01-16.pdf

U.S. Census Bureau. (2003). *Poverty in the United States: 2002* (P60-222). Washington, DC: Author.

U.S. Census Bureau. (2004a). *Table 1. Population by sex and age, for Asian alone or in combination and white alone, not Hispanic: March 2004*. Washington, DC: U.S. Census Bureau, Current Population Survey, Annual Social and Economic Supplement, Racial Statistics Branch, Population Division.

U.S. Census Bureau. (2004b). *Table 8. Foreign-born population by sex, citizenship status, and year of entry, for Asian alone or in combination and white alone, not Hispanic: March 2004*. Washington, DC: U.S. Census Bureau, Current Population Survey, Racial Statistics Branch, Population Division.

U.S. Census Bureau. (2004c). *We the people: Asians in the United States* (CENSR-17). Washington, DC: Author.

U.S. Census Bureau. (2005). *Income, poverty, and health insurance coverage in the United States: 2004* (P60–229). Washington, DC: Author.

U.S. Department of Health and Human Services. (1998). *Tobacco use among U.S. racial/ethnic minority groups—African Americans, American Indians and Alaska Natives, Asian Americans and Pacific Islanders, and Hispanics: A report of the Surgeon General*. Atlanta, GA: U.S. Department of Health and Human Services, Centers for Disease Control and Prevention, National Center for Chronic Disease Prevention and Health Promotion, Office on Smoking and Health.

Weisell, R. C. (2002). Body mass index as an indicator of obesity. *Asia Pacific Journal of Clinical Nutrition, 11*(Suppl.), S681–S684.

Yang, J. S. (2005). *A model to increase access to care for immigrants: Charting the development of San Francisco Chinatown's ethnic-specific health care system*. Ann Arbor, MI: UMI Dissertation Services.

Zane, N. (2002). The use of culturally-based variables in assessment: Studies on loss of face. In K. Kurasaki, S. Okakzaki, & S. Due (Eds.), *Asian American mental health: Assessment methods and theories* (pp. 1–18). Dodrecht, Netherlands: Kluwer Academic.

22

Assessing Needs and Planning, Implementing, and Evaluating Health Promotion and Disease Prevention Programs Among Asian American Population Groups

JUNE GUTIERREZ ENGLISH

RHONDA FOLSOM

Chapter Objectives

On completion of this chapter, the health promotion student and practitioner will be able to

- Explain why combining heterogeneous groups of Asian Americans into the same health promotion and education programs as one aggregated population can result in misleading outcomes for planners as they study program results

(Continued)

AUTHORS' NOTE: The authors wish to extend their appreciation to and thank the following organizations and individuals for their assistance and the use of their materials in preparing this chapter: The Asian American Senior Citizens Service Center; Pathways to Early Cancer Detection for Vietnamese Women Project; Vietnamese Community Health Promotion Project; Division of General Internal Medicine, University of California, San Francisco (UCSF); Dr. Stephen J. McPhee, Principal Investigator and Professor of Medicine at UCSF; Mr. Ahn Le; and the late Mr. Christopher N. H. Jenkins, who served as Project Director at "Suc Khnow La VangA!" The authors also wish to acknowledge the editorial assistance provided by Dr. Michael V. Kline and Dr. Robert Huff.

(Continued)

- Formulate an operational framework for health promotion and education programs for members of Asian American communities, taking into consideration how the diversity among Asian American population groups can affect health outcomes

- Identify, emphasize, and differentiate between key aspects of program planning, program development, program implementation, and evaluation of health promotion and education efforts

- Describe applications of health promotion program planning and implementation efforts intended for Asian American populations and how the differing cultures can influence the focus and design of those efforts

- Identify and define the levels of change sought by programs at the health promotion and health education levels for increasing services to the Asian American communities

Diversity among Asian American groups "in history, cultural practices, language, socioeconomic status, degree of acculturation, and generational differences" (English & Le, 1999) requires providing culturally sensitive and appropriate health programs that target particular populations. Health care planners and practitioners alike must acknowledge and respect these differences when designing and implementing programs serving culturally distinct Asian American populations. As outlined in the prior chapters, key historical, linguistic, religious, and demographic factors and differences in cultural beliefs and practices separate Asian cultures. To some extent, these variables continue in Asian American communities, influencing individual health care choices and behaviors. Owing to space and time limitations, it will not be possible in this chapter to provide a comprehensive review of the range of concerns related to planning and implementing health promotion and disease prevention (HPDP) programs for Asian Americans.

The authors of this chapter are currently working as health educators and administrators in the area of cancer control. The intent of this chapter is to provide a basic orientation to the process of assessing, designing, and implementing health promotion and education programs for Asian Americans. Specific elements of the planning process, including selected health issues and cultural concerns unique to the Asian American experience, are considered. Examples and case studies to illustrate this process have been selectively drawn from the authors' experiences in promoting cancer screening among Asian American women from a variety of cultural backgrounds through tailored health education programs. Health education is the primary mechanism for achieving health promotion goals. Thus, this kind of perspective affords students and practitioners a real-life view from the frontline of community health promotion planning of preventive health programs. The operational constraints of limited funding, time, and resources that face program planners working with Asian American populations are also discussed.

In an earlier work, English and Le (1999) noted the differences in the impact of acculturation and urged health professionals to be sensitive and responsive when working with each ethnic group. There is considerable difference in the approach directed at highly acculturated groups with a long history of American residence as opposed to recent immigrants (also, see Chapters 1 and 21, this volume). In terms of generational differences and the need for effective health communication, learning methods can vary greatly, from an online health education course reflecting the "the digital divide" described (U.S. Department of Health and Human Services, 2000) to tailored, low-literacy materials appropriate for new immigrants.

Planning HPDP programs within the milieu of Asian American target groups requires systematic identification and selection of a particular course of action related to achieving or improving desirable health-related behaviors. Specific elements of the planning process, including selected health issues and cultural concerns unique to the Asian American experience, must be considered. This chapter operates more heavily from a health education vantage point because it is at the health education level, given the realities of financial support in most communities, where most current planning activities that target Asian Americans occur (see Chapter 7, this volume). And in the latter part of the chapter, the authors present case studies on breast and cervical cancer health education for Asian communities in two different regions of California. One program focuses on that region's Vietnamese community, and the other program focuses on a Chinese community in another area. Both programs share commonalities in program design, educational strategies, methods and interventions, and evaluation.

ASIAN AMERICAN HEALTH ISSUES

Program-Planning Consideration. Be aware of problems with the use of aggregate health data.

Ecklund and Park (2005) note that the "public image" of Asian Americans as "model minorities" has been largely dispelled (by scholars). Unfortunately, this stereotype continues in the area of health care due to the application and use of aggregate data in health program planning for Asian Americans. Susan Shinagawa, a breast cancer survivor and advocate, observed in 1997,

> It provided me no comfort when the doctors kept saying that I had nothing to worry about. . . . They said that "Asian women don't get breast cancer." But I was soon to learn that statement to be an absolute fallacy perpetuated by inadequate and aggregate national statistics, which also perpetuated the myth of Asian Pacific Islanders as the "model health minority." (Congressional Asian Pacific Caucus, 1997, p. 31)

Yet, nearly a decade later, S. Shinagawa (personal communication, October 4, 2006) again noted that, at least with respect to Asian American health, this myth persists. She remarked in frustration that a 2006 government document stated that "Asian/Pacific Islander" (API) women are the least likely to get breast cancer among California ethnic groups," while research data published over the past 5 years state that, when disaggregated, certain Asian and all Pacific Islander (PI) women in California are among those most likely to be diagnosed and, in the case of PI women, die of breast cancer.

The U.S. Department of Health and Human Services (2000) in their report titled *Healthy People 2010* noted the difficulties in defining health status, behaviors, and risks specific to each Asian American group, including concerns with diabetes, hypertension, tobacco use, heart disease, stroke, and cancer. Aggregating Asian American health data has masked differences in disease patterns for specific subpopulations and has resulted in portraying the overall Asian American population as healthy and at lower risk for death and illness. In reality, however, after the data are separated by subgroup, studies have identified specific differences in disease patterns for different Asian subpopulations (Association of Asian Pacific Community Health Organizations & National Association of Community Health Centers,

2005; Kagawa-Singer, Wong, Shostak, Raymer, & Lew, 2005). To address the Healthy People 2010 goals for APIs, health services research needs to include API subgroups. Kagawa-Singer et al. (2005) noted that key public health data sources, including the National Cancer Institute Surveillance, Epidemiology and End Results (SEER), Behavioral Risk Factor Surveillance Survey, and the federal CDC Breast and Cervical Cancer Control Program either collect or report Asian American data in the aggregate or in limited subgroups (see also Chapter 21, this volume). Health professionals need to be aware of specific health and health-related problems of different subgroups of Asian Americans.

These difficulties and oversights regarding the identification of health problems in the target groups must be taken into account during the initial assessment phase of the program-planning process. Health promotion planners working in Asian American populations must not assume that health education programs designed for one specific Asian group will work similarly for another.

DESIGNING HEALTH PROMOTION PROGRAMS FOR ASIAN AMERICAN POPULATIONS

Consideration. "Culture and ethnicity are critical . . . when applying theory to a health problem" (National Cancer Institute, 2005).

Kline (1999, this volume) noted that the task of developing and implementing a health promotion program requires planners and participants to work together to accomplish a complex range of activities. These include assessing the needs of the target population, developing appropriate objectives, tailoring target-group-specific strategies and interventions, implementing and monitoring the interventions, evaluating the results, and refining approaches toward greater program effectiveness and efficiency. Planners need to operate from a rational planning framework and not

on the basis of pragmatic, empirical, or expediency considerations. Although there are no perfect health education and health promotion planning models, several have been used widely over time and have served as established frameworks for planning (Kline, 1999, this volume). Regardless of which model is used in planning Asian American health promotion programs, planners must build a *cultural assessment component* into the planning process (see Chapter 6, this volume).

The reader is encouraged to review Chapter 7 (this volume) for an intensive discussion of the health promotion planning process and various planning frameworks, including the PRECEDE-PROCEED and other important frameworks (see also Chapter 4, this volume). The authors of this chapter feel that the diagnostic approach advocated in the PRECEDE model can have major value for the practitioner working with Asian Americans. Another valuable tool for program planners is *Theory at a Glance* (National Cancer Institute, 2005). Regardless of the selected framework, it is helpful to use a simple step-by-step approach to planning to stay on track. Useful sample planning worksheets are found in *Introduction to Health Promotion Program Planning* (The Health Communication Unit at the Centre for Health Promotion, University of Toronto, 2001).

SPECIFIC CONCERNS IN COMMUNITY ASSESSMENT AND THE IMPORTANCE OF SOCIOCULTURAL ISSUES IN PLANNING HEALTH EDUCATION PROGRAMS FOR ASIAN AMERICANS

Conducting a thorough *community and target group needs assessment* is critical to identify community issues and problems, formulate relevant objectives, and determine what educational interventions are appropriate (see Chapter 7, this volume, for detailed approaches to needs assessment). PRECEDE can also be helpful as it guides planners in considering relationships among and between particular health behaviors and their *predisposing, enabling, and reinforcing factors* (Green & Kreuter, 2005). The Pathways Project found that certain predisposing factors among recent Asian immigrants, lacking a preventive orientation and having difficulty understanding medical treatment procedures, can hinder early cancer detection (Hiatt et al., 1996, p. S13). This level of target group assessment can provide convincing evidence regarding the need for early educational interventions designed to positively affect these factors.

Another major consideration of the needs assessment process is development of valid and reliable instruments for obtaining information about the target groups. Pasick, D'Onofrio, and Otero-Sabogal (1996) provided some valuable guidelines for practitioners based on experiences in developing a 101-item core instrument covering demographics, health beliefs and practices, and cultural values in four different languages for four different race/ethnic groups. These include the need to recognize that translation and adaptation constitute a complex process requiring at a minimum (1) an understanding of each language and culture, (2) a commitment to research objectives by all involved, and (3) iterative pretesting in all groups and subgroups (by age, language, ancestry, etc.). (Also, see Chapter 6, this volume, for a detailed Cultural Assessment Framework.)

Needs assessment information should seek to identify local mores and customs. This is particularly true if the target group is located within an ethnic enclave, as in the case of many new Asian immigrants. At the very least, outreach workers who are involved (such as lay health advisors) in obtaining assessment information and who may ultimately introduce the health education program to the community should be perceived as nonthreatening and nonintrusive. They should be drawn from the same ethnic group and preferably be from that community. Ideally, these individuals also have training in health care interpreting to convey health-related concepts accurately and minimize communication barriers (California Healthcare Interpreters Association, 2002).

Contacts during the assessment process should be linguistically appropriate when working in established communities or with recent immigrants. For some groups, such as the Chinese or the Filipinos, the assessment process may lead to staff having to deal with more than one language or several dialects. (The official language of the Philippines, Filipino, is not necessarily the language of choice for all Filipinos, especially those from the southern islands, because it is based on Tagalog, a northern dialect.)

Within a single Asian American ethnic group (e.g. Japanese, Korean, Chinese, Vietnamese), health-related attitudes and behaviors may differ between generations. The assessment must identify such differences and the possible impact of acculturation and biculturalism on persons in a specific community and design interventions accordingly. Survey or interview data with community members of the appropriate demographic breakdown may reveal any significant "generation gap" or the impact of acculturation on values or expressed health beliefs and behaviors.

Acculturation occurs when a person participates in the dominant culture with the corresponding loss of other elements of the ethnic culture. *Biculturalism* occurs when a person participates in both the dominant or majority culture and the subculture. The impact of acculturation on Asian American health behavior is shown in intergenerational differences in rates of smoking (Asian and Pacific Islander Tobacco Education Network & Asian and Pacific Islander American Health Forum, n.d.). Intergenerational differences in health beliefs and behaviors due to biculturalism need to be further explored for Asian Americans groups, particularly in the area of breast health. The study by Chavez, Hubbell, McMullin, Martinez, and Mishra (1995) of how women of different ethnic groups perceive risk factors for breast cancer showed that U.S.-born women of Mexican descent exhibited a collection of beliefs about breast and cervical cancer that were intermediate between the views held by Anglo women and immigrant Mexican women.

Continued affirmation of an Asian American ethnic identity or group affiliation is not predictive of the second (American raised or born) generation's degree of belief or participation in traditional folk medicine. Capps (1994) noted that the effect of abrupt cultural changes among an exclusively Protestant Hmong community in Kansas City has been to introduce medical pluralism, an eclectic medical culture that blends "influences from biomedicine, Christianity, and Chinese medicine" (p. 172), with selective loss of such Hmong medical/religious concepts (including soul loss, shamanism, and animal sacrifice) and practices that no longer "fit" their new situation and collective identity. The local community must be observed for any unique changes or characteristics during the needs assessment part of program planning.

Culture may be loosely defined as shared understandings among members of a corporate group about a wide range of critical life areas, including health and illness issues. These beliefs, values, and practices may be embedded in the traditional social structure and social support system or religion. Illness and pain, thus in part social constructions, may be viewed or treated as a "moral process" by group members, in ways not congruent with that of biomedicine (Good, 1994; Good, Delvecchio, Brodwin, Good, & Kleinman, 1992, p. 172). The general public, medical or legal establishment, or media may regard folk traditions, seen as innocuous by immigrants, with suspicion. One example is the Vietnamese practice of *cao gio*, a cold remedy that entails rubbing coins onto Tiger Balm, which produces the sensation of heat due to the camphor. Because this process may result

in some skin discoloration, this folk tradition has often been misinterpreted as harmful by the dominant society (Dean, 1996).

It may also be difficult to introduce an intervention involving conditions that may be stigmatized in a traditional Asian culture. Various studies of community mental health services for Asian Americans suggest that the low rates of use may be due in part to such stigmatization. Survey or interview data with community members from similar generations may reveal generation gaps in values or expressed health beliefs and behaviors.

Planners must be able to identify such unique changes or characteristics during the needs assessment process and their impact on health education program design. An effective program must address the health needs of the specific segment of the population targeted (e.g., senior smokers, young smokers, women smokers, etc) within the Asian American community. In these instances, program planners must also deal with these specific issues to develop appropriately tailored interventions (Tanjasiri et al., 2007).

HEALTH EDUCATION PROGRAMS IN THE CHINESE AND VIETNAMESE COMMUNITIES

The two health prevention and education case studies to be discussed structure their design and interventions to the different needs of the Chinese and Vietnamese communities they intend to reach. Both focus on increasing cancer screening for Asian American immigrant women (see also Kagawa-Singer et al., 2005). The older Vietnamese case study example (English & Le, 1999), a part of the San Francisco Bay Area Pathways Project, is helpful to review as a well-documented example of how health education planning was incorporated in the area of cancer. This project incorporated portions of the PRECEDE-PROCEED framework as modified for cancer screening

(Walsh & McPhee, 1992) into their program to increase the use of breast and cervical cancer detection practices in four different ethnic populations, including Chinese and Vietnamese.

Program Design Used in Each Program

Hiatt et al. (1996, p. S13) described the development of the Pathway's conceptual framework, using foundations from the PRECEDE-PROCEED framework (Green & Kreuter, 2005) and modifications of that framework for cancer screening, including factors impinging on the patient and physician that could affect cancer screening (Walsh & McPhee, 1992, Ref. 46, p. S26). The framework was used in the needs assessment analysis, as well as other theories, including the Transtheoretical Model of health behavior change (Freudenberg et al., 1995; Prochaska & Velicer, 1997) in the data analysis. Each project associated with Pathways activities made an intensive effort to apply elements of theories appropriate to each population's specific characteristics and goals (Hiatt et al., 1996, p. S13).

Using the PRECEDE-PROCEED framework (Green & Kreuter, 2005), possible influences on the cancer-screening behavior of Vietnamese women were reviewed and analyzed prior to the choice of methodology. These included strong social solidarity (reinforcing factors), cultural and demographic characteristics of the immigrants that contributed to maintaining a social enclave and retention of some traditional values such as modesty (predisposing factors), and knowledge and access issues (enabling factors) (McPhee et al., 1996, p. S62). Because of these challenges for immigrant women, both case studies used the strong social bonds between women through recruitment and training of community health workers who would serve as leaders for facilitating in-language outreach and educational strategies.

Program 1: "Save Life" Breast Cancer Early Detection Program for Chinese Women

For 4 years, the Asian American Senior Citizens Service Center (AASCSC) implemented the "Save Life" Breast Cancer Early Detection Program for Chinese women. The goal of this multifaceted program was to increase awareness and improve breast cancer screening among Chinese American women aged 40 years and older in Orange County. Over the years, progressive improvement was made based on community feedback.

Community Needs Assessment

Breast cancer is the most common cancer among Chinese American women in California (American Cancer Society, 2006). However, the screening rate of breast cancer among Chinese American women is relatively low. To obtain input directly from Orange County women, the Asian and Pacific Islander Task Force (APTIF; 2006) of Orange County and the California State University at Fullerton (CSUF) conducted a local needs assessment survey to determine the breast and cervical cancer-screening behaviors among various Asian and PI women in Orange County. The AASCSC was the lead agency for the assessment of the Chinese community. Survey results revealed that only 47% of women aged 40 and older had had a mammogram within the past year. Even though 85.5% of women aged 40 and older knew what a mammogram was, only 69.7% knew how often a woman at their age should receive a mammogram, and only 33.9% knew the age at which a woman should start getting a mammogram. Furthermore, the most common response that women in the study gave for not having a mammogram was that they had no symptoms (APITF, 2006). These results strongly suggest that more education on breast health, particularly on the importance of getting an annual mammogram even when a woman feels healthy, is greatly needed for Chinese American women aged 40 and older in Orange County.

Based on continuing experiences serving Chinese American women in Orange County, the AASCSC identified language as a major barrier that hinders many women from receiving adequate health care, including cancer screenings. The APITF Needs Assessment indicated that 79% of the Chinese American women in Orange County speak a language other than English at home. Another study found that among Chinese American women in California who speak languages other than English at home, 37.3% cannot speak English well or at all (UCLA Center for Health Policy Research, 2001).

In addition to the language barrier, economic hardship and lack of health insurance are also major reasons that impede some Chinese American women in Orange County from having their mammograms taken. It is estimated that 20.04% of Chinese Americans in Orange County are living under the 200% Federal Poverty Level, and approximately 36% of Asian American women under 65 years of age do not have any form of health insurance (U.S. Census Bureau, 2000). Therefore, it is essential to inform and provide low-income, uninsured/underinsured Chinese American women access to free breast cancer screenings through the Cancer Detection Programs: Every Woman Counts (CDP: EWC), which is funded by the California Department of Health Services, Cancer Detection Section.

Fatalism in traditional Chinese culture also plays an important role in the low screening rate of breast cancer among the Chinese American women. The women who are fatalistic believe that if someone gets cancer, it is meant to be, and nothing can be done. This fatalistic mentality discourages some Chinese American women from receiving regular breast cancer screening.

Methodology and Interventions

One of the essential strategies for the success of the "Save Life" program was the innovative collaboration between the AASCSC and 99 Ranch Markets, a popular grocery store chain frequented by Chinese women. After several months of persistent efforts to get the 99 Ranch Market to collaborate with the AASCSC and promote early-detection screening, the Market's management team finally decided to embark on this new health adventure. The key strategy to attract women's interests and increase the response rate was to reward women with a $10 gift card to the 99 Ranch Market after they received their breast exams.

The AASCSC used broad-based media outreach, such as their own newsletters and flyers, public service announcements (PSAs), and newspaper ads in prominent Chinese newspapers. Outreach booths were set up at four locations of 99 Ranch Markets to promote breast cancer awareness and screening. Through this valuable collaboration, mammogram-promotional booths were set up at these four stores on all Saturdays in October, which is the Breast Cancer Awareness month, and were staffed by volunteers who distributed promotional flyers. These specially designed flyers included response slips with details confirming that a woman has received a mammogram (with the date, site, and technician's signature). Women would mail their response slip to the AASCSC, and on receipt, the AASCSC would mail program participants a $10 gift certificate redeemable at 99 Ranch Markets in Orange County. The 99 Ranch Markets financially contributed toward the gift certificates to further demonstrate their support for this important program.

Mammography screening events held at CDP: EWC provider offices in the community offered Chinese women immediate access to mammograms and clinical breast exams. The AASCSC has assisted low-income, under-insured Chinese women who qualified to receive free breast cancer screenings through CDP: EWC. Bilingual staff and volunteers were on site to help participants complete screening forms and/or act as their language interpreters. Also, the AASCSC served as the bridge between screening providers and Chinese women to overcome any language or cultural barriers. The AASCSC recruited additional Chinese-speaking volunteers to expand their breast health program to a greater number of Chinese women in Orange County. Volunteers were trained on program logistics and implementation and were educated about the basics of breast health and breast cancer.

Tailored education provided women culturally appropriate breast health information in a small-group setting to promote more comfortable discussions. The AASCSC approached existing faith-based organizations, senior centers, and women's groups in the Chinese community with an invitation to hear these educational presentations. Class participants were typically familiar with each other already, and this allowed more honest sharing of sensitive information. Several of these workshops were conducted in a warm and homelike environment. In this comfortable setting, Chinese women listened to a breast health educational presentation and shared their feelings and thoughts casually over a cup of tea and some dessert.

Program success can be very dependent on collaboration with and support from local community partners. The AASCSC maintained successful relationships with the 99 Ranch Markets; the American Cancer Society; the CDP: EWC regional contractor—Orange County Cancer Detection Partnership; Susan G. Komen for the Cure; and the University of California, Irvine Chao Family Comprehensive Cancer Center.

Evaluation

Evaluation tools included a set of pre- and posttests and overall workshop surveys to determine knowledge increase and participant satisfaction for the tailored education sessions, as well as class attendance. Also, the assessment of program success was appraised by the number of women who actually received their mammograms and mailed their response form to the AASCSC. Qualitatively, the success of this project was also illustrated by the enhanced awareness within the Chinese community, increased number of volunteers who assisted with educational outreach and screenings, and continued commitment by local community partners to remain involved.

Program 2: Pathways to Early Cancer Detection for Vietnamese Women

The National Cancer Institute funded the 4-year Pathways to Early Cancer Detection program in four ethnic groups (Hiatt et al., 1996). Although the overall Pathways program included four ethnic groups of women, the breast and cervical cancer detection program targeting Vietnamese women is of main interest in this chapter. The program involved multidisciplinary, multicultural teams concerned with increasing breast and cervical cancer screening among underserved low-income women in the San Francisco Bay Area.

This case study program involved cancer screening among Vietnamese women and took place in the 1990s in the inner-city neighborhoods of San Francisco. The study's goal was to determine whether a neighborhood-based intervention fosters adoption of a preventive health care orientation and increases acceptance and use of the screening test for early cancer detection among Vietnamese women in San Francisco (McPhee et al., 1996). Unless otherwise mentioned, information used in this section is drawn from *Pathways to Early*

Cancer Detection for Vietnamese Women: Suc Khoe La Vang! (Health Is Gold!) (McPhee et al., 1996). Emphasis will be placed on the neighborhood-based intervention aspects of the project dealing with Vietnamese women rather than the methodological and evaluative aspects of the overall project design. Prior to implementation of the interventions, the Pathways survey developed earlier was administered as described in the subsection on evaluation. Readers can find this information in the report of the comprehensive 4-year study *Pathways to Early Cancer Detection in Four Ethnic Groups* (Hiatt, 1996).

Community Needs Assessment

Initially, it is helpful to review the background of this San Francisco community of recent Vietnamese immigrants at the time of the case study. Since the end of the war in Vietnam in 1975, the Vietnamese population has grown to comprise the "fifth largest Asian immigrant group in the U.S., . . . (with) nearly 40% of Vietnamese in California" (Campi, 2005; Chapter 21, this volume). Many came directly to California from Vietnam; others moved to California after settling in other states.

The Vietnamese community in the San Francisco area constitutes an ethnic enclave. However, it reflects diversity in age, education, exposure to urban life and degree of prior acculturation or westernization, English proficiency, and health status. More recent, poorer immigrants tend to be less well educated, in poorer health, and less familiar with Western concepts. (McPhee et al., 1996, p. S61). They are also more likely to experience poverty, cultural conflict, and barriers to the health care system (McPhee et al., 1996).

Vietnamese women in the San Francisco Bay Area have a low rate of screening for breast and cervical cancer. And unfortunately, these are their two most common cancers. The Pathways Vietnamese women project sought to increase breast and cervical cancer screening

and detection in this group by improving their preventive health behavior.

At the outset of a health education/promotion intervention efforts program, baseline data for establishing the scope and seriousness of the problem may not be readily available. In the Pathways study, such information about breast and cervical cancer among Vietnamese women in the study community was limited. The community needs analysis was based in part on demographic data and preliminary California Cancer Registry data for the years 1988 to 1992 concerning age-adjusted incidence rates of breast and cervical cancer among Vietnamese women and on key informant information. Several previous statewide and area-specific studies conducted between 1987 and 1992 helped establish that Vietnamese women were less likely to have had the recommended screening procedures for breast and cervical cancers (McPhee et al., 1996, p. S62).

An extensive baseline survey was later developed (after the intervention had been conducted). The survey, consisting of 101 core questions covering demographics, health beliefs and practices, and cultural values, was administered to each specific project group after an exhaustive effort was made to ensure the appropriateness of each question to that group. Although information from the survey would have been helpful in the formulation of the project intervention, it was administered for later use related to evaluation of the intervention and comparison of differences between each project group.

Methodology and Interventions

A three-phased multifaceted intervention was used to raise the women's awareness concerning the importance of preventive care and breast and cervical cancer screening and then to motivate them to seek screening. The investigators sought to use neighborhood connections as they could provide behavioral modeling and social reinforcement (see Chapter 4, this volume) through familiar communication channels (McPhee et al., 1996, p. S63).

The specific methods selected were informal small-group educational events in private homes and a community health fair centered around the traditional Vietnamese New Year (*Tet*) festival. A multitude of linguistically and culturally appropriate educational materials conveying the desired messages about the need for preventive care and screening included a special training manual for the lay health workers for use in presentations and the following discussions, videotapes, and materials for the participants and Vietnamese physicians (McPhee et al., 1996). The small-group events were organized around the informal educational sessions led by the previously trained neighborhood leaders and similarly recruited individuals.

Evaluation

The primary evaluation tool was the household survey described earlier in the needs assessment section. Project investigators intended to administer the survey, by oral interview, before and after the interventions to assess if there was an increase in screening behaviors following participation in program activities and whether there was a similar positive change in women's knowledge, attitudes, and intentions with regard to preventive care behaviors (McPhee et al., 1996). A control group in a similar Vietnamese neighborhood in Sacramento, California, also received the survey. Readers are encouraged to review the projects' data analysis methods and baseline survey results (McPhee et al., 1996).

Comparison of the Approaches of the Two Programs

Consideration: To provide culturally tailored health education. It is useful for practitioners to examine some of the differences in the planning approaches used by the cancer

education and screening programs described above. Owing to the differing health needs of the respective target groups and different program goals, there was a need to develop and employ different techniques. Common elements in both programs included the use of pre- and postintervention surveys for evaluation, the use of trained community members and health care professionals in outreach, and the development and use of culturally appropriate educational tools and materials in the community's language. Educational materials included brochures, posters, and videotapes. Surveys provided baseline changes in variables associated with the desired health behaviors. The Pathways project's standardized survey questions assessed plans for health screening, acculturation, and insurance among a small sample of women who were presumably more willing to participate in the face-to-face survey conducted by persons visiting their households. The Pathways staff also suggested the use of volunteers to save time and funds.

The neighborhood-based cancer education programs were intended to reach the more socially insulated women of each community. Vietnamese language media was designed to complement a concurrent statewide media program for the general public. This 2-year program provided messages tailored for the community and included billboards, newspapers, and paid television advertisements (Jenkins, McPhee, Le, Pham, Ngoc-The, & Stewart, 1997), complete with videotape. Although this project had the funding to procure paid television advertising, it is often quite costly. Community cable televisions stations will often run materials at no charge, owing to public access requirements, but these may not reach the desired target group. No mention was made of radio spots, which can be had at less expense or for free if public service announcements are prepared and sent out with an appealing cover letter. Any media (print, radio, and television) geared toward serving an Asian American market will of course be more receptive and should be the first contacted.

The techniques used by the cancer education program were created to be more personal and centered on traditional characteristics of social solidarity and mutual assistance using lay health advisors. Neighborhood-based small-group events conducted by trained neighborhood leaders provided short, informal home presentations on preventive health care topics. Health fairs coordinated with community festivities were also used to introduce new concepts in a nonthreatening way. Like the face-to-face survey used in the project, the small-group intervention does require more time and effort than mass media or large presentations, but it is a better way to contact and draw out a cloistered set of individuals. An interpersonal approach, which reinforces information through training or modeling, is much more effective than simply handing out brochures jammed full of information, which may be perceived as overwhelming to read in limited time or irrelevant or may simply be discarded.

Both programs employed a pretest and posttest survey (the Vietnamese program used a control group) as the principal means of evaluation. Evaluation was based solely on the survey, outcome data, and attendance at events or process information (such as the number attending meetings). Although ideally one obtains an objective evaluation of an educational presentation by using a written pretest and posttest to determine its efficacy in changing knowledge, in reality, this can be difficult outside the classroom setting. For informal situations such as the small-group events described above, where participants may have limited test-taking or literacy skills, limited time, or physical difficulties such as poor eyesight or uncomfortable testing conditions, it is probably more appropriate to forego the evaluation of the process beyond a simple head count until such problems can be overcome.

However, evaluation is necessary not only to refine the program process (delivery of services) but also to determine the impact and long-term outcome of the program on an individual's health behaviors and whether objectives are being met. For these two projects, collecting this information by means of an oral survey (via telephone or face–to–face conversation) before and after the intervention proved to be a technique acceptable to the participants and the community, although somewhat labor-intensive. This survey constituted the primary evaluation tool and provided the data necessary to assess the behavioral results of the intervention strategy and, thus, its efficacy in meeting program objectives and mitigating the health concern targeted.

CHAPTER SUMMARY

It is helpful to understand the distinction between the terms *tailoring* and *targeting*. Targeting involves using information about shared characteristics of a population subgroup to create a single intervention approach (National Cancer Institute, 2005). *Targeting* implies the need to clearly identify the specific population subgroup that will be exposed to the intended intervention (Pasick et al., 1996). The authors of the current chapter want to stress to practitioners the need during all segments of the planning process to recognize that Asian Americans encompass many different groups including Chinese, Vietnamese, Japanese, Korean, and those from several countries in Southeast Asia. They reside in many communities, mainstream to small, isolated enclaves. Planners must be acutely aware of the group's and subgroups' diversity in history, cultural practices including health beliefs, language, socioeconomic status, and generational differences. Each of the groups represents varying degrees of acculturation and assimilation in its current country of residence. Once planners have *targeted* (the group), they also need to be able to *tailor*. *Tailoring*, as espoused by Pasick et al. (1996, p. S145), implies the need for planners to be able to adapt the intervention and/or total design to fit the needs and characteristics of a target audience. *Cultural tailoring* indicates that planners develop interventions, strategies, methods, messages, and materials to be adaptable to the specific cultural characteristics of the target group (Pasick et al., 1996, p. S145). In short, health promotion planners working within Asian American populations cannot *tailor* until they have appropriately *targeted* (see also Chapter 7, this volume, for further information on this topic).

The basic strategies and interventions employed in the health education programs described earlier can provide some practical ideas for health professionals concerning how to conduct two different types of health education campaigns. The specific activities employed are geared toward an urban Asian American community of recent immigrants with limited language skills. However, a general understanding of these methods can enable the adaptation of these types of interventions to other types of programs for Asian American community groups in various settings, assuming that careful and culturally sensitive planning and implementation processes are conducted. Use of a comprehensive planning framework such as PRECEDE-PROCEED (or such as the one presented in Chapter 7, this volume) in the process of community assessment should assist planners in designing appropriate services to meet the needs of each community. Health education and promotion programs can play a vital role in helping individuals address various health needs from aging, relocation, or concerns arising from a myriad of other changes all face in life. Given the diverse circumstances that Asian Americans now live and work in, the challenge for health care providers is to appreciate the impact that ethnic and social ties may have on health behavior choices and use these factors effectively in developing programs for communities.

Health promotion professionals working in minority communities need to encourage *cultural competence* among staff working in community health promotion programs (see Chapters 1 and 3, this volume, for more information on this topic). Although staff may possess the language skills and knowledge of the basic customs and cultural beliefs of those they serve, program results may be enhanced if there is a concerted effort to integrate the services into the social framework of the community (Congressional Asian Pacific Caucus, 1997, p. 12). Steckler et al. (1995, p. 314) views the use of social networks as an intervention that can increase access to services among disenfranchised groups through the recruitment of socially significant community members to help convey the program message.

Members of the community for whom the program is intended should participate, either as staff or as volunteers, in the assessment, planning, and implementation process whenever possible. They can provide an insider perspective on issues and insights into local social and cultural norms and structure. This participation increases the likelihood that the project will not conflict with any fundamental cultural values and that it will be credible and well received. At the very least, educational materials and tools such as survey and interview questions should be linguistically and culturally appropriate. Be aware that *key informants* may not have knowledge or represent all elements in the community or group. Certainly if they do and represent the intended program users (or targeted group), or already provide services to the desired users, so much the better. Consistent feedback from community leaders and stakeholders, which was solicited in both of the health education programs discussed earlier, can provide valuable information, guidance, support, and resources for program activities. An important function of these community representatives is to help identify persons in the community already recognized by other community members as sources of assistance and support regarding issues and problems. According to Jackson and Parks's (1997) review of a number of community health promotion programs, the recruitment of indigenous workers based on the collective wisdom of the community and who will serve as the program's lay health advisors taps into the existing social networks and enhances the distribution of the health promotion message to the community. Bowen et al. (1997) used a similar networking technique to obtain informants for the community needs assessment of the mammography project. The Pathways to Early Cancer Detection for Vietnamese Women project used the indigenous model in setting up its small-group interventions among Vietnamese women by using the neighborhood leaders as lay health advisors, who in turn drew other women into the project.

The next chapter presents a case study in which the author tries to emphasize the points made in the overview and planning chapters. The study is concerned with the application of concepts and approaches for bridging the gap between theory and practice. It provides an opportunity for the student and the practitioner to get a "bird's-eye" view of some of the specific methods and techniques of HPDP program planning, application, and problem solving.

DISCUSSION QUESTIONS AND ACTIVITIES

Consider this scenario: Mortality and morbidity from *type 2 diabetes, heart disease, and lung and cervical cancer* have been increasing for the past several years among different Asian American population groups living in a large multicultural metropolitan community.

The local health jurisdiction, private providers, voluntary agencies, and community members are very concerned and want to reduce the number of deaths and illnesses drastically. Local government officials recognize that increased screening, referral, and treatment

programs are critically needed for identifying problems. Limited monies are available for providing cancer-related, diabetes, and heart/disease *health promotion and education programs* to selected multicultural target groups. Select a specific Asian American target group in a specific geographical area in your community as a frame of reference to work from. Then, break up into planning teams and consider the following questions relevant to needed health promotion and education programs designed to increase access and services to that target group:

- Discuss the critical need to be aware of the reasons for not combining heterogeneous groups of Asian Americans into the same health promotion and education programs as one aggregated population. What could be the result in terms of misleading outcomes for planners as they try to assess and interpret program results?
- What kind of operational framework for health promotion and education programs for members of Asian American communities would you use in taking into consideration the diversity of your Asian American target group(s)?
- How would you involve those affected by the above problems?
- How would you assess the needs of specific Asian American target groups in the community or target populations with regard to the above-mentioned diseases?
- What specific health promotion and education program goals and objectives related to target group accessibility to education and treatment programs would be included in the plan?
- What implementation issues should you be aware of for your program(s)?

REFERENCES

American Cancer Society. (2006). *California cancer facts and figures.* Washington, DC: Author.

Asian and Pacific Islander Task Force of Orange County. (2006). *Breast and cervical cancer knowledge and screening behaviors among*

Chinese American women in Orange County: A Needs Assessment. San Francisco: Author.

Asian and Pacific Islander Tobacco Education Network & Asian and Pacific Islander American Health Forum. (n.d.). *Facts on Asians and Pacific Islanders and tobacco.* San Francisco: Author.

Association of Asian Pacific Community Health Organizations & National Association of Community Health Centers. (2005, January). *Health centers' role in reducing health disparities among Asian Americans and Pacific Islanders* (Fact Sheet No. 3105). Retrieved December 19, 2007, from www.aapcho.org/site/aapcho/content.php?type=1&id=9707

Bowen, D., Kinne, S., & Urban, N. (1997). Analyzing communities for readiness to change. *American Journal for Health Behavior, 21,* 289--298.

California Healthcare Interpreters Association, Standards and Certification Committee. (2002). *California standards for healthcare interpreters.* Sacramento, CA: Author.

Campi, A. (2005). *From refugees to Americans: Thirty years of Vietnamese immigration to the United States.* Retrieved December 19, 2007, from www.ailf.org/ipc/refugeestoamericansprint.asp

Capps, L. L. (1994). Change and continuity in the medical culture of the Hmong of Kansas City. *Medical Anthropology Quarterly, 8*(2), 161–177.

Chavez, L. F., Hubbell, F. A., McMullin, J. M., Martinez, R. G., & Mishra, S. I. (1995). Structure and meaning in models of breast and cervical cancer risk factors: A comparison of perceptions among Latinas, Anglo women, and physicians. *Medical Anthropological Quarterly, 9*(1), 40–74.

Congressional Asian Pacific Caucus. (1997). Proceedings of the forum: Cancer crises among Asian Pacific Islanders as articulated by Asian Pacific Islanders. *Asian American and Pacific Islander Journal of Health, 5*(1), 7–36.

Dean, P. (1996, December 13). Culture at the crossroads. *Los Angeles Times,* pp. E1, E4.

Ecklund, E. H., & Park, J. (2005). Asian American community participation and religion. *Journal of Asian American Studies, February,* 1–21.

English, J., & Le, A. (1999). Assessing needs and planning, implementing, and evaluating health

promotion and disease prevention programs among Asian American population groups. In R. Huff & M. Kline (Eds.), *Promoting health in multicultural populations* (pp. 357–373). Thousand Oaks, CA: Sage.

Freudenberg, N., Eng, E., Flay, B., Parcel, G., Rogers, T., & Wallerstein, N. (1995). Strengthening individual and community capacity to prevent disease and promote health in search of relevant theories and principles. *Health Education Quarterly, 22*(3), 290–306.

Good, B. (1994). *Medicine, rationality, and experience.* Cambridge, UK: Cambridge University Press.

Good, M. J., Delvecchio, G., Brodwin, P., Good, B., & Kleinman, A. (1992). *Pain as human experience.* Berkeley: University of California Press.

Green, L. W., & Kreuter, M. W. (2005). *Health education planning: An educational and ecological approach* (4th ed.). New York: McGraw-Hill.

Health Communication Unit at the Centre for Health Promotion, University of Toronto. (2001). *Introduction to health promotion program planning* (Version 3.0). Toronto, Ontario, Canada: Author. Retrieved December 19, 2007, from www.thcu.ca/infoandresources/publications/Planning.wkbk.content.apr01.format.oct06.pdf

Hiatt, R. A. (1996). Preface: Pathways to early cancer detection in four ethnic groups. *Health Education Quarterly, 23*(Suppl.), S7–S9.

Hiatt, R. A., Pasick, R. J., Perez-Stable, E. J., McPhee, S. J., Engelstad, L., Lee, M., et al. (1996). Pathways to early cancer detection in the multiethnic population of the San Francisco Bay Area. *Health Education Quarterly, 23*(Suppl.), S10–S27.

Jackson, E. J., & Parks, C. P. (1997). Recruitment and training issues from selected lay health advisor programs among African Americans: A 20-year perspective. *Health Education & Behavior, 24*(4), 418–431.

Jenkins, C. N. H., McPhee, S., Le, A., Pham, G. Q., Ngoc-The, H., & Stewart, S. (1997). The effectiveness of a media-led intervention to reduce smoking among Vietnamese-American men. *American Journal of Public Health, 87*(6), 1031–1034.

Kagawa-Singer, M., Wong, L., Shostak, S., Raymer, W. C., & Lew, R. (2005). Breast and cervical cancer screening practices for low income Asian American women in ethnic specific clinics. *Californian Journal of Health Promotion, 3*(3), 180–192.

Kline, M. V. (1999). Planning health promotion programs in multicultural populations. In R. M. Huff & M. V. Kline (Eds.), *Promoting health in multicultural populations: A handbook for practitioners* (pp. 73–102). Thousand Oaks, CA: Sage.

McPhee, S., Bird, J. A., Ha, N.-T., Jenkins, C. N. H., Fordham, D., & Le, B. (1996). Pathways to early cancer detection for Vietnamese women: Suc Khoe La Vang! (health is gold!). *Health Education Quarterly, 23*(Suppl.), S60–S75.

National Cancer Institute. (2005). *Theory at a glance: Applications to health promotion and health behavior* (2nd ed.). Washington, DC: National Institutes of Health.

Pasick, R., D'Onofrio, C., & Otero-Sabogal, R. (1996). Similarities and differences across cultures: Questions to inform a third generation for health promotion research. *Health Education Quarterly, 23*, S142–S161.

Prochaska, J., & Velicer, W. (1997). The transtheoretical model of health behavior change. *American Journal of Health Promotion, 12*(1), 38–48.

Steckler, A., Allegrante, J. P., Altman, D., Brown, R., Burdine, J. N., Goodman, R. M., et al. (1995). Health education intervention strategies: Recommendations for future research. *Health Education Quarterly, 22*(3), 307–328.

Tanjasiri, S. P., Kagawa-Singer, M., Foo, M. A., Chao, M., Linayao-Putman, I., Nguyen, J., et al. (2007). Designing culturally and linguistically appropriate health interventions: The "Life Is Precious" Hmong breast cancer study. *Health Education & Behavior, 34*(1), 140–153.

UCLA Center for Health Policy Research. (2001). *California Health Interview Survey*. Los Angeles: Author.

U.S. Census Bureau. (2000). *Asian and Pacific Islander population in Orange County, California*. Washington, DC: Author.

U.S. Department of Health and Human Services. (2000, November). *Healthy people 2010: understanding and improving health* (2nd ed.). Washington, DC: Government Printing Office.

Walsh, J. M. E., & McPhee, S. J. (1992). A systems model of clinical preventative care: An analysis of factors influencing patient and physician. *Health Education Quarterly, 19*, 157–175.

23

Promoting Health Among Asian American Population Groups by Using Key Informants

A Case Study

EVAON C. WONG-KIM

On completion of this chapter, the health promotion student and practitioner will be able to

- Explain how the attitudes and cultural beliefs (concerning health and disease) of newly arrived immigrant Asian American women can affect their obtaining prevention and treatment services for breast cancer

- Develop key informant strategies for collecting specific target group assessment information from which to later tailor breast cancer educational interventions directed toward newly arrived immigrant Asian American women

- Identify and examine some of the other factors and barriers that can restrict access to preventive care and treatment for Asian immigrants

- Identify and discuss how traditional treatments such as complementary and alternative therapies are perceived in the Asian community with regard to treating cancer or dealing with its treatment side effects

- Identify some of the innovative approaches being used in the communities to improve services provided to immigrant target groups of Asian Americans communities in order to meet prevention and treatment gaps

Asian Americans are the fastest-growing population group in the United States and constituted 5% of the total U.S. population in 2000 (Asian "single race" or "in combination of Asian and other race"[1]) (U.S. Department of Commerce, Bureau of the Census, 2000a). Having tripled their numbers in the past two decades, Asian American populations grew 72%, to 11.9 million, in the 10 years between 1990 and 2000 (U.S. Department of Commerce, Bureau of the Census, 2000b). In 2000, 69% of U.S. Asian populations were first-generation immigrants (U.S. Department of Commerce, Bureau of the Census, 2000b). There are more than 30 different Asian ethnic groups originating from areas such as the Far East, Southeast Asia, and the Indian subcontinent. In the aggregate, they speak more than 2,000 distinct languages and dialects—more than 100 of those commonly spoken in the United States (U.S. Department of Commerce, Bureau of the Census, 2000a). Each has its own distinct culture and customs (also see Chapter 21, this volume). The greatest number of first-generation Asian immigrants originate from China, the Philippines, India, and Korea. However, the more recent immigrant groups from Thailand, Korea, Vietnam, Pakistan, and India have the highest percentage of first-generation immigrants (U.S. Department of Commerce, Bureau of the Census, 2000b). The more recent waves of Asian immigrants and refugees introduced many new residents whose socioeconomic status was far lower than those who immigrated in earlier waves, making Asian Americans the only U.S. population group with a bimodal distribution in educational attainment, income, employment, housing, and other social and health indicators (Reeves & Bennett, 2004; U.S. Department of Commerce, Bureau of the Census, 2000b).

IMPORTANT CULTURAL CHARACTERISTICS AND NEEDED AWARENESS

These foreign-born Asian Americans immigrating to the U.S. possess vastly different attitudes and beliefs toward health and disease and certainly differ from the mainstream culture. To provide culturally sensitive and appropriate care to this growing population, an increasing number of studies focused on the differences between Asian and mainstream American culture and their perceptions on health and health care practices (Fadiman, 1997; Mo, 2002; Ro, 2002). These perceptions greatly affect the utilization of health and mental health services among the Asian immigrant population. For example, in mainstream American culture, the body and mind are viewed as dichotomous; therefore, physical and psychological illness are clearly differentiated, while in many Asian cultures, the mind and body are viewed as an integrated whole. By seeking mental health services, the person is no longer viewed as a balanced individual. This perception has greatly stigmatized mental illness and discouraged Asian immigrants from using these services.

The importance of interdependence as reported by Kagawa-Singer (2001) is a family characteristic in Asian culture that affects decision making with regard to health care utilization. The Asian family is usually patriarchal, with clear boundaries concerning roles and structure. Males have dominance over females, and gender roles are rather rigid, with clear boundaries upheld by community expectations. For example, in the Chinese culture, many of the cultural values important to clients are based on the Confucian ideals of filial piety, where the highest regard is held for elders, the parental relationship is foremost, and the greatest authority is given to men (Chang, 2003). The expectation of adult children is to help with care giving for their aging parents.

Grandparents are expected to be involved in caring for the grandchildren. These situations have important implications for staff who work in a health care system with limited resources. Therefore, when working with new or first-generation Asian clients, including family members in decision making and lifestyle modification, program staff will be more effective when they do not assume a rigid, "one-way works" approach to well-being.

Another important cultural characteristic that affects help-seeking behaviors is related to shame, disgrace, and "losing face." Individual action does not just affect the patient or client but also may bring shame to his or her family and relatives. This concept is frequently cited in the literature as a deterrent to Asian clients living in a tight-knit community seeking services when diagnosed with diseases such as HIV and mental illnesses (Fong, 2004).

Although health is considered to be an important part of life for almost all Asian groups, there is a tendency among Asian populations to minimize their own health needs so as to place the needs of others first (President's Cancer Panel, 2002). In a study that compared treatment choice for early-stage breast cancer between Japanese, Chinese, and Anglo-American women, it was found that Asian American women were less likely to choose breast conservation treatment (e.g., lumpectomy) combined with radiation therapy rather than a mastectomy because it would be a burden for others to provide them with transportation to their radiation treatments. Furthermore, the negative aspects of breast conservation treatment are more time consuming and may take them away from fulfilling their family responsibilities. Asian women also tended not to choose oral chemotherapy for breast cancer that was not covered by their insurance. Doing so, they felt, would use money from the family savings (Kagawa-Singer, Wellisch, & Durvasula, 1997).

USE OF KEY INFORMANTS TO OBTAIN ASSESSMENT INFORMATION FROM WHICH TO LATER TAILOR INTERVENTIONS FOR CHANGING ATTITUDES AND BELIEFS TOWARD BREAST CANCER AMONG A TARGET GROUP OF ASIAN AMERICANS

The focus of the case study is using key informants for gathering specific information about the cultural attitudes and beliefs toward breast cancer held by Asian immigrant women living in Hawaii and how their attitudes and beliefs create barriers to cancer prevention and treatment options. Seventy-two percent of the total state population and 80% of the state's total Asian population reside on the island of Oahu. At the time of Census 2000, 41.6% of the state's population was Asian. The total sum of Asians "single race" and "single race or in combination" brings the percentage of Asians living in Hawaii to 58% (U.S. Department of Commerce, Bureau of the Census, 2000a).

Breast cancer was chosen for the case study because it is the main cause of death for Asian American women, while for most other racial/ethnic groups of women, heart disease remains the leading cause of death (Fried, Prager, MacKay, & Xia, 2003). Among Asian women, the incidence of breast cancer is rising rapidly. In a recent 10-year period, incident cases of breast cancer in Los Angeles County doubled for Asian American and Pacific Islanders (AA/PI) overall and among women of Chinese descent specifically (Deapen, Liu, Perkins, Bernstein, & Ross, 2002). However, AA/PI women have the lowest rate of both screening and early detection compared with all other ethnic groups (Kagawa-Singer & Puorat, 2000).

By using findings from studies conducted in other states and information gathered locally from Asian key informants, we examine how cultural attitudes and beliefs significantly influence the ways in which Asian immigrants respond to cancer diagnosis, screenings, and treatment.

Methods

A total of six key informant interviews were conducted in Hawaii from January 2003 to March 2003. Key informants were identified by making community contacts. Names of influential professionals or advocates who worked with the Asian immigrant population in Hawaii were solicited at community meetings and from nonprofit cancer-serving organizations. The final list of participants reflected the diversity of Asian ethnic groups living in Hawaii and the different health care roles they played in the community. The six key informants included (1) a Filipino oncology nurse, (2) a Filipino breast cancer survivor, (3) a Korean physician, (4) a Vietnamese interpreter, (5) a Japanese breast cancer survivor (who also was a volunteer for a national breast cancer foundation), and (6) a Chinese social work director at a private nonprofit hospital.

These key informants were all well connected to the Asian immigrant communities through their provision of important services to community members. All of them were fluent in English and their native language/dialect. Each interview lasted 60 to 90 minutes. A semistructured approach was used to collect qualitative data during the interviews. The content of the interviews was transcribed into English, and the principal investigator and the research assistant extracted themes. These themes were then compared with the studies conducted on Asian Americans and their attitudes and beliefs toward breast cancer.

Findings

The findings from the key informant interviews are categorized and organized into several themes: Attitudes and beliefs toward breast cancer, barriers to screening services, and perception on complementary and alternative medicine (CAM). Taken into context, each of these themes does not act in a vacuum; rather, each theme is intricately interwoven in a way that either helps or hinders cancer screening.

Attitudes Toward Breast Cancer

The most prominent theme relating to the key informant studies was the fear of cancer, which translated to internal barriers in Asian Americans that prevented them from seeking early preventive screening (Wong-Kim, Sun, & DeMattos, 2003). This fear manifests itself in fatalistic views, fear of treatment and costs, fear of pain, and fear of rejection by family, friends, partners, and the community at large. These fears and the lack of accurate information about breast cancer led many to ignore cancer prevention messages, avoid breast cancer screening, and delay breast cancer treatment (President's Cancer Panel, 2002).

Fatalistic views about cancer are salient in some minority populations who believe that if one gets cancer, it is God's punishment, God's plan, or bad karma (Marion & Schover, 2006). One of the Filipino key informants, an oncology nurse who practiced in Hawaii, noted in the interview,

> Once they're told that they have breast cancer and that they're gonna die, it's hard for them to hear. It's hard for them to understand that even though they're diagnosed with breast cancer, if found early, they could still live a long life. They have that sense of fatality of "Bahala Na," by leaving it up to God.

The other Filipino key informant, who is a breast cancer survivor, agreed with the first informant about the same fearful and fatalistic view of breast cancer among Filipinos:

> It's like there's no more hope in your life. It's like you are doomed. It's like all the fun,

the future, and whatever you have is going to be nothing anymore. Some are hopeful, but very rare. And then usually, most of the immigrants, they will hide it. Like, oh, I'm not going to tell my family that I have breast cancer because they feel so bad, so sad. Like there's no future. That's the negative attitude that we have. But we hardly talk about that. They don't want to talk about it in public. It's like a taboo because the moment you have cancer, it's too late.

The Vietnamese key informant in our study also shared the same views of fear in the Vietnamese community in Hawaii. She stated,

They are afraid they will find out something [by screening]. They rather not know. They are shock. They don't want to hear it. They don't want to mention because [cancer] is scary. Like my friend, when I talk to her she only tell me she has a lump. But the doctor who treats her is also my friend who I worked with in Vietnam so I know she has breast cancer. But when we talk, we don't say anything about cancer.

When asked "What does the word cancer mean to the Korean population?" the key informant working in the Korean community stated,

Korean patients are very fearful of the word cancer. That is why they usually are in denial when diagnosed with breast cancer. For example, I have a cousin who was diagnosed with breast cancer and she denies the facts. She doesn't even go for her follow up appointments.

Barriers in Seeking Preventive Services

The Lack of Health Coverage. The lack of health insurance was identified by many key informants as the problem many immigrants stated for not seeking cancer-screening services (Snyder, Cunningham, Nakazono, & Hays, 2000). According to the Korean informant,

Few Korean immigrants have health insurance because of their recent move to the United States. Most of them work as cashiers or receptionists at the restaurants and they have no medical benefits. Very few have access to medical care. They have problems getting cancer screenings or treatment because of health insurance. Also, they don't think about long-term treatment. They don't see cancer screening or treatment as a big problem because they don't put themselves as a priority. For example, many of the families I work with will put their children first and worry about them instead.

Our Filipino cancer survivor informant also agreed that the lack of health insurance was the primary reason why Filipinos do not seek preventive screening services:

Many of them [Filipino] don't have health insurance. I am lucky because I am married to a military guy and I can go to Tripler (a military hospital in Honolulu), almost free, you just pay for Tricare. Some are trying to get health insurance and are being denied because either they had health problems before, they been operated before, their high blood pressure, or they have high cholesterol. And some are denied, and some of them have to pay for medical services. Some are self-employed, and then there are part-timers. Maybe they have three jobs, but it's all part-time so they don't have any coverage.

According to our Vietnamese informant,

Screening and preventive health is a problem since it is secondary. If you don't have insurance, people are only motivated by illness to see a doctor. The people who don't have insurance usually are overlooked and don't get any screenings.

Language and Cultural Barriers

Besides insurance coverage, the barriers to health care for Asians could be attributed to cultural and language differences. Thirty-one million patients in the United States speak different primary languages from their health care providers. Japanese, Korean, and Indian participants experienced similar feelings and problems when trying to seek help and navigate through the unfamiliar Western health care system (Andresen, 2001; Somkin et al., 2004). Also, according to Census 2000, 76% of Hmong, 70% of Cambodians, and 68% of Laotians were limited-English proficient (LEP) compared with 7.5% of LEP persons nationwide (Asian and Pacific Islander American Health Forum, 2002; Leadership Education for Asian Pacifics, 2000). For the first time in 2000, Chinese is the second most common foreign language spoken in the United States. Patients with LEP were often frustrated because they were not able to describe their symptoms effectively to the Western doctors and health care staff they were seeking treatment from.

Another communication problem included using family members as interpreters even though they were not able to adequately translate medical terminology. Using family members as medical interpreters changed the dynamics of the family functioning and caused uneasy feelings between members. Gender, as well as the age of the interpreters, is important to consider when using interpreters because these characteristics of the interpreter might affect the patient's comfort level when discussing sensitive issues such as a diagnosis of cancer relating to sexual organs (Mo, 2002; Ngo-Metzger et al., 2003).

An important study published by the Institute of Medicine found that many health care providers lack the basic sensitivity and cultural competence to serve the diverse patients in the health care system (Haynes & Smedley, 1999). Our Filipino informant, when asked about this barrier, said,

> I asked one of the Filipino patient's "How did you feel approaching the receptionist [at a large hospital]?" She said kind of intimidating. And I said, "Oh, but they always

smile. They seem very friendly." The patient replied: "But then they look at you funny when you could not speak good English. Then it makes me feel stupid."

Besides linguistic barriers, written communication difficulties also created barriers for LEP patients accessing cancer-screening and other health care services. Not all English medical or health terminology has equivalent terms in other Asian languages (Office of Research on Women's Health, 2002). Even when some terminology has equivalent words in English and Chinese, the meaning and context may differ. Linguistic and cultural barriers prevented many Chinese and Vietnamese immigrants from seeking Western health care treatment, and therefore, they are more vulnerable to poor health care (Ngo-Metzger et al., 2003).

Level of Acculturation

Because Asian Americans are a diverse group of people from different backgrounds, it is important to consider the history and cultural characteristics of each subgroup. It is most important to understand the differences between the immigrant generation and the generations born and raised in the United States, who are more acculturated to the mainstream values and norms. Acculturation and English language proficiency significantly affected the utilization of cancer-screening tests. For example, Filipino women who had spent more of their lifetime in the United States were more likely to adhere to cancer-screening procedures than Filipinos who had spent less of their lifetime in the United States (Maxwell, Bastani, & Warda, 2000). This may be due to the fact that Asian American women who have spent more of their lifetime in the United States have higher English proficiency and better skills in negotiating the medical system than more recent immigrants (Juon, Kim, & Shankar, 2004). The findings for newly immigrated Vietnamese women were similar to those for the Filipino women, particularly with respect to lower levels of education, as this group was less likely to learn about preventive screening than those who have lived in the United States for a longer period of time. Each additional year of residence in the United States made a major contribution to the odds of ever having been screened (McPhee, Stewart, et al., 1997). Besides language and attitudes toward cancer, acculturation is also highly correlated with employment. Korean women who were unemployed were less likely to have had a Pap smear than Korean women who were both married and employed because women who are unemployed are less likely to have health insurance (Juon, Choi, & Kim, 2000; Ponce, Gatchell, & Brown, 2003).

Limited or No Knowledge of Services Available

Besides language and cultural barriers, limited or no knowledge of screening services available was another important reason for the lower utilization of such services. According to our Korean informant, "Usually the Korean people come in not because they want a colorectal check but come in when their symptoms have become acute. Even healthy and well-educated people don't come in for preventative care."

The Filipino key informant explained the lack of knowledge of the prevalence of cancer in the community:

It's hard for people to get cancer screening because they think they are so healthy. It's like nothing can happen to me. I eat good. I exercise. They don't go until the last minute, when it's painful and too late. That's why the rate of cancer deaths among Filipinos is so high. It's too late. Why go if there's no pain?"

A study conducted among Vietnamese women in San Francisco and Sacramento found that 31.7% had never heard of a mammogram, 48.6% had never heard of a clinical breast exam, and 73% said they had never heard of a Pap test (McPhee, Bird, et al., 1997). In the same study, women who were not planning on having another mammogram cited, "I'm healthy and don't need one," "I'm worried about the cost," and "I don't have time." Those women who had not had a mammogram reported not needing it because they were healthy, did not have a physician's recommendation, felt it cost too much, or did not have the time for it.

Another study on Koreans and cancer screening found that most of the respondents did not see the need for cancer-screening tests for early diagnosis and treatment. Not having symptoms or health problems was the overriding reason why Korean Americans did not have digital rectal exams or fecal occult blood tests. The lack of screening adherence among Korean Americans can be attributed to a lack of knowledge about screening guidelines and poor understanding of the importance of screening (Kim, Yu, Chen, Kim, & Brintnall, 1998).

Complementary and Alternative Medicine

Our community assessment also found that many Asian patients wanted their physicians to be more knowledgeable about non-Western medical practices because they would like to use both types of medicines. According to the Korean informant,

Koreans still practice traditional methods of healing but it is mostly seen within the older generation. The older generation will seek healing from acupuncturists. They also believe that western medicine does more long-term damage to the body because of side effects or toxins that might be in the medications. With those who have cancer, they will seek treatment from the western doctors, but they will also use traditional interventions such as herbs and acupuncture as well.

Our Chinese informant provided more information about the combination of Western and traditional medicine:

Patients go to the Western doctors to get screening and treatment. Once the patient knows they are diagnosed with cancer, where the cancer is located, and at what stage, they go to an herbalist for treatment. Patients choose to get treated by both doctors (Western and traditional). Chemotherapy is very hard for patients; this type of therapy has many side-effects. Traditional medicine is safer and creates less side-effect. For cancer, some think that herbs are the best for shrinking tumor or treating chemo side-effect. Most patients seemed satisfied with this mixed approach.

However, there were also controversies about using traditional medical practice within the community. According to one Korean informant,

There are problems in getting cancer screening. A lot of immigrants don't know that they should be getting screened [for cancer]. Another problem is with the oriental herb doctors in the Korean communities. There are a lot of these quackeries going on. These quackeries are blatantly advertising in newspapers and radio, claiming that they can cure everything and anything. I have heard of a couple of cases of missed opportunities to actually diagnosing cancer early because some of these herb doctors claim that they can cure cancer and delayed treatment for some patients.

Our Japanese key informant who used CAM provided a more balanced opinion about traditional medicine:

Sometimes the traditional healing methods help and make people feel better. I support using CAM although I do not personally suggest others to get traditional CAM. There are times people do feel better [using CAM] and as long as a patient is not missing any benefit from western medicine, it doesn't hurt to do both. I think we should not exclude either types of medicine but try to use both and see which one works for that individual. In the past I've seen it happen way too many times when patients seek care from a traditional

medicine doctor for lumps in their breast. These people are treated with herbs and eventually breast cancer spreads to a point where it becomes incurable. And then there are others who get CAM that took care of their chemotherapy side effects and felt much better. We must appreciate the people's beliefs in traditional medicine but I wish to see modern medicine combined with holistic therapies. Even if traditional medicine [CAM] is not perfect, it has a lot to offer.

INTERVENTIONS

Many studies have examined intervention strategies that would improve the utilization of cancer screening and treatment in Asian communities; however, different approaches could be taken to reach a larger proportion of LEP and low-income Asian immigrants in Hawaii. Our Filipino informant suggested,

We have to saturate the radio stations and the Filipino newspapers and change the cultural perception of cancer. There's the Filipino Chronicle. Why not have a spot, a PSA on television. We need to identify those key people who have cancer and survive a long time to dispute the myths. We should have posters that show exactly what's going to happen in all the radiation and chemotherapy treatment, that cancer is curable when detected early.

Our Korean key informant suggested,

Many of the people get information from the Korean church. There is also a Chamber of Korean Community Organization that Koreans are connected to once they arrive in Hawaii. Additionally, a Korean yellow page book has lists of Korean restaurants, businesses, and information on "Living in America" (e.g., obtaining driver's license, going to school, visas). Placing an ad in this book will remind Korean people of the cancer screening services.

Health care practitioners can also effectively reach recent, low-income Chinese immigrants with limited English proficiency by using the ethnic language media, such as the widely read national newspapers *Tsing Tao Daily* and *World Journal*, as well as Chinese television and radio stations to disseminate cancer information (Wong-Kim & Wang, 2006).

Health brochures need to improve the way information is delivered by making it culturally sensitive and by having it translated appropriately in other Asian languages. Lay health persons who are fluent in the English language and other Asian languages can serve as the bridge to Asian immigrant communities to provide much needed services.

CHAPTER SUMMARY

The need to identify those in a community who are very familiar with the target group is essential. There is a need to identify and develop a key informant base and strategies for collecting specific target group assessment information from which to later tailor breast cancer educational interventions directed toward newly arrived immigrant Asian American women.

One of the most effective ways to communicate cancer information to varying cultural groups is through culturally relevant, concise, and easily understood educational materials (Susan G. Komen Breast Cancer Foundation, 1997). The likelihood of printed materials being used greatly depends on the format and appropriateness of the illustrations. Proper and accurate translation must also be used. The audience's literacy level must be considered because the more specific and relevant the language and visuals used, the more effective are the materials.

It is critical that programs encouraging health promotion and screening address the economic, social, cultural, and other barriers faced by different Asian populations.

Although there is a correlation between knowledge and more frequent use of cancer-screening tests, knowledge alone was not found sufficient to change behavior (Maxwell et al., 2000), signifying that other factors, identified earlier in this assessment, should also be considered. The use of traditional medicine or healers can either become a facilitator or a barrier to cancer screening, depending on the communication between Western and traditional practitioners.

Community-based program staff must be culturally competent and trained in educational methodologies appropriate for improving cancer attitudes and beliefs relevant to the utilization of cancer-screening networks in Asian communities. Data that accurately illustrate the problems in the Asian communities must be upgraded for accuracy.

Asian researchers also need to begin to create networks of researchers, health care providers, advocates, and cancer survivors who will join in the long-term community effort to improve cancer awareness, research, and training. One such organization is the Asian American Network for Cancer Awareness Research and Training (2004). With the increased number of researchers conducting studies in Asian communities, more culturally appropriate and tailored intervention will likely be available to serve this underserved population.

DISCUSSION QUESTIONS AND ACTIVITIES

Working in small groups, consider the following questions and activities. Be prepared to discuss your responses and/or the results from your activities in full class presentations.

1. What are the immigration rates for Asians into your community, and what Asian cultures are represented within these groups?

2. What are the most prevalent causes of morbidity and mortality within the Asian communities in your community? What do you think are the reasons for these, and what, if anything, is currently being done about these?

3. Design, administer, and analyze a brief survey to ascertain the health beliefs and practices of an Asian American group in

your community, and discuss how this information might help you in designing an intervention focused on a health concern within this community. You may wish to review Chapter 6 before starting this task.

NOTE

1. For Census 2000, individuals were allowed to "mark one or more races," a decision reached by the Office of Management and Budget in 1997 after noting evidence of increasing numbers of children from interracial unions and the need to measure the increased diversity in the United States. Prior to this decision, most efforts to collect data on race (including those by the Census Bureau) asked people to report only one race

REFERENCES

Andresen, J. (2001). Cultural competence and health care: Japanese, Korean, and Indian patients in the United States. *Journal of Cultural Diversity*, 8(4), 109–121.

Asian American Network for Cancer Awareness, Research & Training. (2004). *Who is Asian American?* Retrieved May 5, 2004, from http://aancart.org/Who%20Is%20Asian%20American.htm

Asian and Pacific Islander American Health Forum. (2002). *Asian and Pacific Islander Center for Census Information and Services*. Retrieved December 19, 2007, from www.apiahf.org

Chang, I. (2003). *The Chinese in America: A narrative history*. New York: Viking.

Deapen, D., Liu, L., Perkins, C., Bernstein, L., & Ross, R. K. (2002). Rapidly rising breast cancer incidence rates among Asian-American women. *International Journal of Cancer*, 99(5), 747–750.

Fadiman, A. (1997). *The spirit catches you and you fall down: A Hmong child, her American doctors, and the collision of two cultures*. New York: Farrar, Straus & Girouz.

Fong, R. (Ed.). (2004). *Culturally competent practice with immigrants and refugee children and families*. New York: Guilford Press.

Fried, V. M., Prager, K., MacKay, A. P., & Xia, H. (2003). *Chartbook on trends in the health of Americans. Health, United States, 2003*. Hyattsville, MD: U.S. Department of Health and Human Services, Center for Disease Control and Prevention, National Center for Health Statistics.

Haynes, M. A., & Smedley, B. D. (Eds.). (1999). *Committee on cancer research among minorities and the medically underserved: The unequal burden of cancer: An assessment of NIH research and programs for ethnic minorities and the medically underserved*. Health Sciences Policy Program, Health Sciences Section, Institute of Medicine. Washington, DC: National Academy Press.

Juon, H. S., Choi, Y., & Kim, M. T. (2000). Cancer screening behaviors among Korean-American women. *Cancer Detection and Prevention*, 24(6), 589–601.

Juon, H. S., Kim, M., & Shankar, S. (2004). Predictors of adherence to screening mammography among Korean American women. *Preventive Medicine: An International Journal Devoted to Practice and Theory*, 39(3), 474–481.

Kagawa-Singer, M. (2001). Providing resources for Asian Americans and Pacific Islanders. *Cancer Practice*, 9(2), 100–103.

Kagawa-Singer, M., & Puorat, N. (2000). Asian American and Pacific Islander breast and cervical carcinoma screening rates and healthy people 2000 objectives. *Cancer*, 89(3), 696–705.

Kagawa-Singer, M., Wellisch, D., & Durvasula, R. (1997). Impact of breast cancer on Asian American and Anglo American women. *Culture Medicine and Psychiatry*, 21(4), 449–480.

Kim, K., Yu, E. S. H., Chen, E. H., Kim, J. K., & Brintnall, R. A. (1998). Colorectal cancer screening: Knowledge and practices among Korean Americans. *Cancer Practice*, 6(3), 167–175.

Leadership Education for Asian Pacifics. (2000). *APAs at a glance: Asian Pacific American demographic, labor, and income facts*. Retrieved from www.leap.org

Marion, M. S., & Schover, L. R. (2006). Behavioral science and the task resolving health disparities in cancer. *Journal of Cancer Education, 21*(Suppl.), S80–S86.

Maxwell, A. E., Bastani, R., & Warda, U. S. (2000). Demographic predictors of cancer screening among Filipino and Korean immigrants in the United States. *American Journal of Preventive Medicine, 18*(1), 62–68.

McPhee, S. J., Bird, J. A., Davis, T., Ha, N. T., Jenkins, C. N. H., & Le, B. (1997). Barriers to breast and cervical screening among Vietnamese-American women. *American Journal of Preventive Medicine, 13*(3), 205–213.

McPhee, S. J., Stewart, S., Brock, K. C., Bird, J. A., Jenkins, C. N. H., & Pham, G. Q. (1997). Factors associated with breast and cervical cancer screening practices among Vietnamese American women. *Cancer Detection and Prevention, 21*(6), 510–521.

Mo, B. (2002). Modesty, sexuality, and breast health in Chinese-American women. In *Women of color health data book.* Washington, DC: National Institutes of Health, Office of the Director, Office of Research on Women's Health.

Ngo-Metzger, Q., Massagli, M. P., Clarridge, B. R., Manocchia, M., Davis, R. B., Iezzoni, L. I., et al. (2003). Linguistic and cultural barriers to care: Perspectives of Chinese and Vietnamese immigrants. *Journal of General Internal Medicine, 18*(1), 44–52.

Office of Research on Women's Health. (2002). *Women of Health Color Data Book.* Washington, DC: National Institutes of Health, Office of the Director.

Ponce, N., Gatchell, M., & Brown, E. R. (2003). *Cancer screening rates among Asian ethnic groups.* Los Angeles: UCLA Center for Health Policy Research.

President's Cancer Panel. (2002). *Voices of a broken system: Real people, real problems.* Washington, DC: National Institutes of Health, National Cancer Institute.

Reeves, T. J., & Bennett, C. E. (2004, December). *We the people: Asians in the United States: Census 2000 Special Reports* (CENSR-17). Washington, DC: U.S. Census Bureau, U.S. Department of Commerce. Retrieved December 19, 2007, from www.census.gov/prod/2004 pubs/censr-17.pdf

Ro, M. (2002). Moving forward: Addressing the health of Asian American and Pacific Islander women. *American Journal of Public Health, 92*(4), 516–519.

Snyder, R. E., Cunningham, W., Nakazono, T. T., & Hays, R. D. (2000). Access to medical care reported by Asians and Pacific Islanders in a West Coast physician group association. *Medical Care Research and Review, 57*(2), 196–215.

Somkin, C. P., McPhee, S. J., Nguyen, T., Stewart, S., Shema, S. J., Nguyen, B., et al. (2004). The effect of access and satisfaction on regular mammogram and Papanicolaou test screening in a multiethnic population. *Medical Care, 42*(9), 914–926.

Susan G. Komen Breast Cancer Foundation. (1997). *Asians or Pacific Islanders: Developing effective cancer education print materials.* Kalamazoo, MI: Author.

U.S. Department of Commerce, Bureau of the Census. (2000a, February). *The Asian population: 2000, Census 2000 brief.* Washington, DC: Government Printing Office.

U.S. Department of Commerce, Bureau of the Census. (2000b, March). *The foreign-born population in the United States.* Washington, DC: Government Printing Office,

Wong-Kim, E., Sun, A., & DeMattos, M. (2003). Assessing cancer attitude in a Chinese immigrant community. *Cancer Control, 10*(5), 22–28.

Wong-Kim, E., & Wang, C. (2006). Breast self-examination among Chinese immigrant women. *Health Education & Behavior, 33,* 580–590.

24

Tips for Working With Asian American Populations

MICHAEL V. KLINE

ROBERT M. HUFF

The term *Asian Americans* refers to people of Asian descent who are citizens or permanent residents of the United States. They reside in many communities, mainstream to small, isolated enclaves, and consist of many subgroups, such as Asian Indians, Cambodians, Chinese, Filipinos, Hmong, Japanese, Koreans, Laotians, Thais, Vietnamese, and "other Asian," with 32 linguistic groups. Among this group, the Chinese and Filipinos are the two largest subgroups. There has been a lack of awareness of various health-related problems specific to this population, owing to the convention of aggregating health data. The stereotypes that Asian Americans are hardworking, intelligent, successful, and mentally healthy have masked social, economic, and mental health problems of the Asian American populations. It is critical for the health promoter to recognize the great diversity in cultural beliefs and practices, history, language, and generational differences characterizing each subgroup.

This brief "tips" chapter provides some fundamental information, suggestions, and recommendations for working with these different groups in health promotion and disease prevention (HPDP) activities. These tips have been distilled from the preceding three chapters and other sources (English & Folsom, 2007; English & Le, 1999; Green & Kreuter, 1991, 2005; Hiatt et al., 1996; Inouye, 1999; Ishida, 1999; Kline, 1999; McPhee et al., 1996; Pasick, D'Onofrio, & Otero-Sabogal, 1996; Pasick, Sobogal, et al., 1996; Sobogal, Otero-Sabogal, Pasick, Jenkins, & Perez-Stable, 1996; Chapters 1, 2, 6, 7, and 21–23, this volume). They are offered as general starting points that need to be considered for those involved in assessing, designing, implementing, and evaluating HPDP programs for Asian American population groups.

CULTURAL COMPETENCE

The health promoter needs to develop cultural competency skills for working across multicultural population groups. This is an especially important issue to be considered when working with Asian American populations characterized by such great diversity and differences connected to health practices and health-related problems. The following tips for the health promoter can help facilitate processes that will contribute to more effective HPDP programs:

- Seek to learn the history and immigration patterns of the specific ethnic group you will be targeting for HPDP interventions.
- Be aware that most new immigrants come from homogeneous ethnic countries and have been thrust into heterogeneous surroundings where their self-identity may be threatened and where they must often deal with this "differentness" as well as prejudices and racial bigotry.
- Become familiar with the particular target group's specific cultural values, beliefs, and ways of life. These include forms of address and other verbal and nonverbal communication patterns, food preferences, attitudes towards health and disease, and related cultural characteristics that differentiate this group from other Asian American populations.
- Become familiar with the language differences within each group and how language adjustment was another stress that had to be overcome to function in a new country.
- Engage in active listening (rather than talking) and be alert to nonverbal cues because some Asian American populations tend not to disagree openly with health service providers, thereby avoiding conflict and embarrassment so as to maintain harmony. The nodding of heads might mean they are hearing but not necessarily agreeing with what is being said.
- Be alert to the correspondence between verbal and nonverbal behaviors, being careful to ask open-ended questions that elicit what the individuals or groups think about the situation, resources, or suggestions, as well as how comfortable they are with the available choices in terms of what they want and can live with.

- Be aware that although in many Asian American families one adult might be the spokesperson for the family, all members should be encouraged to voice their opinions.
- Be aware of the dynamics within the Asian American family. Because problems are generally handled within the confines of the family, concerns may not be shared with the health care provider unless there is a trusting relationship established.
- Seek to incorporate or assist planners in incorporating these cultural values, beliefs, and ways of life into the HPDP program or service where appropriate.
- Be aware that many different Asian American groups refer to their generational differences according to the arrival or birth in the United States and are, with your exploration, distinguishable by their various ages, experiences, languages, beliefs, and values.
- Recognize that acculturation is a critical factor in explaining risk behavior and health status. The more traditional the individual or group, the less likely the individual or group is to know about, understand, or practice Western approaches to HPDP.
- Be aware that for many Asian American subgroups, immigration caused a number of adjustment and acculturation stresses that might be related to their overall health and health practices, such as being forced to leave their homes, facing political exile, or being separated from family members.
- Seek to learn how differences in beliefs and values among different subgroups may help identify some of the possible areas of conflict and frustration experienced by new immigrants and sometimes later generations.
- Be aware that all the groups represent varying degrees of acculturation and assimilation in their current country of residence.
- Be aware that beliefs and values play an important role in acculturation and integration of Asian Americans into Western culture and that the process of integration differs for each of the Asian groups.
- Acknowledge that the measurement of acculturation is an important activity for understanding how traditional, acculturated, and

assimilated a specific ethnic group may be. There are a variety of scales that can be used, and the reader is urged to read Chapters 1, 6, 7, and 8 for a more detailed discussion of this process.

- Be aware that two beliefs that are prominent in Asians, especially those from Southeast Asia, are *kinship solidarity* and *equilibrium* or *balance*. Kinship solidarity refers to the view that the individual is subservient to the kinship-based group or family.

- Be aware that most Asian family patterns are characterized by filial piety, male authority, and respect for elders and that this pattern sometimes determines decision-making practices relating to health care for recent immigrants.

- Appreciate that family support is one of the most important core values among Asian American population groups. Be aware how devastating separation from family members can be to a culture that values the nuclear and extended family.

- Remember that decisions associated with seeking medical care and/or participating actively in a prescribed treatment or health program might involve the head of the household or other family members, whose decisions will be based on what they feel is best for the family.

- Be aware that avoiding conflict and achieving harmony in interpersonal relationships is a strong cultural value among Asian Americans.

- Show respect for Asian American beliefs and values because they are an extremely important factor in all relationships and especially in HPDP encounters.

- Recognize that the diverse circumstances under which Asian Americans live and work require you to appreciate the impact that ethnic and social ties might have on health behavior choices and the need to use these factors effectively in developing HPDP programs or services.

HEALTH BELIEFS AND PRACTICES

There are a variety of health beliefs and practices that characterize the many different Asian population groups residing in the United States.

The health promoter needs to understand and be sensitive to the differences he or she is likely to encounter. The health promoter needs to be aware of how to use this knowledge and how to incorporate these differences into HPDP programs and services. The health promoter should keep the following tips in mind:

- Recognize that belief in folk illnesses still is a strong cultural characteristic among many traditional Asian population groups. Developing an understanding of some of these illnesses and their traditional treatments can help you to be more effective in the design of specific HPDP intervention and treatment services.

- Remember that it is often assumed by health care workers that everyone embraces the Western biomedical model. However, within Asian cultures, traditional or cultural beliefs of spiritual or supernatural forces and balance with nature are often overlooked, and traditional practitioners may assist the individual in achieving this energy balance.

- Understand that there are a number of explanatory models used to make sense of health and disease and that these are generally associated with the social, psychological, and physical domains. Recognize that although health is defined in the United States as a state of complete physical, mental, and social well-being, and not merely the absence of disease, Asians view it as a state of harmony with nature or freedom from symptoms or illness.

- Remember that the need to achieve a harmonious relationship with nature might be a central concept of the traditional health care system still used today. This system often is the first one used when an illness or other disorder is detected in a family member, and those who use this system are generally not inclined to discuss this with a Western health care practitioner.

- Be aware that beliefs and expectations about health care treatment may enhance or impede Asian groups' participation in the health program or service. There is a need to explore these beliefs and expectations in the assessment or initial health care encounter phase.

- Be aware that although there are wide variations in health beliefs and practices shaped by cultural values in determining what is important in one's life, many Asian groups may share some similarities based on their religious background and on the influence of Chinese culture throughout Asia.
- Recognize that the prominence of Confucian ideology, Buddhism, and Taoism in Asian culture focuses on the upholding of a public facade and against public admission of mental or physical illness or any admission of personal weakness.
- Be aware that, to a large extent, culture and language influence how one conceptualizes etiology, symptoms, and treatment of illnesses and may influence how one is to interact with health care providers and organizations.
- Recognize that because of language difficulties and cultural differences, many Asians, especially the newer immigrants, might still prefer the traditional forms of Chinese and native medicine and seek help from Chinatown "physicians" or "masters," who treat them with traditional herbs and other methods.
- Be aware that Asians often do not seek help from the Western system of medicine because of painful diagnostic tests and lack of information and understanding about what is being done to them.
- Be sensitive to the effect of abrupt cultural changes among an immigrant community introduced to medical pluralism. An eclectic medical culture that blends influences from biomedicine, Christianity, and Chinese medicine could result in a selective loss of medical or religious concepts and practices that no longer "fit" their new situation and collective identity.

PROGRAM-PLANNING CONSIDERATIONS

The health promoter must be aware that planning HPDP programs or services for Asian American population groups, given their tremendous diversity, requires systematic identification and selection of tailored courses of action related to achieving or improving health-related behaviors. Such programming also will require the planner to be culturally competent and sensitive to the differences in how the planner views and operates in the world and how his or her target group sees this same process. Thus, the health promoter should consider the following comments and suggestions relevant to the program-planning process:

- Be sensitive to indiscriminately applying health care and programs to all groups in the same manner. Also, recognize that because all Asian Americans do not have similar beliefs and health practices, health professionals cannot assume that programs for one Asian group will work for another similar group.
- Be sure that the program or service being developed will be culturally acceptable to the target group and will not come into conflict with the target group's values, beliefs, attitudes, or knowledge about the problem.
- Clearly identify potential barriers that might be encountered that would impede participation in the HPDP program or service and identify how you might overcome these.
- Wherever possible, seek to eliminate obstacles to participation in the HPDP program or service. This may involve simplifying how the target group enrolls in or accesses the service or program, bringing the program or service to the target group, making sure that the program or service is offered in the language of the target group, and making sure that any follow-up activities that the participants might need to do are simplified, relevant, and easily understood.
- Consider employing the principles of *relevance* and *participation* when designing the program or service—that is, starting your program or service where the target group is and involving its members' active participation throughout the entire process, from design through evaluation.
- Make sure that the organization or agency involved in designing the program or service has a mission, goals and objectives, policy, procedures, an organizational structure, and staff that reflect a sense of cultural competence

and sensitivity to the target group on which the program or service is being focused.

NEEDS ASSESSMENT

The extensive data that serve as the foundation of Asian American HPDP programs and services can assist the HPDP planner to better understand and address the specific health needs and interests of the planner's target population. It is critical that the health promoter take the time to adequately determine the characteristics of the target group he or she will be serving, including factors such as morbidity and mortality, historic and immigration patterns, specific cultural characteristics, demographics, health care access and use patterns, and related variables. Huff and Kline in Chapter 6, this volume, present a Cultural Assessment Framework that can help provide guidelines for the assessment areas that should be considered when preparing to develop the needs assessment component of the program-planning process. In addition, the following suggestions may be useful in the needs assessment process:

- Remember that conducting a thorough needs assessment is critical to identify community issues and problems in the Asian American communities, formulate relevant objectives, and determine what educational interventions are appropriate.
- Be aware that regardless of the planning model used (e.g., PRECEDE-PROCEED) for Asian American health promotion programs, you must be extremely conscious and sensitive to the need for building a cultural assessment component into the planning process.
- Be aware that aggregating Asian American health data might mask differences in disease patterns for specific subpopulations and could result in an erroneous portrayal of the overall Asian American population as healthy and at lower risk for death and illness.
- Remember that needs assessment information should seek to identify local mores and customs. This is particularly true if the target

group is located within an ethnic enclave, as in the case of many new Asian immigrants.

- Where possible, involve community representatives who can function to help identify persons in the community already recognized by other community members as sources of assistance and support regarding issues and problems.
- Where possible, train and use community members to assist in the data collection process because this can help facilitate community ownership of the program or service being developed and can provide perspectives that might have otherwise been missed by a non–community member.
- Recognize that, at the very least, outreach workers (e.g., lay health advisors) who are involved in obtaining assessment information and who may ultimately introduce the health education program to the community should be perceived as nonthreatening and nonintrusive. They should be drawn from the same ethnic group and preferably be from that community.
- Be aware that contacts during the assessment process should be linguistically appropriate when working in established communities or with recent immigrants. For some groups, such as Chinese or Filipinos, the language of the assessment process might have to deal with more than one language or several dialects.
- Be sure to include key community members (both formal and informal) in the community needs assessment process.
- Recognize that survey or interview data with community members from similar generations may reveal "generation gaps" in values or expressed health beliefs and behaviors.
- Consider including acculturation measures in the needs assessment instrument.
- Be sure to assess the types of media used within the community because this might be a critical factor when the program or service is ready to go online and marketing activities are being planned. It also relates to acculturation levels in the community.
- Be sure that assessment and evaluation efforts reflect the needs, interests, and values of the stakeholders within the community.

- Be aware that at the outset of an HPDP program, baseline data for establishing the scope and seriousness of the problem might not be readily available. Initial assessment information might need to be based in part on demographic data, morbidity and mortality data, and (in large part) key informant information.
- Be aware that key informants might not have knowledge of or represent all elements in the community or group. If these persons represent the intended program users (or targeted group) or already provide services to the desired users, then so much the better.
- Understand that an extensive baseline survey consisting of core questions covering demographics, health beliefs and practices, and cultural values might need to be administered to target groups after an exhaustive effort is made to ensure the appropriateness of each question to that group.
- When designing questions for survey instruments or interviews to be administered to Asian American subgroups in a language other than English, recognize that translation and adaptation are part of a complex process that requires an understanding of each language and culture and might require iterative pretesting in all groups and subgroups (by age, language, ancestry, etc.).
- Focus groups can be a useful and effective approach to determining the knowledge, attitudes, behaviors, and felt needs of the community.
- The PRECEDE model can be helpful because it guides you to consider relationships between and among particular health behaviors and their predisposing, enabling, and reinforcing factors and can provide convincing evidence regarding the need for early educational interventions designed to affect these factors positively.

INTERVENTION CONSIDERATIONS

Well-planned and culturally appropriate interventions are critical to the successful implementation of HPDP programs and services for Asian American population groups. *Cultural tailoring* urges the planner to develop interventions, strategies, methods, messages, and materials to be adaptable to the specific cultural characteristics of the target group (Pasick, D'Onofrio, et al., 1996). The health promoter might wish to consider the following comments and suggestions as he or she begins the design phase of the program-planning process:

- Be aware that new immigrants may differ on many social and health-related issues. You also should be aware that those at high risk will more likely include individuals with the following characteristics: low socioeconomic status, uninsured, limited English proficiency and/or linguistically isolated, foreign born or recently immigrated, and rigid adherence to certain cultural health beliefs and traditions that might conflict with some proven effective Western practices.
- Understand that an effective program must specifically address the health needs of the segment of the population targeted (e.g., women at risk for cervical or breast cancer, male smokers) within the Asian American community. You also need to deal with these needs as they result from the target group's diversity and collective history and culture.
- Recognize that the development of culturally appropriate interventions requires consideration of available community resources and inclusion of important cultural themes of the target group. For example, *family* is one of the strongest core values of traditional Asian culture, so interventions that have a family focus may prove more effective than those that focus on the individual.
- Remember that members of the community for whom the program is intended should participate, and they can help provide an "insider's" perspective on issues and insights into local social norms and structure. This participation increases the likelihood that the project will not conflict with any fundamental cultural values and that it will be credible and well received.
- Recognize that a formal community advisory board used earlier in the planning stages also can provide valuable information, feedback, support, and resources during the educational intervention activities.

- Be aware that program results may be enhanced if there is a concerted effort to integrate the services into the social framework of the community.
- Be aware that interventions such as role modeling and use of community social networks may be useful approaches for demonstrating and reinforcing individual behavior change.
- Consider that developing partnerships with the local media (e.g., radio, television, newspapers) for the dissemination of health education and health promotion information can be a valuable and effective approach for both marketing programs or services and reinforcing the successes of program participants who may be recruited as role models for the community in which the program or service has been targeted.
- Be aware that the utilization of behavioral theory to guide development of intervention approaches is central to well-conceived and appropriately designed intervention strategies (see Chapter 4, this volume).
- Be aware that a multiphased and multifaceted intervention might need to be used, for example, to (a) initially raise the awareness concerning the importance of preventive care and screening, (b) help motivate the target group to seek screening, and (c) use neighborhood connections because they can provide behavioral modeling and social reinforcement through familiar communication channels.
- Recognize that the recruitment and training of a group of community peer networkers who can distribute program materials and reinforce messages can be an extremely effective method for maintaining community involvement and support for the HPDP program or service.
- Recognize that employing and training community members to facilitate educational programs in the community is a valuable and effective approach for implementing an HPDP program or service.
- Seek to develop interventions that focus on positive health changes rather than on negative or fear-arousing consequences.
- Remember that development of educational materials must reflect relevant the cultural values, themes, and learning styles of the target group for which they are designed.

- Recognize that all materials used in the HPDP program that are written in a language other than English must be *back translated* and pilot tested to ensure that they say what is meant and that the messages are clear and understandable to the target group.
- Always assess the cultural appropriateness of any pictures, models, dolls, manuals, videotapes, messages tailored for the community (e.g., billboards, newspapers, radio, and paid television advertisements), or other educational materials prior to their inclusion in the program because some materials may make the target group uncomfortable.
- Be aware that special training manuals can be developed for participating physicians and lay health workers for use in presentations and the subsequent discussions, videotapes, and other material for the participants and physicians. These should be linguistically and culturally appropriate.
- Consider selecting methods and events led by trained neighborhood leaders or similarly recruited individuals. Such events could involve informal and small-group educational events in private homes and community health fairs centered on the traditional New Year's festivals.
- Consider techniques that are more personal and centered on traditional characteristics of social solidarity and mutual assistance.

EVALUATION CONSIDERATIONS

Evaluation is central to understanding how well a program or service is doing in meeting the needs of the clientele it is serving. For this reason, the health promoter is urged to consider the following recommendations:

- Evaluation of HPDP programs and services should include culturally relevant measures for evaluating the impact of the program or service on the target group.
- Assessment and evaluation items must be tailored to the educational and linguistic capabilities of the target group for which they are intended. Here, again, back translation of items will be an important consideration in

the development of the assessment and evaluation instruments.

- Be aware that evaluation and assessment are processes that frequently are difficult to gain support for, even from the most sophisticated of groups. Efforts to explain the underlying assumptions governing these processes, as well as the methods and anticipated outcomes from these activities, can help make explicit what is often unclear to those inexperienced in evaluation and can help motivate increased interest and support for evaluation and assessment methods and procedures.

- Providing evaluation and assessment training for community members who will be involved in the provision of the HPDP program or service can help promote increased input and support for evaluation efforts. This also can extend the number of staff and community supporters who can be involved in data collection activities related to assessment and evaluation activities.

- Consider administering surveys or conducting oral interviews before and after the interventions to assess whether there was an increase in screening or other target behaviors following participation in program activities or there were positive changes in target group knowledge, attitudes, and intentions toward the target behaviors. In reality, this can be difficult outside a classroom setting.

- Be aware that participants might have limited test-taking and literacy skills or time, or physical difficulties such as poor eyesight or uncomfortable testing conditions. Thus, it might be more appropriate, in some instances, to forgo a time- and item-intensive evaluation of outcomes and process until such problems can be overcome.

The next section of the book considers Pacific Islander population groups. This section includes three chapters followed by a customized "tips" chapter. The first chapter in this section presents an overview devoted to understanding this special population from a variety of perspectives and includes terms used to define the subgroups within the broader population, historical and demographic characteristics, immigration patterns, health and disease issues and concerns, and health beliefs and practices. The second chapter of the section is concerned with how to assess, plan, implement, and evaluate programs for Pacific Islander population groups, including tips, models, and suggestions for more effective program design. The third chapter in this section presents a case study to emphasize points made in the overview and planning chapters. This section begins with Chapter 25.

REFERENCES

English, J. G., & Le, A. (1999). Assessing needs and planning, implementing and evaluating health promotion and disease prevention programs among Asian American population groups. In R. M. Huff, & M. V. Kline (Eds.), *Promoting health in multicultural populations: A handbook for practitioners* (357–374). Thousand Oaks, CA: Sage.

Green, L. W., & Kreuter, M. W. (1991). *Health promotion planning: An educational and environmental approach*. Mountain View, CA: Mayfield.

Green, L. W., & Kreuter, M. W. (2005). *Health program planning: An educational and ecological approach* (4th ed.). New York: McGraw-Hill.

Hiatt, R. A., Pasick, R. J., Perez-Stable, E. J., McPhee, S. J., Engelstad, L., Lee, M., et al. (1996). Pathways to early cancer detection in the multiethnic population of the San Francisco Bay Area. *Health Education Quarterly, 23*(Suppl.), S10–S27.

Inouye, J. (1999). Asian American health and disease: An overview of the issues. In R. M. Huff & M. V. Kline (Eds.), *Promoting health in multicultural populations: A handbook for practitioners* (pp. 337–356). Thousand Oaks, CA: Sage.

Ishida, D. N. (1999). Promoting health among Asian American population groups: Case study from the field. In R. M. Huff & M. V. Kline (Eds.), *Promoting health in multicultural populations: A handbook for practitioners* (pp. 375–381). Thousand Oaks, CA: Sage.

Kline, M. V. (1999). Planning health promotion and disease prevention programs in multicultural populations. In R. M. Huff & M. V. Kline (Eds.), *Promoting health in multicultural populations: A handbook for practitioners* (pp. 73–102). Thousand Oaks, CA: Sage.

McPhee, S. J., Bird, J. A., Ha, N. T., Jenkins, C. N. H., Fordham, D., & Le, B. (1996). Pathways to early cancer detection for Vietnamese women: Suc Khoe La Vang (health is gold!). *Health Education Quarterly, 23*(Suppl.), S60–S75.

Pasick, R. J., D'Onofrio, C. N., & Otero-Sabogal, R. (1996). Similarities and differences across cultures: Questions to inform a third generation for health promotion research. *Health Education Quarterly, 23*(Suppl.), S142–S161.

Pasick, R. J., Sabogal, F., Bird, J. A., D'Onofrio, C. N., Jenkins, C. N. H., Lee, M., et al. (1996). Problems and progress in translation of health survey questions: The pathways experience. *Health Education Quarterly, 23*(Suppl.), S28–S40.

Sabogal, F., Otero-Sabogal, R., Pasick, R. J., Jenkins, C. N. H., & Perez-Stable, E. J. (1996). Printed health education materials for diverse communities: Suggestions learned from the field. *Health Education Quarterly, 23*(Suppl.), S123–S141.

PART VI

Pacific Islander Populations

25

Pacific Islander Health and Disease

An Overview

JOHN CASKEN

> ### Chapter Objectives
>
> On completion of this chapter, the health promotion student and practitioner will be able to
>
> - Explain how the diversity among Pacific Islander population groups within and outside the United States affects health outcomes
>
> - Provide general background information to help other students and practitioners become more familiar with the many ethnic subgroups of Pacific Islander Americans
>
> - Identify and give specific examples of traditional health beliefs and practices of the many different subgroups of Pacific Islander Americans
>
> - Compare the patterns of the major diseases of Pacific Islanders in their rates and health effects among the other racial/ethnic groups living in the United States
>
> - Describe how culture can influence both the focus and the design of health promotion and health education efforts in the Pacific American populations

This chapter is designed to introduce the health practitioner to the current health status of Pacific Islander Americans in the United States. For the health professional, these populations can be unknown territory, primarily because their numbers are so small. There is a tendency to group the various subpopulations together, making the assumption that all have the same problems and can be expected to respond to health concerns in similar ways. This chapter examines the overall problems that can be encountered when dealing with these populations, lays out some specific health and medical problems, and discusses the pitfalls to be avoided when dealing with these populations.

PACIFIC ISLANDER AMERICANS IN THE UNITED STATES

Defining Terms and Describing the Diversity of Subgroups

Turning the globe to the Pacific Ocean reveals the small specks of land that create the island territories that make up the Pacific Islands, the home base from which most Pacific Islanders moved to become Pacific Island Americans. Just as finding the individual specks of land on the face of the Pacific Ocean can be a difficult task, so too can finding the small groups of Pacific Islanders who have moved to take up residence in the continental United States. The term *continental United States* is used among many Native Hawaiians, who see the expression *the mainland* as reinforcing the "colonialist" approach of the non–Native Hawaiians (Trask, 1985).

The problem of small, widely scattered numbers is one of the key issues encountered when examining the health status of Pacific Islanders. In effect, most of the data on these populations are very limited. Prior to the 1980 census, all Pacific Islanders except Native Hawaiians were included in the Asian and Pacific Islander (API) classification. Since the 1980 census, Pacific Islanders have been separated out from the API group. Native Hawaiians have been separated out since the 1960 census. Work prior to the 2000 Census has increased the possibility of more precise information on these groups. In 1997, the Office of Management Budget (OMB) released

new standards for the classification of federal data on race and ethnicity. In the standards, the OMB determined that there should be five racial categories: (1) American Indian or Alaska Native, (2) Asian, (3) Black or African American, (4) Native Hawaiian or Other Pacific Islander (NHOPI), and (5) White. The 2000 Census also allowed respondents to use a sixth category: Some Other Race. The new standards were to be used in the 2000 Census and then implemented by all federal agencies by January 1, 2003.

Based on the OMB regulations, the NHOPI category now can be broken down into 12 racial and ethnic groups. Under the classification "Polynesian" are found (1) Native Hawaiian, (2) Samoan, (3) Tongan, and (4) Other Polynesian. Under the classification "Micronesian" are found (1) Guamanian or Chamorro and (2) Other Micronesians. Under the classification "Melanesian" are found (1) Fijian and (2) Other Melanesians. A fourth major category is "Other Pacific Islander."

This richness of classification is a major improvement over the previous situation when all the groups were placed in one category. Problems still remain, however. In general, the numbers in any of the groupings are so small that it is often difficult to draw meaningful conclusions from the data collected regarding these groups. Thus, sampling can be very difficult or can be skewed.

Finally, it should be noted that this chapter is dealing with American Pacific Islanders and so is not directly concerned with the non-America-linked groups including Samoans from Western Samoa, Tongans, Tahitians, and all the Melanesian groups, though data from those groups will be noted in the figures. To prevent confusion, however, *NHOPI* will be used throughout the chapter with the understanding that we are primarily referring to Native Hawaiians and those Pacific Islanders who are linked to the United States by a variety of political relationships.

A related issue is that even within groups of NHOPIs, there can be confusion as to what the name implies. How representative of a specific NHOPI community is any individual NHOPI? This confusion arises from the current fashion of determining ethnicity. Just as in the 18th and 19th centuries any drop of African American blood was sufficient to label a person as a member of that racial/ethnic group, now the current fashion often is to describe as an NHOPI anyone who has even the slightest blood claim to that designation. The fashion has been legalized, as one can see in the definition of Native Hawaiian used in this chapter. Public Law 100-579, the Native Hawaiian Health Care Act of 1988 states,

> The term *Native Hawaiian* means any individual who has any ancestors who were Natives, prior to 1778, of the area that is now the state of Hawai`i as evidenced by (a) genealogical records, (b) *Kupuna* (elders) or *Kama'aina* (long-term community residents) verification, or (c) birth records of the state of Hawai'i. (Section 8.3, italics added)

With this, as with other racial/ethnic definitions, there is a major caution. In many cases, demographic information in the data sets that are used for health purposes includes self-definition of race/ethnicity. This permits those who have no blood line claim or title to appropriate a racial/ethnic designation to which other members of that ethnic group might not feel they are entitled. Such an approach has been legitimized by the 1980, 1990, and 2000 censuses, which allowed self-identification.

As discussed in Chapter 1 (this volume), there often is confusion between the terms *race* and *ethnicity*. Some authors suggest that there are more differences within a given population than between populations that claim distinction (Young, 1994). Other authors have suggested that ethnicity is, in fact, a useless variable because it never can be clear exactly

what is meant by the term. The argument goes that it is better to use socioeconomic descriptors that can be quantified (Navarro, 1989).

A subtheme of this chapter is to raise this issue of ethnicity as a variable, even though it appears that ethnicity will continue to be used as a descriptor for some time to come, despite the fact that errors in ethnic classification can affect health data (Dearing, 1996). The reason for raising this issue is that if, for example, a person is classified as a Samoan, then what does that mean? To the individual, it means one thing; to the observer, it means something else. However, it is rare for the observer to clearly lay out the parameters of the description. Does the term *Samoan* include Western Samoans as well as American Samoans? Does it include recent Samoan immigrants to the United States as well as those Samoans who were born in the United States? Implicit in the use of ethnic variables, it seems, is that ethnicity can form the basis from which to judge the health status of the person. Yet the four groups just mentioned, although classified as Samoans, probably would exhibit different health status, based not so much on their ethnicity as on their socioeconomic status. Having raised the issue, this chapter will continue to accept the ethnicity descriptor. Still, it is very important for the health professional to be aware of the discrepancies involved in data and not accept data at face value but rather recognize that what includes also excludes (Stone, 1988).

If it is difficult to determine in general the NHOPI population, then the difficulties are compounded when examining the health problems specific to the NHOPI population. Pacific Islanders who have moved from their home islands to the continental United States, or even to the state of Hawaii, begin a subtle process of transformation as they adopt the habits of their new neighbors (Barringer, Gardner, & Levin, 1993). Although ties are kept with the islands—for some, the remittances at home form an important part of the home island's economy, diets change, approaches to education change, jobs change, recreational activities change, and housing situations change, all of which can lead to major changes in health outcomes (Hall, 1990; Pouesi, 1994).

ORIGINS OF PACIFIC ISLANDER AMERICANS

The NHOPIs come from the Polynesian, Micronesian, and Melanesian groupings of islands in the North and South Pacific. This tripartite division is based primarily on genetic, linguistic, and sociocultural analysis (Bellwood, 1979). The U.S. Census Bureau (2001a) reports a total of 874,414 persons identifying themselves as Native Hawaiian or Other Pacific Islander alone or in combination with one or more other races (Figure 25.1). Among the NHOPIs reported in the 2000 census, the largest group numerically was made up of Polynesians, including Native Hawaiians (401,162), followed by Samoans (133,281), Tongans (36,840), followed by Tahitians (3,313) and 8,796 respondents who identified

themselves as Polynesian "not specified." The second largest NHOPI group is made up of Micronesians, which includes Guamanians or Chamorros, who alone make up 92,611; Marshallese (6,650); and Palauans (3,469). The final group, Melanesians, is represented primarily by the Fijians, with a 2000 population of 13,581. The Fijian population also includes Indians from the Asian subcontinent, many of whom had immigrated to Fiji during the late 19th and early 20th centuries and then emigrated from Fiji following the Fijian constitutional changes designed to give more power to the ethnic Fijians.

Because the Native Hawaiian population forms about 46% of the NHOPI population, this chapter concentrates on this subpopulation. Reasons other than size also suggest such an emphasis. First, the Native Hawaiian population's health status has been more thoroughly researched than has that of the remaining subpopulations (Wegner, 1989). Then, too, there is the consideration that NHOPIs genetically not only could be considered as three different subgroups but also could have major ethnic differences even within the

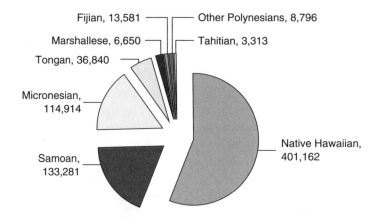

Figure 25.1   NHOPI Populations, 2000
SOURCE: U.S. Census Bureau (2001a).

subgroups. This would include the ethnic differences between the Tahitians, who have been dominated by the French for nearly 200 years, and the Tongans, who remained under British rule for more than 100 years. Most important, there are political issues that demand different approaches to health for Native Hawaiians and other NHOPIs. Many Native Hawaiians are seeking to redefine the political structure in Hawaii with calls for sovereignty, and Native Hawaiian health status is being linked with these calls (Blaisdell, 1993; Trask, 1993).

As might be expected, the majority of NHOPIs live in the state of Hawaii, primarily because the state is home to approximately 239,655 Native Hawaiians, a number that included nearly 80,137 pure Hawaiians in 2000. The state also is home to many of the other NHOPI groups, partly because the climate and lifestyle are similar to those of the other Pacific Islands.

However, no NHOPI group has more than 50% of its numbers living in Hawaii. As of 2000, approximately 50% of Samoans and Guamanians lived in California, 80% of Fijians also lived in California, and Utah was home to approximately 20% of Tongans living in the United States, reflecting the missionary influence in the South Pacific of the Church of the Latter Day Saints. In the continental United States, NHOPIs are found predominantly in the West Coast urban areas of Seattle, the San Francisco Bay Area, Los Angeles, and San Diego and in sizable numbers in New York and Utah (U.S. Census Bureau, 2001b).

The final reason for placing emphasis on Native Hawaiians is that Hawaii is the first foreign destination for many of the other Pacific Islanders as they begin their journey to the continental United States. The state of Hawaii also provides the closest medical assistance for the Pacific Islands in a cultural context that feels more familiar to the Pacific

Islanders. Janes (1990) suggests that in Hawaii, it is easier for NHOPIs to retain their familiar lifestyles and traditions. For example, Samoans are able to keep many Samoan habits and traditions while they are in Hawaii, but when they move to California, the typical traditional patterns disappear.

As noted earlier, the legal U.S. status of NHOPIs varies depending on the political relations between the United States and the individual territory. For example, Native Hawaiians are full citizens. American Samoans carry U.S. passports and can freely take up jobs in the United States, but they are classified as U.S. nationals, not U.S. citizens. American Samoa however sends a representative to the House of Representatives in the U.S. Congress. Western Samoa is an independent state with close political links to New Zealand and close familial links to American Samoa.

Since the Organic Act of Guam in 1950, Guamanians have been full U.S. citizens. Guam is now seeking commonwealth status similar to that of Puerto Rico. After spending a number of years under U.S. political control, many of the other Polynesian and Micronesian territories have become independent states, although they still have very close connections to the United States politically and also to the state of Hawaii through family and medical support. With this independence, came the loss of U.S. citizenship and, in many cases, fiscal support. No Melanesian state has been under the direct control of the United States.

HISTORICAL PERSPECTIVES: A BRIEF OVERVIEW OF PACIFIC ISLANDER AMERICANS IN THE UNITED STATES

The NHOPIs' history of interaction with the United States is very different from that of most of the population groups discussed in this book. There was no large-scale immigration of Pacific Islanders for specific purposes, such as the importation of West Africans to work as slaves on plantations or the importation of Chinese to work on the California railroads. This was partly due to the small population base in all of the islands, which ruled out such a move. So Japanese, Chinese, and Filipinos were imported to work on the sugar plantations in Hawaii because the Hawaiians were not considered sufficiently industrious to work on the plantations (Daws, 1968). These immigrant groups however were working as free men. As the small number of NHOPIs indicates, there has been very little permanent immigration from the Pacific Islands into the continental United States. Key routes for many have been through the military and through education (Barringer et al., 1993).

From a Hawaiian viewpoint, it would be more historically correct to talk about the history of the United States in Hawaii (Kame'eleihiwa, 1992). At the time the Declaration of Independence was being signed in the United States, King Kamehameha I, from the Big Island of Hawaii, was embarking on a set of conquests designed to bring all the inhabited islands of the Hawaiian chain under his rule, a task he had almost accomplished by the time of his death in 1819 (Howe, 1984). From then until the overthrow of Queen Lili'uokalani in 1893 (Budnick, 1992; Dougherty, 1992), Hawaii remained a separate kingdom that signed formal treaties with the United States and various European powers. In 1898, the islands were annexed by the United States. Though President McKinley declared that the annexation was illegal, he made no attempt to rectify the situation, and so Hawaii remained a territory until 1959, when it became the 50th state (Daws, 1968).

During the past two decades, the calls for sovereignty for Native Hawaiians have become increasingly strong. It is now generally accepted that Native Hawaiian sovereignty will become a reality, although there are a wide variety of opinions among the Native Hawaiians as to the form that sovereignty should take. The state of Hawaii funded and set up a Hawaiian Sovereignty Elections Council to ask the following question of Native Hawaiians: "Should the Hawaiian people elect delegates to propose a Native Hawaiian government?" This seemingly simple procedure was challenged by many of the groups seeking sovereignty, on the ground that it should be the Native Hawaiians themselves who should decide what questions should be asked in this matter as well as when and how they should be asked, instead of the state (even with some Native Hawaiian input) trying to determine those issues. Most recently, the question of how Native Hawaiians should relate to the state was addressed in the "Akaka Bill," first introduced in the U.S. Senate by Senator Daniel Akaka (D-HI) in 2000. This bill, in a variety of formats, proved divisive for Native Hawaiians, and the final demise of the bill in 2006 presented the opportunity for a fresh look at the political question. Senator Akaka reintroduced the bill in 2007, but with a threatened veto from the White House, the final outcome is still unknown.

SOCIO-DEMOGRAPHIC CHARACTERISTICS OF PACIFIC ISLANDER AMERICANS IN THE UNITED STATES

Age

Based on the 2000 census and examining the differences in age breakdowns between NHOPIs (Harris & Jones, 2005) and the total U.S. population (U.S. Census Bureau, 2006), it is clear that NHOPIs are a young population group, with 10.1% of the population being under 5 years of age, compared with 6.8% for the U.S. population overall. Only 64.1% of NHOPIs are aged 18 years or over, compared with 74.3% for the U.S. population overall. The largest difference is found in the population aged 65 years or over—5.0% for NHOPIs versus 12.4% for the U.S. population overall. The median age of the U.S. population overall is 35 years, compared with 25.0 years for NHOPIs. The youthfulness of the NHOPI population group has important considerations, especially in the areas of maternal and child health. For example, 18.3% of Native Hawaiians, 16.4% of Guamanians, and 10.7% of Samoans have children between the ages of 15 and 19 years, compared with 5.3% for the U.S. population overall.

Education

Western education is highly respected among most NHOPI population groups (Barringer et al., 1993). In 2000, NHOPIs had about the same percentage of the population with high school diplomas as the U.S. population overall (78% vs. 80%). That advantage is quickly dissipated, however, as the figures were reversed at the undergraduate level. That is, only 14% of NHOPIs had undergraduate degrees, compared with 24% for the U.S. population overall (Harris & Jones, 2005, p. 12).

As suggested earlier, even though NHOPIs comprise a small population group, these overall figures hide specific problems, such as the extremely low numbers among Native Hawaiians living in rural areas. One such area is the Wai`anae district of Oahu, which has a high concentration of Native Hawaiians living in the four census tracts that make up the district.

Even the figure of 8.2% of NHOPIs holding undergraduate degrees suggests an imbalance tied to other low socioeconomic indexes including jobs and housing. Health problems for low-socioeconomic-status groups, regardless of their ethnic backgrounds, can be considerably different from those for others from the same ethnic background who have a higher socioeconomic status (Montgomery, Kiely, & Pappas, 1996).

Ability to Use the English Language

The ability to use the English language is a crucial predictor of employment status and is useful for activities of daily living that can affect overall health. The ability to use English also is critical in terms of health promotion activities, especially when much of the material is based in English. Even when educational material is prepared in another language, the amount of such material normally is very restricted. It also can be difficult to find a native speaker who can correctly deal with health promotion and disease prevention activities in another language. Thus, it is critical that NHOPIs have the ability to use English. The 2000 census data suggested that approximately 15% of Pacific Islanders could not speak English very well (Harris & Jones, 2005, p. 11). Given that people's judgment on this matter might well err on the high side, a secondary finding is perhaps more relevant—that of linguistic isolation. This refers to households in which no one aged 14 years or over speaks only English and no one who speaks a language other than English speaks English very well. Among Pacific Islanders, Tongans had a problem in this category, with nearly one third claiming to be linguistically isolated. Samoans were the next highest, at 19.5%. These percentages should be expected given the high proportion of NHOPIs who completed their high school educations (normally conducted in English) (Harris & Jones, 2005, p. 11).

Occupational Status

NHOPIs are more likely to be in management, professional, and related occupations (23.3%); service (20.8%); sales and office (28.8%); construction, extraction, and maintenance (9.6%); and production, transportation, and material moving (16.5%) (Harris & Jones, 2005, p. 14). Because job status is a critical component of a person's socioeconomic status, the health problems of NHOPIs would be expected to differ more on occupation and overall socioeconomic status than on membership in a specific ethnic population group (Navarro, 1989). For example, in occupations related to construction, extraction, and maintenance and production, transportation, and material moving, Tongans (36.7%) and Samoans (30.5%) were more likely than any other group to be involved (Harris & Jones, 2005, p. 14).

The author has observed on the Wai`anae Coast that only a small number of people are employed as managers or professionals, compared with higher employment rates for the state population as a whole. That the imbalance is continuing is suggested by the observation that only a small minority of firms and businesses in Hawaii are owned by NHOPI, whereas the large majority of them are owned by Asians.

Income and Poverty Status

Income, although used as a general indicator of economic status, is a limited tool because it fails to take into account wealth, which provides the basis on which so many other demographic variables depend (Greenberg, 1989). Income also can give a false reading if one looks at total family income rather than at per capita income, because for NHOPIs the family income can include the amounts from the extended family as well as a variety of entitlements.

Median earning figures (dollars) based on a sample of Native Hawaiians and Other Pacific Islanders Population-Alone in 1999 (Harris & Jones, 2005, p. 20) indicated that median annual earnings for NHOPI men were $31,030 and for NHOPI women, $25,694. Median income for NHOPI families amounted to $45,915. These figures do give a broad indication of the economic status of a group. This is especially likely when considered against

figures showing percentages of families below the poverty level, although many (e.g., Schram, 1995) argue that the poverty level index is totally arbitrary and does not fully indicate the real extent of poverty. For example, an NHOPI family of five living in Hawaii in the year 2000, on a combined income of $22,950, in light of the above median income figures would be considered as living below the poverty level as defined by the U.S. Department of Health and Human Services (Federal Register, 2000). In fact, about 18% of NHOPI are living below the poverty level (Harris and Jones, 2005, p. 20). This certainly suggests the difficulties that those individuals and families would have in obtaining health insurance or even an adequate level of preventive health care.

A key issue to bear in mind when dealing with these demographic data is that the socioeconomic status of a person can have a major effect on his or her health status. Looking at the data examined in this section can be more revealing about a person's health status and possible health problems than can looking at specific health data. If a person's income level is known and if his or her job, living situation, housing, and educational level also are known, then it will be less difficult to calculate what the person's health status will be like.

ACCULTURATION, INTEGRATION, AND GROWTH OF PACIFIC ISLANDER AMERICANS IN THE UNITED STATES

This section begins with one major caveat. As suggested earlier, the history of Native Hawaiians demonstrates that the health professional must exercise caution in presuming that all the ethnic groups that came to the United States are now becoming acculturated to the mainstream culture and growing as a population group within the United States. Native Hawaiians, American Indians, and Alaska Natives claim that they are the indigenous inhabitants, and we should not be examining how they have acculturated. The health professional must be cautious not to inhibit access to health care because of an attitude suggesting that they should meet American standards.

We can now look at the growth and acculturation of other NHOPIs in the United States. As always for this group, it is difficult to document any growth until recently. With a total population in the 2000 census of only 874,414 (reported earlier), of whom 401,162 were Native Hawaiians (most of whom resided in the state of Hawaii), the growth obviously is not going to be spectacular. In addition, with the recent attempts at the federal and state levels to reduce legal and illegal immigration, the prospects of more rapid growth are not good. The author does not foresee an explosion of growth and natural fertility of this population. Some of the recent growth probably came from the way in which the 1990 census rephrased the race question on the census form as well as from improvements in the collection and processing procedures in the 1990 census. Individual immigrant groups also were very active in 1990, ensuring that all their members completed the application, with the knowledge that the key to more resources was in increased numbers.

Because very few Pacific Islanders were "foreign born," using the 1990 census language, acculturation is a relatively easy process for this group. For Native Hawaiians, acculturation is not the big deal it might be for, say, the Asian American population (after all, only 1% of the Native Hawaiian population are foreign born, and Hawaii had been a territorial possession of the United States for about three generations before it acquired statehood in 1959). Samoans and Guamanians also had low percentages of members who were foreign born, suggesting that for them, as well, acculturation should be a relatively easy process. Because the Tongan population in 1990 was approximately 61% foreign

born, acculturation has been a more difficult process. Embedded in the concept of acculturation, however, is the suggestion that the new arrivals take on the culture of the established population. When a Samoan travels to the continental United States but settles in with family members who already have established themselves, questions arise as to what culture is adopted. The new arrival might pick up only the minimal skills necessary to survive in the United States but continue to follow most aspects of the Samoan culture of the new Samoan group he or she has joined (Barringer et al., 1993). Acculturation also is more difficult if the move to the United States is not seen as a permanent move and there is a constant returning to the islands as the real home. Thus, acculturation is a very difficult concept to measure for NHOPIs.

For most Pacific Islander populations, such as the Samoans, the move to live in the continental United States has led to a change in attitude toward work and the workplace (Filoialii, 1980). The reality of living in a cash-based economy forces changes that can be avoided in the homeland, even when the cash economy there is powerful (Bousseau, 1993). The ties of the family ensure that no one goes hungry or homeless. However, even though relationship ties still are very strong, it is becoming increasingly difficult for Samoans living in large cities in a cash economy to support relatives in the way they would be supported in Samoa (Franco, 1991).

CAVEATS WHEN GENERALIZING ABOUT PACIFIC ISLANDER AMERICANS IN THE UNITED STATES

The main caveat has been repeated many times in this and other chapters of this book; that is, *any generalizations about an ethnic group should be avoided*. Ethnicity as a variable is too ill defined to be used with precision.

Another major caveat that has been emphasized early and will be dealt with again is the suggestion that NHOPIs are, on the whole, healthier than the general population and so do not need any special care. As will be seen, it is a myth that APIs are healthier than the U.S. population overall (Chen, 1996; Chen & Hawks, 1995), and it is even more of a myth that NHOPIs are healthier than the U.S. population overall.

A third caveat, which might almost fall into the realm of myths, is that NHOPIs are too tied to their traditional health beliefs to be concerned with Western medicine, so any approach to these population groups must be done only in a traditional form. As will be seen, NHOPI populations do have very specific traditional beliefs about health practices, but these are primarily for illnesses that are vague and ill defined. For illnesses that are clearly Western in nature, such as accidents, surgical procedures, and AIDS, help usually is sought from Western practitioners, although help also can be sought from traditional healers in the same way as folk remedies also will be used by many people in urban America (MacPherson & MacPherson, 1990).

HEALTH AND DISEASE

Health and Disease Patterns Among Pacific Islander Americans: An Overview of the Issues

Myths and Historical Background

The 1985 report of the Secretary's Task Force on Black and Minority Health suggested that the "Asian/Pacific Islander minority in aggregate is healthier than all other racial/ethnic groups in the United States, including whites" (p. 6). This naturally led to the general idea that API populations had no health problems that needed special attention—the myth of healthy APIs (Chen & Hawks, 1995; see

also Chapter 21, this volume for an excellent discussion concerning the fallacy of this "healthier" myth). Even worse, the Asian population treated as one whole was seen as superior to the white population on a wide variety of socio-demographic indicators, as can be seen, for example, in the various attempts to limit the number of Asian Americans obtaining entrance into the University of California. Even though the NHOPI population has been separated from the Asian American population since 1980, the myth of a healthy population still persists, partly because the numbers of Pacific Islanders are so small that, when they are disaggregated, it is difficult to paint a clear picture of their strengths and weaknesses. The base conclusion has to be that because of the weighting of Native Hawaiians and their poor health indexes, NHOPIs have some of the poorest health statistics in the United States (Blaisdell, 1996).

If it is a myth today that the Pacific Islander population is unhealthy, this certainly was not the case when Captain Cook first landed on the Big Island of Hawaii in 1778. He described the Hawaiians in words that he could not have used about his own crew or his own countrymen at that time:

> The Native men are above middle size, strong, muscular, well made of dark copper colour . . . walk gracefully, run nimbly and are capable of great fatigue . . . The women . . . have handsome faces . . . are very well made . . . very clean, have good teeth and are perfectly devoid of any disagreeable smell. (Beaglehole, 1967, pp. 1178, 1180)

Similar statements from the eyewitness accounts of the earliest travelers to Hawaii, including physicians on board the ships of Cook, Vancouver, and Perouse, all comment on the excellent health status of Hawaiians.

Although for many years the Hawaiian population in 1778 had been estimated at approximately 300,000, new approaches have estimated that the population in 1778 could have been around 1,000,000 (Stannard, 1989). Despite the Hawaiians' excellent health in 1778, by the 1840s their demise was being predicted. This claim is becoming increasingly more real, as demonstrated by the small number of pure Hawaiians. The Office of Technology Assessment report attached to the Native Hawaiian Health Care Act of 1988 predicted that the number of pure Hawaiians would dwindle during the early 21st century and that the number of Native Hawaiians with an increasing percentage of Hawaiian blood also would decline (U.S. Congress, Office of Technology Assessment, 1987).

Although none of the other Pacific Islander populations that were investigated by the Europeans during the 18th century could claim to be as healthy as Cook and other early visitors found the Native Hawaiians to be, most of the Pacific Islander populations certainly were at least as healthy as the European populations of that time, and the status of the lowest members of the Pacific Island societies undoubtedly was better than that of similarly placed Europeans (Howe, 1984).

E Ola Mau: The Native Hawaiian Health Needs Study (Native Hawaiian Health Research Consortium, 1985) was commissioned by Senator Daniel Inouye (D-HI) to respond to the 1984 report on the poor health of Native Hawaiians. Although the five-volume study recognized the part played by poor access to health and medical resources, the study stressed throughout that emphasis should be placed on the role played by the loss of land, literature, religion, culture, and sovereignty. The study concluded that

the historical and cultural basis for our health plight must be the major consideration, and not merely concern for proximal casual factors such as specified in the currently fashionable government model of

lifestyle, environmental factors, access to health care and genetic factors, with problems only in terms of physical health promotion, disease prevention and intervention. (p. HC-4)

The Native Hawaiian Health Care Act of 1988 was designed to respond to the issues raised by the E Ola Mau study. Instead, using the framework of *Healthy People: The Surgeon General's Report on Health Promotion and Disease Prevention* (U.S. Department of Health, Education, and Welfare, 1979), the act placed nearly all its emphasis on the health promotion and disease prevention aspects of *Healthy People* rather than on dealing with issues of loss of land, sovereignty, religion, and culture (Casken, 1994). Similarly, McCubbin's (1983) culture loss/ stress hypothesis suggests that the current maladaptive behaviors of Native Hawaiians are due to the rapid and severe loss of culture by Native Hawaiians with Westernization and Western values.

The Office of Hawaiian Affairs presented an aggregation of health status data on Native Hawaiians in their *Databook 2006* (Reynolds, 2006). These health data on Native Hawaiians are being presented here not to suggest that these figures are representative of all NHOPIs but rather to emphasize the health status of the largest group of NHOPIs in the United States. Discussions on these Native Hawaiian data also could promote among other groups of NHOPIs the approaches to improving health status that are being used among Native Hawaiians.

It is generally acknowledged that the occurrence of disease—with corresponding mortality, morbidity, and disability—is strongly linked to individuals' lifestyle and risk factors. Interestingly, this report noted that

of all racial groups living in Hawai'i, Native Hawaiians are the racial group with the highest proportion of risk factors leading to illness, disability, and premature death. Statistics reveal a high risk profile for Native Hawaiians, with the bulk of them having one of the following risk factors: sedentary life, obesity, hypertension, smoking, and acute drinking. (Reynolds, 2006, p. 97)

Databook 2006 presents alarming data showing that Native Hawaiians are experiencing high rates of heart and other circulatory diseases and malignant neoplasms (particularly in digestive and respiratory sites). These life-threatening conditions are undoubtedly related to risk factors such as smoking, alcohol consumption, obesity, diabetes, and sedentary lifestyles (Reynolds, 2006).

While our focus is on the Native Hawaiian population, the user must also note that a few minority populations mirror our data. What is not in the data collected is information on Native Hawaiian health as compared with that of other Hawaiians. By understanding the current data on Native Hawaiians and the events that have an impact on Hawaii's host culture, policymakers and program developers may use the information to make system changes in service delivery and plan for the availability and distribution of health care services to ensure their accessibility to Native Hawaiians and others.

Chronic Health Conditions

As noted above, diseases that are of increasing concern to Native Hawaiians are malignant neoplasms, circulatory disease, heart disease, cerebrovascular disease, chronic obstructive pulmonary disease, arthritis, and asthma. Of decreasing concern are atherosclerosis, congenital abnormalities, perinatal conditions, and hypertension. Diabetes has also increased among Native Hawaiian males.

Acute and Infectious Conditions

Two conditions are of importance here for the NHOPI population. The first is AIDS and the second, injuries and accidents. Discussions with Hawaii State Department of Health officials suggest that the potential problem with tuberculosis is primarily among the Asian populations and not Pacific Islanders. Officials did caution, however, that some of the housing conditions for NHOPIs could indeed be seen as a danger for this population.

As of December 31, 2005, a cumulative total of 2,847 AIDS cases had been reported to the STD/AIDS Prevention Branch, Hawaii State Department of Public Health. Of these patients, 1,542 (54.2%) have died. By the end of 2005, 1,305 persons were still known to be living with AIDS, resulting in a prevalence rate of 102.3 AIDS cases per 100,000 population. Also, 109 cases (11% females and 89% males) were reported during 2005 (an AIDS report rate of 8.5 per 100,000 population). In 2005, breakdown of cases by county included Honolulu County, 58 cases; Maui County, 18 cases; Hawaii County, 12 cases; and Kaua`i County, 21 cases (STD/AIDS Prevention Branch, 2005).

When the data for AIDS are examined, one can see a repeat of the pattern noted previously in terms of keeping ethnic groups separate. The state of Hawaii STD/AIDS Prevention Branch maintains data on 23 subgroups in the NHOPI category, which in theory should at least allow researchers to make predictions about the populations under study. Part of the difficulty is that although the data are broken down by these 23 subgroups, regulations forbid dissemination of the data on any ethnic group where there are four or fewer entries in a particular ethnic cell. Thus, apart from noting that the new cases coming into the system in 1994 and 1995 total 50 for Native Hawaiians, the Polynesian count cannot be broken down among the other Pacific

Islander groups, and one can say only that there have been four new cases reported during the years 1994 and 1995 among Micronesians and none among Melanesians in the state. The count cannot be broke down further because the numbers in the individual ethnic cells are four or less; to report them could lead to a breach of confidentiality lawsuit. The California HIV/AIDS data are simply broken down into the usual Office of Management and Budget five-part ethnic categories.

The Hawaii State Department of Health, Injury Prevention and Control Program, in their 2005 report "Hawaii Injury Prevention Plan 2005–2010," note that

> injuries are responsible for more deaths of children and young adults from the first year of life through age 39 than all other causes combined, including heart disease, stroke and cancer . . . and . . . Among all ages, injury is the fourth leading cause of death and disability. (Injury Prevention and Control Program, 2005, p. 4)

Within the injury category, fewer than 0.8% are fatal injuries. Thus, the majority of injuries are nonfatal, often require long-term treatment and rehabilitation, and therefore have higher-level public health implications (Injury Prevention and Control Program, 2005)

Interestingly, not all injuries are accidents. They can often be understood and predicted through the application and analysis of epidemiological data. Once understood, many of these accidents can be prevented by looking at the "who, what, and where" of how these accidents and injuries occur (Injury Prevention and Control Program, 2005, p. 4).

All these issues are amenable to a variety of interventions. One key issue, however, is whether the attempts to improve the health status of NHOPIs by simply using standard Western approaches, even those that are culturally acceptable, can fully answer the question of land and sovereignty raised by Blaisdell (1993). Blaisdell agrees with the standard of a Maori (Polynesian) physician, Mason Durie, who notes,

> More effective utilization of land and retention of tribal lands as measures in the broad sense may prove more effective in the long run [to improve Maori health] than advice about diet or early cancer detection. (Durie, 1987, p. 212)

HEALTH BELIEFS AND PRACTICES: THE EFFECTS OF PACIFIC ISLANDER AMERICAN DIVERSITY ON ACCESS AND USE OF HEALTH RESOURCES IN THE UNITED STATES

Just as data on individual ethnicities are difficult to obtain, so too information on health beliefs is not as widespread as statisticians and authors would like it to be. One difficulty with health beliefs is in pinpointing what is original and what is the result of an interweaving of customs and beliefs (Linnekin, 1983).

Blaisdell (1989), Bushnell (1993), and Chun (1994) all have documented Native Hawaiian health beliefs that were operational prior to 1778. The key belief was the spiritual aspect of a sickness and the relationship between sickness and the breaking of rules (*kapu*). Second was the link between the sickness of the individual and the community; sickness was not the Western individual focus but rather involved the whole community. These beliefs have been carried down till today. It is difficult, however, to clearly demonstrate how these beliefs affect the practice of medicine and people's access to health care. With the resurgence of all things Native Hawaiian, there has been a resurgence too in Native Hawaiian approaches to health and medical care, especially in the Native Hawaiian health care system. E Ola Mau, an organization of Native Hawaiian health professionals, has been organizing workshops and forums to investigate the extent of traditional healing practices. One of the key issues, however, has been the question of reimbursement. Native Hawaiian health beliefs suggest that the healer cannot be reimbursed directly for his or her healing work. Such a skill is not a question of learning but rather a question of righteousness (Blaisdell, 1989). However, some healers have been seeking compensation, and insurance companies are interested in reimbursement. Discussions with Native Hawaiians suggest that, as in most cultures, traditional health beliefs are used along with standard allopathic medical practices.

The issue of determining what is truly a traditional health belief also can be clearly seen in the Samoan medical beliefs and practices. In contemporary Samoa, there are two coexisting systems, traditional and Western, based on the determination as to whether the sickness is indigenous (*ma'i Samoa*) or foreign (*ma'i Palagi*) (MacPherson & MacPherson, 1990). Depending on the sickness, treatment is sought from a traditional healer (*fofo*) or an allopathic practitioner. MacPherson and MacPherson (1990) suggest that these systems will continue because there are many illnesses that continue to be regarded as indigenous. They suggest, however, that as Samoan communities assimilate into the United States, these differences will disappear. This approach of dealing with indigenous sickness with indigenous care and dealing with introduced sickness with Western care is found in nearly all the other NHOPI groups.

There is no simple generic description that covers health beliefs. It is essential to know the geographic area one is dealing with as well as the ethnic group. Even the assertion that beliefs are subordinate to economics is debatable. If an NHOPI is living in what

might be called a typical middle-class situation, with a regular job that carries health insurance, this does not ensure that he or she is going to find it easier to access standard Western professionals for all health care. Health beliefs and practices held by that individual will continue to play a role in determining whether Western medical care is accessed.

Tied in with the individual's health beliefs and practices will be his or her opinion of the appropriateness of access to available medical care services. If the person believes that he or she will be given inferior service because of the negative way in which the medical care providers might perceive the person (in spite of having the economic means to successfully complete the medical care encounter), then the person might not complete the encounter. The principle or strategy for improving this situation is based on providing medical care through professionals who are of the same ethnicity as the patient so as to make the patient feel more comfortable with the Western medical model.

Two issues fall out from this solution. The first is that finding the appropriate professionals often is very difficult. Even if one finds the appropriate professionals, there often is very little with which to persuade the professionals to serve in that medical setting. The second is the more precise question of what constitutes an appropriate professional. Is it simply being ethnically linked to that clinic in the broadest sense? For example, will any Pacific Islander be appropriate for a Samoan population–based clinic, must it be someone who was born in American Samoa of the correct family but whose knowledge of Samoan may be very limited, or should it be someone who speaks Samoan well and has some understanding of Samoan beliefs and practices regarding health and disease but might not have been born there (or indeed might not even be a Pacific Islander by ethnicity)? As the Indian Health

Service discovered, simply being an American Indian did not necessarily mean that an American Indian health professional would be welcomed in a specific medical clinic. Of course, the key difficulty with this approach to access for Pacific Islanders is again the small, scattered numbers, which makes it very difficult to provide appropriate medical care in easily accessible areas.

Finally, there is the economic issue hinted at earlier but made more direct in the words of the director of the Native Hawaiian Health Clinic, Hui Malama Ola Na 'Oiwi. In an interview in 1994, he remarked that almost the only Native Hawaiians who had used his clinic were those who had no jobs or no health insurance (Casken, 1994). Ethnically based clinics that appear to be primarily designed to provide medical care to those who cannot afford to receive it through their family physicians will become segregated institutions that have appeal only to members of that ethnic group who do not have other resources.

BARRIERS TO HEALTH PROMOTION AND DISEASE PREVENTION AMONG PACIFIC ISLANDER AMERICANS IN THE UNITED STATES

> Faced with Western medicine and a health care system that is unfamiliar, Americans of Asian and Pacific Island Heritage experience unique access barriers to primary care. In addition to linguistic and cultural differences, financial problems beset many subgroups, especially recent immigrants and refugees. (U.S. Department of Health and Human Services, 1990, p. 37)

The barriers to health promotion and disease prevention have been touched on throughout this chapter and in many ways replicate the problems faced by all ethnic groups discussed in this book. An immigrant family, unless well provided with economic resources, will be in a second-class situation with regard to medical care and health activities (Mokuau, 1996). Although the family's or individual's economic situation in the natal territory might have been no better than that in the immigrant territory, the lack of viable economic resources was more than compensated for in the former by the invisible social commitments that support communities in their home territories.

Coming to the United States, especially to the continental United States, is a radical change for many NHOPIs (Wong, 1996). In addition to the obvious barriers, the more subtle barrier is the political and socioeconomic climate of the United States. In contrast to all the Pacific Islander jurisdictions, the United States is basically a classical liberal society (Greenberg, 1989). It is a society that prizes the rights of private property above the property rights of the community; that stresses that the individual is responsible for himself or herself rather than being part of a responsible community; that views the free market as the best way in which to distribute goods and values as opposed to the needs of the community; and that believes the government should play a very limited role and should not try to control the free market, or even try to level the playing field. Above all, the government should not take over an individual's own responsibilities, including those in the health field. NHOPIs thus have to contend with a social system that, although it initially might seem familiar, is in reality a contradiction to the one in which they were raised. When one thinks of the role of individual responsibility that has been built into health promotion and disease prevention activities since the first publication of *Healthy People* (U.S. Department of Health, Education, and Welfare, 1979), the barriers to successful implementation of these activities among most NHOPIs are immense.

CHAPTER SUMMARY

The health professional who is working with or plans to work with NHOPIs must consider a number of key issues as he or she designs an approach. The overall understanding must be that it is a myth that this is a healthy population. The myth has arisen in part because of the extremely limited amount of data available on this population. We know very little about the size of the population, the exact locations, the health needs, and the overall socioeconomic status. We do know that the population is extremely small in comparison with the rest of the U.S. population or, indeed, in comparison with any other ethnic group within the U.S. population. As noted earlier, NHOPIs form only about 5% of the Office of Management and Budget API classification and thus are totally swamped in any data that are used to describe the API population.

It was suggested that even within this comparatively small population, there are major differences among the three main groups: Polynesians, Micronesians, and Melanesians. Perhaps even more noticeably, within those subgroupings, there are further differences based on socioeconomic status. Thus, the task of the health professional working with these populations becomes increasingly difficult. An additional factor is that the definitions that are used to determine who is a member of each subgroup are so vague that almost anyone could claim to be a member of any subgroup.

Because Hawaii is the state in which the majority of NHOPIs live, this chapter has suggested that one approach should be to examine the situation in Hawaii as a first step in approaching other NHOPI populations. At least two of the subpopulations are broken down within the Hawaii State Department of Health's data reports. Yet even in Hawaii, the same problems present in the continental United States are present in the state as well.

A temporary solution would be to ensure that more of the data collected are broken down into sets that are applicable to this population. As we saw in the Hawaiian data, results that suggest that NHOPIs are reasonably healthy can hide major problems for those NHOPIs at the lower end of the socioeconomic scale. Perhaps the first charge of the concerned health professional would be to deal with issues of education, language use, and employment because these can be key to improving a person's health status.

Paraphrasing Pukui (1983), perhaps today one could say that "now is the right time to work for the good health of Native Hawaiians and Other Pacific Islanders."

DISCUSSION QUESTIONS AND ACTIVITIES

Working in small groups, consider the following questions and activities and then be prepared to present your responses and activity outcomes for full classroom discussion:

1. What are the demographics of NHOPIs living in your community? Are they blended into the other API data? How could you actually determine the numbers and Islander affiliations of the NHOPIs in your community?

2. What are the major causes of morbidity and mortality in the NHOPI populations in your community?

3. Design, implement, and evaluate a brief survey to identify the major health concerns of your NHOPI populations, including their health beliefs and practices associated with these concerns. Based on your survey results, discuss the interventions you might employ to do something to reduce these concerns.

REFERENCES

Barringer, H., Gardner, R., & Levin, M. (1993). *Asians and Pacific Islanders on the United States*. New York: Russell Sage.

Beaglehole, J. C. (Ed.). (1967). *The journeys of Captain Cook on his voyages of discovery, 1776–1780*. Cambridge, UK: Cambridge University Press.

Bellwood, P. (1979). *Man's conquest of the Pacific: The pre-history of Southeast Asia and Oceania*. New York: Oxford University Press.

Blaisdell, R. K. (1989). Historical and cultural aspects of Native Hawaiian health. In E. Wegner (Ed.), *Social process in Hawai'i: Vol. 32. The health of Native Hawaiians: A selective report on health status and health in the 1980s* (pp. 1–21). Honolulu: University of Hawai'i Press.

Blaisdell, R. K. (1993). The health status of Kanaka Maoli (indigenous Hawaiians). *Asian American and Pacific Islander Journal of Health, 1*(2), 116–160.

Blaisdell, R. K. (1996). 1995 update on Kanaka Maoli (indigenous Hawaiians') health. *Asian American and Pacific Islander Journal of Health, 4*(1–3), 160–165.

Bousseau, S. J. (1993). *Fa'a Samoa: Yesterday and today—A resource guide*. Sacramento, CA: California Office of Criminal Justice Planning.

Budnick, R. (1992). *Stolen kingdom: An American conspiracy*. Honolulu, HI: Aloha Press. Bushnell, O. A. (1993). *The gifts of civilization: Germs and genocide in Hawai'i*. Honolulu: University of Hawai'i Press.

Casken, J. (1994). *Bringing culture into health? The Native Hawaiian Health Care Act of 1988*. Unpublished doctoral dissertation, University of Hawai'i.

Chen, M. A. (1996). Demographic characteristics of Asian and Pacific Islander Americans: Health implications. *Asian American and Pacific Islander Journal of Health, 4*(1–3), 40–49.

Chen, M. S., & Hawks, B. L. (1995). A debunking of the myth of healthy Asian Americans and Pacific Islanders. *American Journal of Health Promotion, 9*, 261–268.

Chun, M. N. (Trans.). (1994). *Native Hawaiian medicine*. Honolulu, HI: First People's Productions.

Daws, G. (1968). *Shoal of time*. Honolulu: University of Hawai'i Press.

Dearing, E. C. (1996). Asian American and Pacific Islander identity and classification. *Asian American and Pacific Islander Journal of Health, 4*(1–3), 82–87.

Dougherty, M. (1992). *To steal a kingdom*. Waimanalo, HI: Island Style Press.

Durie, M. H. (1987). Implications of policy and management decisions on Maori health. In M. W. Raffel & N. K. Raffel (Eds.), *Perspectives on health policy; Australia, New Zealand, and the United States*. New York: Wiley.

Federal Register (2000, February 15). *HHS poverty guidelines: One version of the (U.S.) federal poverty measure* (Vol. 65, No. 31, pp. 7555–7557). Washington, DC: U.S. Department of Health and Human Services.

Filoialii, L. A. (1980). *Attitudes towards the traditional Fa'a Samoa as a problem of adjusting to urban life in America*. Unpublished master's thesis, Pepperdine University, Malibu, CA.

Franco, K. W. (1991). *Samoan perceptions of work: Moving up and moving around*. New York: AMS Press.

Greenberg, E. (1989). *The American political stem: A radical approach* (5th ed.). Boston: Little, Brown.

Hall, S. (1990). Cultural identity and diaspora. In J. Rutherford (Ed.), *Identity: Community, culture, difference* (pp. 222–237). London: Lawrence & Wishart.

Harris, P. M., & Jones, N. A. (2005). *We the people: Pacific Islanders in the U.S., Census 2000* (2000 Special Reports, CENSR-26, pp. 1–21). Washington, DC: U.S. Census Bureau.

Howe, K. K. (1984). *Where the waves fall: A new South Sea Islands history from first settlement to colonial rule*. Honolulu: University of Hawai'i Press.

Janes, C. R. (1990). *Migration, social change, and health: A Samoan community in urban California*. Stanford, CA: Stanford University Press.

Kame'eleihiwa, L. (1992). *Native lands and foreign desires*. Honolulu, HI: Bishop Museum Press.

Linnekin, J. S. (1983). Defining tradition: Variations on the Hawaiian identity. *American Ethnologist, 10,* 241–252.

MacPherson, C., & MacPherson, L. (1990). *Samoan medical belief and practice.* Auckland, New Zealand: Auckland University Press.

McCubbin, H. (1983). Cultural loss and stress among Native Hawaiians. In *Native Hawaiian educational assessment project.* Honolulu, HI: Kamehameha Schools/Bernice Pauahi Bishop Estate.

Mokuau, N. (1996). Health and well-being for Pacific Islanders: Status, barriers and resolutions. *Asian American and Pacific Islander Journal of Health, 4*(1–3), 55–67.

Montgomery, L. E., Kiely, J. L., & Pappas, G. (1996). The effects of poverty race, and family structure on U.S. children's health: Data from the NHIS, 1978 through 1980 and 1989 through 1991. *American Journal of Public Health, 86,* 1401–1406.

Native Hawaiian Health Research Consortium. (1985). *E Ola Mau: The Native Hawaiian health needs study* (5 vols.). Honolulu, HI: Alu Like.

Navarro, V. (1989). Race or class or race and class. *International Journal of Health Services, 19,* 311–314.

Pouesi, D. (1994). *An illustrated history of Samoans in California.* Carson, CA: KIN Publications.

Pukui, M. K. (1983). *Olelo No'eau.* Honolulu, HI: Bishop Museum Press.

Reynolds, A. (2006). *Databook 2006* (health section, pp. 96–110). Honolulu, HI: Office of Health Affairs.

Schram, S. F. (1995). *Worlds of welfare: The poverty of social science and social science's poverty.* Minneapolis: University of Minnesota Press.

Secretary's Task Force on Black and Minority Health. (1985). *Executive taskforce on black and minority health* (Vol. 1). Washington, DC: U.S. Department of Health and Human Services.

Stannard, D. (1989). *Before the horror: The population of Hawai'i on the eve of Western contact.* Honolulu: University of Hawai'i Press.

STD/AIDS Prevention Branch. (2005). *HIV/AIDS surveillance semi-annual report: Cases to December 31, 2005* (pp. 1–4). Honolulu, HI: Hawaii State Department of Health.

Stone, D. A. (1988). *Policy paradox and political reason.* Glenview, IL: Scott, Foresman.

Trask, H. K. (1985). Hawaiians, American colonization and the quest for independence. In C. Sullivan & G. Hawes (Eds.), *Social process in Hawai'i: Vol. 31. The political economy of Hawai'i.* Honolulu: University of Hawai'i Press.

Trask, H. K. (1993). *Notes from a native daughter: Colonialism and sovereignty in Hawai'i.* Monroe, ME: Common Courage Press.

U.S. Census Bureau. (2001a). Table 4: Native Hawaiians and other Pacific Islander populations by detailed group: 2000. In *Briefs and special reports: The Native Hawaiian and other Pacific Islander populations 2000* (p. 9). Retrieved January 23, 2008, from www.census.gov/prod/2001pubs/c2kbr01-14.pdf

U.S. Census Bureau. (2001b). Table 3: Ten largest places in total population and in Native Hawaiian and other Pacific Islander population: 2000. In *Briefs and special reports: The Native Hawaiian and other Pacific Islander populations 2000* (p. 7). Retrieved January 23, 2008, from www.census.gov/prod/2001pubs/c2kbr01-14.pdf

U.S. Census Bureau. (2006). Table 11: Residential population by age and sex: 1980 to 2004. In *Statistical abstract of the United States* (125th ed.). Washington, DC: Government Printing Office.

U.S. Congress, Office of Technology Assessment. (1987). *Current health status and population projections of Native Hawaiians living in Hawai'i.* Washington, DC: Government Printing Office.

U.S. Department of Health, Education, and Welfare. (1979). *Healthy people: The surgeon general's report on health promotion and disease prevention.* Washington, DC: Public Health Service.

U.S. Department of Health and Human Services. (1990). *Healthy people 2000: National health promotion and disease prevention objectives*

(DHHS Publication No. [PHS] 91-50213). Washington, DC: Government Printing Office.

Wegner, E. (Ed.). (1989). *Social process in Hawai'i: Vol. 32. The health of Native Hawaiians: A selective report on health status and health care in the 1980's.* Honolulu: University of Hawai'i Press.

Wong, D. (1996). Access, barriers, and problems of present working models of API com-munity health centers. *Asian American and Pacific Islander Journal of Health, 4*(1–3), 88–96.

Young, I. K. (1994). *The health of Native Americans: Toward a biocultural epidemiology.* New York: Oxford University Press.

26

Health Promotion Planning in Pacific Islander Population Groups

GREGORY P. LOOS

Chapter Objectives

On completion of this chapter, the health promotion student and practitioner will be able to

- Identify and discuss how to assess cultural-related differences among Pacific Islander populations relevant to their unique health risk problems on their own respective islands and on the U.S. mainland, where at times they might also reside

- Discuss how foldback analysis can be used as a tool to assist in the planning and intervention development process, in general, and specifically among other target groups

- Discuss the kinds of activities you would select for assisting different Pacific Islander populations to empower themselves for later program development (e.g., Native Hawaiians, Samoans, Guamanians) and how empowerment activities might differ by Pacific Islander populations

- Identify and discuss the range of possible activities for obtaining the participation of the Pacific Islander target community under study when planning social marketing campaigns

- Identify the advantages of the different research methods useful for planning social marketing campaigns with the target community—for example, formative evaluation

- Describe how social marketing research and the activities presented in this chapter can be used to facilitate change at various stages of program development

There are numerous groups of Pacific Islanders, and although they might share certain commonalities (e.g., value orientations, colonization experiences, migration, and development patterns), use of the collective term *Pacific Islander* is in no way meant to imply that these populations or communities are homogeneous in nature. Realizing this, complex concepts such as health and its promotion and disease and its prevention will vary across and within Pacific Island societies. Within this and other logical restrictions to Pacific Islander uniformity and comparability, this chapter discusses general approaches to the topics of health promotion and disease prevention (HPDP) that the author believes to be accurate based on his own circumscribed familiarity with the many different Pacific Islander populations.

This chapter is directed at Pacific Islanders in the aggregate. That is, the focus of HPDP is on social action for health rather than on individual behavior change. Furthermore, although the author's experience with Pacific Islander populations is limited to specific culture groups in the Pacific Basin and Pacific Rim jurisdictions, the approaches to health behavior change advocated herein are applicable to most Pacific Islander groups, including migrant populations from the islands of the Pacific that have relocated to the U.S. mainland and elsewhere outside their home jurisdictions.[1] The President's Advisory Commission on Asian American and Other Pacific Islanders Addressing Health Disparities (U.S. Department of Health and Human Services, 2003) recognizes that the leading causes of death among Pacific Islander populations closely parallel those in the mainland United States—that is, cardiovascular diseases, cancer, and injuries. Also, endocrinologic/nutritional and respiratory diseases rank quite high as causes of death in the Pacific Islander population.

To be effective among Pacific Islander populations, social actions that contribute to HPDP must use a variety of strategies, including (a) advocacy that generates public interest in, and political and economic support for, health; (b) social systems that encourage healthy lifestyles as a social norm and that foster community action for health; and (c) the instillation of attitudes, knowledge, and skills in Pacific Islander communities, which enable them to act effectively within culturally accepted parameters to prevent health problems (Stevenson & Burke, 1992). To make these strategies operational, it is clear that socially appropriate health communication and social mobilization strategies are required to foster community action for health.

The approaches to community-based health behavior change discussed in this chapter rely heavily on aspects of well-known models of behavior change, such as the importance of predisposing, enabling, and reinforcing factors espoused by Green and Kreuter (2005); the Health Belief Model (Janz, Champion, & Strecher, 2002); the Theory of Reasoned Action and the Theory of Planned Behavior (Montano & Kasprzyk, 2002); the Transtheoretical Model and Stages of Change (Prochaska, Redding, & Evers, 2002); and Diffusion of Innovations (Oldenburg & Parcel, 2002; Rogers, 2003). These models and concepts are discussed in greater depth in Chapter 4 of this volume. The health promotion and disease prevention (HPDP) methods discussed in this chapter help operationalize these theories for the student and practitioner in an effort to facilitate more effective health interventions among Pacific Islander populations. Three approaches are distinguished and presented in some depth: community involvement/empowerment, foldback analysis, and social marketing.

Used individually or in sequence, each of these approaches is culturally appropriate for HPDP work with Pacific Islander communities. For example, because clan groupings are central to Pacific Islander cultures, community empowerment can be used effectively throughout the HPDP campaign process (i.e., from needs assessment, to HPDP campaign planning and intervention, to evaluation). On the other hand, foldback analysis, although useful throughout, is particularly valuable in reducing outsider bias and, therefore, is most functional at the front and tail ends of campaigns (i.e., to assess needs and to plan and evaluate interventions). Finally, given the geographic and increasing socioeconomic and intergenerational variations across Pacific Islander groupings, social marketing is recommended as the best approach for tailored interventions with targeted groups of Pacific Islanders.

The levels of HPDP planning may be comprehensive, incremental, and mixed in scope and may be systems based with an epidemiological, environmental, or ecological perspective. Different planning models are discussed in Chapter 7 of this volume. In this chapter, no one focus is championed more than another. What is advocated, no matter which planning perspective is used, is that the views of the Pacific Islander community must be engaged throughout if the HPDP campaign is to be successful. That is, no intervention planned and imposed in Pacific Islander communities will achieve the desired ends unless it is self-imposed. As such, it is more important to invest time to involve the Pacific Islander community from the onset than to rush into planning interventions that will not be supported or sustained.

This may be referred to as an indigenous planning model. Such an approach is emphasized for all phases of HPDP programs—assessment, planning, intervention, and evaluation. Each phase is discussed separately in what follows. To appreciate the recommendations made, however, it is necessary to establish some parameters for Pacific Islander populations as a whole and as they are discussed in this chapter.

EMPOWERMENT AS A PREMISE FOR HEALTH PROMOTION AND DISEASE PREVENTION AMONG PACIFIC ISLANDERS

Emerson states that "the secret of education is respecting the pupil" (quoted in Peter, 1980,

p. 162). A fundamental principle of HPDP planning and activity is the need to keep in mind the perspectives of the target community and to evaluate people's health behavior in terms of a holistic concept of health. In this context, this chapter considers possible strategic parameters designed to improve HPDP efforts with Pacific Islander populations through methods that are politically, economically, and socioculturally acceptable to Pacific Islander populations.

Included in most models analyzing health behavior is a consideration of health beliefs and attitudes (e.g., the seriousness and causes of disease and one's degree of perceived susceptibility). In addition, health behavior models often include structural parameters such as the availability of resources and social factors known to influence service use such as demographic differences (e.g., income, age, ethnicity, sex). In a like manner, these same factors are also hypothesized to influence Pacific Islander health behavior and readiness to use formal health services. That is, for Pacific Islanders, multiple internal and external influences combine to determine health behavior, health status, and the potential for positive outcomes resulting from HPDP interventions. As presented in this chapter, health is not only a biomedical status but also one influenced by demographic, economic, and political parameters related to Pacific Islanders as well as to more conventional medical factors.

In addition to being easier to perceive population, political-economic, and material differences within and across Pacific Islander groups, perceptions of health and achieving qualitative standards of life for Pacific Islanders are also inclined to differ and to be influenced significantly by several distinct but interrelated psychosocial and cultural dimensions. Some of the more important dimensions, when considering Pacific Islander populations, include (a) a historical dimension (e.g., cultural heritage, colonial legacy, predominant religion), (b) a political-ideological dimension (e.g., organization of social rank, social value differences, different views about the importance of material or spiritual goods, different metaphysical interpretations of human life), (c) a psychological dimension (e.g., self-concept and roles of individuals in society, attitudes toward authority and cooperation, different readiness for change and experiment, the importance of "secondary" virtues such as punctuality and hygiene), and (d) a cognitive dimension (e.g., the perception, interpretation, and labeling of reality; the ability to express complex concepts in purely symbolic form as abstract, linguistic, logical, or mathematical principles that can be used without concrete objects or imagery).

An added overlay is the growing difference between traditional values and social structures and the expectation to share the benefits and enticements of modern consumption-oriented lifestyles. Differences in these views are creating increasingly dualistic societies in Oceania. This is particularly evident in those island communities with close and migrational relationships with former colonizing nations and/or advanced communication media (e.g., television, the Internet). Young adults and youths, seduced by consumption orientations and vestiges of wanting to emulate lifestyles of former colonizers, are torn most by these dichotomous circumstances.

This situation can create health-related concerns in the islands that differ between generations. Among Cook Islanders, for example, many teens wanting to migrate to New Zealand make the economic decision to give birth to children whom they can leave behind with their parents. The teens then feel capable of leaving the islands to pursue employment and experiential opportunities elsewhere. In exchange, the grandparent-caretakers receive social services from the New Zealand government to care for the children who remain behind and are left with emotional surrogates for the departed children. The result is a high teen pregnancy rate, the youngest population in the Pacific (50.1% under 15 years of age), and the potential for intergenerational psychosocial problems (World Health Organization [WHO], 1990, p. 2). The result is a high teen pregnancy rate and the creation of more intergenerational conflict and psychosocial problems. Although there is a downward trend, New Zealand's pregnancy rate in 2001 was the third highest in the developed world (Boddington, Khawaja, & Didham, 2003).

From another perspective, population growth, economic growth, and the increasing use of more technology-intensive production methods are threatening to result in a serious degradation of the fragile physical environment of the islands. As a result, direct and indirect environmentally related health problems will likely escalate. For example, the continued sale of old growth timber by the Solomon Islanders to purchasing agents from Asian countries such as Malaysia and Japan threatens sustainable development and the health of the people through loss of native flora and fauna as well as indirectly through the loss of topsoil for crop production.

Although the economic need in the islands is easy to intuit for most Pacific Islanders, the actual and potential negative environmental impacts, along with the possible concomitant impacts on health and nutrition, might be less easy to comprehend because they are frequently without precedent in the islands. Such negative impacts also might threaten Pacific Islanders' harmonic accord with the land that is central to their health belief system and psychic balance.

To address such complex issues effectively requires forethought and the development of intersectoral preventive health strategies. Such strategies, however, might compete for political priority with economic necessity in many of the island nations.

At a minimum, fostering successful HPDP strategies will require the ability of Pacific Islanders to visualize abstract concepts such as the long-term impacts of development and its potential negative influence on their social, health, and psychological welfare, that is, the ability to not only solve problems but also comprehend problems before they occur.

Development of such well-functioning and advanced cognitive capacities (i.e., the ability to understand abstract issues without prior experience) might not be fully possible among individuals in societies that are grounded in concrete life circumstances (e.g., the gathering, farming, and fishing societies found on many of the islands) and that lack precedent experiences of a similar type.

Furthermore, it is proposed (Arlin, 1975) that the ability to find health problems before they occur is an advanced cognitive ability that can only build on a history of sophisticated "problem solving." Such "sophistication" might not be established in many of the island jurisdictions that are only now encountering complex environmental and health problems for the first time or that have little understanding of Western causative theories of health, relying more on animistic or fatalistic explanations for disease and environmental catastrophes.

Therefore, effective social action for HPDP in the islands and on the mainland will require both basic and advanced health literacy, which in turn will depend on culturally effective health communication strategies. To accomplish these ends, social culture must be considered and local vocabulary must be employed rather than professional health jargon and Western values (Loos, Hatcher, & Shein, 1994).

Many Pacific Islanders, however, might not have the means to establish communication and trust with health care providers and, because of this lack of trust, might be hesitant to share their traditional beliefs (Kumabe, Nishida, & Hepworth, 1985). Kim (1990) conducted focus group interviews in Hawaii with several ethnic groups (e.g., Hawaiians, Filipinos, Samoans) regarding prenatal care. Men and women in this study complained that doctors did not speak their languages, did not verify their statuses, and did not share the same explanatory models for pregnancy.

Similar results (i.e., identifying cultural insensitivity among health care workers and language barriers for Pacific Islanders) have been found repeatedly in other studies (Loos

et al., 1994). Thus, a major access barrier to health service use for Pacific Islanders is the general lack of health professionals who come from these ethnic groups, who can comprehend their cultural values, and who can speak their languages.

Outside health workers' ignorance of Pacific Islander cultures can interfere with effective communication. Furthermore, "communication," for Pacific Islander populations, must be considered in a broad context, including language and choice of illustrations used as well as tone, topic and context, body language, eye contact, and order of speaking (or when not to speak).

In addition, Pacific Islander deterministic attitudes toward health and disease (i.e., that poor health is a naturally occurring integral part of life resulting from a variety of forces) can cause Pacific Islanders not to seek health care or take part in HPDP strategies based on the Western view of health. Many Pacific Islanders lack familiarity with Western diagnostic techniques and treatments and, therefore, are apprehensive or outright disbelieving.

Information-seeking behavior is also different for Pacific Islanders. It frequently is less direct than that of Westerners; this is especially true when the information is coming from an "outsider." Relevance of the HPDP message to the beliefs, needs, and desires of the target audience is vitally important to engage Pacific Islander interest in an HPDP campaign.

Furthermore, investigation of certain subjects is inappropriate for Pacific Islanders, whereas investigation of other subjects is not only appropriate but also expected. Therefore, fundamental cultural characteristics must be kept in mind during the introduction, design, and administration of HPDP assessments; the implementation of interventions; and the conduct of evaluation, not only out of consideration for the people but also for accuracy in the interpretation of their responses.

For these many reasons, for HPDP interventions across Pacific Islander culture groups to be successful, they must be based on a biopsychosocial model of health that includes consideration of the origins and causes of health behavior in relation to economic, demographic, social, and cultural changes affecting health. As such, the primary goal of HPDP planning and intervention with Pacific Islander populations must be to engage the target community through the promotion of participatory processes.

Success in HPDP for Pacific Islanders will require both "bottom-up" and "top-down" planning and action. That is, learning from people, valuing their views, and listening rather than lecturing will be essential for successful community-based health promotion among Pacific Islanders. For these people, the methods selected must empower the target community to be centrally involved in the entire HPDP campaign process (Minkler, 2004; Minkler & Wallerstein, 2002; Wallerstein, 1992).

Empowerment is a concept, a philosophy, a set of organized behavioral practices, and an organized program (Raeburn, 1992). As a concept, empowerment is the vesting of decision making or approval authority in members of the target Pacific Islander community. Empowerment as a philosophy and set of behavioral practices means allowing the members of the community to be in charge of their own lives while working on a cooperative basis for the betterment of the community Empowerment as an organizational program involves providing the framework and giving permission to all members of the community to unleash, develop, and use their skills and knowledge to their fullest potential for the good of the community. Given this perspective of empowerment, the following should be kept in mind regarding Pacific Islanders:

- It is necessary to have community participation, not merely representation, throughout the HPDP process.
- The community must share responsibility in defining the HPDP problem and for its solution.
- For the HPDP campaign process to be successful, all influential stakeholder public in the Pacific Islander community must be consulted

and, to the degree possible, engaged to work together (Cronbach, 1982; see also Chapter 4, this volume).

- This social connectedness is very important to the integrative dimension of a comprehensive approach to HPDP and to continued community support for the planned intervention.
- Although the HPDP project focus should consider long-term effects, it is more important to stress interim short-term objectives. The immediacy of short-term success will better ensure the Pacific Islander community participation in the HPDP process and sustain its members' interest in the longer-term horizon.
- HPDP interventions under consideration must be relative to a historical understanding of the specific Pacific Islander community. In this way, the selected HPDP campaign will work through existing community structures and in congruence with the people's ways of operating. That is, it is important to focus on the context of the target population and to be aware of the conditions that will inhibit or facilitate HPDP interventions as these may exist in individual communities.

For Pacific Islanders, *empowerment* of people and community also implies an interconnected worldview with nature and the larger cosmos.

PACIFIC ISLANDER WORLDVIEW AND NOTIONS OF HEALTH AND DISEASE

A well-known Maori proverb says,

> If you tear the heart from the flax bush, where will the bellbird sing from?
>
> If you ask me, "What is the most important thing in the world?"
>
> I will say to you, "It is people, it is people, it is people."

Perhaps the most valuable result of all HPDP is the ability to make people do what they should do to preserve health when it ought to be done, whether they like it or not. As such, then, the aim of HPDP activity is not the knowledge of fact but rather the knowledge of values. When working cross-culturally to promote health and prevent disease, especially (perhaps) with Pacific Islander groups, it is important to determine where "health" is considered in their life views and also what their beliefs are about, and their attitudes are toward, preserving health (Kamehameha Educational Research Institute, 1983).

Before suggesting new knowledge, attitudes, and behaviors, HPDP personnel need to empower Pacific Islander groups to express what health and disease mean to them. That is, how do Pacific Islanders define illness, what disorders do they recognize and which do they feel are susceptible to cure using modern methods, what are their notions of prevention and cause, what knowledge do they have of curing techniques, and how is illness tied to other aspects of culture? Such knowledge is gained during project assessment and planning and is foundational to the acceptance and success of HPDP interventions among Pacific Islanders.

To understand the minds of Pacific Islanders, Western notions of selfhood and individualism must be replaced with "a contextual perspective in which person, family, nature, and spiritual world are interconnected and interdependent" (see Chapters 1, 2, and 25). That is, there is a "psychic unity" that binds the physical, mental, emotional, social, and spiritual being of the person with the ecological and cosmological, and the well-being of the individual (e.g., health) cannot be ensured unless the individual parts and the greater firmament are in harmony.

The distinguishing feature of indigenous island cultures is that they think of themselves as an integral part of the natural order that is a balanced relationship of people, Earth and its resources, and the greater infinite whole. In this context, the occurrence of disease signals disharmony that could be taking place at any point in the overall balance, and the promotion of health can best be achieved by redressing identified imbalances. For Pacific Islanders, becoming ill often is viewed as a naturally

occurring process for redressing a social wrong as part of a larger cosmic order (Kinloch, 1985).

For example, among Hawaiians, the word *ola* alternately means *life, health, well-being, livelihood, salvation, curable, healed, saved, to save,* and *to heal* and is expected to be a way of living (i.e., in total life harmony). *Ma'i* (the wrong way of living) is the opposite of *ola*. *Ma'i* can be caused by bacteria or a virus, by an accident or injury, by spirits or ghosts, or through retribution or revenge by someone else or the supernatural.

The Hawaiian word *lokahi* means healthful harmony and refers to overall equilibrium among all life forces and entities. *Ho'ola* (to do *ola*) refers to all the healing arts, including salvation, consultation, cure, and convalescence. As such, the concepts of HPDP align with *lokahi,* whereas health care services align more with *ho'ola*. Within most Pacific Islander groups, there are concepts and words similar to *ola, ma'i, lokahi,* and *ho'ola* (Hawaii State Department of Health, 1991).

HPDP for the Pacific Islander is never an individual situation but always a collective concern. Among Pacific Islander groups, the family is the basic unit of social structure, consisting of several nuclear families related by blood or marriage as well as adopted members (Kamehameha Educational Research Institute, 1984; Kamehameha Schools, 1985). The extended family system is usually headed by a designated "chief." This chief is sought for counsel, advice, and approval on any familial or personal matter, and the family as a whole is typically involved in both disease prevention and disease cure (Palafox & Warren, 1980; Pan Asian Parent Education Project, 1982).

Obedience to the family as a whole, family heads, and elders is a primary responsibility of all family members. The family is the key to the "island way" and has structure, meaning, duties, and pervasiveness that go beyond the meaning of family held in much of the West. The values of the family unit have retained their importance with Pacific Islander populations even as they migrate (Ablon, 1971; Janes, 1990). Because of this kinship allegiance, there is a sense of cooperation and responsibility among members to support and assist new migrants among expatriate populations (Labarthe, Reed, Brody, & Stallones, 1973; Prior, 1974; WHO, 1975).

For Pacific Islanders, ecological and cosmic harmony and reliance within the kinship group are central to the maintenance of health and are core to their belief systems. As such, these concepts must be incorporated throughout HPDP activity with Pacific Islander groups, from assessment to intervention and including evaluation. Fortunately, the communal focus of all activities among Pacific Islanders affords a basis for social action for health. Unlike many Western populations, in which the notion of "community" has to be created, the basis for healthy community initiatives is well established among Pacific Islanders.

COMMUNITY ANALYSIS FOR HEALTH PROMOTION AND DISEASE PREVENTION PLANNING

The process of analysis used to plan and prepare HPDP campaigns should consider multiple perspectives of need from key data sources to determine where the different perspectives converge and where the greatest consensus can be established (see Chapter 7, this volume). The professional health community typically relies on normative perspectives of need such as those prescribed by professional health service and epidemiological standards (e.g., the *Healthy People 2010* objectives for the nation, U.S. Department of Health and Human Services, 2000; see also Ghosh, 2003, who discusses the difficulties of defining baselines for Asian Americans/Pacific Islanders in "Healthy People 2010 and Asian Americans/ Pacific Islanders"). Health professionals usually collect data related to these standards (e.g., vital statistics, mortality, morbidity,

service use rates) to compare relative need across communities and to select targets for HPDP activity

Although professional perspectives of need are important to identify health issues and target communities requiring HPDP activity, they are not necessarily adequate to explain how best to intervene, especially when the health professional and target community differ culturally. To empower and involve the Pacific Islander population in the HPDP process, means must be employed to also assess the felt needs of the community. Whereas some criteria of need for the layperson might be consistent with professional values, others might not be and still others might be outside the range of professional interests (Kamehameha Educational Research Institute, 1985).

For lay members of any target community, there are multiple life issues of importance, and where "health" falls among competing priorities should be a starting point for HPDP investigations. Given the particular worldview and deterministic perspectives related to health and disease held by Pacific Islanders, HPDP might not be a high-ranked life issue (Hawaii State Department of Health, 1988).

In an effort to determine whether the value structures of Hawaiians and other ethnic groups living in Hawaii differ significantly, the author developed and compared three-dimensional value maps for Hawaiians and Caucasians/Japanese (non-Hawaiians) living in Hawaii in response to the question "What are the important things in life?" (the study methodology, foldback analysis, is discussed later; Loos, 1998). Figure 26.1 presents these two maps.

For illustration of the value differences between Hawaiians and non-Hawaiians, it is interesting to note the dissimilarities in the two value maps. The important life issues for Hawaiians, generated by the community itself, tend to cluster together more than for non-Hawaiians. Indeed, the largest Hawaiian cluster joins five life issues ("me [1], knowing self

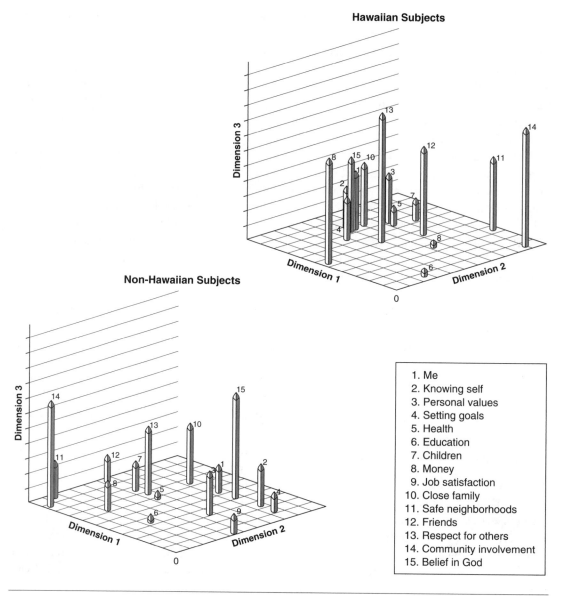

Figure 26.1   Three-Dimensional Value Plots: What Are the Important Things in Life?

[2], setting goals [4], close family [10], and belief in God [15]"). For non-Hawaiians, the largest cluster couples only two items ("safe neighborhoods [11] and community involvement [14]"). These visual cluster differences may epitomize the interconnectedness of life issues for Hawaiians (Pacific Islanders) more than for non-Hawaiians.

These value maps also locate the relationship of "health (5)" among other identified "important things in life" for both groups. Determining this relationship, as we will see, provides vital information for the HPDP planner to design interventions that will be effective to influence community attitudes toward health.

For now, what is important to note is that the worldviews and connectedness of health *are* likely very different for Pacific Islander and non-Pacific Islander populations. To empower

Pacific Islanders, HPDP methods must be used that will accurately record and precisely measure the study population's health values and beliefs without them being distorted by the biases of an outsider. This is the precise value of foldback analysis.

Foldback analysis is a multimethod research that interweaves qualitative data collection and data analysis strategies to develop and explain survey research and community value maps (Loos, 1995). The method includes open-ended interviewing, nominal group dialogue, survey and attitude scaling techniques, and multidimensional and cluster analyses (see Figure 26.2).

These study methods are used in sequence where each procedure is "folded back" into the interpretation of results from the other methods. This sequenced approach combines the assets and helps overcome the weaknesses of each method. As such, it is useful for cross-cultural studies in which inadvertent misinterpretation of data must be minimized.

The combination of techniques into a single, combined approach affords both a richer and a more usable database than does any of the procedures used alone. Therefore, it is recommended that the individual techniques be used in full sequence rather than in part. When this is not possible, segments of the overall sequence may be used; however, the full benefit of foldback analysis will be compromised.

Although the entire foldback process might require time upfront in the analysis phase of HPDP planning, it is time well spent because it (a) serves to engage and empower the Pacific Islander community in assessment, planning, and (later) evaluation; (b) provides guidance for HPDP campaigns and social marketing messages; and (c) reduces the chance of developing misguided HPDP interventions that will not be used or sustained by the Pacific Islander community. It is possible to adapt the foldback process for rapid analysis by replacing the large random sample (Step 4 in Figure 26.2) with a representative sample of key informants.

The statistical processes for foldback analyses are not complex and are available with several commercial software programs that are affordably priced.[2] These programs are available for use with personal computers, thus permitting greater use for the field health practitioner. The result is a bountiful database of community perception that can be used throughout all phases of the HPDP process.

Foldback Data Collection Process

The analysis of issues key to the local community is started during initial interviews (Step 1 in Figure 26.2) and then targeted, developed, and refined during the first nominal group process (Steps 2 and 3). This information provides the foundation for the development of the survey instrument used with a larger sample of community respondents (Step 4) and later for the interpretation of survey results and value maps developed from survey data (Steps 5 and 6).

The survey instrument is formed by the community in large part using vernacular drawn directly from the original interview transcripts and nominal group dialogue. The target community also defines the sampling frame for the survey and helps collect the data.

The survey instrument is constructed using attitude scales in whole or in part. Rank-order and modal score data are then made available to a second nominal group to analyze. These data are also submitted for further analysis using multidimensional scaling (MDS) and cluster analysis.

MDS is a procedure for transforming community ratings of similarity among, or preference for, identified "key issues" into a multidimensional graph or map (see Figure 26.1). In this manner, large and complex data sets can be reduced to two- and three-dimensional images for easier comprehension and interpretation.

Cluster analysis, on the other hand, groups key issues according to how similar or near in preference survey respondents scored them

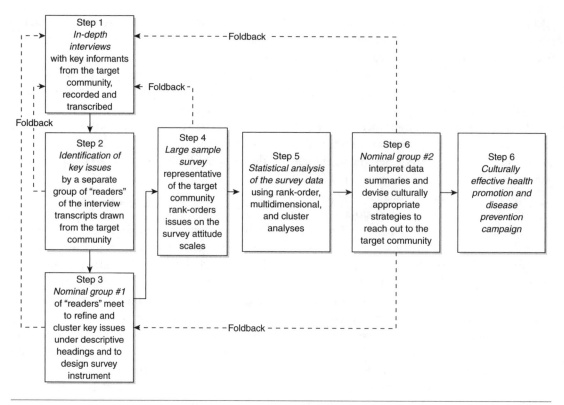

Figure 26.2   Sequence of Direct and "Foldback" Processes Involved in Foldback Analysis

across the sample (see Table 26.1). In so doing, it permits the HPDP planner to identify which issues frequently cluster with which other issues and to determine concepts that are connected in thought among the target population.

Using Foldback Analysis for Planning Health Promotion and Disease Prevention Campaigns

Because the foldback process begins with a series of open-ended interview questions, it is important to direct these questions toward the HPDP issues of concern from the onset. Generally, however, it is productive to initiate interview responses with very general questions that most people can easily answer (e.g., "In your opinion, what are the important things in life?" "Tell me about a typical day"). Answers to such questions generally afford opportunities to explore more specific questions

that might be crucial to HPDP intervention planning (e.g., community health beliefs about the target issue, barriers to HPDP use, HPDP interests and concerns, preferred channels of and locations for communication, how to craft messages to be most effective). Subsequent use of the nominal group and survey data can confirm community preferences among alternative HPDP strategies raised during the interviews.

All the issues identified on the survey instrument and analyzed in Step 5 of the process (Figure 26.2) are important because they arose from interviews with members of the target community (Step 1) and were singled out for in-depth attention by them (Steps 2 and 3). Rank-order survey data, however, permit researchers to distinguish issues of greater and lesser importance among all the community-identified key issues.

On the other hand, MDS permits HPDP planners to visualize the structure of community

Table 26.1 Cluster Analysis: What Are the Important Things in Life?

Cluster 1	Cluster 2	Cluster 3	Cluster 4	Cluster 5
(a) Hawaiian subgroup				
Me (1)	Me (1)	Knowing self (2)	Close family (10)	Safe neighborhood (11)
Knowing self (2)	Knowing self (2)	Personal values (3)	Job satisfaction (9)	Friends (12)
Setting goals (4)	Personal values (3)	Setting goals (4)	Respect for others (13)	Community involvement (14)
Job satisfaction (9)	Setting goals (4)	Health (5)	Belief in God (15)	
Close family (10)	Health (5)	Education (6)		
Respect for others (13)	Close family (10)	Children (7)		
Belief in God (15)	Friends (12)	Money (8)		
	Belief in God (15)			
(b) Non-Hawaiian subgroup				
Me (1)	Me (1)	Setting goals (4)	Personal values (3)	Belief in God (15)
Knowing self (2)	Health (5)	Education (6)	Children (7)	
Personal values (3)	Education (6)	Money (8)	Close family (10)	
Close family (10)	Children (7)	Job satisfaction (9)	Safe neighborhood (11)	
Respect for others (13)	Safe neighborhood (11)		Friends (12)	
	Friends (12)		Respect for others (13)	
			Community involvement (14)	

NOTE: Table shows inclusive items and item numbers, as in Figure 26.1.

values that underlie the identification of key issues and the rank ordering in importance of these issues by the community. MDS value maps afford multiple insights into community values that underlie and shape decision making in the target population and that will be vital to planning successful HPDP campaigns (see Figure 26.1).

First, MDS provides an estimate of how much variance in community opinion underlies each dimension in the value map. Therefore, by labeling, understanding, and stressing these value dimensions in HPDP campaigns, the planner can better reach more of the target community

For example, the first dimension in Figure 26.1 (left to right, contrasting "knowing self [2] and money [8]") accounts for 57.9% of the variance in opinion among Hawaiians.[3] Therefore, HPDP messages focused on this dimension alone could, in theory, attract the interest of three out of five residents in the Hawaiian community.

Second, interpretation and labeling of dimensions, and how best to use this information for HPDP communication within the target community, should be undertaken by the community itself. The planner should merely facilitate the process. Labeling dimensions is accomplished, first, by considering the items at the extremes of each dimension (e.g., "knowing self [2]" vs. "money [8]") and deciding what opposing constructs these items might represent (in this study, they were viewed as contrasting the "subjective" and the "material") and, second, by using these and other items along the same dimension but progressively less at the extremes (e.g., "belief in God [15], close family [10], and setting goals [4]" on the left and "community involvement [14], safe neighborhoods [11], and education [6]" on the right). The process of labeling tries to determine what common factor links all these items in their displayed progression from one end of the continuum (dimension) to the other.

In this study, the Hawaiian community labeled the first dimension "the good and successful life." By emphasizing this motto in outreach messages, the planner could better secure the interest of the Hawaiian community in the HPDP message being delivered.

Third, MDS permits the planner to understand more how individual value subsets (e.g., "health" and "belief in God") are juxtaposed in the community's overall structure of values.

To increase the importance of a targeted issue (e.g., "health"), HPDP campaign messages should link the target issue with other issues of high importance to the community (e.g., "belief in God" was the highest ranked issue by Hawaiians in this study). By developing HPDP messages that discuss the target issue ("health") and the high-ranked issue ("belief in God") in the same communication, the target issue will increase in importance.

In addition, by using interconnecting items that lie between the target and the high-ranked issues on the value maps (e.g., "personal values [3]" and "close family [10]") (i.e., a line connecting "belief in God" to "health" would pass nearest these two intermediate items on the value map displayed in Figure 26.1), the importance of a lesser valued issue ("health") can be edged progressively toward the higher valued issue ("belief in God") and elevated in importance.

For example, by using HPDP messages that couple first *personal values*—"health," then *close family-personal values*—"health," and finally *"belief in God"-close family-personal values*—"health," the concept of "health" is aided gradually toward higher importance ("belief in God") among Hawaiians.

Fourth, together with MDS, cluster analysis permits researchers to understand best how to connect most effectively issues key to the community in HPDP campaign messages. Together with the MDS results, this information can be used to tailor further HPDP outreach messages to generate maximum interest in the target community.

Cluster data can also be used to locate HPDP services (e.g., at sites in the community delivering services appearing in the same cluster as "health." For example, in Table 26.1, "health" for Hawaiians is alternately clustered with "education" and "belief in God." Therefore, to reach the Hawaiian community, it might be preferable to locate HPDP services in church and educational facilities.

Fifth, the process of creating health campaign messages that are important to the community can be enhanced further by rereading the original interview transcript data for more in-depth understanding of the rank-order survey, MDS, and cluster analyses data. That is, by using the precise words and phrases of the target community drawn from the interview transcripts, culturally tailored HPDP messages can be created.

Sixth, by conducting a second follow-up survey after intervention as part of the HPDP impact evaluation, it is possible to determine whether the targeted issue (e.g., "health") did increase in importance (i.e., was higher ranked) and move in the preferred direction on the MDS value map.

Rank-order survey data, MDS, and cluster analyses all provide means to better understand the values of the Pacific Islander community (Carroll & Green, 1997). For the second nominal group, these data are more interpretable by returning to the original focus group interview transcripts and the work of the first nominal group. Using all the foldback data, effective HPDP campaigns can be planned efficiently to have the greatest impact.

Strengths and Weaknesses of Foldback Analysis for Health Promotion and Disease Prevention

HPDP planning grounded in the values of the target community promises to have great potential for improving health promotion research, theory, and practice. Unfortunately, commonly used quantitative community assessment methods (e.g., aggregate rates of disease occurrence; knowledge, attitude, and practice survey research) seldom include in-depth "felt need" data from the subjective experience of the target population (Eakin & Maclean, 1992).

What is needed is a study approach that marries the cold preciseness of quantitative data with the richness of qualitative data in a systematic manner, that is, a study method that will focus on culturally sensitive HPDP interventions. This is particularly crucial in developing countries and with minority populations in which health service resource allocations are limited and health status needs are often greater.

Foldback analysis offers both information-rich qualitative data and objective and measurable quantitative categories that can be easily manipulated to establish priorities and to assess, plan, and evaluate HPDP outcomes from the perspective of the service community The foldback process engages (empowers) the target population throughout HPDP interventions and in the design, implementation, and analysis of the results. To date, however, the process has had limited use among Pacific Islander populations (e.g., with Hawaiians and Samoans in several studies).

The foldback analytical research model explains health behaviors in rational terms with minimal external bias but with no lack of procedural rigor. The analytic results are rich with information useful for crafting culturally appropriate campaign messages to plan improved HPDP interventions; and follow-up use of foldback analysis can serve as part of the evaluation process.

Conduct of all steps in the foldback process, however, does require an investment of time and resources. This is especially true at the front end of the project. Although possible, the adaptation of foldback analysis for rapid assessment has not yet been tested.

Although not a quick solution to HPDP planning, foldback analysis does afford a wealth of information and permits numerous opportunities for the planner to integrate with the target community. To date, the process has been used very successfully with some Pacific Islander populations.

PLANNING TARGETED PACIFIC ISLANDER HEALTH PROMOTION AND DISEASE PREVENTION CAMPAIGNS

Identification of Health Promotion and Disease Prevention Intervention Goals and Objectives

Because of the variation in economic, social, educational, and intergenerational parameters across and within Pacific Islander groups (e.g., between the main and outer islands, between home and migrant groups), it is best to tailor HPDP interventions for the greatest impact. Generally speaking, given the cognitive simplicity and heavier use of emotive strategies, it is believed that social marketing techniques would be more effective than detailed health education campaigns. Furthermore, social marketing, in addition to tailoring the message of the HPDP campaign, can use alternate delivery media and information dissemination media tailored to the infrastructure of the community and interests of the target group.

Most important, social marketing messages can be modified to the different stages of behavior change found across groups for the greatest progressive impact (Maibach, Rothschild, & Novelli, 2002). Social marketing provides a framework for looking at health decisions from the point of view of the client and enables the design of interventions that address particular issues from the client's perspective, particularly because it employs (a) population segmentation and (b) a staged approach to behavioral change (see Table 26.2).

Social marketing, in contrast to other HPDP intervention approaches, employs more emotional (e.g., making the individual "feel good" about the message) than cognitive parameters. Given the likely great variability in cognition (e.g., worldview that can vary by location, social influence, income access, and other factors) among Pacific Islander populations, emotive continuity might be greater across publics. The author believes this to be true based on the continuity of value maps he has created using foldback analysis across several Pacific Islander groups (Loos, 1994).

Furthermore, because social marketing is based on classical marketing strategies, the intention is to repeatedly capture the attention of the community segment with short, succinct fragments of information rather than long-term engagement in detailed educational strategies. Given the community segment selected,

different informational outreach tactics can be employed across settings (e.g., multiple communication media used more by the target group, in places frequented regularly such as church, work, and school) in an effort to reach the target group repeatedly and "drive home" the HPDP message.

Such announcements can be crafted from the information provided by foldback analysis and developed by the community segment itself. Short, culturally appropriate, catchy informational bits would be easier for the lay Pacific Islander public to develop and digest than would detailed HPDP educational curricula or other more cognitive-based approaches (see also Weinreich's [1999] *Hands-On Social Marketing*).

The hallmark of social marketing responsiveness is the needs, issues, and unique situations of consumers in creating programs or interventions, because otherwise there is a risk of developing programs that are not effective. Putting the consumer first (i.e., empowerment) on a continuing basis is what separates social marketing from health education or information programs. In fact, if consumers are kept in the center of the program with continuing dialogue (e.g., by using ongoing focus group processes), then the results always are a program built from the bottom up.

At the onset of the project, HPDP personnel, in collaboration with the Pacific Islander community, can target health issues of importance to the community and determine which segments of the community are at greatest risk. Once these are identified, representatives from those community segments can be engaged in a foldback analysis to identify their HPDP parameters of importance and preferred social marketing strategies,

Foldback analysis also can be used to determine the target group's current stage of behavior change, so intervention objectives and goals can be identified (see Table 26.2). The objective of social marketing is to move the behavior of the community segment from its

Table 26.2 Schematic Overview of Stages of Behavioral Change and Social Marketing Strategic Issues

Stage	Precontemplation	Early Contemplation	Later Contemplation	Preparation to Act	Action Initiated	Commitment to Act	Maintenance of Action
Message issue	Make TP aware of new behavioral possibility and that it is not antithetical to TP's values	Persuade and motivate selected TP market segments to undertake new behavior by stressing its benefits	Persuade and motivate selected TP market segment to undertake new behavior by stressing its lower costs compared with status quo	Encourage self-efficacy of target and heighten social desirability of and support for new behaviors	Orchestrate TP opportunity for successful first experience	Determine whether new behavior is a onetime or repeated but finite action, situational action, or permanent lifestyle change	Anticipate what might thwart continued use and expansion of new behavior
Marketing goal	Increase TP's awareness and interest; change inhibiting TP values; identify barriers; overcome TP's ignorance and presumed irrelevance for TP	Create TP's perception of benefits and positive consequences of new behaviors and negative consequences of status quo	Create TP's perception of lower personal costs associated with new behaviors and higher costs for continuance of status quo	Instill TP's personal belief that its members have the capacity to change and that TP's social milieu will support new behaviors versus the status quo	Make TP's first experience as rewarding as possible	Make continued action possible (i.e., reduce task complexity and time required); increase TP's priority for new behavior among competing behaviors	Create a win-win experience (e.g., prescribed social behavior change is adopted, and target is happy with change)
Prime strategy	Provide education and propaganda to increase TP's perceived personal risk for status quo	Create a superior exchange of new behavior for old behavior that TP finds socially desirable, is easily undertaken, and affords TP added benefits	Create belief that perceived costs related to new behaviors are less than status quo costs and/or are manageable costs	Overcome TP's perceived lack of personal capacity and presumption of social opposition	Organize external environment to permit behavior to occur; it is urgent to get TP commitment to desired action on the spot	Make opportunities for behavior as convenient and painless as possible for TP commitment to desired action on the spot	Afford constant reminders and TP-appropriate reinforcers

(Continued)

Table 26.2 (Continued)

Stage	Precontemplation	Early Contemplation	Later Contemplation	Preparation to Act	Action Initiated	Commitment to Act	Maintenance of Action
Study caution	Consumers see few benefits and many costs at this stage	Use a single core strategy; emphasize benefits, not costs; focus on likelihood that benefits will occur and their value and importance to TP	Focus on short-term costs and cost reduction and efficiency-enhancing strategies TP can use	Cultural norms and values will differ for different TP segments	For major changes in behavior or lifestyle, "sequential approximation" of the ideal, repeated steps that are socially reinforced, might be required for TP to adjust slowly	Make the complex simple; success breeds success; some outcomes are less wonderful than TP imagined or are hard for TP to detect	Old habits die hard, especially when new behaviors are not as easy, convenient, and rewarding as TP expected (i.e., negative consequences can become excessive)
Research questions	What are TP's preferred media for communication? Times, places, and circumstances TP is receptive to message. Do different TP segments require different messages?	What benefits does TP believe will occur? How important are these things to TP? Focus on precise benefits and values, not benefit attributes or long-term outcomes.	What are perceived costs related to new behavior, and why is each cost important to TP? What are TP's preferences among combinations of benefits and costs?	Who are TP's opinion leaders? identify TP's social networks and who its members turn to for advice; who are TP's role models?	What are TP's personal rewards? Is TP's locus of control internal or external?	What are TP's barriers and triggers to action? What are new behavior's intrinsic and extrinsic rewards?	How can one improve delivery system, enlist social support, make benefits more visible, control TP expectations, and provide TP with skill training as needed?

SOURCE: Adapted from Andreasen (1995).

NOTE: TP = target population.

members' current stage of behavior to the next (more preferred) stage of behavior, with the long-term goal that HPDP behavior is sustained in an ongoing manner.

Selecting Appropriate Implementation Strategies

To implement strategies successfully in any culture group, it is important to be sensitive to its members' life view and learning and teaching styles. The need for such sensitivity is no less true for Pacific Islanders. How these people project, accept, and react to new ideas being proposed by "health experts" is filtered through their values, which influence how they perceive issues and what to seek, avoid, or ignore. Pacific Islander values may be subject to modification, provided that new ideas are presented through accepted social channels and processes. Therefore, these mechanisms must be identified and employed appropriately if HPDP campaigns are to be effective.

The ideas that follow, in large part, are drawn from (and might be limited by) the author's 20 years of professional experience in the areas of education and public health in the Pacific Basin and Pacific Rim. They are not meant to be fully inclusive.

Conceptions of Knowledge

In many Pacific Islander cultures, illness is considered the result of some moral transgression or the "hot" or "cold" nature of things. Presented without sensitivity, modern disease theory does not make sense to people with such beliefs.

Thus, it is crucial that the HPDP change agent understand that his or her advice might be misunderstood or ignored by people who operate with another concept of reality and understanding for cause and effect. The change agent must also appreciate that his or her values (e.g., the high value placed on good health and the maintenance of personal and environmental cleanliness) might not be mutually or similarly held across publics.

For Pacific Islanders, the learning of knowledge must incorporate both intellect and emotion—both head and heart. The power of the word must go hand-in-hand with a wholeness and connectedness to life. This final point is very different from the compartmentalization of Western thought.

Furthermore, among Pacific Islanders, knowledge is viewed as precious, something that should be aspired to but not too easily attained. Barriers to learning knowledge should be high enough to test learners' commitment and perseverance as well as appreciation once knowledge is attained. Holders of knowledge deserve respect so long as they earn it and deserve to be abandoned if they do not.

Knowledge also belongs to the group, not to the individual. As repositories of knowledge, individuals are (as trustees) expected to use it for the good of all. On the other hand, experts should not teach all that they know, thus forcing learners to hypothesize and invent as they learn. As such, the "problem-based" approach to teaching often is productive with Pacific Islander groups because of its heuristic aspects, in contrast to instruction that is solely didactic.

Traditional communities have numerous opinion leaders whom the change agent should engage in his or her HPDP efforts. For many Pacific Islander communities, these opinion leaders include family chief, church, and village leaders; traditional healers and birth attendants; or even local schoolteachers and postal workers. Less formal leaders might include local area recognized storytellers, market hawkers, and any area vendors where select publics might congregate (e.g., barber).

Furthermore, it is important to remember that many island cultures are matriarchal and that women remain important, although perhaps less formal, leaders of community opinion. It also should be remembered that socialization in many Pacific Islander communities, more than in the West, is still centered on strong gender-related roles in domestic and select public domains and that some topics might be taboo by gender.

Learning Styles

Whereas individuation and individual performance is fostered early in life in most Western cultures, communal behavior and learning is fostered early in the lives of Pacific Islanders. During the formative years, families assign chores to sibling groups, the eldest child usually taking the lead. This group approach to learning remains pervasive throughout life and across Pacific Islander groups.

For example, in controlled studies (Kamehameha Schools, 1985) conducted at the Kamehameha Early Education Program during the early 1980s, it was discovered that Hawaiian children taught using Western and indigenous study methods differed in performance. Both groups of children performed equally and on par with other ethnic groups on entry to the study. The children who were permitted continued use of group learning strategies, similar to child-rearing strategies found in Hawaiian homes, performed much better throughout their early academic years. In contrast, students who were required to adopt the Western instructional style (e.g., individualized seating, performance, and grading) fell behind progressively.

These studies suggest that group assessment, intervention, and evaluation strategies (e.g., focus group interviews) are apt to be more successful than is work with individuals. Furthermore, individualized assessments (e.g., testing such as the use of questionnaire forms) are typically less palatable to Pacific Islanders.

Much learning for Pacific Islanders is informal and semiconscious (e.g., through observation or embedded in the ongoing life of the community). Many lessons are conveyed indirectly in the course of doing something else (e.g., during chance social encounters or meetings of groups for entirely other purposes such as women's weaving).

For example, quilt making is popular among many Pacific Islander women, and successful HPDP communication can occur during such times. The Kamehameha Educational Research Institute used designs created by the target community and related to child growth and development as panels for quilts; as each quilt was constructed, the quilters discussed the importance of the information depicted in each panel.

Typically, prospective learners are put into group activity situations with a range of expertise and are "seeded" with experts, where participation is required. Newcomers are given assistance to develop skills and understanding but are largely left to observe, "pick things up," and hone their capacities for themselves. Sometimes, apprentice-like or tutorial strategies are employed such as when a more competent worker is paired with someone less skilled and they work on projects together.

As such, there is much emphasis on the learners looking, listening, and imitating with a minimum of verbal exchange. Groups of learners work side by side learning by demonstration, trial and error, and joint effort. Moreover, certain things should be done only in context and for real rather than just practiced (i.e., learning by doing tasks in their proper setting). Therefore, learning work site injury prevention is done on the job rather than discussed in a classroom removed from the work site.

Among Pacific Islanders, the "medium *is* the message" because it helps shape and control the search and form of their associations and actions. Considering the isolation and lack of utilities on many of the Pacific Islands, especially the outermost ones, use of advanced media (e.g., television, videos, the Internet) is less prudent. Instead, "talk story" in "under the tree" small groups, radio broadcasts, the use of folk media (e.g., music, song, drama, dance, storytelling, proverbs), role-playing, and the use of pictorial presentations (e.g., wood carvings, paintings, shaded drawings [National Development Service, 1976, pp. 12–18], as well as cartoons and comic books) are preferable. All these vehicles are accessible and acceptable communication modes and media (Maibach & Parrott, 1995).

Appropriate learning materials are essential tools for community health promotion and health communication. The above-listed ways of conveying health messages to island publics are also good ways to involve the local community. That is, local composers, musicians, dancers, artists, actors, storytellers, and comedians should be involved in developing culturally appropriate health messages.

The best promotional materials should combine expert knowledge presented by peer instructors and materials producers. The risk of stating a message using incorrect "phraseology" and/or in terms that appear condescending or preachy is lessened when peer language and peer art are used.

Selection of credible spokespersons and recognized artists also strengthens the message. In addition, it is prudent to deliver HPDP messages at locations typically frequented by Pacific Islander groups (e.g., churches, sports clubs, community festivals) rather than more formal settings (e.g., clinics).

It is best to reinforce general or abstract ideas with specific, concrete examples or illustrations. Indeed, it is often best to use learners' own statements and productions in the promotional materials (e.g., these can be drawn from foldback interview transcripts).

Be specific and concise; do not use idioms unless they are well-known (e.g., soda and chips vs. junk foods). Use common terminology rather than professional jargon (e.g., baby shots vs. vaccinations). Use direct, positive statements rather than complex, negative sentences (e.g., "You get vitamin A and fiber when you eat fruits and vegetables" vs. "Studies show that if you don't eat fruits and vegetables, then needed nutrients and roughage required for good health will be absent").

Teaching Styles

Several "lessons" are often imparted at once (e.g., through storytelling that may or may not be directed at participants but rather at eavesdroppers nearby). Those who have knowledge to depart frequently make it difficult for learners to comprehend easily. For example, snippets of information are "thrown out," often without context or detail.

Pacific Islander trainers often refuse to give reasons or explanations for why things must be done and generally discourage questions. Stress is laid on memorization of the "right" way in which to do something. The responsibility for learning is placed on learners rather than teachers.

Sometimes, teachers tease learners for mistakes, but praise and blame are typically addressed to the group, and singling out of individuals in public is avoided. Disciplining is shared; it is done by whoever is closer. Correction can be heated, even physical, but sustained punishment is not condoned.

"Experts" favor the modest and withhold instruction from the arrogant. More important than individual attainment is learning to work with others and the skills of interpersonal relations and cooperation.

The teaching of certain types of knowledge is restricted on the basis of gender, descent, ability, and maturity, and these parameters can vary across Pacific Islander groups. It is best to permit the community to select the appropriate type of trainer for each topic taught.

EVALUATION OF HEALTH PROMOTION AND DISEASE PREVENTION STRATEGIES

Strengths and Weaknesses of Current Evaluation Methods

One obstacle to successful evaluation has been the way in which many HPDP activities are planned using an orientation to problems (instead of strengths) and that emphasize the medical model (e.g., natural sciences in the study of illnesses, which isolates individuals from their environment). The medical model is appropriate for linking a certain behavior to a specific disease (justifying the demand for HPDP), but its focus is too narrow to understand the social, economic, and cultural factors that underlie the behavior.

Increasingly, health promotion planning frameworks (e.g., the PRECEDE model, Green & Kreuter, 2005) direct attention at solutions (not just problems) and at intervention processes (not just program inputs). These same models focus correctly on intervening parameters (e.g., predisposing, enabling, and reinforcing factors) that can influence beliefs and attitudes and behavioral outcomes. As advocated throughout this chapter, these models must extend this same focus to program implementation strategies and the evaluation of program outcomes among Pacific Islanders.

The planner and the community participants must be involved in the evaluation process. Each wants to know what the program accomplished without being influenced by subjective judgments or political motives. The participation of the community in this process helps empower *them* to determine if the program met their needs toward achieving optimal health (see Chapter 7, this volume).

Disaggregative and reductionist views created by Western models of medicine are not adequate to assess HPDP programs for Pacific Islanders given their all-inclusive ecological, cosmic view of health and disease. To evaluate the contribution of HPDP initiatives, the opinion of lay publics of Pacific Islanders should be included using criteria of import to the Pacific Islanders themselves.

Good HPDP results among Pacific Islanders will require careful preparation to account properly for socioeconomic or cultural factors and variations. To accomplish this, the community must be involved. Indeed, the direct involvement of the target group in all HPDP project phases—assessment, planning, implementation,

and evaluation—might be the most crucial aspect for project success. This is true because only Pacific Islanders can accurately view their HPDP issues holistically. This advocacy is appropriate regardless of whether a target population resides in the Islands or has migrated.

Provided that the targeted Pacific Islander community segment has been involved throughout the HPDP process (e.g., from analysis to intervention), its members should determine the evaluation process as well. That is, it is *their* determination of HPDP need, HPDP project goals and objectives, and intervention design that is being evaluated. Therefore, it is best that they should determine how well these needs, goals, and objectives were met and how well intervention processes were conducted.

Process and Summative Evaluation Strategies

Community involvement may be critically important to successful HPDP among Pacific Islanders and is advocated throughout this chapter. Suggestions previously presented have related to culturally sensitive HPDP analysis, and intervention strategies apply equally to the development of process and summative evaluation methods.

Because HPDP initiatives with Pacific Islanders *must* include community involvement throughout, it is also crucial to evaluate the community's acceptance of these processes of involvement (e.g., the nature and scope of community participation, how it was initiated and sustained, whether it was productive and satisfying to the participants). Process evaluations among Pacific Islanders are better conducted using action-participatory research (e.g., employing ongoing focus group and talk-story strategies more than using paper-and-pencil activities).

Summative aspects of the project (e.g., the improvements in health awareness, policy and advocacy, health status, and health services use) can employ community participation as well. For example, a follow-up foldback assessment can be used to demonstrate whether targeted attitudes and values changed in the preferred direction, and observation strategies can be used to evaluate targeted behavior change.

The use of objective secondary analysis of extant data and project records by the researcher can be also employed because it need not involve the target community to gather and tabulate the data. The interpretation of these data, however, should be discussed with the community to better understand the meaning behind the numbers.

Health Promotion and Disease Prevention Materials Evaluation

Specific to printed materials used for HPDP campaigns (e.g., text, pictorial), it is recommended that they be tested using the Cloze Test (Folmer, Moynihan, & Schothorst, 1992, pp. 37–39). By deleting every nth word or picture segment, the Cloze Test ascertains how much of the message is still understood by the target population. That is, the more familiar the target population is with the subject, the easier it is to convey messages.

When materials are written in the native language, deleting every 5th through 7th word is suggested; when the materials are in a second language, it is recommended that every 10th through 12th word be left out.[4] A modified approach can be used for pictorial information (e.g., leaving out selected lines in a drawing).

Readability analysis should also consider the number of syllables per word and the number of words per sentence. Text that uses fewer syllables and words is generally easier to read.[5] Conrath, Doak, and Root (1996) have written an excellent text that incorporates many helpful examples and tools concerning assessing readability and for teaching individuals with low literacy skills (see also

Zarcadoolas, Pleasant, & Greer (2006, pp. 287–313).

Finally, it is crucial to assess the materials directly, through solicited feedback from the target audience, by questionnaire or (preferably) by focus group interviews.

CHAPTER SUMMARY

To achieve significant improvements in the health status of Pacific Islanders, HPDP must become a priority. Although Pacific Island groups are sensitive to maintaining health and staving off disease, their perceptions of how best this is accomplished might be based on belief patterns and value structures that are uniquely their own.

For Pacific Islanders, the design, conduct, and evaluation of HPDP intervention strategies will be most successful when they employ "local" involvement in the production, implementation, and analysis. For Pacific Islanders, it is crucial for communities to make and follow up on their own conclusions.

Consumer-oriented perspectives, such as those provided by community empowerment, foldback analysis, and social marketing, are viewed as crucial to promoting health and preventing disease among Pacific Islanders. This is especially true because these methods are focused on and employ social groups as a whole and facilitate social action that is fundamental to the willing engagement of Pacific Islander populations.

To achieve healthy outcomes in the islands themselves and among expatriate populations of Pacific Islanders, it is essential that they be empowered to direct the HPDP process throughout (i.e., from assessment and planning, to intervention, to evaluation). Otherwise, Pacific Islanders will not engage HPDP concepts or sustain HPDP practices if they are not their own. Perhaps this is true for other ethnic groups as well, but it is central to Pacific Islander cultures.

Historical deductive methods, popular with the professional health community, cannot guarantee that they will identify needs and prescribe interventions that are supported by the Pacific Islander community. These methods emphasize professional hypothesis testing, with little attention devoted to inductive approaches aimed at generating culturally based health and disease hypotheses and concepts.

Foldback analysis, as a method of behavioral research, is particularly appropriate for engaging Pacific Islander communities in their own behavioral health analyses. Because foldback processes use the target community throughout—employing the researcher as a process facilitator—the results are highly meaningful locally

The foldback process empowers the community in its own behavior analysis. To the extent possible, the researcher also becomes a participant and is viewed less as an outsider because he or she works *with* the community to assess HPDP needs and to plan and evaluate HPDP interventions.

Because of its tailored and paced approach to change based on the wants of the target audience and involving its members centrally throughout, social marketing HPDP intervention strategies are apt to work best with Pacific Islander populations. This is particularly true when considering the great variability of Pacific Islander group context, individual circumstance, and diversity of experiences found among the different groups and across subgroups. Because social marketing emphasizes stages of behavior change, HPDP strategies may be refined for different population segments and paced for progressive success.

On many of the islands, especially those of the South Pacific, the traditional collective responsibility system remains vital to the delivery of community services. This system also should be effective for promoting healthy community HPDP habits and lifestyles encouraged in this chapter (WHO, 1993).

The fundamental essence of HPDP for Pacific Islanders lies in community involvement for social action. The community

empowerment, foldback assessment, and social marketing frameworks presented in this chapter should help create a receptive environment among Pacific Islanders for HPDP materials and programs.

NOTES

1. Relatively speaking, among cultural groups, there is strong continuity of social practices across Pacific Islander populations and consistency across settings within groups. Even when Pacific Islander populations relocate, social protocols and practices remain very much intact—even if other populations (e.g., coworkers, non-Pacific Islander groups) are engaged as surrogates for the familial and social groups left behind (see Ablon, 1971; Hanna, Fitzgerald, Pearson, Howard, & Hanna, 1990; Loos, Hatcher, & Shein, 1997).

2. Most common statistical software packages (e.g., SPSS) include the appropriate analyses for foldback analysis procedures. One very affordable package, however, is by Borgatti (1992).

3. The first dimension for the non-Hawaiian group accounted for only 42.1% of the variance in opinion, implying that (a) this group is significantly less collective in its opinion (this makes sense given that its members are less uniform culturally) and (b) more dimensions would have to be considered to craft health promotion messages to reach as much of the non-Hawaiian community (i.e., the first dimension, at more than 40%, could address the primary value structures of only two of every five non-Hawaiians).

4. To calculate a readability score, the number of missing words correctly identified by the test population is divided by the total number of words deleted and then multiplied by 100. When 60% or more of the missing words are correctly identified, the language is correct. Scoring lower than 60% suggests that the text should be rewritten.

5. One approach, the Rudolph Flesch method, uses the following formula: Reading ease = 206.835—(.846 × Average number of syllables per 100 words)—(1.015 × Average sentence length). Scores under 60 are increasingly difficult, scores 60 to 70 are standard, and scores more than 70 are increasingly easy.

DISCUSSION QUESTIONS AND ACTIVITIES

1. Identify and weigh the costs and benefits of taking time up-front to engage the target community when planning social marketing campaigns. Are the benefits you identify always worth the costs at each stage in behavioral change?

2. Explain the benefits of scaling methods over other statistical procedures when developing community value maps. Why are these benefits important when working with different stakeholder groups?

3. Suggest three ways the author should measure the effectiveness of the social marketing campaign with the Native Hawaiian community he describes.

The next chapter presents a case study where the author tries to emphasize points made in the overview and planning chapters. The study is concerned with the application of concepts and approaches for bridging the gap between theory and practice. They provide an opportunity for the student and the practitioner to get a "bird's-eye" view of some of the specific methods and techniques of HPDP program planning, application, and problem solving.

REFERENCES

Ablon, J. (1971). Retention of cultural values and differential urban adaptation: Samoans and American Indians in a west coast city. *Social Forces, 49,* 385–393.

Andreasen, A. R. (1995). *Marketing social change: Changing behavior to promote health, social development, and the environment.* San Francisco: Jossey-Bass.

Arlin, P. (1975). Cognitive development in adulthood: A fifth stage. *Developmental Psychology, 11,* 602–606.

Boddington, B., Khawaja, M., & Didham, R. (2003). Teenage fertility in New Zealand. In *Key Statistics, September 2003* (pp. 9–13). Wellington, New Zealand: Statistics New Zealand, Demographic Division.

Borgatti, S. P. (1992). *ANTHROPAC 4.0.* Columbia, SC: Analytic Technologies.

Carroll, J. D., & Green, P. E. (1997). Psychometric methods in market research. II: Multidimensional scaling. *Journal of Marketing Research, 34,* 193–204.

Conrath, C., Doak, L. G., & Root, J. H. D. (1996). *Teaching patients with low literacy skills* (2nd ed.). Hagerstown, MD: J. B. Lippincott.

Cronbach, L. J. (1982). *Designing evaluations of educational and social programs.* San Francisco: Jossey-Bass.

Eakin, J. M., & Maclean, H. M. (1992). A critical perspective on research and knowledge development in health promotion. *Canadian Journal of Public Health, 83*(Suppl.), S72–S76.

Folmer, H. R., Moynihan, M. N., & Schothorst, P. M. (1992). *Testing and evaluation manuals: Making health learning materials more useful.* Amsterdam: Royal Tropical Institute.

Ghosh, C. (2003). Healthy people 2010 and Asian Americans/Pacific Islanders: Defining a baseline of information. *American Journal of Public Health, 93*(12), 2093–2098.

Green, L. W., & Kreuter, M. W. (2005). *Health program planning: An educational and ecological approach* (4th ed.). New York: McGraw-Hill.

Hanna, J. M., Fitzgerald, M. H., Pearson, J. D., Howard, A., & Hanna, J. M. (1990). Selective migration from Samoa: A longitudinal study of pre-migration differences in social and psychological characteristics. *Social Biology, 37,* 204–214.

Hawaii State Department of Health. (1988). *Timely prevention: The key to healthy children.* Honolulu, HI: Department of Health, Office of Research and Statistics.

Hawaii State Department of Health. (1991). *Ka Papahana O Ka 'Ohana Ola Hawai'i.* Honolulu, HI: Department of Health, Office of Research and Statistics.

Janes, C. R. (1990). *Migration, social change, and health: A Samoan community in urban California.* Stanford, CA: Stanford University Press.

Janz, N. K., Champion, V. L., & Strecher, V. J. (2002). The Health Belief Model. In K. Glantz, B. K. Rimer, & F. M. Lewis (Eds.), *Health behavior and health education: Theory, research, and practice* (3rd ed., pp. 45–66). San Francisco: Jossey-Bass.

Kamehameha Educational Research Institute. (1983). *Life views of Hawaiians and non-Hawaiians: What are the important things in life?* Honolulu, HI: Author.

Kamehameha Educational Research Institute. (1984). *The "important things in life," for Hawaiians and non-Hawaiians.* Honolulu, HI: Author.

Kamehameha Educational Research Institute. (1985). *The perceived service needs of pregnant and parenting teens and adults on the Wai'anae Coast.* Honolulu, HI: Author.

Kamehameha Schools. (1985). *Developmental risk indicators and early childhood education services for Native American Hawaiians.* Honolulu, HI: Author.

Kim, U. (1990). *Culture, health care system and prenatal care: An analysis of three ethnic communities in Hawai'i.* Unpublished manuscript, University of Hawaii.

Kinloch, P. (1985). *Talking health but doing sickness: Studies in Samoan health.* Wellington, New Zealand: Victoria University Press.

Kumabe, K. T., Nishida, C., & Hepworth, D. H. (1985). *Bridging ethnocultural diversities in social work and health.* Unpublished manuscript, University of Hawaii.

Labarthe, D., Reed, D., Brody, J., & Stallones, R. (1973). Health effects of modernization in Palau. *American Journal of Epidemiology, 98,* 161–174.

Loos, G. P. (1994). A blended qualitative-quantitative assessment model for identifying and rank-ordering service needs of indigenous people. *Journal of Evaluation and Program Planning, 18,* 237–244.

Loos, G. P. (1995). Foldback analysis: A method to reduce researcher bias in health behavior research. *Qualitative Inquiry, 1,* 465–480.

Loos, G. P. (1998). *Value differences among Hawaiians and non-Hawaiians.* Unpublished manuscript, National Institute for Occupational Safety and Health.

Loos, G. P., Hatcher, P., & Shein, T. (1994). *Preventive health behaviors of Samoans in Hawai'i and American Samoa: A behavioral health research study.* Unpublished manuscript, University of Hawaii.

Loos, G. P., Hatcher, P., & Shein, T. (1997). Health behavior strategies to improve rates of immunizations among Samoans. *Pacific Health Dialog, 3*(2), 166–177.

Maibach, E., & Parrott, R. L. (Eds.). (1995). *Designing health messages: Approaches from communication theory and public health practice.* Thousand Oaks, CA: Sage.

Maibach, E. W., Rothschild, M. L., & Novelli, W. D. (2002). Social marketing. In K. Glantz, B. K. Rimer, & F. M. Lewis (Eds.), *Health behavior and health education: Theory, research, and practice* (3rd ed., pp. 437–461). San Francisco: Jossey-Bass.

Minkler, M. (2004). *Community organizing and community building for health* (3rd ed.). Piscataway, NJ: Rutgers University Press.

Minkler, M., & Wallerstein, N. B. (2002). Improving health through community organization and community building. In K. Glantz, B. K. Rimer, & F. M. Lewis (Eds.), *Health behavior and health education: Theory, research, and practice* (pp. 279–311). San Francisco: Jossey-Bass.

Montano, D. E., & Kasprzyk, D. (2002). The Theory of Reasoned Action and the Theory of Planned Behavior. In K. Glantz, B. K. Rimer, & F. M. Lewis (Eds.), *Health behavior and health education: Theory, research, and practice* (3rd ed., pp. 67–98). San Francisco: Jossey-Bass.

National Development Service. (1976). *Communicating with pictures in Nepal.* Kathmandu, Nepal: United Nations Children's Fund.

Oldenburg, B., & Parcel, G. S. (2002). Diffusion of Innovations. In K. Glantz, B. K. Rimer, & F. M. Lewis (Eds.), *Health behavior and health education: Theory, research, and practice* (3rd ed., pp. 312–324). San Francisco: Jossey-Bass.

Palafox, N., & Warren, A. (Eds.). (1980). *Cross-cultural caring: Transcultural health care forum.* Honolulu: University of Hawaii, John A. Burns School of Medicine.

Pan Asian Parent Education Project. (1982). *Pan Asian child rearing practices: Filipino, Japanese, Korean, Samoan, Vietnamese.* San Diego: Author.

Peter, L. J. (1980). *Ideas for our time.* New York: Bantam Books.

Prior, I. A. (1974). Cardiovascular epidemiology in New Zealand and the Pacific. *New Zealand Medical Journal, 80,* 245–252.

Prochaska, J. O., Redding, C. A., & Evers, K. E. (2002). The Transtheoretical Model and Stages of Change. In K. Glantz, B. K. Rimer, & F. M. Lewis (Eds.), *Health behavior and health education: Theory, research, and practice* (3rd ed., pp. 99–120). San Francisco: Jossey-Bass.

Raeburn, J. (1992). Health promotion research with heart: Keeping a people perspective. *Canadian Journal of Public Health, 83*(Suppl.), 20–24.

Rogers, E. M. (2003). *Diffusion of innovation* (5th ed.). New York: Free Press.

Stevenson, H. M., & Burke, M. (1992). Bureaucratic logic in new social movement clothing: The limits of health promotion research. *Canadian Journal of Public Health, 83*(Suppl.), S47–S52.

U.S. Department of Health and Human Services. (2000, November). *Healthy people 2010: Understanding and improving health* (2nd ed.). Washington, DC: Government Printing Office.

U.S. Department of Health and Human Services, President's Advisory Commission on Asian Americans and Pacific Islanders. (2003). *Asian Americans and Pacific Islanders addressing health disparities: Opportunities for building a healthier America.* Washington, DC: Government Printing Office.

Wallerstein, N. (1992). Powerlessness, empowerment, and health: Implications for health promotion programs. *American Journal of Health Promotion, 6,* 197–205.

Weinreich, N. K. (1999). *Hands-on social marketing: A step-by-step guide.* Thousand Oaks, CA: Sage.

World Health Organization. (1975). *The prevention and control of cardiovascular disease.* Manila, the Philippines: Western Pacific Regional Office, WHO.

World Health Organization. (1990). *Western Pacific region data bank on socioeconomic and health indicators.* Manila, the Philippines: Western Pacific Regional Office, WHO.

World Health Organization. (1993). *Implementation of the global strategy for health for all by the year 2000* (Vol. 7). Manila, the Philippines: Western Pacific Regional Office, WHO.

Zarcadoolas, C., Pleasant, A. F., & Greer, D. S. (2006). *Advancing health literacy: A framework for understanding and action.* San Francisco: Jossey-Bass

27

Promoting Health in Pacific Islander Populations

Case Studies

D. WILLIAM WOOD

CLAIRE K. HUGHES

Chapter Objectives

On completion of this chapter, the health promotion student and practitioner will be able to

- Identify and discuss at least five factors that would be important to consider when working with Pacific Islander population groups

- Identify and discuss the long-term health effects of shifting from a traditional islander diet to a more Western diet

- Identify and discuss at least three culturally sensitive and appropriate intervention strategies one can use when working with Pacific Islander population groups

The dramatic improvements in health care and social conditions in many developed countries have resulted in the near eradication of many infectious diseases. This epidemiological transition has meant that these nations are now faced with new diseases as the focus of attention for their health systems. These chronic diseases do not respond to treatment as did the infectious diseases; Dr. Ehrlich's "magic bullets" (Brandt, 1987, p. 40) seem ineffective in fighting these diseases, leaving both the medical system and the patients powerless to attain cures. With improved understanding of the etiology of these chronic conditions, prevention becomes the first line of defense against the pandemic.

As a chronic disease, type 2 diabetes (non-insulin-dependent diabetes mellitus [NIDDM]) is a particularly insidious condition.

> The complications of Type II diabetes take root long before diagnosis is made. Type II diabetes is a "silent disease" that does not have the dramatic clinical onset characteristic of Type I diabetes. Several studies show that among Type II [diabetes] patients, 10%–20% already have complications such as retinopathy or neuropathy. (Zimmet & McCarty, 1995, p. 8)

Often taking as long as 10 or 20 years to manifest, the sequelae of the untreated condition are devastating to the patient. The peripheral neuropathies often lead to amputations, retinopathies often lead to blindness, and renal failure often leads to end-stage renal disease, with dialysis and death its all too common outcome. In part because of the insidious nature of the condition, its lack of initially clear signs and symptoms, and the fact that the academic preparation of medical practitioners often has less focus on chronic diseases than perhaps it should, it is estimated that the best of prevalence rates underestimate the condition by more than 50%.

Paul Zimmet, an internationally noted expert on diabetes, reports,

> By the year 2010, the global number of people with diabetes could have risen from 100 million to 240 million. . . . We expect the prevalence of diabetes in Latin America to double to 19 million. . . . The numbers could increase to 28 million in Europe and to 14 million in the former U.S.S.R., but the regions with the greatest potential increase by far are Asia and Africa. (Zimmet & McCarty, 1995, p. 16)

Data for the islands of the Pacific are less reliable but suggest similar patterns. In Hawaii, no seroprevalence studies have been completed, but a recent monograph on diabetes suggests that not only are the rates increasing, they are doing so differentially across ethnic groups (Wood, 1994). Evidence from the islands of the Pacific also points to a rapid change in prevalence and a serious problem emerging with the disease (Federated States of Micronesia [FSM], 1997).

In fact, a suspected problem exists across the Pacific and among most indigenous peoples of the world. As is evidenced elsewhere—Native Americans, Aborigines in Australia, Chamorros in Guam, Samoans in both American Samoa and Western Samoa—all are affected. This chapter focuses on diabetes prevention among Pacific Islanders in their natural settings, with the hope that interpretation of what seems to work "at home" will be possible for those Pacific Islanders resident in the continental United States.

The authors' expectation, within any of the literature searches performed for this chapter, was that many discussions about cultural competence and health programs for minority groups would emerge. This turned out, in general, not to be the case, meaning that discussions of minority populations did not necessitate discussions about cultural competence for health programs. Because the authors' initial review of the literature did not yield all the information in which they were interested, the authors broadened the search to include cultural competence issues that were not necessarily associated with health activities.

What are the factors that the health promoter must consider if he or she were to develop a culturally sensitive health promotion program for minorities? The recent literature suggests the following.

Sinclair (1991) suggests that when considering minorities, age, education, economics, and community also should be considered or controlled in the development of a culturally sensitive program that is to be effective. Avila and Hovell (1994) found that exercise and diet modification training among Latinas was effective in decreasing obesity and increasing fitness within the targeted group, Mexican American women of low socioeconomic status ($N = 44$). The Shintani et al. and Hawaii-based Traditional Hawaiian Diet (THD) programs represent a Native Hawaiian, community-based activity developed as a response to the high rates of obesity and chronic illness associated with this ethnic affiliation (Shintani, Beckham, O'Connor, Hughes, & Sato, 1994). The THD is a 3-week program that relies on eight interventions: a noncaloric restricted weight loss program, dietary clinical intervention, cultural sensitivity, a transition diet, a whole-person approach, group support, community intervention, and role modeling.

Obesity often is associated with NIDDM. Auslander, Haire-Joshu, Houston, and Fisher (1992) worked with obese African Americans of lower socioeconomic status, as one example. Their intervention was community based, focusing on four community organization strategies: integrating community values into health messages, facilitating neighborhood decision making, making use of formal and informal networks, and empowering.

In addition, outreach strategies are suggested to reach the African American population, as shown by Nakyonyi's (1993) work in Canada. A community-based outreach AIDS information program was presented that relies on educational material and media contacts. Educational material was suggested on various subjects, including misconceptions, marriage, sexuality, confidentiality, basic HIV/AIDS information, condoms, homophobia, and the use of videos.

Other health promotion programs also are culturally sensitive. Whereas Auslander's et al. (1992) and Nakyonyi's (1993) previous efforts focused on the African American population, the work of Samolsky, Dunker, and Hynak-Hankinson (1990) focused on the major health problem associated with the Hispanic population. Their work focused on energy, fat

and salt diet modification, and the importance of considering both cultural and demographic influences in helping this population. Heath, Wilson, Smith, and Leonard (1991) state that cardiovascular disease also is a problem for the Zuni Indians and suggest participation in a community-based exercise program and the benefits associated with weight loss competitions.

Forety (1994) observed in a study that the Mexican American participants in their family-oriented approach were divided among three groups: a booklet-only comparison group, an individual group that received the booklet and 1 year of classes, and a family group that received the booklet and 1 year of family classes. Not surprisingly, their unsurprising results were that those in the individual and family yearlong group sessions had greater weight losses than did those in the pamphlet-based, information-only group.

Alternatively, Rogler, Cortes, and Malgady (1994) suggest that a culturally sensitive program for Puerto Ricans (in New York City) would reflect and consider idiomatic phrases associated with anguish. Their work started with focus groups, then solicited important volunteers from the community, and finally compared the information obtained with the views of community-based mental health professionals. Their work suggested that sensitivity to idiomatic expressions more often was associated with an increase in the use of services.

Similarly, de Leon Siantz's (1990) work, predominantly with Mexican American migrant farm workers (but also with Cubans and Puerto Ricans), emphasized lifestyles, problems, and strengths and needs often associated with depression. Important cultural characteristics pertained to religion, familial perspective, male dominance, machismo, and the roles of women and children, among others. de Leon Siantz suggests that for an assessment to be culturally sensitive, it has to include health status, education level, a measure of acculturation, degree of participation in traditional culture, and length of stay in the United States.

Schwab, Meyer, and Merrell (1994) report interesting work in their effort to design a culturally sensitive instrument that measured the health beliefs and attitudes of Mexican Americans with diabetes. This is of special interest because of the well-acknowledged relationship between diabetes and diet. They relied on the Health Belief Model because of its potential predictive value regarding health behaviors. Their work suggests that the model was effective for two of the five subscales: barriers and benefits. To ensure cultural sensitivity, they added the acculturation and fatalism subscales.

Alternatively, Castro de Alvarez's (1990) work on AIDS prevention among Puerto Rican women considered the cultural factors that contribute to the perception of risk and associated behavioral changes in examining culturally sensitive AIDS prevention programs. Castro de Alvarez suggests that such programs need to be culturally sensitive to gender-role expectations and the role of motherhood. These Latinas may benefit from a health promotion program that assists them in executing self-protective behaviors. Such a program would consider that a Latina population expects a program to be sensitive to respect and modesty; therefore, suggestive clothing in a heterogeneous exercise class would be difficult for such a population.

What is the relationship between health promotion and empowerment? McFarlane and Fehir (1994) relied on the concepts often associated with empowerment—unity, validation of key health promoters, and acceptance of a community's ability to identify and reestablish its own health needs. In this case, volunteer mothers were paired with mothers vis-à-vis community coalitions (with health clinics, social service agencies, local businesses, schools, churches, elected officials, and the media) to facilitate increasing access to health care.

From a more general perspective, Braithwaite, Bianchi, and Taylor (1994), relying on ethnographic procedures, suggest advocating for empowerment of disadvantaged populations by participating in the planning, assessment, and implementation of community-based health initiatives that have been identified as necessary for health promotion and disease prevention programs. Their research suggests that we rely on the intersection of three concepts: development of community-owned plans, community organizations, and ethnographic procedures. They suggest that consideration of these concepts is the most effective way in which to plan health intervention programs.

One of the problems among minority groups is the question of access to appropriate medical services, especially at an early stage of diagnosis. When cancer is detected in its earlier stages (Stages 1 and 2), the survival rates are much greater than with the diagnosis of more advanced cases (Stages 3 and 4). Michielutte, Sharp, Dignan, and Blinson (1994) report that cancer is the third leading cause of mortality among Native Americans. They note that the presently existing intervention programs for Caucasians are not culturally relevant for the American Indian population. Their work explores fundamental differences between Caucasians and American Indians in both behaviors and values. Furthermore, van Breda (1989) notes that Native American children are products of their surrounding society, in this case often associated with poverty and alcoholism and its associated problems—diabetes, gastroenteritis, accidents, and fetal alcohol syndrome.

What are the issues and difficulties associated with culturally sensitive exercise programs? Lewis, Raczynski, Heath, Levinson, and Cutter (1993) and Lewis, Raczynski, Heath, Levinson, Hilyer et al. (1993), among others, note that low-income and minority groups, in this case African American communities, tend to be less physically active than the general population. To facilitate participation, Lewis and colleagues collected data from focus group interviews and then conducted a random survey of Alabama residents' exercise practices, beliefs, and barriers to and facilitators of physical activity They found that trained community leaders with intervention expertise were more likely to be associated with participation in physical activity.

In a broader sense, Campinha-Bacote (1994) suggests that we consider a culturally sensitive model, the culturally competent model of care, which includes awareness, knowledge, skill, and encounter as critical parts of a culturally sensitive model for those considering psychiatric nursing. The model views competence as a process, not as a static characteristic that ought to be incorporated into the provision of services.

In general, the culturally sensitive literature has focused on the groups mentioned heretofore, although the authors did find some interesting work by Watt, Howel, and Lo (1993) for the Chinese population. These researchers suggest that the Chinese have a lack of knowledge about health care possibilities in England. They asked this sample of 30 Chinese who frequented shops to fill out a questionnaire about their knowledge, use, and experiences associated with primary health care and health promotion. With a 71% return rate, it was determined that the Chinese were not making optimal use of health services. This population uses some services inappropriately (e.g., emergency clinics), whereas they underuse preventive health programs. The suggested reasons for either the inappropriate use or the underuse of services were language and communication difficulties.

What role does health promotion play among immigrant populations? The Levin-Zamir, Lipsky, Goldberg, and Melamed (1993) case study of Ethiopian immigrants to Israel found that the immigrants relied on an anthropological approach to bridge the gap between the skills brought from the existing country and the skills expected in Israel. Their work relied on educating the immigrant population about health services, nutrition, medication, the prevention of accidents, first aid, and the use of personal hygiene. Their program relied on visual tools, reflecting concern about the development of module tools, and was well accepted.

Jeffery's (1991) work best summarizes the section of literature focusing on culturally relevant health promotion programs for minority groups. He argues that obesity among minority groups is better understood and intervened from a larger, cultural-theme perspective. The environment is assumed not to provide the necessary access to appetizing food at a low cost for underserved populations, and one needs to understand that for many underserved populations, exercise is not a sought-after activity.

PROPOSALS FOR PREVENTION

In examining the potential of various interventions for type 2 diabetes, several factors emerge that need to be examined. First, tradition in health education would suggest that for this type of condition (asymptomatic), some sort of Health Belief Model–based (Rosenstock, 1974) intervention would be appropriate. Unfortunately, many programs designed around these theoretical parameters (e.g., American Diabetes Association Prevention programs) have been unsuccessful among minority populations. Interestingly, the literature has been especially silent on the fact that for many minority populations, the salience of the threat of the disease is considerably lower than that of more immediate life threats from other external stimuli (e.g., violence, poverty, drugs). In fact, in reviewing the many theoretical proposals for the modification of human behavior with respect to disease, one finds the issue of overall or global risk and the salience of the particular risk to be avoided sadly missing.

This chapter does not deal with the theoretical development of health promotion and disease prevention programs. However, as can be seen in the several case studies that follow, the theme of multiple risk and intervention is continued.

LEVELS OF PREVENTION

Because of the long and complex etiology of most chronic diseases, the fact that the disease goes undiscovered for many years, and the fact that many of the sequelae of the disease often do not manifest for many years after diagnosis, prevention programs must differentially focus on several distinct population groups, each with specific prevention needs. For the asymptomatic, undiagnosed, high-risk population, awareness of the disease as a "real" life threat that can be avoided and controlled is essential; for these individuals, the adoption of healthy diets, lifelong exercise programs, and the periodic monitoring of blood glucose and general health are needed. For those diagnosed but as yet without the serious sequelae of the disease evident (e.g., neuropathy, retinopathy, renal dysfunction), the regimen for prevention shifts to one of more direct actions that will reduce the risk of the diabetes-related outcomes. More rigid control of diet, compliance with drug regimens, increased exercise, controlled weight loss programs, and (above all) regular monitoring of blood sugar and monitoring for the signs of advancement of the disease are essential. Finally, for those already symptomatic with the sequelae of the disease, the regimen shifts to one of attempting to slow the inevitable processes. Close monitoring of the blood sugar levels, more aggressive drug therapy, and increased emphasis on dietary control, exercise, and weight loss usually are an essential part of the effort. All these levels of prevention are amply infused with education about the disease, its etiology, and the ways in which the individual can alter the course of the disease.

DESCRIPTION OF CASE STUDIES

The case studies that follow are brief descriptions of efforts by local people to solve local problems. They are this way because this is what has been shown to work best in the islands of the Pacific. For the reader intent on adopting and adapting these programs to his or her own local setting on the mainland, a note of caution is in order. These programs were not externally derived. They arose from the bottom up, from seeds sown over the years, and finally began to bloom after the local people acquired the necessary skills to make them happen. They are the essence of community development and community participation. They are "from the people."

As a general description, the Kosrae Gardening Project and the THD program are presented in two different ways. First, each is described on the basis of its central features as a sort of overview of the project. Then, each is presented systematically across the same variables to allow for comparison of the two projects.

In the Pacific, distances are enormous. The many island states and nations cover a portion of the Earth that is equivalent in size to the continental United States but with virtually no land and few people (Figure 27.1). With Hawaii anchored as the easternmost point, the distance to Guam and Palau is approximately the same as that from Boston to Los Angeles. The population of this entire region (including Hawaii), however, is well under 1.5 million. Island life creates special demands on the health systems of the region. Prevention, although logically beneficial to the health of the people, is not always well defined by the various health departments. This section of the chapter speaks of the role of the community in developing culturally appropriate disease prevention strategies and promoting them in Micronesia.

The Kosrae Gardening Project

Summary

The island of Kosrae has seen the occurrence of many cases of type 2 diabetes, with the negative sequelae resulting in the island

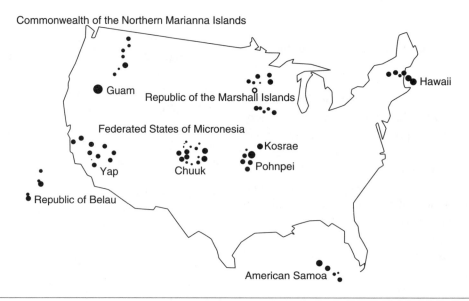

Figure 27.1   The Pacific Islands of Micronesia

population having a burden of disease costing more than the inhabitants can meet using conventional treatment paid by local resources. For those who have been medically referred to other islands or to Hawaii for renal dialysis, the cost is so prohibitive that it cannot be borne in the long run. The Department of Health in Kosrae state always has had a strong public health program using public health nurses as both educators and outreach workers as well as for the provision of care in the community From within this group, a simple plan to make affordable a better diet for those with diabetes and their families was begun.

The Kosrae Gardening Project has no official sanction from the government or health department, and it has essentially no budget— just people caring for people. The administrator for public health is a nurse in the Department of Health and was the instigator of the project, starting with patients who seemed amenable to taking some sort of concrete action to control their diabetes and eventually expanding that net to those families with an interest in learning about gardening and diabetes prevention at the same time.

The structure of the program is simplicity at its finest in that it calls on the basic cultural values of the population of Kosrae—namely, independence and respect for the land. The skills development phase was quite short because the initial participants were older and had previous experience with gardening. The health education phase began immediately with the choice of produce to grow and was followed through with preparation tips and actual demonstrations. The program had a natural duration, one cycle of growing (about 3 months), and allowed for ample discussion time with the public health nurse regarding diabetes control, dietary exchange, and the importance of exercise. In addition, the program duration was sufficient to establish the extent to which the diabetes was in control in the participants.

The second round of the project used those already participating in the project to work with others with minimal intervention by the public health nurse. Materials were provided for the educational component, and several special sessions also were held by the nurse; however, in general, the project was self-operating. Initially, 6 individuals participated. The second round saw 4 more join in. After 3 years, a total of 14 persons with diabetes had participated in this community project.

The Setting

Kosrae is the easternmost state in the FSM, located about 2,500 miles west of Hawaii at approximately 5′ 19″ North latitude and 163° East longitude. It is the smallest of the four states of the FSM, with a land mass of 43.2 square miles, a population of 7,435, and no outer islands. Because of the size and the fact that Kosrae is the only state within the federation without outer islands, accessibility to health is ideally excellent. The economy is rural subsistence, with an annual average per capita domestic product of $1,989 (U.S.).

The population of Kosrae increased from about 4,305 in 1973 to 7,354 in 1994, an increase of 70% over the past two decades. The age and gender composition of the population also has changed over the past two decades. In general, the gender ratio has remained in excess of 100, indicating that there are more males than females in Kosrae. However, as is shown in the following population pyramids, the reverse (more females than males) is true for the 15- to 19-year, 20- to 24-year, and 55- to 59-year age groups (State of Kosrae, 1996).

The proportion of the younger generation has shown a gradual decline, whereas that of the adult population has gradually increased. For example, the proportion of the population under 10 years of age declined from a high of 34.4% to a low of 27.3%, whereas the proportion of those aged 15 years or over increased from 63.3% to a high of 72.6%. The median age increased from 15.9 years in 1973 to 18.8 years in 1994, about a 3-year increase over the past two decades. These figures indicate that the population is gradually getting older. The reason for this gradual aging is mainly due to a decline in fertility, a continued low level of mortality, and age-selective migration.

This sets the stage in which the epidemiological transition (Gribble & Preston, 1993) found in many developing countries should be occurring, and in Kosrae we see a rapid increase in chronic disease, while the burden of infectious disease remains. Over the past two decades, the causes of both morbidity and mortality have changed from essentially sanitation-based problems to more chronic and lifestyle-related problems (State of Kosrae, 1996, Appendix B). Over the same two decades, dependence on imported food has become very high, with canned goods being the main source of produce and protein. Type 2 diabetes is a major concern for the population of this small island. In 1994, there were no patients abroad for renal dialysis, but there were an estimated 277 individuals identified as diabetics on the island.

Kosraeans are a proud people with a strong religious affiliation (Ridgell, 1988). The island is without bars and without dancing. On Sundays in Kosrae, there is no shopping, no television, no beachgoing, and no parties; there is only church attendance. Alcohol is consumed by permit only, with visitors required to obtain a permit after 3 days if they wish to purchase and consume alcohol. With the traditional culture almost destroyed through the disease of modernization during the late 19th and early 20th centuries, the missionaries re-created the culture using their own interpretation. Thus, while more stringent and appearing more traditional than some, the real Kosraean culture is weak and poorly recalled.

Nonetheless, as one seeks culturally relevant interventions, those of Kosrae are appropriate to include in the listing because they have been derived from local traditions by local practitioners to be used with local people. Because of fiscal constraints, the government of Kosrae reduced the number of weekly hours for employment to 32 a few years ago. The day on which people (except emergency staff) were without work was to be used for agricultural activities and fishing for food for their families. About 1 year later, the people of Kosrae started a venture—that of agricultural self-sufficiency Beginning with poultry, bananas and other fruits, and then vegetables, the efforts under way in Kosrae targeted the year 2000 as the one in which major signs of progress would be visible to the people in terms of locally raised, locally appropriate foods being readily available. This project was set within that context as well as within the fact that type 2 diabetes, primarily a nutrition- and lifestyle-related disorder, had become a problem of significance to this small island state.

The Objectives

Within the constraints of the culture of Kosrae, and in keeping with the goals and objectives of the government's self-sufficiency program while supporting positive diabetes education and control, this project attempts to assist persons with type 2 diabetes in living better lives, more healthfully and with more stringent glycemic control.

The Design

The project has a start-up phase, in which some skill building occurs in terms of choice of crop and methods of cultivation and soil preparation. The next phase has to do with the actual planting and growing of the gardens. Here, exercise such as weeding and turning the soil is promoted to ensure good crops. At the same time, the public health nurse begins some diabetes education efforts with the diabetics and their families. Beginning with the importance of maintaining glycemic control and the processes of testing for glucose levels, the importance of exercise and a proper diet, the importance of good foot and eye care, and dietary exchanges all are part of the education provided. As the gardens grow, the educational emphasis transfers to preparation of the produce and the use of fresh fruits and vegetables along with poultry and fish at the dinner table.

The problems with canned goods, such as bully beef and turkey tails, also are emphasized.

The final phase of the project involves instilling pride in the participants through photographs of produce grown, awards, and the like. At this time, the most successful gardeners are recruited to assist with the next group to be brought into the process.

The Issues Around Implementation

The initial recruiting of participants was thought to be a problem for the Department of Health. However, after the effort got under way, that concern quickly disappeared as individuals with type 2 diabetes came forward to volunteer. The second concern was that of attrition. Here, the community itself served as a social pressure force, encouraging and recognizing the efforts that were being made. The gardens were used as examples of people taking initiative on their own, without government money, to solve their own food problems. Finally, concerns were expressed about the sustainability of the process. Here, the jury is still out. The project has been operational for only about 3 years, and it is too early to see whether things will revert to former times or whether they can be maintained in the Kosrae of the future.

The Evaluation

A very real problem exists with the evaluation of this project. Ideally, the measures for evaluation should target the objectives of the project. However, Kosrae is a very poor state, often having few (if any) medications at the hospital and having equipment that is outdated and not able to be maintained or repaired locally. Thus, assessing the glucose levels of participants, although an easy task in Hawaii or on the mainland, is an impossibility because the Department of Health cannot afford the test strips or the meters with which to do the testing.

Assessment can be made of the success of the gardens; the photographs do that. And success can be measured on the basis of the participants, both their numbers and their duration and subsequent participation as trainers/educators. The major evaluation of the effort, however, will come over time as one sees whether the Kosrae Gardening Project will be sustainable.

Results and Discussion

The fact that the project has remained operational for 3 years is a suggestion that it seems to be working. The years of abuse to which the endocrine systems of the people of Kosrae have been subjected cannot be expected to show immediate improvement. However, for what it is worth, the gardeners appear to have lost weight (this is a sensitive subject, and data are not readily available), appear to be fitter, and (according to the public health nurses) are healthier.

The likelihood that this intervention will be sustainable is quite high. It is a variation on a popular theme in the culture—living off the land. It also is in harmony with other community efforts and, while targeting a specific subgroup of the population, allows these individuals to take a leadership role within the community. The key to everything with the program will be the success it is able to generate in transferring the knowledge, attitudes, and practices of one group of participants to another.

Hawaii: The Traditional Hawaiian Diet

Summary

The THD program is now well established as part of the health resources available to providers within the state of Hawaii. It is used under medical supervision and otherwise and has been amply described in two separate publications (O'Connor, Teixeira, Tan, Beckham, & Shintani, 1995; Shintani & Hughes, 1992). This diet program, however, is more than just a diet designed to assist people in managing their hypertension and diabetes. It is essentially a plea to the people for a lifestyle change.

The initial work for the diet came from Moloka'i, where a 1985 cardiovascular risk study (Curb et al., 1991) of 247 Moloka'i homesteaders was completed. The results revealed a population with significant diseases present, including high cholesterol (45% of the sample), obesity (60%), hypertension (36%), and diabetes (23%). The subsequent dietary intervention led researchers to believe that the use of traditional Hawaiian foods (e.g., taro, fish, sweet potato, poi, banana) resulted in a reduction in nearly all indicators of the diseases mentioned.

As time has passed, the THD (the packaging of the Moloka'i Diet), with its additional features of exercise and health education, has been adopted by many in the state. In 1997, the state governor and 20 colleagues went on the diet for a 3-week period. The results were similar, and the publicity greatly assisted in spreading the word about a "local way" in which to manage some of the most devastating diseases in Hawaii.

Setting

Hawaii is known as the "Aloha State," and more recently has become known as the "Health State" (Figure 27.2 and Table 27.1). Longevity is the greatest of any state in the union, and the health status indicators are, in general, better than the U.S. average. With a warm healing climate and ready access to medical care (96% of the population have some form of health insurance), the people of the state boast short lengths of stay in hospitals for most conditions as well as the lowest admission rates.

However, in examining the situation further, one finds that within this generally healthy population there are subgroups for whom life is not so healthy Most notable of these is the indigenous Hawaiian population. Initially resulting from studies of Native Hawaiians completed in 1985 (Native Hawaiian Health Research Consortium, 1985), the picture of the health of Native Hawaiians has become clearer over the past decade. With that clarity has come the Native Hawaiian Health System, funded by Congress in 1988 and now present on all major islands of the state.

It has been well established in the literature that Westernization of the Native populations of the Pacific has caused deleterious effects on their health status (Blaisdell, 1988, 1993; Hankin & Dickinson, 1972; Prior, 1971; Reed, Labarthe, & Stallones, 1970; Ringrose & Zimmet, 1979; Shintani & Hughes, 1994; Taylor et al., 1992; Taylor & Zimmet, 1981; Zimmet, Arblaster, & Thoma, 1978). Similar declines in health conditions have occurred among Native Americans and immigrants to the continental United States (Boyce & Swinburn, 1993; Flegal et al., 1991; Howard, Abbot, & Swinburn, 1991; Kumanyika, Morssink, & Agurs, 1992; Swinburn, Boyce, Bergman, Howard, & Bogardus, 1991). Dietary change is the most prominent factor

among the environmental and urbanization adaptations that negatively affect these populations, followed by decreased exercise and qualitative aspects of the diet (Prior, 1971; Taylor et al., 1992; Taylor & Zimmet, 1981; Zimmet et al., 1978). The change from traditional diets to high-fat, high-calorie, low-fiber, refined and canned foods has resulted in an increasing prevalence of overweight, obesity, cardiovascular disease, and glucose intolerance and the eventual occurrence of type 2 diabetes in these groups (Blaisdell, 1988, 1993; Flegal et al., 1991; Howard et al., 1991; Reed et al., 1970; Ringrose & Zimmet, 1979; Shintani & Hughes, 1994; Sloan, 1963; Taylor et al., 1992; Taylor & Zimmet, 1981). Ethnic Hawaiians exhibited alarming diabetes prevalence rates in 1963, when full-blooded Hawaiians were found to have a prevalence rate of 48.8% and part Hawaiians a rate of 26.6%, compared with the overall state rate of 18.4% (Sloan, 1963). Recent screening programs among Native Hawaiians, using newer technology and standards, have established a diabetes prevalence rate of 18.5% and an impaired glucose tolerance rate of 34% (Beddow & Arakaki, 1997; RCMI: The Native Hawaiian Research Project, 1994).

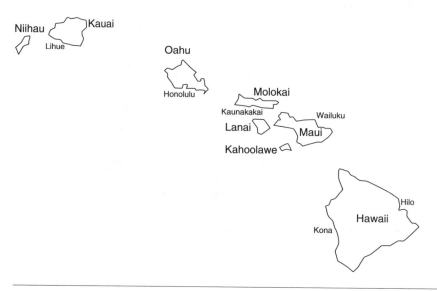

Figure 27.2   State of Hawaii

Table 27.1   General Health Data for Hawaii: All Ethnicities

(a) Ten leading causes of death, by sex (1993)			
Condition	*Total*	*Male*	*Female*
1. Heart disease	2,204	1,287	917
2. Malignant neoplasm	1,717	1,006	711
3. Other diseases	741	389	352
4. Cerebrovascular disease	546	276	270
5. Influenza/pneumonia	303	163	140
6. Accidents	272	204	68
7. Chronic obstructive pulmonary disease	259	166	93
8. Other infective diseases	255	199	56
9. Diabetes mellitus	175	81	94
10. Suicide	123	104	19

(b) Chronic conditions (1992)		
Condition	*Total*	*Run per 1,000*
1. Hypertension	92,182	80.9
2. Impairment of back/spine	72,017	63.2
3. Hay fever	63,853	56.1
4. Chronic sinusitis	57,805	50.8
5. Asthma	53,863	47.3
6. Hearing impairment	50,882	44.7
7. Arthritis	47,125	41.4
8. Skin condition	44,558	39.1
9. Heart disease	35,197	30.9
10. Diabetes	25,448	22.3

SOURCE: State of Hawaii (1996).

This impaired glucose tolerance rate is nearly twice the overall U.S. rate (Beddow & Arakaki, 1997). Among the Native populations of Micronesia and Polynesia, rural Natives were leaner and healthier compared with urbanized Natives and were much healthier than the highly modernized Native Nauruans and Hawaiians (Taylor et al., 1992; Taylor & Zimmet, 1981; Zimmet & Whitehouse, 1981). Diabetes prevalence ranged from 4.6% in rural Samoans to 42.1% in urbanized Nauruans (Prior, 1971; Taylor et al., 1992; Taylor & Zimmet, 1981).

Whereas the negative health status of urbanized Native populations is well documented, information about health interventions and prevention efforts is noticeably lacking in the literature. Medically competent providers who are culturally uninformed and thus treat clients ineffectively (Aluli, 1991; Blaisdell, 1993; Hughes & Aluli, 1991; Mokuau, Hughes, & Tsark, 1995; Zimmet & Whitehouse, 1981) and the prevailing lack of knowledge about the relationship between chronic health conditions and lifestyle choices within Native populations are frequent obstacles to care (Aluli, 1991; Aluli & Hughes, 1994; Blaisdell, 1993; Curb et al., 1991; Hughes & Aluli, 1991; Hughes, Tsark, & Mokuau, 1996; Mokuau et al., 1995). Other serious health care barriers are accessibility to health services, including geographic distances and cost, and the acceptability or compatibility of health programs to the cultures they serve (Blaisdell, 1993; Mokuau et al., 1995).

The community-based THD program is an innovative, culturally competent approach to improving the health status of Native Hawaiians who suffer from diet-related chronic conditions such as obesity, hypertension, hypercholesterolemia, hyperlipidemia, diabetes, and other cardiovascular conditions (Blaisdell, 1993; Mokuau et al., 1995). The THD program integrates traditional foods, cultural values, and components of the traditional lifestyle of Hawaii into a 3-week group intervention (Aluli & Hughes, 1994; Blaisdell, 1993; Hughes et al., 1996; Hughes & Aluli, 1991; Mokuau et al., 1995; Shintani et al., 1994). Traditional values such as spirituality, outreach to others, and unique cultural communication style are incorporated into the THD programs along with cultural preferences for group-focused affiliation, developing close bonds among peers, and reliance on personal networks in coping with problems (Blaisdell, 1993; Hughes et al., 1996; Hughes & Aluli, 1991; Mokuau et al., 1995; Pukui, Haertig, & Lee, 1972). THD program participants are self-selected and agree to participate fully in the 21-day program, which includes a diet of traditional foods, dining at a congregate site for breakfast and dinner, packing a take-out lunch and snacks, participation in health and cultural education, and monitoring by a physician and trained health personnel (Blaisdell, 1993; Hughes et al., 1996). The Moloka'i Diet study of 1987, sponsored by Na Pu'uwai (a Native Hawaiian advocacy organization), implemented the first THD program to study the remediation of hyperlipidemia as a cardiovascular risk factor in Native Hawaiians and employed the traditional communication style for health and cultural education (Aluli, 1991; Aluli & Hughes, 1994; Blaisdell, 1988, 1993). The THD meals incorporate traditional foods, including mainly fish with occasional chicken, taro (a starchy tuber), sweet potato, yams, breadfruit, seaweed, bananas, taro leaves, and several Native greens (Mokuau et al., 1995; Shintani et al., 1994). Since 1987, numerous community-based THD programs have been sponsored by a variety of agencies, schools, and individuals, many in collaboration with the Hawaii State Department of Health (1992, 1993a, 1993b; see also Hawaii State Department of Education, 1994; Kamehameha Schools/Bernice Pau'ahi Bishop Estate, 1993).

Evaluation

The Wai'anae Diet Program (WDP), which started in 1989, is the best known of the THDs (Blaisdell, 1993; Shintani et al., 1994). It is customary for 20 individuals who are obese, based on body mass index (at least 27.2 for men and 26.9 for women), to participate for a 21-day period. Among the first WDP group of 10 men and 10 women, the average body mass index was 39.6 and ranged from

27.7 to 49.7 (Blaisdell, 1993; Shintani et al., 1994). The participants were encouraged to eat to satiety ad libitum amounts of pre-Western-contact Hawaiian foods, except for protein foods, which were controlled at 5 ounces per day for each participant (Blaisdell, 1993; Shintani et al., 1994; T. Shintani, personal communication, November 5, 1997). This traditional diet is low in fat (7%), high in complex carbohydrates (78%), and moderate in protein (15%). The major protein foods were fish and occasionally chicken. The energy intake decreased from about 10.85 microjoules (2,594 kilocalories) pre-WDP to 6.57 microjoules (1,569 kilocalories) during the WDP (Blaisdell, 1993; Shintani et al., 1994).

The average weight loss experienced by the first group was 7.8 kilograms, and the average serum cholesterol decrease was 0.81 millimoles per liter, from 5.76 to 4.95 millimoles per liter. The group blood pressure decreased an average of 11.5 millimeters hemoglobin systolic and 8.9 millimeters hemoglobin diastolic (Blaisdell, 1993; Shintani et al., 1994). Diabetic medications were cut dramatically for some within the first few days of the THD program, and eventually two of the six diabetics gave up all medication, maintaining dietary control of serum glucose levels (T. Shintani, personal communication, November 5, 1997). Another unexpected health benefit noted was a marked improvement among asthmatic participants (T. Shintani, personal communication, November 5, 1997). The health status improvements noted in the first program were repeated in the 14 WDPs that followed. The other community-based programs have mirrored these impressive results (Hawaii State Department of Education, 1994; Hawaii State Department of Health, 1992, 1993a, 1993b; Kamehameha Schools/Bernice Pau'ahi Bishop Estate, 1993).

There is great similarity in the nutrient composition of the diets of early American Indians, Pacific Islanders, and Asians (Blaisdell, 1988, 1993; Boyce & Swinburn, 1993; Shintani & Hughes, 1994; Swinburn et al., 1991). Although the THD is slightly lower in protein (Blaisdell, 1988), the nutrient composition is very similar to the traditional Pima Indian diet, which has been estimated to be 70% to 80% carbohydrates, 8% to 12% fat, and 12% to 18% protein (Boyce & Swinburn, 1993; Howard et al., 1991; Swinburn et al., 1991). The traditional diet of Hawaiians has been assessed at 78% carbohydrates, 12% to 15% protein, and 8% to 10% fat (Blaisdell, 1988). The Pima diet has changed to one that is about 47% carbohydrates, 35% fat, 15% protein, and 3% alcohol (Boyce & Swinburn, 1993; Howard et al., 1991). The adapted diets of Pacific Islanders reflect changes in percentages of nutrients similar to those of Westernization (Taylor et al., 1992; Zimmet et al., 1978). Researchers consistently have suggested that it is this shift in dietary nutrient and food composition, along with decreasing physical activity, that is responsible for increases in diabetes, hypertension, and other cardiovascular conditions that previously were rare in these populations (Blaisdell, 1993; Flegal et al., 1991; Howard et al., 1991; Reed et al., 1970; Ringrose & Zimmet, 1979; Taylor & Zimmet, 1981).

The THD approach of modeling and demonstrating healthy food choices, appropriate serving sizes, cooking methods, and cultural food customs and values is a culturally competent teaching method for the Native Hawaiian community (Pukui et al., 1972). For diabetics, the THD method reduces the stress and frustration of using measuring spoons and cups to serve each meal and memorizing correct serving sizes from the diabetic diet exchange lists to manage dietary intake. This culturally appropriate THD supplants the regimen of rigidly controlled daily living, adherence to a restrictive diet, and compliance with a controlled medication schedule demanded by Western treatment methods. Prescribed exchange diets can be confusing and tedious to plan and execute and are frustratingly limiting. THD participants take part in group meals at least twice a day and in evening educational sessions that foster bonding and group support, and, by the end of the 3-week period, there is successful change in behavior and improved self-esteem among participants. Some community THD programs encourage family participation and offer three group meals daily. This fosters a family support system for dietary change. The THD programs, with their holistic approach, treat the whole individual (spiritual, emotional, and physical self), validate the importance of traditional practices and cultural values, and inculcate an understanding and acceptance of cultural health practices such as *lomilomi* (massage) and *ho'oponopona* (family-centered problem solving) (Blaisdell, 1993; Hughes et al., 1996; Hughes & Aluli, 1991; Mokuau, 1990; Pukui et al., 1972). The contrast between the THD programs (Aluli, 1991; Blaisdell, 1993; Hughes & Aluli, 1991; Mokuau, 1990) and Western treatment methods reflects the vast difference between these cultures (Prior, 1971; Zimmet et al., 1978).

The THD program is one that is locally driven. The impetus to do something has come from within the culture and is promoted as part of the rediscovery of the culture in which Hawaiians have been participating for the past two decades. The fact that the program is locally planned and implemented removes many of the barriers of acceptability. The program is a natural fit with the Native Hawaiian Health System and is medically linked to obesity-related diseases.

EVALUATION

Analysis of the Case Studies

Although the Kosrae Gardening Project and the THD project both are about nutrition and at least partially focused on better dietary lifestyle and diabetes control, they differ in their levels of sophistication and application. The former is elegant in its simplicity. People used to grow gardens, and in the latter half of the 20th century, modern foods and beverages such as Coca-Cola, Pringles potato chips, and frozen turkey tails (to name but three) lined the shelves of the local market. With a return to former ways, the people affected by type 2 diabetes as well as by hypertension and other lifestyle-related diseases live healthier lives.

The THD project, on the other hand, focuses attention not on the growing of the foods but rather on the preparation and composition of the diet itself. Here, a relatively traditional Hawaiian diet is resurrected along with the culture in which it was used. The results of the diet are tracked and monitored intensively to see what effects occur within the diabetic and hypertensive populations participating. In both cases, the lessons are from the past, and the applications and implications clearly are for a healthier future.

Recommendations

Although it is important that programs at the community level be scientifically valid and do no harm to the participants, it is equally important that the programs have roots that are firmly entrenched within the community. The Kosrae Gardening Project and the THD project both are of this type. In examining these two projects, the following recommendations are made.

The roots of the program need to be in the community and its culture to ensure investment on the part of potential participants. The contents of the program need to be of relevance to those who will participate, and the health benefits of the program need to be recognized as valid by the health professionals in the community and those associated with the program. The predefined and desired health outcomes of the program should be explicit and known to participants. Participants should be involved in establishing those desired outcomes, again to enhance the quality and commitment of participation.

The levels of complexity of the programs are not as important as the levels of clarity in what is to be done and with what expected outcomes. The notion of comfort, of harmony with program methods and objectives, is the essential ingredient for success. Although important, cost is of somewhat lesser importance. In considering cost, the broadest of definitions must be used. That is, participant time, inconvenience, discomfort, and the like all must be considered.

From the two case studies examined, as well as from the literature reviewed, community participation in the planning, implementation, and evaluation of disease prevention interventions is a critical element in the process of development of these strategies. Focusing attention on discrete segments of the population seems a wise strategy as well. Finally, drawing from the familiar—that which is recalled from the past—affords each program an "instant history."

Implication

The fact that, in spite of Hawaii's multicultural society, the THD project focuses its efforts on Hawaiians is not accidental. This population is at extreme risk for the many conditions outlined in this chapter, and because much of this risk is reduced with improved diet and weight loss, the intervention is appropriate. That others are not excluded and in fact are encouraged to participate, and have participated, in the program suggests that it has a multicultural potential for application.

Kosrae, on the other hand, is the antithesis of a multicultural society. Here, the focus of the program is on the activity and process and on its relevance to Kosraeans.

As more of America becomes multicultural, and as immigration from the Pacific continues, models such as these might become even more important as models to adapt to local populations. That they have risen from within the cultures of the Pacific makes them competent in terms of their cultural content. That they seem to work makes them of value to those trying to prevent disease and promote the health of the population.

REFERENCES

Aluli, N. E. (1991). Prevalence of obesity in Native Hawaiian population. *American Journal of Clinical Nutrition, 53,* S1556–S1560.

Aluli, N. E., & Hughes, C. K. (1994, Spring). Cardiovascular risk and Native Hawaiians. *NIH-NHLBI Heart Memo,* pp. 19–21.

Auslander, W. F., Haire-Joshu, D., Houston, C. A., & Fisher, E. B., Jr. (1992). Community organization to reduce the risk of non-insulin-dependent diabetes among low-income African-American women. *Ethnicity and Disease, 2,* 176–184.

Avila, P., & Hovell, M. F. (1994). Physical activity training for weight loss in Latinas: A controlled trial. *International Journal of Obesity and Related Metabolic Disorders, 18,* 476–482.

Beddow, R., & Arakaki, R. (1997). Non-insulin-dependent diabetes mellitus: An epidemic among Hawaiians. *Hawaiian Medical Journal, 56,* 14–17.

Blaisdell, R. K. (1988, July). Ka ho'ok 'ai: Mokuna 'elua. *Ka Wai Ola OHA,* p. 28.

Blaisdell, R. K. (1993). The health status of Kanaka Maoli (indigenous Hawaiians). *Asian American and Pacific Islander Journal of Health, 7*(2), 117–162.

Boyce, V. L., & Swinburn, B. A. (1993). The traditional Pima Indian diet. *Diabetes Care, 16*(Suppl.), 369–371.

Braithwaite, R. L., Bianchi, C., & Taylor, S. E. (1994). Ethnographic approach to community organization and health empowerment. *Health Education Quarterly, 21,* 407–416.

Brandt, A. M. (1987). *No magic bullet: A social history of venereal disease in the United States since 1880.* New York: Oxford University Press.

Campinha-Bacote, J. (1994). Cultural competence in psychiatric mental health nursing: A conceptual model. *Nursing Clinics of North America, 29*(1), 1–8.

Castro de Alvarez, V. (1990). AIDS prevention program for Puerto Rican women. *Puerto Rican Health Science Journal, 9*(1), 37–41.

Curb, J. D., Aluli, N. E., Kauz, J. A., Petrovitch, H., Knutsen, S. E., Knutsen, R., et al. (1991).

Cardiovascular risk factor levels in ethnic Hawaiians. *American Journal of Public Health, 81*, 164–167.

de Leon Siantz, M. L. (1990). Maternal acceptance/ rejection of Mexican migrant mothers. *Psychology of Women Quarterly, 14*, 245–254.

Federated States of Micronesia. (1997). *Healthy Nation 2001: A five year plan.* Palikir, Pohnpci State: Government of the Federated States of Micronesia, Department of Health and Human Services.

Flegal, K., Ezzati, T. M., Harris, M. I., Haynes, S. G., Juarez, R. Z., Knowler, W. C., et al. (1991). Prevalence of diabetes in Mexican Americans, Cubans and Puerto Ricans from the Hispanic Health and Nutrition Examination Survey, 1982–84. *Diabetes Care, 14*(Suppl.), 628–638.

Forety, J. P. (1994). The impact of behavior therapy on weight loss. *American Journal of Health Promotion, 8*, 466–469.

Gribble, J. N., & Preston, S. H. (Eds.). (1993). *The epidemiological transition: Policy and planning implications for developing countries.* Washington, DC: National Academy Press.

Hankin, J. H., & Dickinson, L. E. (1972). Urbanization, diet, and potential health effects in Palau. *American Journal of Clinical Nutrition, 25*, 348–353.

Hawaii State Department of Education. (1994). *Ho'oulu Kailua 'opio: Kailua traditional Hawaiian eating experience.* Honolulu, HI: Author.

Hawaii State Department of Health. (1992). *The Kaua'i Native Hawaiian diet program: An evaluation.* Honolulu, HI: Author.

Hawaii State Department of Health. (1993a). *Maui Traditional Hawaiian Diet program* (La'au no ka mea 'ai: Summary report). Honolulu, HI: Author.

Hawaii State Department of Health, School Health Nursing Branch. (1993b). *Native Hawaiian Traditional Diet project at Kaimuki Intermediate School.* Honolulu, HI: Author.

Heath, G. W., Wilson, R. H., Smith, J., & Leonard, B. E. (1991). Community-based exercise and weight control: Diabetes risk reduction and glycemic control in Zuni Indians. *American Journal of Clinical Nutrition, 53*(Suppl.), S1642–S1646.

Howard, B. V., Abbot, W. G. H., & Swinburn, B. A. (1991). Evaluation of metabolic effects of substitution of complex carbohydrates for saturated fat in individuals with obesity and NIDDM. *Diabetes Care, 14*, 786–795.

Hughes, C. K., & Aluli, N. E. (1991). A culturally sensitive approach to health education for Native Hawaiians. *Journal of Health Education, 22*, 387–390.

Hughes, C. K., Tsark, J. A., & Mokuau, N. K. (1996). Diet-related cancer in Native Hawaiians. *Cancer, 78*, 558–563.

Jeffery, R. W. (1991). Population perspectives on the prevention and treatment of obesity in minority populations: *American Journal of Clinical Nutrition, 53*(Suppl.), S1621–S1624.

Kamehameha Schools/Bernice Pau'ahi Bishop Estate. (1993). *Hawaiian cultural foods athletic project.* Honolulu, HI: Author.

Kumanyika, S. K., Morssink, C., & Agurs, T. (1992). Models for dietary and weight change in African-American women: Identifying cultural components. *Ethnicity and Disease, 2*, 166–175.

Levin-Zamir, D., Lipsky, D., Goldberg, E., & Melamed, Z. (1993). Health education for Ethiopian immigrants in Israel, 1991–92. *Israeli Journal of Medical Science, 29*, 422–428.

Lewis, C. E., Raczynski, J. M., Heath, G. W., Levinson, R., & Cutter, G. R. (1993). Physical activity of public housing residents in Birmingham, Alabama. *American Journal of Public Health, 83*, 1016–1020.

Lewis, C. E., Raczynski, J. M., Heath, G. W., Levinson, R., Hilyer, J. C., Jr., & Cutter, G. R. (1993). Promoting physical activity in low-income African-American communities: The PARR project. *Ethnicity and Disease, 3*, 106–118.

McFarlane, J., & Fehir, J. (1994). De Madres à Madres: A community, primary health care program based on empowerment. *Health Education Quarterly, 21*, 381–394.

Michielutte, R., Sharp, P. C., Dignan, M. B., & Blinson, K. (1994). Cultural issues in the development of cancer control programs for poor, underserved American Indian populations. *Journal of Health Care, 5*, 280–296.

Mokuau, N. (1990). A family-centered approach in Native Hawaiian culture. *Families in Society:*

Journal of Contemporary Human Services, 71, 607–613.

Mokuau, N., Hughes, C. K., & Tsark, J. U. (1995). Heart disease and associated risk factors among Hawaiians: Culturally responsive strategies. *Health and Social Work, 20,* 46–51.

Nakyonyi, M. M. (1993). HIV/AIDS education participation by the African community. *Canadian Journal of Public Health, 84*(Suppl.), S19–S23.

Native Hawaiian Health Research Consortium. (1985). *'E Ola Mau: The Native Hawaiian health needs study.* Honolulu, HI: Author.

O'Connor, H. K., Teixeira, R. K., Tan, M., Beckham, S., & Shintani, T. (1995). *Wai'anae Diet cookbook: 'Elua.* Wai'anae, HI: Wai'anae Coast Comprehensive Health Center.

Prior, I. A. M. (1971, July–August). The price of civilization. *Nutrition Today,* pp. 2–11.

Pukui, M. K., Haertig, E. W., & Lee, C. A. (1972). *Nana I Ke Kumu* [Look to the source] (Vol. 2). Honolulu, HI: Queen Lili'uokalani Children's Center.

RCMI: The Native Hawaiian Research Project. (1994). Diabetes mellitus and heart disease risk factors in Hawaiians. *Hawaiian Medical Journal, 53,* 340–364.

Reed, D., Labarthe, D., & Stallones, R. (1970). Health effects of Westernization and migration among Chamorros. *American Journal of Epidemiology, 92,* 94–112.

Ridgell, R. (1988). *Pacific nations and territories: The islands of Micronesia, Melanesia, and Polynesia.* Honolulu, HI: Bess.

Ringrose, H., & Zimmet, P. (1979). Nutrient intakes in an urbanized Micronesian population with a high diabetes prevalence. *American Journal of Clinical Nutrition, 32,* 1334–1341.

Rogler, L. H., Cortes, D. E., & Malgady, R. G. (1994). The mental health relevance of idioms of distress: Anger and perceptions of injustice among New York Puerto Ricans. *Journal of Nervous and Mental Disorders, 182,* 327–330.

Rosenstock, I. M. (1974). The Health Belief Model and preventive health behavior. *Health Education Monographs, 2,* 354–386.

Samolsky, S., Dunker, K., & Hynak-Hankinson, M. T. (1990). Feeding the Hispanic hospital patient: Cultural considerations. *Journal of the American Dietary Association, 90,* 1707–1710.

Schwab, T., Meyer, J., & Merrell, R. (1994). Measuring attitudes and health beliefs among Mexican-Americans with diabetes. *Diabetes Education, 20,* 221–227.

Shintani, T., Beckham, S., O'Connor, H. K., Hughes, C., & Sato, A. (1994). The Wai'anae Diet Program: A culturally sensitive, community-based obesity and clinical intervention program for the Native Hawaiian population. *Hawaiian Medical Journal, 53*(5), 136–147.

Shintani, T., & Hughes, C. K. (Eds.). (1992). *The Wai'anae book of Hawaiian health: The Wai'anae Diet Program manual.* Wai'anae, HI: Wai'anae Coast Comprehensive Health Center.

Shintani, T. T., & Hughes, C. K. (1994). Traditional diets of the Pacific and coronary heart disease. *Journal of Cardiovascular Risk, 1,* 16–20.

Sinclair, M. A. (1991). A revised weight loss program in Manitoba Native communities. *Arctic Medical Research* (Suppl.), 97–98.

Sloan, N. R. (1963). Ethnic distribution of diabetes mellitus in Hawai'i. *Journal of the American Medical Association, 183,* 419–424.

State of Hawaii. (1996). *The state of Hawai'i data book, 1995: A statistical abstract.* Honolulu, HI: State Department of Business, Economic Development, and Tourism.

State of Kosrae. (1996). *Healthy Kosrae 2001: State health plan.* Kosrae, Federal States of Micronesia: Department of Health.

Swinburn, B. A., Boyce, V. L., Bergman, R. N., Howard, B. V., & Bogardus, C. (1991). Deterioration in carbohydrate metabolism and lipoprotein changes induced by modern, high fat diet in Pima Indians and Caucasians. *Journal of Clinical Endocrine Metabolism, 73,* 156–165.

Taylor, R., Badcock, J., King, H., Pargeter, K., Zimmet, P., Fred, T., et al. (1992). Dietary intake, exercise obesity and noncommunicable disease in rural and urban populations of three Pacific island countries. *Journal of the American College of Nutrition, 11,* 283–293.

Taylor, R. J., &. Zimmet, P. Z. (1981). Obesity and diabetes in Western Samoa. *International Journal of Obesity, 5,* 367–376.

van Breda, A. (1989). Health issues facing Native American children. *Pediatric Nursing, 15,* 575–577.

Watt, I. S., Howel, D., & Lo, L. (1993). The health care experience and health behaviour of the Chinese: A survey based in Hull. *Journal of Public Health and Medicine, 15,* 129–136.

Wood, D. W. (1994). *Diabetes: A monograph on prevalence rates in Hawai'i.* Honolulu, HI: University of Hawai'i, International Center for Health Promotion and Disease Prevention Research.

Zimmet, P., Arblaster, M., & Thoma, K. (1978). The effect of Westernization on Native populations: Studies on a Micronesian community with a high diabetes prevalence. *Australia and New Zealand Journal of Medicine, 8*(2), 141–146.

Zimmet, P., & McCarty, D. (1995). The NIDDM epidemic: Global estimates and projections—A look into the crystal ball. *IDF Bulletin, 40,* 8–16.

Zimmet, P., & Whitehouse, S. (1981). Pacific islands of Nauru, Tuvalu and Western Samoa. In H. C. Trowell & D. P. Burkitt (Eds.), *Western diseases: Their emergence and prevention.* Cambridge, MA: Harvard University Press.

28

Tips for Working With Pacific Islander Populations

ROBERT M. HUFF

MICHAEL V. KLINE

There are numerous groups of Pacific Islander peoples living in the continental United States and on islands scattered throughout the Pacific. As might be expected, these groups do share some common characteristics but also reflect significant diversity with respect to cultural beliefs, values, and ways of life. Thus, the term *Pacific Islander or Pacific Islander American* (PIA) in no way adequately begins to describe this diversity. In fact, the use of this term as a category for describing peoples in census tracts and health databases often functions to obscure this diversity by lumping and combining the specific issues, health problems, and needs of these PIA population groups into one overall category. In addition, PIA groups often are combined under the much broader category of *Asian or Pacific Islander*, which further serves to mask specific issues and problems of each of these PIA groups. Thus, as a general rule of thumb, the health promoter is encouraged to use the descriptor that is used by the particular PIAs in describing themselves and to learn, as much as possible, about the specific populations groups with whom the health promoter may be working. This "tips" chapter, although intentionally broad-based, seeks to provide some general considerations and tips for working with PIAs in health promotion and disease prevention (HPDP) programs. These tips have been drawn from the preceding three chapters (Chapters 25, 26, and 27, this volume) and other sources (Ishida, Toomata-Mayer, & Mayer, 1996; Chapters 1, 2, 4, 6, and 7, this volume) and are meant only as a starting point for the practitioner involved with providing HPDP programs or services to PIA population groups.

CULTURAL COMPETENCE

As has been noted in all the "tips" chapters, the need to develop increasingly higher levels of cultural competence—with respect to the many multicultural groups health promoters

549

are confronted with today—is of paramount importance. Thus, the health promoter should heed the following tips:

- Devote time to learning the history and patterns of migration and immigration of the specific PIA population with which you will be working.
- Seek to discover the specific cultural values, beliefs, and traditions of your target group.
- Remember that every PIA group will have its own unique traditions and patterns of life and that these may be very different from yours and those of the agency that is providing the HPDP program or service to this group. It will be critical to develop the skill of suspending your own judgments, biases, and stereotypes because these can act to block sensitive and mutually respectful interpersonal relationships among all involved parties.
- Remember that there is likely to be a range of acculturation levels, from the very traditional to the very acculturated. Therefore, there is a need to assess these levels before beginning the planning process for delivering the HPDP program or service to the target group. Do not assume that because your target group is residing in the continental United States, its members are acculturated and assimilated into the mainstream culture.
- Be very cognizant of both the verbal and nonverbal communication patterns and cultural taboos of your target group.
- Take the time to make multiple visits to the community in which the target group resides. Talk with community leaders and members, visit important sites in the community where appropriate, sample local cuisine, participate in local events where the public is invited, and otherwise become familiar with the community's ways of life.
- Seek to establish early and continuing support from the community for any HPDP program or service that is to be offered.
- Be aware that there might be major discrepancies in the health data that are available about the target group. Here, again, assessment of your target group using available

data from the agency providing a program or service to your specific target group, as well as information derived from the community in question, will be essential.

HEALTH BELIEFS AND PRACTICES

An understanding of the health beliefs, practices, and health care use patterns of any cultural group is an essential component of the formative evaluation process one would use to increase one's understanding of a specific target group. The following tips might prove useful to the health promoter in this early needs assessment process:

- Identify the explanatory model(s) used by the target group to define health and disease, including preferences for traditional, Western, or a combination of both types of health care services when seeking help with illness or sickness states.
- Expect that there will be a range of explanatory models that are employed across this broad multicultural population group, ranging from very traditional folk beliefs and practices to those reflective of the current biomedical model.
- Seek to ameliorate and work with differences in explanatory models where these are in opposition between the target group and yourself.
- Seek to become more familiar with traditional healing practices of the community because these may provide opportunities to bring beneficial health practices into the biomedical framework.
- Identify perceptions related to personal control and responsibility for promoting individual health and well-being—that is, locus of control, interest, needs, and activities used for promoting or maintaining one's health.
- Identify the health care access issues, including usual patterns of use, types of care generally sought, barriers to care, social assistance services accessed by the target group, and other sources related directly or indirectly to the target group.

- Be aware that, in general, PIA population groups recognize that there are indigenous illnesses that must be treated with traditional remedies and Western illnesses that are more amenable to treatment using Western medical approaches.
- Recognize that there is no simple generic description for describing the health beliefs and practices of a PIA group. You must know the geographic locale and ethnic group to begin to understand these differences.
- Recognize that in matters of disease prevention and illness management, the whole family will be involved in the process.
- Consider that modesty, taboos, and traditional healing practices must be respected when providing the HPDP program or service.
- Consider involving traditional healers in the planning and delivery of the HPDP program or service.
- Where the HPDP program or service is focused on specific Western clinical conditions, be sure to identify and compare the expectations of the PIA individual or group to ensure that both sides understand and agree with what is to be provided for that particular problem or condition.
- Recognize that cultural sensitivity to other points of view about health and disease will be a critical factor to consider when learning about your target group's health beliefs and practices.

- Review all previous and current programs or services offered to the target group to identify intervention strategies and resources that have been found to enhance or impede the successful adaptation of programs and services by the target group.
- Develop positive alliances with the leadership of the community as you begin the program-planning process.
- Be sure to include traditional healers as well as spiritual, cultural, and other important community members in the planning, implementation, and evaluation process.
- Be sure that the goals, objectives, and intervention processes target the felt needs of the target group and not just those of the sponsoring agency. Otherwise, this becomes a case of *doing to* rather than *doing with* the target group.
- Remember that successful HPDP programs for PIAs will employ a top-down and bottom-up approach to the planning and implementation process—that is, starting where the people are and involving them in every aspect of program development and delivery.
- Be aware that the program or service must fit within the cultural context of the community's values, beliefs, and health practices.
- Consider incorporating an indigenous model for planning, implementation, and evaluation of the HPDP program—that is, employing members of the target group to help plan, implement, and evaluate the program or service to be offered to the target group.

PROGRAM-PLANNING CONSIDERATIONS

Comprehensive and well-informed program planning is one of the most important tasks for designing a high-quality and successful HPDP program and/or service. Planning will require that the health promoter be culturally competent and sensitive to the differences in worldviews and ways of life of the target group. Keeping in mind the suggestions that have been made by others in this book, the health promoter also is encouraged to consider the following recommendations:

NEEDS ASSESSMENT CONSIDERATIONS

Needs assessment is the foundation of any successful HPDP program or service and should never be overlooked or superficially conducted. The data from this process are what will be used to identify the real and potential health issues and problems as well as the felt needs of the target group. Huff and Kline, in Chapter 6, this volume, present a Cultural Assessment Framework that can be used for identifying information and health data about the target group under consideration. In addition to the assessment areas and questions presented in this framework (Chapters 7 and 26, this volume), the following suggestions may also prove useful to the health promoter:

- Be aware that most census and health data lump the many diverse PIA groups together under the broad heading of *Asian Pacific Islander*. It will be critical to try and tease out the data directly applicable to the specific target group with which you will be working.
- Where possible, provide opportunities for PIA communities to conduct or be as involved as possible in conducting their own needs assessments because this can help build community capacity and a sense of community empowerment with respect to defining and solving their health and social problems.
- Recognize that needs assessment instruments need to reflect the linguistic, literacy, and cultural symbols and values of the community.
- Be aware that standardized needs assessment instruments designed for the mainstream culture might have little meaning for some PI population groups. Thus, instruments will need to be shaped and validated to reflect the community in which they are to be used.
- Consider including acculturation measures in the community assessment process.
- Consider that foldback analysis, as described in Chapter 26, this volume, may be a very effective approach to defining the real and felt needs of the community.
- Remember that any needs assessment process conducted with PIA population groups should employ a variety of approaches including interviews with key informants, focus groups, community surveys, and other approaches that actively involve the target group in defining its members' health issues and concerns.
- Be sure to include assessment of the media resources and channels that are used by members of the community, because these might play an important role in the marketing of the HPDP program or service to be offered in the community.
- Be sure that questions to be asked of the target group reflect appropriate and relevant

cultural values and expectations, and be aware that some question areas might not be appropriate with respect to cultural taboos and other social conventions.

INTERVENTION CONSIDERATIONS

As has been demonstrated throughout this book, well-planned interventions that employ behavioral theory in association with cultural themes, values, beliefs, and other cultural characteristics are key to the successful implementation of any HPDP program or service. The health promoter is encouraged to consider these factors as well as the following suggestions in the planning of intervention strategies:

- Remember that the most effective HPDP interventions are built on the community's strengths, resources, and assets and include significant involvement of the target group in the design process.
- When designing interventions, focus on the family system rather than on the individual. This recognizes the value and interpersonal dynamics of the family, which is very important to PIA groups.
- Be aware that because many island cultures are matriarchal, involving women in all aspects of the planning, implementation, and evaluation process can be a very effective strategy.
- Remember that intervention planning must start where the people are and must fit within the context of the community's values, beliefs, and cultural practices.
- Remember that HPDP learning experiences for PIA populations should reflect concepts of wholeness and interconnectedness because these are central features of the cosmology of many PIA population groups.
- Be aware that the use of theory to support intervention design is an important feature of successful HPDP programming.
- Be aware that social marketing approaches can be highly effective in working with PIA population groups.
- Recognize that professional health jargon and Western values can impede HPDP processes among PIA population groups.

Seek to include the cultural values and vocabulary of the target group because these have been found to enhance the potential for successful HPDP programs or services.

- When designing HPDP interventions, use short and culturally appropriate messages that present new ideas through accepted social channels and processes.

- Consider developing partnerships with the local media to disseminate information about the HPDP program or service being planned by and for the community.

- Consider that "talk-stories," folk media (e.g., music, dance, song), role-playing, and pictorial presentations are very culturally acceptable and appropriate strategies to employ in HPDP programs or services for PIA population groups.

- Recognize that using multiple channels for the communication of HPDP messages, such as through churches, schools, and work settings, is an effective way in which to work with PIA populations. This also should include family chiefs, church and village leaders, and traditional healers as message sources for HPDP activities.

- Focus health messages on the positive health benefits of change rather than on the negative or fear-arousing consequences of the issue being addressed.

- Where possible, employ and train peer educators from the target community because this can help enhance the credibility and acceptance of the HPDP program or service within the community in which it is being offered.

EVALUATION CONSIDERATIONS

As has been stressed in many of the chapters in this book, evaluation and assessment throughout the planning and implementation of HPDP programs or services are vital to understanding how well these activities functioned to facilitate the health changes that were intended by the programs or services. With this idea in mind, the health promoter should consider the following suggestions when preparing evaluation and assessment plans:

- Seek to develop evaluation strategies, methods, and instruments that reflect an understanding of current theory and practice from the evaluation and research literature.

- Understand that evaluation and assessment processes are often difficult to gain support for, even from the most sophisticated of target groups. Thus, efforts to explain these processes and to involve the target group in evaluation and assessment planning and implementation activities can do much to enhance the successful accomplishment of this component of the HPDP program or service process.

- Evaluation of the HPDP program or service must include culturally relevant measures for assessing the impact of the program or service on the target group.

- Assessment and evaluation methods and questions must be tailored to the educational and linguistic capabilities of the target group.

- Evaluation processes must include the participation of the community, and criteria for evaluation should be sought from the community because its members are the ones who know what is important to them.

- Recognize that HPDP participants might have limited test-taking abilities and skills. Thus, efforts to design evaluation methods and tools should be matched to the relevant experiences, interests, and needs of the target group.

- Wherever possible, provide opportunities for staff members from the community to be trained in evaluation and assessment processes, including the implementation of these processes throughout the life of the program or service.

- Be sure to set up and use evaluation- and assessment-reporting mechanisms to ensure that the target community receives feedback on how well the program is functioning to improve the health issue or problem for which it was designed.

REFERENCE

Ishida, D. N., Toomata-Mayer, T. F., & Mayer, J. F. (1996). Samoans. In J. G. Lipson, S. L. Dibble, & P. A. Minarik (Eds.), *Culture and nursing care: A pocket guide* (pp. 375–381). San Francisco: UCSF Nursing Press.

PART VII

Conclusions

29

Closing Thoughts and Emerging Issues

Multicultural Health Promotion and Disease Prevention

MICHAEL V. KLINE

ROBERT M. HUFF

The U.S. Census Bureau News (2006) reported that the nation's population would reach a historic milestone of 300 million on October 17, 2006. The United States has always been a country of diverse peoples and cultures, from its first indigenous inhabitants to the later throngs of immigrants who arrived from all over the world. In the past 30 years or so, immigrants (and their first and second generations through natural increase) continue to account in great part for driving the current population growth of the United States. And with the increasing volatility in many parts of the world, there most likely will be further increases of people representing many origins, cultural orientations, and social situations. Existing and new groups will continue to make up an increasing and significant part of the urban and rural population of the United States—mainland, islands, reservations, and territories. This ongoing growth of diverse groups has made, and will continue to

make, organized efforts and activities for promoting health and preventing disease in the United States a formidable task!

The purpose of this book was to highlight the importance of multicultural influences and their effects on health problems, determinants of health, health status, and health disparities as these relate to encouraging the health-promoting and disease-preventing behaviors of target populations. A further intent was to increase the awareness of students and health practitioners who are or will be involved in planning health promotion and disease prevention (HPDP) programs. The outcomes of those programs are, to a large extent, shaped by a unique combination of different cultural orientations and influences from the target populations they will be working in. Students and practitioners also are reminded that their own sociocultural orientations can play a role in these outcomes. And it is important to gain increasing awareness of how powerful the interplay and role of environmental factors can be in supporting or discouraging positive health behavior at the individual and community levels. The present chapter provides some final thoughts on some important issues raised in this volume.

GROWING MULTICULTURAL DIVERSITY

America is a *multicultural* society, and the American culture is very diverse. Lawrence Green (1999), in the Foreword to the first edition of this book, noted a major paradox that is faced by nations, states, communities, and institutions seeking to create multicultural societies, especially where equity is the central value of multiculturalism. There is an effort to maintain a respect for differences while recognizing that differences conspire against equity. Multiculturalism, as its use attempts to relate equity to equality, uniformity, and sameness, poses a difficult dilemma: "People cannot be simultaneously different and equal on all counts of living" (p. ix). Some of these dimensions include such basic determinants of health as living conditions, income, education, nutrition, access to health care, and protection from environmental hazards. It is clear that those who are poor, regardless of race/ethnicity or culture, tend to experience more health problems in general over the course of their lives than do their more socioeconomically advantaged counterparts.

A major dilemma, given our levels of knowledge and expertise at any given time, political affiliations, cultural-related orientations, and resources, will always be how to (1) accurately identify the health needs and concerns of all members and groups within our population—vulnerable target groups and others regardless of ethnicity or culture and (2) how to respond—that is, in terms of assessment, design, financing, and implementation of the array of effective HPDP programs that even begin to meet the tremendous diversity of needs represented in nearly all areas of this country. The health promotion student and practitioner working in multicultural settings will be increasingly confronted with difficulties related to the issues mentioned above, which in large part stem from the substantial and growing heterogeneity within groups in terms of culture, racial/ethnic background, social norms, and generational and acculturation differences. Many groups representing many origins and social situations will continue to make up an increasing and significant part of the urban and rural population of the United States—mainland, islands, reservations, and territories. These are some of the main issues that have been dealt with in this book.

COMPLEXITIES IN DESCRIBING DIVERSITY

Data collection systems that have evolved for the purpose of classifying individuals by ethnicity/race have increased our overall information base. But this has also further complicated our ability to accurately define target groups. For example, the U.S Census Bureau (2006, p. 4) now collects information using six race categories: white; black or African American; American Indian or Alaska Native; Asian; Native Hawaiian or other Pacific Islander; and a category termed "some other race." Under this format, the Census 2000 question on race included 15 possible self-report response categories and three areas where the respondent could write in a more specific race group or race groups (U.S. Census Bureau, 2006, p. 4)—that is, choose one race alone (e.g., Black or African American) or in combination (e.g., white and black, white and Asian). An additional change in the 2000 Census is that data on Hispanic (Spanish/Hispanic/Latino) origin were collected by using a self-identification question that asked the respondents to classify themselves in the specific Hispanic origin category (i.e., Mexican, Puerto Rican, Cuban) or in the Other Spanish/Hispanic/Latino origin category (origins from

Spain, the Spanish-speaking countries of Central or South America, or the Dominican Republic) (U.S. Census Bureau, 2006, p. 5). Thus, the data collection and classification methodology treats race and Hispanic origin as two separate concepts. That is, people who are Hispanic may be any race, and people in each race group may be either Hispanic or Not Hispanic (U.S. Census Bureau, 2006, p. 5). For an explanation of the race modification procedure, the reader is referred to U.S. Census Bureau Population Estimates (2003).

These categorizations, as they attempt to differentiate more accurately between the various populations, actually create further challenges and difficulties for planners in defining cultural differences in what might seem like a homogeneous target group. The effective response to this predicament will depend to a great extent on the quality of the needs and cultural assessment performed (this is further discussed in Chapters 6 and 7, this volume). The social marketing practice of segmenting target audiences (discussed in Chapter 7, this volume) to identify common and different needs in health settings could have great value in the health promotion practitioner's armamentarium. The complexity of identifying target groups and their multicultural health promotion needs *will force the planner to discover new ways to become involved and more intimately familiar with the specific membership and cultural characteristics of the target group, their problems, the settings, and the interventions selected.*

POPULATION TRENDS AND ISSUES WITH IMPLICATIONS FOR MULTICULTURAL HPDP

The overview chapters (9, 13, 17, 21, and 25, this volume) provided information about population growth and trends. They also examined a great variety of health problems and health promotion and education needs of several different population groups. In general, most individuals

in multicultural populations are seeking and receiving appropriate health care. Most are working and are relatively well educated, and most are striving to improve the quality of life for themselves and their families. However, many individuals and families continue to be at higher risk of poor physical, psychological, and/or social health. Findings and projections from the U.S. Census Bureau (2006) and the National Center for Health Statistics (NCHS) (2005) are helpful in identifying target groups within multicultural population groups that are at greater risk for particular health problems.

The bulleted entries presented below have been extracted from selected U.S. population and health-related statistics. The information can give planners a glimpse of what the trends and projections of future health care and health promotion and education-related program needs will be. Certainly, these will influence the present and future scope of needs related to the health of multicultural populations:

- The population of the United States reached over 300 million in 2006 (U.S Census Bureau News, 2006) and is projected to steadily increase to over 336 million by 2020 (U.S. Census Bureau, 2006, Table 3, p. 9).
- If current immigration patterns and policies hold (nearly 1 million people every year could be admitted under a number of classes), then a possible 20 million immigrants could be added between 2000 and 2020, contributing further to the numbers and diversity of the population (U.S. Census Bureau, 2006, Table 6, p. 10).
- In 2004, nearly one fifth (19.61%) of the total population belonged to a racial group other than white (U.S. Census Bureau, 2006, Table 14, p. 16).
- In 2002, at 65 years of age, the average life expectancy for males and females was over 80 years (17 years for males and 20 years for females, respectively) (NCHS, 2005, p. 64).
- Approximately 51% of the U.S. population is women, and 43% of all women were between 15 and 44 years of age (U.S. Census Bureau, 2006, Table 11, p. 13). U.S. Census

Bureau (2006) projections for the percentage of women between 15 and 44 years for 2005 and 2010 will remain similar (41.2% and 39.52%, respectively) (Table 12, p. 14).

- In 2004, children from 5 to 14 years of age constituted over one fifth (21.4%; over 60 million) of the total population (U.S. Census Bureau, 2006, Table 11, p. 13). The racial and ethnic diversity of America's children continues to increase over time.

- In 2003, 60% of U.S. children were white-alone, non-Hispanic; 16% were Black-alone; and 4% were Asian-alone. The proportion of Hispanic children has increased faster than that of any other racial and ethnic group, growing from 9% of the child population in 1980 to 19% in 2003 (Federal Interagency Forum on Child and Family Statistics, 2005, p. vii).

- Individuals 55 years and over (this includes baby boomers) totaled over one fifth (59 million) (21.05% of the U.S. population) (U.S. Census Bureau, 2006, Table 14, p. 16) and will total over 76 million (or nearly a quarter of the total population (24.7%) by the year 2010 (U.S. Census Bureau, Table 15, p. 17).

- In 2003, 12.5% of Americans lived in poverty (10.5 % of the white population, 24.4% of the black population, 11.8 % of the Asian and Pacific Islander population, and 22.5% of the Hispanic population (U.S. Census Bureau, 2006, Table 693, p. 472).

- In 2001 to 2003, about 23.2 % of American Indians and Alaska Natives were below the poverty level (DeNavas-Walt, Proctor, & Mills, 2003; see also NCHS, 2005, p. 11).

- The census statistics for 2003 disclosed that 17.2% of American children under 18 live below the poverty level (33.6 % of African American children and 29.5% of Hispanic children) (U.S. Census Bureau, 2006, Table 694, p. 472).

- Furthermore, in 2003 about 2 million black families (22.3%) and about 2 million Hispanic families (20.8%) were living below the poverty level (U.S. Census Bureau, 2006, Table 698, p. 474).

Regardless of race/ethnicity, generational status, citizenship status, residential status, employment status, educational level, and health status, each population group has an appreciable number of members whose health behaviors and risk factors have important effects on their health and that of their families. Many individuals and target groups within multicultural settings have single or multiple health risk factors that can be reduced through HPDP efforts. It is very clear, given the trends anticipated, that there will be increasing needs to effectively identify and expand multicultural HPDP activities among these target groups to try to reduce their disproportionate levels of individual risks of illness and disability. Several years ago, Blane (1995) noted the consistency in the distribution of mortality and morbidity among social groups: "The more advantaged groups, whether expressed in terms of income, education, social class, or ethnicity, tend to have better health than the other members of their societies" (p. 903). Pamuk, Makuc, Heck, Reuben, and Lochner (1998) further note that the worse health experienced by those with low income is a result of many factors, including a higher prevalence of health risk factors, poor nutrition and housing, occupational and environmental hazards, and other social ills. Aday (2001) also comments, "The poor and those with less education tend to experience more health problems in general over the course of their lives, based on an array of indicators of need, than do their more socioeconomically advantaged counterparts" (p. 54). And, finally, the NCHS (2005), in their most recent *Chartbook on Trends in the Health of Americans*, affirm, "People with low income are more likely to be in poor health and have a higher prevalence of many serious chronic diseases than those with higher incomes" (p. 74; see also Tables 56, 57, 60, 61, and 85).

Shi and Stevens's (2005) recent text provides an excellent source of information concerning the vulnerable populations and focuses on three key risk factors that are powerful predictors of poor health care access and health and "therefore vulnerability" (p. 28).

These key risk factors are race/ethnicity, socioeconomic status (SES), and health insurance coverage (Shi & Stevens, 2005; see also Chapter 5, this volume). Social injustice in all its overt and subtle and diabolical manifestations also plays a major role in sustaining disproportionate health risks in multicultural settings, vulnerability, and disparities in our country. Levy and Sidel (2006) in their book *Social Injustice and Public Health* lament, "Social injustice leads to increased rates of disease, injury, disability, and premature death because of increased risk factors and decreased medical care and preventive services" (p. 10).

NEED FOR GREATER UNDERSTANDING OF THE CONCEPTS OF HPDP: A MAJOR PREREQUISITE FOR APPLICATION

There is a critical need for health care reform in America that makes quality health care services, health promotion services, and disease prevention activities accessible and available to all residents and at the same time helps contain costs. Chapters 1 and 7, this volume, provided definitions and discussion concerning the concepts of HPDP. These definitions emphasized the importance of being able to conduct a range of HPDP efforts involving a combination of activities at multiple levels of change in order to reduce risks. The practitioner might find that the most immediate need of a planning or educational endeavor is to prepare participants with at least a basic level of understanding of the different levels of health promotion and education strategies and activities and how they can help increase the community's capacity to design and implement effective disease prevention and health programs. Within their own cultural milieu, planning participants need to recognize that any HPDP interventions contemplated must consider the personal experiences, knowledge, health practices, and problem-solving methodologies that are acceptable within the framework of the group

or community. At one level, programs might concentrate on facilitating the voluntary acquisition of specific health-related knowledge, attitudes, and practices to achieve behavior related to improving or promoting health where people live and work. And at a more complex level, program efforts will be needed to seek social or environmental changes (supportive structures) in the form of policy changes, regulations, and new or increased organizational arrangements for encouraging, enabling, and reinforcing the practice of certain health-related behaviors for reducing health risk (Green & Kreuter 1991, 2005). It is important to recognize that interventions designed to achieve change on only the individual level will not be as effective as those that can achieve change on the broader, community level.

Another very important area of needed understanding was discussed in the opening chapter of this book—the concept and levels of *disease prevention*, which include the *primary prevention level* (providing specific protection that prevents the onset of the disease itself), *the secondary prevention level* (providing activities related to early diagnosis and prompt treatment of a disease that is present), and *the tertiary level* of prevention (activities to minimize disability from existing illness through treatment and rehabilitation efforts). All participants should understand the relationship between the levels of disease prevention activities and *health promotion and education* efforts at the individual, family, community, and policy levels. And this understanding must be built on a foundation that considers differing cultural beliefs and practices concerning matters of individual, family, and community health.

MULTICULTURAL HPDP: GROWING NEEDS FOR PARTICIPATION, EMPOWERMENT, AND OWNERSHIP

There are many reasons why people become involved and stay involved in multicultural health promotion planning efforts. The challenge, of course, is to be able to identify and initiate appropriate approaches for securing and maintaining involvement. Chapter 7 stressed the importance of identifying the distinct cultural protocols and styles that may lead the practitioner to better recognize where the possible points of securing and maintaining involvement might lie. The *principle of participation* is discussed in Frankish, Lovato, and Shannon (1999, p. 61, and Chapter 4, this volume; see also Kline, 1999, pp. 79–80, and Chapter 7, this volume), where the people—the participants—should have a part in the planning to make the situation one in which there is planning *with* not *for* the people. Frankish et al. (Chapter 4, this volume) observe that when people participate in a program, they feel greater ownership of the program and a sense of "responsibility for and control over promoting changes in their behavior and health status." Community organization and development approaches are built on the principle of participation, which stresses that an HPDP program is likely to be more successful when the community at risk identifies "its own health concerns, develops its own prevention and intervention programs, and forms a decision-making board to make policy decisions and identify resources for program implementation" (Braithwaite, 1992, p. 327; see also Braithwaite, Taylor, & Austin, 1999; Minkler, 2004; Minkler & Wallerstein, 2002).

The planner and participants must also work together to become "community competent." Cottrell (1983) defines community competence as evidenced in the context of various component parts of the community that are able to (1) collaborate effectively on identifying the problems and needs of the community, (2) achieve a working consensus on goals and priorities, (3) agree on ways and means to implement the agreed-on goals, and (4) collaborate effectively in the required actions. Goodman and others (1998) studied the concept of community competence further, as reflected in two earlier definitions of "community capacity":

1) the characteristics of communities that affect their ability to identify, mobilize, and address social and public health problems, and 2) the cultivation and use of transferable knowledge, skills, systems, and resources that affect community- and individual-level changes consistent with public health-related goals and objectives. (p. 259)

People do not empower other people. However, through the process of developing a community coalition, participants are able to gain the knowledge and skills to *empower* themselves to participate and ultimately assume control and ownership over their own programs, assessments, and planning and evaluation activities.

There are difficulties and complexities, however, in the use of cooperative endeavors, such as the building of coalitions for accomplishing mutually identified health-risk-related problems in the community. Participants can hold unrealistic expectations about what a coalition can actually accomplish with the limited time and resources. The planner must assist the coalition participants to build their coalition framework according to a sound planning model (as discussed in Chapter 7, this volume) that helps assess, diagnose, and develop appropriate coalition objectives, appropriate interventions, and a sound evaluative framework. And this is a complex and difficult endeavor (see also Butterfoss & Kegler, 2002; Kreuter, Lezin, & Young, 2000). The planner, who is strategically located in this dynamic process, has an awesome task working in partnership with participants toward achieving mutual goals.

In essence, as Lawrence Green points out in the Foreword of this volume, "One overriding lesson, principle, or prediction to be drawn from the multicultural experiences reflected in this handbook would be that promoting health in multicultural populations must ultimately begin from within the cultures intended to benefit from the health promotion." Green advocates the need for collaboration in the spirit of participatory research and comments,

"Practitioners working cross-culturally can only participate in the self-study, learning, and action process effectively if the population affected by the issues is actively engaged in all three."

THE NEED FOR PRACTITIONERS TO USE THEORIES, MODELS, AND PRINCIPLES AS GUIDES TO PRACTICE

Chapters 4 and 7 of this volume discussed the value of organizing frameworks for planning and intervention development. Certainly, in too many instances, empirical or pragmatic considerations have guided health promotion program planning and intervention efforts. It becomes frustratingly clear to most practitioners that *there is no one magic prepackaged HPDP program guaranteed to work in all situations, in all settings, and for all multicultural groups or subgroups*. In fact, many times the planner is not even quite sure why some programs work or why some of the interventions achieve their desired effect. It is known, however, that each program or intervention design situation should require intensive thought and analysis and that each requires consideration of established guides to practice. What has made planning and intervention design and selection such a complex task for the practitioner working with specific target groups, settings, and health issues is the overwhelming number of theories, principles, and models that guide health promotion and health education professionals. The usefulness of many is questionable, whereas other frameworks have been well established over time and are of immense value to the field of health promotion. Frankish et al. (1999, and Chapter 4, this volume) observe that theoretical frameworks provide program developers "with a perspective from which to organize knowledge and to interpret factors and events" (Frankish et al., 1999, p. 42). They discuss the need and rationale for using a theoretical framework; differentiate among theories, models, and principles;

and present many of the dominant theories used in health promotion and health education. Also, it should be stressed that effective intervention designs need to be conducted by practitioners who understand the theories of behavioral change and who have the ability to use them skillfully in practice (Glanz, Lewis, & Rimer, 1997; Glanz, Rimer, & Lewis, 2002). Intervention development will be discussed later in this chapter (see the section Multicultural Health Promotion Intervention Development and Design).

CULTURAL ASSESSMENT: A KEY COMPONENT OF PLANNING HEALTH PROMOTION PROGRAMS IN MULTICULTURAL POPULATIONS

It may very well be that the most needed skill of the planner is to conduct well-thought-out target group needs and cultural assessments. This skill, coupled with knowledge of theory, best practices, and best experiences (see the section The Notion of Best Practices and Best Experiences), can greatly increase the planner's capability to develop and refine more effective health promotion and education interventions. Gaining knowledge that will enable tailored health promotion programming that is congruent with each group's needs is critical. It requires the practitioner and participants from the target community to accurately assess cultural differences, beliefs, and practices in the contexts of social conditions, such as rural/urban, social class, country of origin, language, generational aspects, and historical experiences with the wider society. The challenges of multicultural target group assessment and programming are increased when several culturally diverse groups live within the same community sharing common geographical boundaries. In these situations, it becomes critical to identify group differences and similarities related to specific cultural positions, norms, and practices held within each population or subpopulation. The practitioner will have to be more aware of the need to carry out an accurate assessment of each subgroup's particular or unique set of risk factors and to understand how these should relate to the design and implementation of prevention programs and interventions that will be more congruent with the cultural uniqueness of a community or group. Tools such as the Cultural Assessment Framework (described in Chapter 6, this volume) can facilitate a more complete assessment of important cultural characteristics.

In Chapter 1, Huff and Kline discussed *culture* as the repository of devices needed for a group's (or subgroup's) adaptation that evolves over many generations. A health promotion planning group contemplating the development of health promotion and education activities within a first-generation group of immigrants to the United States, regardless of where they came from, needs specific information concerning differences in health-related belief systems and cultural practices. Issues such as the impact of degrees of acculturation would be of equal importance if one were assessing differences in program needs related to the second, third, or even fourth generations of the first-generation immigrant. These types of considerations will challenge health promotion programmers for many years to come given the current immigration trends.

Issues of *acculturation* and *assimilation* also become important variables. Although closely related, awareness of these important cultural variables may provide key areas with which to more specifically assess and segment intra-ethnic groups (Chapter 1, this volume; see also Padilla, 1980). A methodology such as that developed by Balcazar, Castro, & Krull (1995) can provide the planner with a tool for assessing key factors such as acculturation and educational status in various subgroups of Hispanics. The value of such a tool is that its method can be transferred and used in other ethnic group settings—for example, to help identify information for planning more

culturally appropriate cancer risk reduction programs. Huff and Kline in Chapter 1 of this volume and Castro, Cota, and Vega (1999) discussed the use and value of these types of assessment tools. Also, Abraido-Lanza, Armbrister, Florez, and Aguirre (2006) provide excellent discussion of the need for a more theory-driven model of acculturation in public health research.

Ethnicity, which was discussed in Chapter 1 (this volume) has many referents—a sense of identity based on a common ancestry: national, religious, tribal, linguistic, or cultural origins (Nunnally & Moy, 1989; Paniagua, 1994); feelings of belonging and continuity through time; shared meanings and traditions; and self-ascribed genealogical and social affiliations, including related forms of family and group affect (Keogh, Gallimore, & Weisner, 1997). Whereas ethnic identity tends to persist through time, *culture* changes when individuals and groups modify their beliefs and practices to survive and adapt. Although ethnicity and culture are correlated in many ways, the practitioner needs to understand that there are cultural differences among groups with the same ethnic backgrounds (Chapter 1, this volume). The complexities of health education and health promotion planning are increased when groups share common health-related problems but, owing to culturally unique factors, approach solutions to the problems in different, culturally prescribed ways.

One of the dilemmas of a multicultural society is how to effectively take into account issues of cultural or ethnic diversity, particularly in working with, planning, and implementing health promotion and education programs. The planner must be extremely sensitive to diversity, without stereotyping subgroups within the same ethnic/racial groups. For example, Keogh et al. (1997) observe that it is imprecise and inaccurate to use identification labels such as *Hispanic, Asian, African American, Native American, and Anglo-American or Euro-American* as substitute terms for culture. Rather, it is much more precise to use the terms that these different cultural or ethnic groups use to describe themselves.

MULTICULTURAL HEALTH PROMOTION INTERVENTION DEVELOPMENT AND DESIGN

Several chapters in this book dealt specifically with aspects of program assessment, design, implementation, and evaluation in culturally specific settings. Underlying these efforts was an attempt to focus program design in a way that built in a more culturally competent and responsive approach, needed for reaching and influencing the health behavior of the target group. Most of the contributors to these chapters agreed that program design and development should intensively capitalize on the strengths of the community in which the participants and programs are located (Ashley, 1999, Chapter 14, this volume; Castro et al., 1999, Chapter 10, this volume). However, the professional literature is relatively meager when it comes to agreement on what the "best" approach is or even what approach or direction to use for designing effective health promotion and education programs directed at culturally specific ethnic populations or subpopulations.

Intervention development and design is a complex issue, as discussed throughout this volume (see the discussion in Chapter 7 of the very important issues of tailoring and targeting concerning intervention development). Students and the planner, therefore, should be aware of some of the different viewpoints or positions concerning the direction the program can take. For example, one school of thought suggests that if a program for a particular ethnic group in the community is organized traditionally (i.e., in terms of the time-tested components of health education program planning, such as those discussed in Chapter 7),

then with appropriate modification, the program approach should be transferable to other ethnic groups in their specific community settings. However, built into this approach is an intentional separation of factors from their cultural context or setting, even though such a program is focused on changing specific behaviors in the target group (e.g., diet, exercise, smoking, periodic screening visits). That is, culture is viewed in more neutral terms but as an important factor to be considered in addition to other social, psychological, epidemiological, physical, and environmental factors. Montes, Eng, and Braithwaite (1995) observe,

> Separation of factors from their cultural context is largely a function of (1) developing programs that can be replicated on a wider scale and (2) the assumption that changes in the cultural context will occur as increasing numbers of people change their behaviors. (p. 248)

Program designs that use, for example, the PRECEDE framework use a sequential approach to program planning, starting with the proposition acknowledging that health behaviors are very complex, are multidimensional, and may be influenced by a variety of factors (Gielen & McDonald, 1997, 2002). Castro et al. (1999) and Ashley (1999) provided good examples of this type of program approach, even though the respective target group settings were within heavy Hispanic or African American/black communities.

Another school of thought concerning the direction to be taken in health promotion and education program design advocates the need to emphasize the cultural aspects of the particular racial/ethnic population for which the program is being planned. In contrast to the previous view, this approach acknowledges that there are significant differences in cultural worldviews and norms within each minority group. According to this approach, these differences derive from particular social conditions within urban or rural settings, social class, country of origin, and historical experiences with the larger society. Adherents to this viewpoint maintain that the practitioner must be able to intensively assess the need for differences in program direction by clearly and sensitively understanding each group's cultural uniqueness. This understanding, it is maintained, can help the programmer become more knowledgeable about and culturally sensitive to the way in which the specific group defines health problems and needs, how that relates to group members' personal experiences, the knowledge required and the context in which that knowledge must be acquired, health practices, and how group members undertake and participate in problem-solving processes that are acceptable within the framework of that group or community.

There are those who believe that, in many instances, if a program is targeted only at the needs of the general population, then it might not be effective in reaching or achieving the desired behavioral changes within underserved groups. They also cite the need for health education programs to target and consider the unique conditions experienced by underserved groups owing to their specific cultural characteristics or to the fact that they have been underserved (Marin et al., 1995). Fredericks and Hodge's (1999) "Talking Circle" health education program is still a good example of this second viewpoint because rather than using a well-defined traditional health education planning and intervention model, it was built from the ground up in an attempt to ensure a culturally unique program response. The importance given to culture in this school of thought is "largely a function of (1) developing prevention programs that can be tailored to each community and, hence, may not be transferable and (2) assuming that behavioral change must be sustained through concomitant social change and adaptation to cultural context" (Montes et al., 1995, p. 248).

Another very important ingredient in the area of intervention development is that social/ecological/environmental interventions are having a profoundly positive effect on creating health-promotive environments designed to change risk behaviors toward the use of mandated effective safety practices (Stokols, 2000a, 2000b). In some instances, smoking has been banned in workplace environments as a result of local or state regulations. There are even more powerful applications of these concepts. Stokols (2000a) views the environment "as *an enabler of health behavior* [italics added], exemplified by the installation of safety devices in buildings and vehicles, geographic proximity to health care facilities, and exposure to interpersonal modeling or cultural practices that foster health-promotive behavior" (pp. 147–148). He also observes that

> the environment serves as a *provider of health resources*, such as high-quality community sanitation systems, organizational and community health services, and legislation protecting the quality of physical environments and ensuring citizens' access to health insurance and community-based health care. (p. 148)

The Institute of Medicine's Committee on Capitalizing on Social Science and Behavioral Research to Improve the Public's Health speculates that it "may be more cost-effective to prevent many diseases and injuries at the community and environmental levels than to address them at the individual level" (Smedley & Syme, 2000, p. 3).

THE NOTION OF BEST PRACTICES AND BEST EXPERIENCES

The preceding section pointed out many different viewpoints concerning the design of multicultural program interventions within specific target groups. Studying other interventions that have been successful in particular settings and target groups can strengthen the rationale for the selection of an intervention approach. In fact, the notion of "best practices" implies that ideally the intervention used has been subjected to rigorous research and evaluation review, which substantiate its repeated effectiveness in a particular target population or group (e.g., as to achieving the behavioral outcomes sought). Furthermore, it has been used in other populations and circumstances with similar outcomes. If this were the case in reality, we would have some definitive *evidence-based practice* menus of best-practice interventions to choose from in particular settings and situations. We are not at this stage yet but are slowly moving toward it (DiClemente, Crosby, & Kegler, 2002).

Lawrence Green (2001), in his American Academy of Health Behavior Research Laureate address, pondered the need to think about replacing our emphasis from "best practices" to "best processes" during the task of intervention development in health promotion and health behavior research (p. 165). Green and Kreuter (2005) observed later that "we find ourselves using these notions of best practices more cautiously and preferring a notion of best processes" (p. 193). They define "best processes" as

> The processes of assessing the population and the local circumstances for a program . . . [to] provide a more appropriate basis for the selection of interventions than does the testing of specific interventions in dissimilar populations and circumstances. But together, *the combination of best processes of diagnosis* and *best practices of intervention* can produce the best *program* for a particular population and circumstance. (p. 193)

This would underscore the importance of conducting an intensive assessment and diagnosis process (as covered in Chapter 7, this volume, Subtasks B, C, D, and E) that would yield the quality of information enabling a best-process intervention. Glanz et al. (2002) report that the U.S. Task Force on Community Preventive Services ultimately aims to define, categorize, summarize, and rate the quality of evidence on the effectiveness of population-based interventions for disease prevention and control (see Briss et al., 2000).

So, it appears that regardless of the level or direction in which a program is focused, it will have to be reached through a very intensive process of target-group-specific needs assessment and diagnosis and community familiarity. And regardless of which direction the program design takes with regard to achieving specific individual behavior change or community-wide change through the establishment of health risk reduction environments, there is the need to view the cultural uniqueness of the population or group under focus as it relates to the way in which group members define health problems, how they identify proposed solutions to those problems, how they select the types of activities to be initiated, and how favorable behavioral change, once achieved, can be sustained in that population. Those involved in health promotion and education activities might be hard-pressed to have the range of staff or other resources available that will be able to deal with the needs of each culture in the most appropriate ways. In either case, the practitioner should not adhere rigidly to one approach or the other because the approach should depend on a thorough assessment of the situation and the particular target group. Each approach also requires an explicit recognition of different cultural groups and their diversity, the need for cultural competence, and the need for effective skills in intercultural communications. This topic is discussed in the next section.

ISSUES OF CULTURAL COMPETENCE: PREPARING TO WORK IN MULTICULTURAL POPULATIONS

The health promotion practitioner will increasingly be working in multicultural program settings and will need to possess cultural awareness and knowledge about the target group, cultural skill, and cultural encounter. In short, the practitioner must be culturally competent. *Cultural competence* was discussed in Chapters 1 and 3. There is a need, in this final chapter, to reinforce the importance of the concept. Cultural competence has been defined as "a process for effectively working within the cultural context of an individual or community from a diverse cultural or ethic background" (Campinha-Bacote, 1994, pp. 1–2). Thus, the health promotion practitioner who is expected to function in multicultural settings must be aware and accepting of cultural differences, culturally knowledgeable about the target group, and able to adapt to diverse situations (see Chapter 3, this volume). Kreps and Kunimoto (1994) emphasize that the system in which we work is "a cultural melting pot, comprising individuals from different combinations of national, regional, ethnic, racial, socioeconomic, occupational, generational, and health status cultural orientations" (p. 5). Planning, initiating, and implementing HPDP activities in this complex system of cultural differences and points of view requires great thoughtfulness. If participants are not sensitive to each other's cultural orientations, beliefs, and practices in the variety of possible planning and program scenarios involving different populations, settings, health issues, and levels of program focus, then the health promotion processes could be seriously jeopardized.

Brislin and Yoshida (1994) recognized that lack of knowledge concerning health beliefs and practices, as well as competing cultural values, beliefs, and norms among different population groups, can seriously undermine the credibility of the health professional working with these groups and can disrupt the provision of services. The notion of cultural competence, particularly in health promotion planning interactions, needs to be built on a two-sided partnership with the expectation that individuals need to work together in planning situations or health program settings and that each needs to be aware of the other's

cultural values, beliefs, and norms. Collaboration between the planner and participants is possible only if each understands the other's values, has mutual respect for the agenda to be accomplished, and accepts the other party as integral to the approach to the problem.

MULTICULTURAL HEALTH PROMOTION: THE ETHICAL DIMENSION

Kachingwe and Huff in Chapter 3 (this volume) intensively discussed the ethics of health promotion intervention in multicultural populations. As a final thought, there is a need to briefly consider some further aspects of the ethical dimension likely to be encountered by the practitioner. And this involves situations where the practitioner works in multicultural health promotion and education settings on a broader community level rather than on a narrower client level. For example, there always have been and always will be many points of view held and espoused by practitioners and participants concerning what should be the "right" methods of assessment, approaches, priorities, and interventions to be used in particular HPDP activities. Questions then are raised as to who should have access to assessment data that are collected? Who should be involved in the interpretation of the information? To what degree should planning information be kept confidential?

When peoples of different cultures representing a variety of knowledge and skill areas work together, there will always be different points of view about how programs or activities should be implemented, maintained, and evaluated. In reality, these diverse points of view (cultural or otherwise) held by the parties involved ultimately bring creativity, rationality, and progress to the health promotion undertaking. However, when a point of view becomes subject to dispute, it becomes an *issue* to the parties involved. The issues usually arise from the social and cultural values people hold about something that gives meaning and purpose to their lives. Values also provide the means by which the practitioner and participants alike judge or compare the relative worth or the rightness or wrongness of certain ideas, practices, or approaches. Many times, the conflict caused by these issues emanate from differing points of view as to rightness; fair play, and justice; respect for one's cultural, personal, or group autonomy; subtle or blatant misrepresentation of one's position or professional skills; and issues of legality. In many instances, the practitioner is told that he or she has an obligation to behave ethically. What does that mean?

Health promotion endeavors are complex because they deliberately focus on making judgments concerning the elimination or modification of some aspect of community health risk or risk behavior of individuals. The practitioner and participants are encouraged to engage in intensive processes of problem identification, select a course of action, and make decisions concerning resource acquisition and use. However, should their desire to enhance personal freedom and self-determination override their desire to modify an environment to shape more healthful behavior? These efforts might involve directing educational interventions at high-risk individuals, families, groups, or whole communities with the intent of facilitating the voluntary acquisition of specific health-related knowledge, attitudes, and practices related to improving or promoting health where people live and work. To what extent can the practitioner impose his or her values on a community? Are the program or activities designed to further social ends? Whose? Who decides what is a proper social end? The majority? If yes, then what if the majority is wrong? Thus, in an ethical context, any interventions used should seek voluntary behavior and should be supported by an informed and consenting public. At another level, health promotion efforts may seek to bring about social or environmental changes (supportive structures) in the form of policy changes, regulations, or new and increased organizational arrangements

for encouraging, enabling, and reinforcing the practice of certain health-related behaviors (Green & Kreuter, 1991, 2005). Interventions to be used in these instances might be for purposes of fostering economic, political, legal, and organizational changes. The intent of these changes is to support individual or community actions favorable to achieving health behaviors associated with protecting health or lowering risks including the organization and equitable distribution of preventive health care services. All these levels of change confront practitioners with complex ethical issues and decisions, especially when the practitioner and the target group have differing cultural beliefs and practices. When change is needed and sought in certain individual or collective health behaviors for reducing risk, ethical issues invariably will be raised concerning what the appropriate actions should be of the people whose health is in question and what the actions should be of community decision makers, health practitioners, teachers, employers, parents, and others who may influence health behaviors, resources, or services in the community. Implied in this process is the element of participation in the design of programs and interventions that are intended, what the changes will be, how they will be affected, and how that will influence them or the target community. What level of participation should be solicited, and should it be voluntary and encouraged?

The health promotion practitioner has the awesome responsibility of helping individuals, families, and communities make health decisions directed toward improving the quality of their lives. It is the health promoter's obligation to pursue this outcome with moral and ethical conduct and at the highest level of professional competence.

CHAPTER SUMMARY

There is a need to close the chapter by reminding the reader that throughout this book, he or she has been exposed to an extensive range of subjects, thinking, and approaches that illustrates the richness and scope of health promotion and health education activities in multicultural settings. What has characterized each chapter, particularly the case study chapters and the assessment, design, and evaluation chapters, has been the reliance of the practitioner on frameworks for organizing knowledge and thinking. The frameworks used, whether brand new or traditional, have been derived, over time, from a myriad of health promotion and health education theories, principles, and practice models. Earlier chapters presented health behavior and health promotion conceptual foundations, behavioral change theories from the individual to the community levels, models, and cultural assessment frameworks. Major aspects of culture and cultural diversity among African Americans/blacks, Latinos/Hispanics, American Indians/Native Americans, Alaska Natives, Asian Americans, and Pacific Islanders were also examined. The concepts of ethnicity, race, assimilation, acculturation, and health and health care disparities were studied from a multicultural perspective, and the barriers and problems frequently encountered by the health practitioner seeking to design HPDP programs were outlined.

Several chapters were devoted to the demanding and complex topics of HPDP assessment, design, implementation, and evaluation aspects in the context of specific cultural settings. Case study chapters were provided after each major section to illustrate and discuss important aspects of application. "Tips" chapters were offered after each major section to help summarize and highlight major points.

In the final analysis, there is a need for practitioners to become culturally competent and sensitive to the populations with which they are working and to use current theories, models, and principles of health promotion and education in their program designs. Given the broad tapestry of cultures that surround us, health promoters must strive to improve on their own individual and collective learning

curves through thoughtful, informed, and considerate HPDP programming. This must include reflection on what they see, experience, and feel if they are to gain perspective and skill in working with the diversity of peoples they are encountering in this multicultural world.

REFERENCES

Abraido-Lanza, A. F., Armbrister, A. N., Florez, K. R., & Aguirre, A. N. (2006). Toward a theory-driven model of acculturation in public health research. *American Journal of Public Health, 96*(8), 1342–1346.

Aday, L. (2001). *At risk in America: The health and health care needs of vulnerable populations in the United States* (2nd ed.). San Francisco: Jossey-Bass.

Ashley, M. (1999). Health promotion planning in African American communities. In R. M. Huff & M. V. Kline (Eds.), *Promoting health in multicultural populations* (pp. 223–240). Thousand Oaks, CA: Sage.

Balcazar, H., Castro, F., & Krull, J. (1995). Cancer risk reduction in Mexican-American women: The role of acculturation, education, and health risk factors. *Health Education Quarterly, 22*(1), 61–84.

Blane, D. (1995). Social determinants of health: Socioeconomic status, social class, and ethnicity [Editorial]. *American Journal of Public Health, 85*(7), 903–904.

Braithwaite, R. L. (1992). Coalition partnerships for health promotion and empowerment. In R. L. Braithwaite & S. E. Taylor (Eds.), *Health issues in the black community* (pp. 321–337). San Francisco: Jossey-Bass.

Braithwaite, R. L., Taylor, S. E., & Austin, J. N. (1999). Building health coalitions in the black community. Thousand Oaks, CA: Sage.

Brislin, R. W., & Yoshida, T. (Eds.). (1994). *Improving intercultural interactions: Modules for cross-cultural training programs.* Thousand Oaks, CA: Sage.

Briss, P., Zaza, S., Pappaioanou, M., Fielding, J., Wright-de Aguero, L., Truman, B. I., et al. (2000). Developing an evidence-based guide to community preventive services: Methods. *American Journal of Preventive Medicine, 18*(Suppl. 1), 35–43.

Butterfoss, F. D., & Kegler, M. C. (2002). Toward a comprehensive understanding of community coalitions. In R. J. DiClemente, R. A. Crosby, & M. C. Kegler (Eds.), *Emerging theories in health promotion practice and research: Strategies for improving public health* (pp. 157–193). San Francisco: Jossey-Bass.

Campinha-Bacote, J. (1994). Cultural competence in psychiatric mental health nursing: A conceptual model. *Nursing Clinics of North America, 29*(1), 1–8.

Castro, F. G., Cota, M. K., & Vega, S. C. (1999). Health promotion in Latino populations: A sociocultural model for program planning, development, and evaluation. In R. M. Huff & M. V. Kline (Eds.), *Promoting health in multicultural populations* (pp. 137–168). Thousand Oaks, CA: Sage.

Cottrell, L. S., Jr. (1983). The competent community. In R.Warren & L. Lyon (Eds.), *New perspectives in the American community* (pp. 398–432). Homewood, IL: Dorsey Press.

DeNavas-Walt, C., Proctor, B., & Mills, R. (2003). *Income, poverty, and health insurance coverage in the United States: 2003* (p. 11, see Health U.S. 2005). Retrieved April 24, 2006, from www.census.gov/prod/2004pubs/p60-226.pdf

DiClemente, R. J., Crosby, R. A., & Kegler, M. C. (Eds.). (2002). *Emerging theories in health promotion practice and research: Strategies for improving public health.* San Francisco: Jossey-Bass.

Federal Interagency Forum on Child and Family Statistics. (2005). *America's children: Key national indicators of well-being, 2005.* Washington, DC: Government Printing Office.

Frankish, C. J., Lovato, C. Y., & Shannon, W. (1999). Models, theories, and principles of health promotion with multicultural populations. In R. M. Huff & M. V. Kline (Eds.), *Promoting health in multicultural populations* (pp. 41–72). Thousand Oaks, CA: Sage.

Fredericks, L., & Hodge, F. S. (1999). Traditional approaches to health care among American Indians and Alaska Natives: A case study. In R. M. Huff & M. V. Kline (Eds.), *Promoting*

health in multicultural populations (pp. 313–326). Thousand Oaks, CA: Sage.

Gielen, A. C., & McDonald, E. M. (1997). The PRECEDE-PROCEED planning model. In K. Glanz, F. M. Lewis, & B. K. Rimer (Eds.), *Health behavior and health education: Theory research and practice* (2nd ed., pp. 359–383). San Francisco: Jossey-Bass.

Gielen, A. C., & McDonald, E. M. (2002). Using the PRECEDE-PROCEED planning model to apply health behavior theories. In K. Glanz, B. K. Rimer, & F. M. Lewis (Eds.), *Health behavior and health education: Theory, research and practice* (3rd ed., pp. 409–436). San Francisco: Jossey-Bass.

Glanz, K., Lewis, F. M., & Rimer, B. K. (Eds.). (1997). Linking theory, research, and practice. In *Health behavior and health education: Theory research and practice* (pp. ix–xi). Thousand Oaks, CA: Sage.

Glanz, K., Rimer, B. K., & Lewis, F. M. (Eds.). (2002). Theory, research, and practice in health behavior and health education. In *Health behavior and health education: Theory, research and practice* (3rd ed., pp. 22–39). San Francisco: Jossey-Bass.

Goodman, R., Speers, M., McLeroy, K., Fawcett, S., Kegler, M., Parker, E., et al. (1998). Identifying and defining the dimensions of community capacity to provide a basis for measurement. *Health Education & Behavior, 25*(3), 258–278.

Green, L. W. (1999). Foreword. In R. M. Huff & M. V. Kline (Eds.), *Promoting health in multicultural populations* (pp. 73–102). Thousand Oaks, CA: Sage.

Green, L. W. (2001). From research to "best practices" in other settings and populations (American Academy of Health Behavior Research Laureate address). *American Journal of Health Behavior, 25*(3), 165–178.

Green, L. W., & Kreuter, M. W. (1991). *Health promotion planning: An educational and environmental approach.* Mountain View, CA: Mayfield.

Green, L. W., & Kreuter, M. W. (2005). *Health program planning: An educational and ecological approach* (4th ed.). New York: McGraw-Hill.

Keogh, B. K., Gallimore, R., & Weisner, T. (1997). A sociocultural perspective on learning and learning disabilities. *Learning Disabilities Research & Practice, 12*(2), 107–113.

Kline, M. V. (1999). Planning health promotion and disease prevention programs in multicultural populations. In R. M. Huff & M. V. Kline (Eds.), *Promoting health in multicultural populations* (pp. 73–102). Thousand Oaks, CA: Sage.

Kreps, G. L., & Kunimoto, E. N. (1994). *Effective communication in multicultural health care settings.* Thousand Oaks, CA: Sage.

Kreuter, M. W., Lezin, N. A., & Young, L. A. (2000). Evaluating community-based collaborative mechanisms: Implications for practitioners. *Health Promotion Practice, 1*(1), 49–63.

Levy, B. S., & Sidel, V. W. (Eds.). (2006). The nature of social injustice and its impact on public health. In *Social injustice and public health* (pp. 5–21). New York: Oxford University Press.

Marin, G., Burhansstipanov, L., Connell, C. M., Gielen, A. C., Helitzer-Allen, D., Lorig, K., et al. (1995). A research agenda for health education among underserved populations. *Health Education Quarterly, 22*(3), 346–363.

Minkler, M. (2004). *Community organizing and community building for health* (3rd ed.). Piscataway, NJ: Rutgers University Press.

Minkler, M., & Wallerstein, N. B. (2002). Improving health through community organization and community building. In K. Glanz, B. K. Rimer, & F. M. Lewis (Eds.), *Health behavior and health education: Theory, research and practice* (3rd ed., pp. 279–311). San Francisco: Jossey-Bass.

Montes, J. H., Eng, E., & Braithwaite, R. L. (1995). Commentary on minority health as a paradigm shift in the United States. *American Journal of Health Promotion, 9*(4), 247–250.

National Center for Health Statistics. (NCHS) (2005). *Health, United States, 2005: With chartbook on trends in the health of Americans.* Hyattsville, MD: Government Printing Office.

Nunnally, E., & Moy, C. (1989). *Communication basics for health service professionals.* Newbury Park, CA: Sage.

Padilla, A. M. (1980). *Acculturation: Theory, models and some new findings.* Boulder, CO: Westview.

Pamuk, E., Makuc, D., Heck, K., Reuben, C., & Lochner, K. (1998). *Socioeconomic status and health chartbook, Health United States, 1998.* Hyattsville, MD: National Center for Health Statistics.

Paniagua, F. A. (1994). *Assessing and treating culturally diverse clients: A practical guide.* Thousand Oaks, CA: Sage.

Shi, L., & Stevens, G. D. (2005). *Vulnerable populations in the United States.* San Francisco: Jossey-Bass.

Smedley, B. D., & Syme, S. L. (Eds.). (2000). *Promoting health: Intervention strategies from social and behavioral research.* Washington, DC: National Academy Press.

Stokols, D. (2000a). Creating health promotive environments: Implications for theory and research. In M. S. Jamner & D. Stokols (Eds.), *Promoting human wellness: New frontiers for research, practice, and policy* (pp. 135–162). Berkeley: University of California Press.

Stokols, D. (2000b). The social ecological paradigm of wellness promotion. In M. S. Jamner & D. Stokols (Eds.), *Promoting human wellness: New frontiers for research, practice, and policy* (pp. 21–37). Berkeley: University of California Press.

U.S. Census Bureau. (2006). *Statistical abstract of the United States* (125th ed.). Washington, DC: Author.

U.S. Census Bureau News. (2006, October 12). *Nation's population to reach 300 million on October 17.* Retrieved December 21, 2007, from www.census.gov/Press-Release/www/releases/archives/population/007616.html

U.S. Census Bureau Population Estimates. (2003). *Methodology: U.S. population estimates by age, sex, race, and Hispanic origin: July 1, 2003.* Retrieved November 28, 2006, from www.census.gov/popest/topics/methodology/2003_nat_char_meth.html

Author Index

Subject Index

About the Editors

Michael V. Kline is Emeritus Professor of Public Health at California State University, Northridge. He taught undergraduate and graduate courses involved with training students and practitioners to design, implement, and evaluate health promotion and education programs within a variety of health settings, population groups, and public sector and community organizations. Through the years, he has been actively involved in community organization activities relevant to assisting special populations to plan and organize health programs in their neighborhoods.

He served in the capacities of editorial consultant, associate editor, and executive coeditor of the *Journal of Drug Education*. He continues his long association as Behavioral Sciences Consultant with the Research and Evaluation Section, Planning Division, Alcohol and Drug Program Administration, Department of Public Health, County of Los Angeles. He has worked in several areas: alcohol prevention and education consultation, assistance in the development of data management and information systems, alcohol client tracking activities, and alcohol and drug program evaluation systems. He formerly was the executive director of several alcohol and drug treatment programs in Los Angeles, including the Edgemont House social model program and the Golden State Community Mental Health Center Comprehensive NIAAA (National Institute on Alcohol Abuse and Alcoholism) alcohol treatment program. He was the director of the Los Angeles County

Alcohol Training Consortium and Associate State Director of the California Alcohol Foundation. He also has been involved in providing extensive technical consultation and education in the development and evaluation of drinking driver programs. He formerly was the district director of health education, Southeast Region, Department of Health Services, County of Los Angeles. He also served as the medical care organizer for the Department of Health Services, Department of Hospitals, and Department of Mental Health, County of Los Angeles in the early development of the Hubert Humphrey Health Center in South Los Angeles. He also was the director of public health education at the Orange County (California) Department of Public Health. He received his MPH degree in public health education and behavioral sciences from the University of California, Berkeley, School of Public Health. He received his DrPH degree in medical care organization and health administration from the University of California, Los Angeles, School of Public Health.

Robert M. Huff is Professor of Public Health Education at California State University, Northridge (CSUN). Prior to joining the faculty at CSUN, he was a health education practitioner for the Charles Drew Postgraduate Medical School in Los Angeles, where he was actively involved in community hypertension education, screening, referral, and follow-up activities and in the Martin Luther King, Jr.,

General Hospital, where he directed patient education programming in the Department of Internal Medicine. He later moved to the Ventura County Health Care Agency–Public Health Services and the Ventura County Medical Center, where he established and directed the Department of Patient Education for inpatient and outpatient services and was the health education consultant for the hospital's Family Practice Residency Program. He also organized and managed an agency-wide teleproduction facility; codeveloped and managed a countywide health promotion center; and consulted on a variety of public health programs, including chronic disease prevention, family life education, and HIV/AIDS awareness and prevention, where he was also an HIV Alternative Test Site Counselor for Public Health Services.

He currently teaches both undergraduate and graduate courses in public health education in the areas of program planning and evaluation; health behavior change; communications and media; cross-cultural issues in public health; holistic health; and other related courses. He has been an evaluation consultant for a variety of organizations and projects, including the V.A. Hospital in Sepulveda, California; the Violence Prevention Project with Ventura County Public Health Services; an alcohol and drug project in the student health center at CSUN; and the Youth Wellness Village Project funded by the California Wellness Foundation in Ojai, California. He also was an editorial consultant and coeditor for the *Journal of Drug Education*.

His research interests combine his undergraduate training in anthropology with his graduate training in public health education to focus on multicultural health promotion and disease prevention programs in a variety of settings. He has a special interest in traditional medicine, shamanism, and complementary and alternative medical practices. He received his MPH. degree in health education from CSUN and his PhD in confluent education from the University of California, Santa Barbara, Graduate School of Education.

About the Contributors

Mary Ashley, BSN, PHN, MPH, MBA, is a retired assistant professor from the Department of Family Medicine at the Charles Drew University of Medicine and Science in Los Angeles. She has spent the majority of her career working in low-income and underserved communities. She has served as Principle Investigator and Director of Community Public Health programs for the University, where she has been actively involved in promoting community HIV/AIDS outreach and intervention efforts in the African American community.

Hector Balcazar, MS, PhD, is a professor of health promotion and behavioral sciences and Regional Dean of the El Paso Regional Campus at the University of Texas-School of Public Health at Houston, Texas. He also serves as the codirector of the Hispanic Health Disparities Research Center, a National Cancer Institute–funded initiative in collaboration with the College of Health Sciences at the University of Texas at El Paso. His research focus is in the study of public health problems of Latinos/Mexican Americans, and he currently serves as a member of the editorial board of the American Public Health Association and is a member of the Board of Trustees of the Society for Public Health Education.

Betty Geishirt Cantrell, MSSW, is program administrator for the CANFit Program, a nonprofit nutrition and fitness education and leadership program in Oakland, California. She has extensive experience as a researcher and administrator in multicultural educational programs. She served as Project Director for the diabetes research program held on the Sioux and Winnebago reservations and has served as a consultant to various minority programs offering child welfare services to communities.

John Casken, RN, MPH, PhD, is an associate professor and director of the Office of International Affairs at the School of Nursing and Dental Hygiene at the University of Hawaii at Manoa. His major interest is in the health of Pacific Islanders and Native Hawiians but has now expanded to include the countries bordering on the Eastern and Southeastern Pacific Basin.

Felipe G. Castro, MSW, PhD, is a professor of clinical psychology in the Department of Psychology at Arizona State University. His research areas include the study of cultural factors in the design and evaluation of health promotion programs for Hispanic/Latino(a) and other racial/ethnic minority populations. He is also interested in resiliency and how it may protect individuals from disease and disorder, including drug abuse and addiction. He was awarded the 2005 Community, Culture, and Prevention Science Award from the Society of Prevention Research, and he serves as an associate editor for *Prevention Science* and the *American Journal of Public Health*.

Patricia Chalela, DrPH, is an assistant professor in the Department of Epidemiology and Biostatistics at the Institute for Health Promotion Research at the University of Texas Health Science Center at San Antonio, Texas. She has developed and coordinated international outreach programs, personal training, and communications for the prevention of eye disease and coordinated international workshops in ocular health. Her research interests are in health disparities, health promotion, and health communications.

Marya Cota, MA, PhD, is a clinical psychologist and certified school psychologist at St. Joseph's Hospital in the Children's Rehabilitation Services and Pediatric Ambulatory Care clinics in Phoenix, Arizona. She has been a Peace Core Volunteer in Central America and has served as core faculty at the University of Arizona, Phoenix campus for the past 6 years. Her clinical emphasis is in the areas of health and educational psychology, working primarily with Hispanic children, adolescents, and their families.

Michael R. Cousineau, DrPH, is an associate professor of research in the Department of Family Medicine and Director of the Center for Community Health Studies at the University of Southern California, Keck School of Medicine. His primary research interests are health policy and health services evaluation research, access to care for low-income and uninsured families, governance and operation of safety-net providers, and health needs of vulnerable populations including the homeless.

Bonnie M. Duran, DrPH, is an associate professor in the School of Public Health and Community Medicine at the University of Washington. She also directs the Center for Indigenous Health Research at the Indigenous Wellness Research Institute.

She conducts alcohol, drug, and mental health services research with Native communities.

Rhonda Folsom, MPH, CHES, is a program supervisor at the County of Orange Health Care Agency in Orange County, California. She manages a statewide program that provides breast and cervical cancer education and screening services and conducts tailored outreach to Asian American, Pacific Islander, American Indian, and African American women.

C. James Frankish, PhD, is the Director of the Centre for Population Health Promotion Research and is a Professor in Health Care and Epidemiology (Medicine) and the College for Interdisciplinary Studies at the University of British Columbia. He has authored numerous papers on community participation, mental health and population health, health impact assessment, and participatory research. His prior work includes research on regional health boards and national studies of measures of health communities, health goals, and health promotion in primary care. His current projects focus on health promotion and homelessness, health literacy, and poverty and nutrition. He is on the board of the Lookout Homeless Shelter Society, and is chair of the Impact of the Olympics on Communities Coalition.

Kipling J. Gallion, MA, is an assistant professor in the Department of Epidemiology and Biostatistics and Deputy Director of the Institute for Health Promotion Research at the University of Texas Health Science Center at San Antonio, Texas. He is currently the National Program Coordinator for the National Cancer Institute–supported Redes En Acción, the National Hispanic/Latino Cancer Network, and directs several other national and local programs. He has played a lead role in the creation of award-winning national cancer-related media and promotional educational materials.

June Gutierrez English, MPH, MA, is a program administrator at Santa Barbara County Public Health Department in Santa Barbara, California. Trained as a medical anthropologist, she currently serves as a regional coordinator for one of the State of California's women's health services programs, where she oversees provider, professional education, and public education services. She and her staff work with Asian American, American Indian, and African American communities to provide health education focused on breast and cervical cancer early detection services.

Jung Hee Han, BS, has worked with Dr. Marjorie Kagawa-Singer at the UCLA School of Public Health and at the Orange County Korean American Health Information and Education Center, a small community-based organization providing resources and services to the Korean American community in Orange County, California.

Maya Harris, MEd, an active community organizer, works in the Research and Evaluation Department of a publicly funded organization serving children aged 0 to 5 years and their families. She formerly worked at the Charles Drew University of Medicine and Science in Los Angeles, where she was involved in offering program and evaluation training as well as capacity-building services to organizations providing HIV/AIDS prevention and intervention services to at-risk African American communities.

Patti (Rosa Patricia) Herring, RN, MA, PhD, is an associate professor in the Department of Health Promotion and Education at Loma Linda University, Loma Linda, California. She is a codirector and co-investigator for the Adventist Health Study-2 and consults in a variety of roles, including the San Bernardino County Head Start Program, The Inter-American Improvement Association, and the Moreno Valley Unified School District grant

to serve underserved, minority, and disadvantaged children's academic and social development—a service learning project.

Christopher Elliott Hodge is currently in a master's degree program in forensic psychology at the Chicago School of Professional Psychology. His work entails the cultural constructs of behaviors, childhood trauma, and maladaptive behaviors.

Felicia Schanche Hodge, DrPH, is a professor in the School of Nursing and School of Public Health at the University of California, Los Angeles. She has over 30 years of experience working in American Indian communities and has developed the Talking Circle intervention as a method of delivering education targeted at a variety of health issues and problems including cancer, diabetes, and smoking cessation.

Joyce W. Hopp, PhD, MPH, CHES, RN, is Dean Emeritus, School of Allied Health Professions and Emeritus Distinguished Professor, Health Promotion and Education, School of Public Health, Loma Linda University, Loma Linda, California. She has worked internationally and cross-culturally in diverse locations, including the Navaho Reservation in Utah, Saudi Arabia, China, Myanmar, and Tanzania. Her interests are in school health education and HIV/AIDS.

Claire K. Hughes, DrPH, RD, is administrator for the Office of Parity within the Hawaii State Department of Heath. She is of Native Hawaiian ancestry and continues to write regularly on Native Hawaiian culture and past achievements as well as on improving Native Hawaiian nutrition and health.

Ted Jojola, PhD, is a tribal member of the Pueblo of Isleta, where he resides with his family. He is a Regents' Professor of Planning at the University of New Mexico and holds a joint appointment as a Visiting Distinguished Professor at Arizona State University. He is also the cofounder and chair of the Indigenous Planning Division, American Planning Association.

Aimie F. Kachingwe, PT, EdD, OCS, F.A.A.O.M.P.T., is an assistant professor in the Department of Physical Therapy at California State University, Northridge. She is an American Physical Therapy Association Board Certified Clinical Specialist in orthopedics and a fellow of the American Academy of Orthopaedic Manual Physical Therapists. Her research interests include the promotion of ethnic diversity in the profession of physical therapy and the incorporation of multiculturalism into the health care educational curriculum.

Marjorie Kagawa-Singer, PhD, MA, MN, RN, is a professor in the Department of Asian American Studies at the UCLA School of Public Health in Los Angeles, California. Her clinical work has been in oncology and on the etiology and elimination of disparities in physical and mental health care outcomes for communities of color, with a primary focus on Asian American and Pacific Islander communities. She serves on multiple local, state, and national committees addressing the impact of ethnicity on health care and health outcomes and is the principal investigator of the Los Angeles site for the National Cancer Institute–funded national Asian American Network on Cancer Awareness Research and Training.

Gregory P. Loos, EdD, MPH, MS, is Division Chief for Basic Education at the United States Agency for International Development (USAID). He has trained as a learning theorist and public health planner. He has extensive international experience in Southeast Asia and the Pacific Islands, where he was involved in community assessment activities, community health education, and health administration. He has been on the faculties of the University of Hawaii and East Stroudsburg University and has worked with the State of Hawaii and the Kamehameha Research Institute.

Chris Y. Lovato, PhD, is an associate professor in the Department of Health Care and Epidemiology at the University of British Columbia where she teaches program evaluation to graduate students. She is also director of the Evaluation Studies Unit for the Faculty of Medicine at UBC. Her primary areas of expertise are population health and program evaluation. Much of Dr. Lovato's research has focused on youth tobacco control including the evaluation of smoking cessation interventions. She has extensive experience in program evaluation and has provided consultation to numerous government and nongovernment agencies evaluating health-related programs.

Alfred L. McAlister, PhD, is a professor at the University of Texas, Houston School of Public Health. He was the lead member of the research teams of the Stanford 3-Community Study in California and the North Karelia Project in Finland. He has been involved in the CDC's AIDS Community Demonstration Projects, led several international research studies in Europe and Latin America, and participated in teaching and research in a variety of countries in Europe and Central and South America.

Iraj Poureslami, PhD, is a senior research associate at the Human Early Learning Partnership and Centre for Population Health Promotion Research at the University of British Columbia. He is a WHO (EMRO) mentor of health promotion, WHO Early Childhood Development Knowledge Network consultant, and member of the Canadian Council on Learning's health literacy expert panel. His research interests are in the sociocultural determinants of health and quality of life within ethnocultural communities in Canada. He has extensive knowledge and expertise on developing community-based health literacy information, audio-visual materials, and working with newcomer communities and their families in British Columbia.

Amelie G. Ramirez, MPH, DrPH, is an assistant professor of epidemiology and biostatistics at the University of Texas Health Science Center at San Antonio, where she is also the director of the new Institute for Health Promotion Research. She holds the Dielmann Chair in Health Disparities Research and Community Outreach and the newly created Max and Minnie Tomerlin Voelcker Endowed Chair in Cancer Health Care Disparities. Over the past 25 years, she has directed numerous state, federal, and privately funded projects focusing on health disparities affecting Hispanics/Latinos and other populations.

Sarah Rodriguez'G, BS, is a health educator whose research interests are in the areas of community health education, program planning, and evaluation.

Gregory D. Stevens, PhD, is an assistant professor of research in the Department of Family Medicine and Center for Community Health Studies at the University of Southern California, Keck School of Medicine. His research has focused on primary health care quality for vulnerable children, racial/ethnic and socioeconomic disparities in care, and patient-provider relationship issues involved in the delivery of well-child care and developmental services.

Nathania T. Tsosie, MCRP, is a research coordinator at the University of New Mexico Master's in Public Health Program. Her research interests are in community building and health promotion planning in indigenous communities.

Luis F. Vélez, MD, PhD, MPH, has worked in health promotion since 1991. He has taught at the Universidad del Valle schools of medicine and public health in Cali, Colombia, and at the Health Science Institute in Medellin, Colombia, and is now at the Baylor College of Medicine in Houston, Texas. He has served as an advisor to the World Health Organization, the Inter-American Development Bank, and the World Bank. He is actively involved in Latino health issues, health disparities, health communications, and community empowerment.

Nina Wallerstein, DrPH, is Professor and Director of the Master's in Public Health Program, School of Medicine, University of New Mexico. Her research focus is on developing participatory research methodologies and empowerment intervention research. She has worked in North American and Latin American contexts, in healthy city initiatives, adolescent and women's health research, and community health development.

Gina M. Wingood, ScD, MPH, is the Agnes Moore Endowed Faculty in HIV/AIDS Research; an associate professor in the Department of Behavioral Sciences and Health Education; and Director, Social and Behavioral Science Core, Emory Center for AIDS Research at the Rollins School of Public Health at Emory University. She currently serves as the principal investigator on four National Institutes of Health–funded studies. Her research focuses on assessing the efficacy of gender and culturally congruent HIV prevention intervention for adult women.

Evaon C. Wong-Kim, PhD, LCSW, MPH, is an associate professor in the Department of Social Work at California State University at East Bay, where she chairs the Children, Youth, and Families concentration and the Research Curriculum. She is an advocate for minority and low-income cancer patients, and her research interests are focused on cancer survivorship and quality-of-life issues confronting Chinese immigrants. She is a founding member of the Intercultural Cancer Council and a member of the Minority Women's Health Panel, Office on Women's Health.

D. William Wood, MPH, PhD, is professor and chair of the Department of Sociology in the College of Social Sciences at the University of Hawaii at Manoa. He teaches research methods and statistics, social epidemiology, and drugs in America. He has served as director of the International Center for Health Promotion and Disease Prevention Research and as senior investigator for the Hawaii Medical Service Association Foundation. His research interests include patterns of substance abuse, stress, organization of health care systems, operational research, and health care system outcomes.

Soheila Yasharpour, MPH, is Project Coordinator of the Infoshare Project at the David Geffen School of Medicine at the University of California, Los Angeles. She has been involved in a variety of health education projects addressing the needs of underserved communities and is currently working on a project focusing on information technology and bioinformatics in local hospitals and clinics in Los Angeles.